Pitfalls, Variants, and Artifacts in Body MR Imaging

Pitfalls, Variants, and Artifacts in Body MR Imaging

Scott A. Mirowitz, M.D.

Associate Professor of Radiology,
Washington University School of Medicine
Radiologist-in-Chief,
Jewish Hospital of St. Louis
Co-Director of Body Magnetic Resonance,
Mallinckrodt Institute of Radiology
St. Louis, Missouri

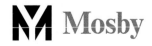 Mosby

St. Louis Baltimore Boston Carlsbad Chicago Naples New York Philadelphia Portland
London Madrid Mexico City Singapore Sydney Tokyo Toronto Wiesbaden

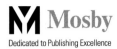

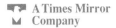

Vice President and Publisher: Anne S. Patterson
Developmental Editor: Sandra Clark Brown
Production Editor: Chuck Furgason
Design Coordinator: Renée Duenow
Manufacturing Manager: Theresa Fuchs

Printed in the United States of America
Composition by the Clarinda Company
Printing/binding by Maple Vail

Mosby–Year Book, Inc.
11830 Westline Industrial Drive
St. Louis, Missouri 63146

Library of Congress Cataloging in Publication Data

Mirowitz, Scott A.
　　Pitfalls, variants, and artifacts in body MR imaging / Scott A. Mirowitz
　　　　p.　cm.
　　Includes bibliographical references and index.
　　ISBN 0-8016-7670-3
　　1. Magnetic resonance imaging.　I. Title.
　　[DNLM: 1. Magnetic Resonance Imaging.　2. Technology, Radiologic.　3. Quality
Assurance, Health Care.　WN 185 M676p 1995]
　　RC78.7.N83M54　1996
　　616.07'548--dc20
　　DNLM/DLC
　　for Library of Congress 　　　　　　　　　　　　　　　　　95-12769
　　　　　　　　　　　　　　　　　　　　　　　　　　　　　　　　CIP

96 97 98 99 00 / 9 8 7 6 5 4 3 2 1

This book is dedicated to my wife, Jacki,
to our children Jessica, Melanie, and Adam,
and to my parents Carl and Helene,
for their understanding, support, and inspiration

Foreword

As a relatively recent initiate into the world of MRI, I have longed for a book that would deal with the kinds of problems illustrated in this work. Certainly before one can accurately define pathology, he or she must eliminate all sources of error including normal anatomic variation, artifacts, and technical pitfalls. A compilation of these distracting entities represents an enormous benefit to those who are attempting to attain competence in MRI.

In my own work in plain film radiography, I have attempted to correlate plain film variants with their MR explanations and have been able to elucidate their nature to better advantage. I suspect that the converse may occur as more experience is accumulated in MR interpretation. As MR technology evolves, many of the technical artifacts will disappear and new ones will arise. I foresee many future editions that will deal with these new issues as they become apparent.

I congratulate Dr. Mirowitz for taking the initial step in this endeavor. I believe that he will find it increasingly intriguing, as I have. I am delighted to at last see this publication. It is sorely needed.

Theodore E. Keats, M.D.
Professor of Radiology
Professor of Orthopedics
University of Virginia Health Sciences Center
Charlottesville, Virginia

Foreword

Rapid progress has been made in the field of magnetic resonance imaging (MRI) since its initial introduction into clinical practice over a decade ago. Although the first applications of MRI focused on the brain because of its size and lack of respiratory and other physiologic motion, developments of better coil technology, cardiac triggering, various motion suppression techniques, and fast imaging sequences have made it possible to use MRI for other parts of the body. MRI has replaced computed tomography (CT) as the imaging procedure of choice for evaluating many brain and spinal diseases because of its superior soft tissue contrast sensitivity and its direct multiplanar imaging capability. Likewise, MRI has become the preferred imaging modality for evaluating many of the musculoskeletal disease processes. Furthermore, the clinical utility of MRI in the cardiovascular system, the abdomen, the pelvis, and the thorax continues to be expanded and better defined.

The rapid growth and complexity of this technology has made it difficult for practicing radiologists to keep up with new developments and to decide what is relevant for their daily practice. Furthermore, MRI opens up a wide range of pitfalls and artifacts that are unique to this imaging modality and are often unfamiliar to the users. As clinical indications for extracranial MRI continued to expand, it is becoming increasingly important for practicing radiologists to be well versed in the artifacts and pitfalls that may masquerade as disease processes.

This book on *Pitfalls, Variants, and Artifacts in Body MR Imaging* is timely and practical. Combining his own vast experience in body MR imaging with those of the other leading researchers in this field, the author introduces each pitfall and variant in its appropriate anatomic compartment. Each subject is closely coupled with a clinical example and the attendant explanation is succinct and easy to understand. Such an approach makes it clinically relevant and will be warmly received by all of us who use MRI for patient care.

Joseph K.T. Lee, M.D., F.A.C.R.
Professor and Chairman
Department of Radiology
University of North Carolina
School of Medicine
Chapel Hill, North Carolina

"You cannot imagine, Old Scout, the number of unique and bizarre types of pitfalls that are ever yawning their abysmal depths to medical men, ready to gulp the unwary physician or surgeon, much in the manner of 'Lisbon Town, when she saw the earth open and gulp her down'."

Pitfalls
A.J. Caffrey, M.D.
The Gorham Press, Boston
1921

Preface

The objective of this book is to familiarize the reader with the wide range of pitfalls, variants, and artifacts that may be encountered on MR images. It may be useful to review the meanings of these terms. Webster's dictionary defines them as follows.* A *pitfall* is "a hidden or not easily recognized . . . error . . . into which one that is unsuspecting . . . may fall." A *variant* is "one that varies from the original or archetype"; in the context of this book this usually refers to anatomic variation. An artifact is "a product of artificial character due to extraneous agency . . . not indicative of actual structural relationships"; this usually relates to artificial appearances created by technical aspects of the MR imager. Each of these entities, of course, is closely related in that each may result in the simulation of lesions that do not exist, failure to identify lesions that do exist, or mischaracterizing the nature of lesions encountered on MR images.

Magnetic resonance (MR) imaging is subject to a wide range of pitfalls and artifacts. Some of these entities are familiar from experience with plain radiography or other cross-sectional imaging techniques (such as computed tomography), while many others are unique to MR images. The large number of these entities is in part related to the wide variety of pulse sequences and techniques that are available in MR imaging. Unfamiliarity with these pitfalls may result in overdiagnosis, underdiagnosis, or misdiagnosis of abnormalities. In the first case, the patient may undergo unnecessary further testing or treatment, at increased expense and risk, on the basis of spurious findings. In the second situation, appropriate further testing and treatment may not be provided to the patient on the basis of a false-negative report. In the third scenario, the wrong course of treatment—whether it is passive or active—may be chosen. The ability to recognize and avoid pitfalls and artifacts on imaging examinations has always had major importance for patient care. However, it has perhaps assumed even greater significance in the context of the current health care environment, where quality assurance and containment of unnecessary costs are emphasized.

It is my hope that readers will be able to use this text to "short-circuit" the learning process by gaining from the experience of others. The book will probably be most useful to those in training (i.e., residents and fellows) and to those relatively new to MR interpretation. Although many experienced MR readers will have already navigated their way around many of the pitfalls discussed here, the book can hopefully be of value to them as well. The book may also be helpful to some clinicians who refer patients for MR studies so that they can better understand some of the limits and constraints of this technology, and for MR technologists who encounter these pitfalls and artifacts on a daily basis.

The book has been prepared with a distinctly clinical orientation. There are several excellent references that provide technical descriptions of MR artifacts; it is not my intention to reproduce such material here. Rather, my goal was to emphasize the significance of such artifacts from a clinical perspective. At the same time, I have attempted to not only describe these pitfalls and artifacts, but also to discuss potential remedies for alleviating them. It should be emphasized that this book is not intended to serve as a complete text on MR imaging. It is meant to supplement existing texts by focusing on issues that represent current challenges or boundaries for MR imaging.

The rapid march of MR technology should help radiologists to avoid some of the entities discussed in this book, by providing images of improved resolution and quality. On the other hand, as new MR techniques become available, they too will present previously unencountered pitfalls and artifacts. This book discusses entities encountered using state-of-the-art MR techniques in general use at the time of publication; it is anticipated that discussion of new techniques will be provided in future editions. I would also welcome examples of documented MR pitfalls, variants, and artifacts that readers of this book might encounter in their own practice, for possible inclusion in future editions.

*Webster's Third New International Dictionary; G & C Merriam Co, Springfield, Mass. USA 1976.

In preparing this book I have emphasized those pitfalls and artifacts that have been described to date in the radiologic literature. I am indebted to the many authors who have made these contributions to the literature, so that others may benefit from their experience. Their contributions have been critically important in advancing the level of patient care that is provided on the basis of MR imaging.

ACKNOWLEDGMENTS

It is a pleasure to have the opportunity to express my great appreciation to many individuals who have contributed in various ways to this book. I am fortunate to work with a group of outstanding MR technologists; they include Robert Kowalik, Michelle Onder, Mary Watkins, and Carrie Sullivan. Many thanks are due to Camy Piper, Marilyn Crawshaw, and Amisue Rasnic for their assistance in the preparation of the materials for this book.

At Mosby–Year Book I thank Anne Patterson for her enthusiasm for this project in its conceptual stage, and for the overall guidance that she and Susan Gay provided. Maura Leib and Sandy Clark Brown were very helpful in the editing and overall coordination of this book, as were Peggy Fagen, John Rogers, and Chuck Furgason with the production process.

I am indebted to two outstanding radiologists for contributing forewords to this book; their participation is particularly meaningful to me. Dr. Joseph Lee introduced me to MR research, and has served as an outstanding mentor. Dr. Theodore Keats has pioneered the description of radiographic entities that may simulate disease in his classic work *Atlas of Roentgenographic Variants That May Simulate Disease* and in related publications. His efforts have stimulated my interest in the material presented in this book.

I am very appreciative of the support of Dr. Ronald Evens, Director of the Mallinckrodt Institute of Radiology, as well as of the many outstanding colleagues—faculty, residents, and fellows—at this Institute, which I have the great fortune to work with. Most importantly, I wish to thank my family for their unending support and understanding, without which this book could not have been possible.

Scott A. Mirowitz, M.D.

Contents

Section Four
MUSCULOSKELETAL SYSTEM

Section Five
SPINE

Pitfalls, Variants, and Artifacts in Body MR Imaging

Section One

CHEST/ CARDIOVASCULAR SYSTEM

1

Thorax

MEDIASTINUM

Lymph Nodes

Normal lymph nodes

The presence of mediastinal lymphadenopathy is of critical importance in staging the extent of lymphoma and metastatic carcinoma. Small mediastinal lymph nodes can be visualized in normal individuals.[52] The most frequent locations for both normal and pathologic mediastinal lymph nodes include the right paratracheal region, precarinal or subcarinal space, and region lateral to the aortic arch. However, lymph nodes may also be present in more unusual mediastinal locations. Normal mediastinal nodes are small and few in number, with well-defined margins and homogeneous signal intensity. The accepted upper limit of normal size for mediastinal lymph nodes is 1 cm in diameter. An exception to this general rule is retrocrural nodes, which should be no larger than 6 mm in diameter in normal subjects.

Lymph node characterization

The use of size criteria alone as a method for distinguishing normal from abnormal lymph nodes can result in diagnostic errors. These criteria do not allow for recognition of early tumor involvement that has not yet led to nodal enlargement.[39,69] Conversely, marked enlargement of mediastinal lymph nodes can result from granulomatous or infectious processes, among other entities, and is not specific for malignancy.

It had been hoped that magnetic resonance imaging (MR) would allow for distinction between enlarged reactive lymph nodes and neoplastic lymphadenopathy on the basis of different signal intensity characteristics. However, this distinction remains difficult, since both entities display similar signal intensity features on all pulse sequences.[34,77,88,90] In general, all lymph nodes appear moderately hypointense on T1-weighted images and moderately hyperintense on T2-weighted images. The use of quantitative measurement of T1 and T2 relaxation times has also been attempted and has again proved un-

reliable in distinguishing between benign and malignant lymph nodes.

Improvement in the ability to characterize lymph nodes on MR is expected with the introduction of reticuloendothelial contrast agents, such as ultrasmall superparamagnetic iron oxide particles. These agents, it is hoped, will allow for visualization of tumor replacement within nonenlarged nodes and also allow enlarged reactive nodes to be distinguished from neoplastic nodes.

Another factor that may render size criteria unreliable for characterization of mediastinal lymph nodes is the potential for a cluster of small nodes to appear as a single larger nodal mass on MR images[76] (Fig. 1-1). This phenomenon most often occurs in the pulmonary hila; it is related to the limited spatial resolution of MR images and to image blurring, which is due to respiratory motion and to pulsatile motion of adjacent vascular structures. Consequently, this pitfall can be minimized when a higher resolution imaging matrix is prescribed and when methods for suppressing respiratory and vascular motion artifacts are employed.

Chemical shift misregistration artifact may also contribute to artifactual increase or decrease in apparent nodal size. This artifact occurs at interfaces between fat and water, such as at the border between lymph node and mediastinal fat. Because of the different precessional fre-

---

DIFFICULTIES IN LYMPH NODE CHARACTERIZATION

- Unreliable size criterion
- Unreliable signal intensity criterion
- Cluster nodes appear as single mass
- Chemical shift misregistration
- Heterogeneity caused by hilar fat
- Heterogeneity resulting from calcification
- Active tumor vs. posttherapeutic fibrosis
- Heterogeneity caused by motion artifacts

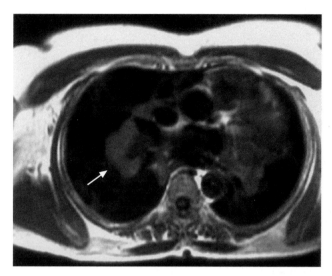

Fig. 1-1. A cluster of enlarged lymph nodes in the right hilar region *(arrow)* appears as a single confluent nodal mass on this transaxial T1-weighted image (TR 714, TE 12, 4 Nex) image in patient with sarcoidosis.

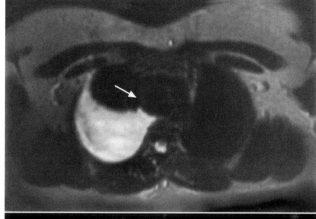

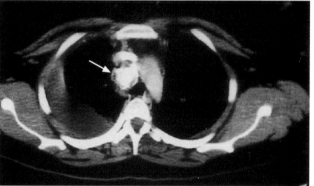

Fig. 1-2. (A) Transaxial T2-weighted image (TR 3400, TE 80, 2 Nex) demonstrates middle mediastinal mass characterized by signal void *(arrow)*. This appearance is suggestive of a vascular lesion. However, this actually represents a cluster of calcified lymph nodes, as verified on corresponding CT image (B). Note large right pleural effusion, with associated ghosting artifacts.

quency of fat and water protons, a mismapping of signal intensity occurs along the frequency encoding direction of the image. Chemical shift misregistration is generally more severe on T2-weighted than T1-weighted images. T1-weighted images also provide more reliable depictions of lymph node size than T2-weighted images because of their relative improved signal-to-noise ratio and motion artifact resistance. Chemical shift misregistration can be further minimized with the use of a high-resolution matrix, decreased slice thickness, and increased receiver bandwidth. However, each of these will contribute to reduction in signal-to-noise ratio, which is usually more detrimental to image quality than the achieved reduction in chemical shift effects.

Normal lymph nodes usually demonstrate homogeneous signal intensity, as mentioned before. However, a central focus of aberrant signal intensity can be observed in normal lymph nodes, as a result of fat within the nodal hilum. This focus appears slightly hyperintense on T1-weighted images and slightly hypointense on T2-weighted images relative to the remainder of the node. This contrasts with the appearance of nodal necrosis, which is a strong indicator of malignant involvement. Necrosis is usually manifested as a central focus of relative decreased signal intensity on T1-weighted images and increased signal intensity on T2-weighted images. Unfortunately, the ability of MR to depict central nodal necrosis has been somewhat limited on standard pulse sequences. The use of contrast-enhanced T1-weighted images assists in the detection of such necrotic foci.[82] In the absence of necrosis, however, enhancing lymph nodes and other masses can be difficult to detect following paramagnetic contrast material administration, because of the isointensity with surrounding mediastinal fat.

The presence of coarse calcifications within mediastinal and hilar lymph nodes indicates old granulomatous involvement. Calcifications may be observed on MR images as foci of relative decreased signal intensity on all pulse sequences. This may lead to an inhomogeneous appearance of the affected lymph node, raising suspicion for neoplastic involvement. Diffuse hypointensity of a mediastinal mass caused by calcification can also simulate the flow void of a vessel or vascular lesion (Figs. 1-2, *A* and *B*). More important than these situations, however, is the relative insensitivity of MR for depiction of calcification.[76,81] As a result, we are deprived of a valuable diagnostic criterion of benign nodal enlargement. Gradient echo images are considerably more sensitive than spin echo images for depiction of calcification and should be utilized when nodal calcifications are sus-

---

SIMULATION OF ENLARGED LYMPH NODES

- Slow flow/thrombosis in mediastinal vessels/aneurysms
- Partial volume averaging vessels with mediastinal fat
- Partial volume averaging pericardial fluid with mediastinal fat
- Atrial appendages
- Ectopic thyroid/parathyroid tissue
- Bronchogenic/duplication cysts
- Normal convexity azygoesophageal recess
- Vertebral osteophytes
- Esophagus, hiatal hernia
- Dilated azygos/hemiazygos veins
- Extramedullary hematopoiesis

---

pected. Phase reconstructions of gradient echo images have been advocated as a means of further increasing the conspicuousness of calcifications.[38] Surgical clips appear as hypointense foci that can potentially simulate mediastinal calcifications.

Simulation of enlarged nodes

Several entities may simulate the appearance of enlarged lymph nodes or other mediastinal masses on MR images. Slow flow within mediastinal vessels often results in intermediate signal intensity within the vascular lumen, similar to that of a soft tissue mass. The use of radiofrequency presaturated spin echo images or flow compensated gradient echo images usually allows blood flow to be recognized as hypointense or hyperintense relative to soft tissues, respectively. However, a thrombosed mediastinal vessel can appear similar to a soft tissue nodule on all sequences. In this situation, the tubular course of the lesion and its continuity with adjacent patent vessels should suggest vascular thrombosis. Thrombosed aneurysms are another related entity that can mimic a mediastinal soft tissue mass.[35] Continuity with the parent vessel may be difficult to establish, particularly in the case of thrombosed saccular aneurysms.

Transversely oriented vascular structures such as the pulmonary arteries or aortic arch can undergo partial volume averaging with surrounding mediastinal fat, thereby simulating a mediastinal mass (Figs. 1-3, *A* and *B*). Volume averaging can also affect tortuous mediastinal vessels, such as the brachiocephalic artery, with similar results. The use of reduced slice thickness and multiplanar image acquisition usually allows these entities to be recognized.

A small amount of fluid is frequently present within the superior recess of the pericardium, even in the absence of pericardial effusion. This fluid, located immediately dorsal to the aortic root, can undergo partial volume averaging with mediastinal fat simulating adeno-

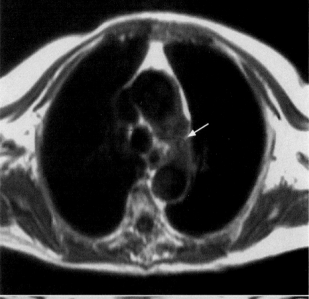

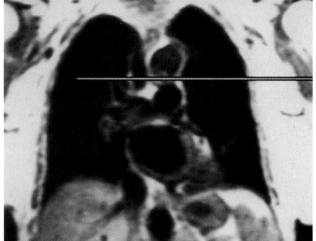

A

B

Fig. 1-3. Transaxial T1-weighted image (TR 960, TE 12, 4 Nex) demonstrates apparent mediastinal lymphadenopathy in the region of the aorticopulmonary window **(A)** *(arrow)*. This is due to partial volume averaging of mediastinal fat with the undersurface of the aortic arch. This is depicted on coronal image **(B)**, in which the position of image **A** is noted.

pathy.[92] A small collection of epicardial fat can be located along the pericardial recess below the main pulmonary artery and can simulate mediastinal lymph nodes, particularly on coronal T1-weighted images.[21] The atrial appendages contain prominent trabeculated soft tissues and are also a site of relatively slow blood flow. These factors can both contribute to the appearance of an intermediate signal intensity mediastinal mass (Fig. 1-4). This is most likely to occur when the atrial appendages are enlarged on the basis of regurgitant cardiac valvular lesions. Partial volume averaging of the atrial ap-

Fig. 1-4. The right atrial appendage simulates a juxtacardiac mass on this transaxial T1-weighted image (TR 600, TE 11, 4 Nex).

pendages with adjacent mediastinal fat can also simulate a mediastinal mass.

Ectopic parathyroid adenomas can be found in the mediastinum, where they may simulate enlarged lymph nodes.[49] Thyroid tissue can also extend into the superior mediastinum, simulating adenopathy or other mediastinal masses. Substernal goiter can be recognized by its connection with the cervical thyroid gland on coronal images (Figs. 1-5, *A* and *B*).

Assessment of lymph node response to therapy

MR is frequently used to monitor the effects of chemotherapy and/or radiotherapy on mediastinal lymph nodes and other masses. A diagnostic dilemma is presented when residual mediastinal lymph nodes are observed in patients who have undergone such treatment because neoplastic tissue within lymph nodes may be replaced by fibrotic tissue following therapy, without such nodes undergoing significant decrease in size. Therefore, nodes that have been successfully treated and no longer harbor neoplastic tissue can simulate sites of residual or recurrent mediastinal neoplasm.

This phenomenon renders size of mediastinal lymph nodes on serial examinations somewhat unreliable for determining the success of previous therapy. Consequently, attention has been directed toward the use of signal intensity criteria in this determination. It has been observed that T2-weighted images may allow for distinction between neoplastic and fibrotic lymph nodes. Fibrotic (i.e., inactive) nodes characteristically demonstrate reduced signal intensity because of their paucity of mobile protons, whereas tumor involvement usually results

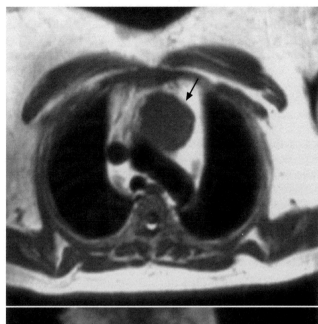

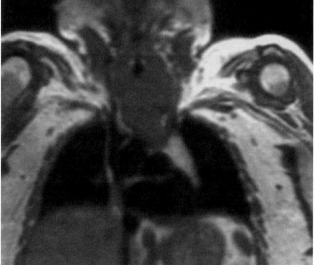

Fig. 1-5. A, Transaxial T1-weighted image (TR 460, TE 12, 4 Nex) depicts large anterior mediastinal soft tissue mass *(arrow)* suspicious for lymphadenopathy. **B,** Coronal T1-weighted image (TR 630, TE 12, 4 Nex) indicates continuity of the mediastinal lesion with enlarged thyroid gland, thus documenting that it represents substernal thyroid tissue.

in moderately increased signal intensity on T2-weighted images.

These criteria may be useful in selected patients, though several important pitfalls should be recognized. The diagnosis of posttherapeutic mediastinal fibrosis requires that the "mass" demonstrate uniform, low signal intensity on T2-weighted images. The presence of any subtle focus of increased signal intensity or any signal heterogeneity should be viewed with suspicion. Respiratory and vascular motion may generate high signal intensity ghosting artifacts, which can appear to represent intrinsic increased signal intensity within a mediastinal mass. Evaluation of such masses mandates the use of artifact reduction techniques such as respiratory ordered phase encoding, spatial presaturation, and others as available.

Even when a mediastinal mass demonstrates uniform signal intensity, diagnostic difficulties can arise. A major source of difficulty relates to ambiguity regarding the degree of hypointensity that is sufficient to consider a mediastinal lesion benign. The use of an internal signal intensity reference, such as paravertebral muscle, can be helpful in this regard. When the apparent mass appears uniformly isointense or hypointense with reference to skeletal muscle, it is likely to represent posttherapeutic fibrosis. However, when the signal intensity of such a lesion exceeds that of muscle—and particularly when it approaches that of mediastinal fat—residual/recurrent tumor should be suspected.

In the evaluation for lymph node activity, it is critical to use sequences having sufficient T2-weighted characteristics to allow for distinction between the signal intensity of different soft tissues. The use of a weak or moderate T2-weighted sequence will render neoplasm and fibrosis isointense with one another. Therefore, an echo time (TE) of at least 70 msec should be prescribed.

Following successful tumor eradication, the involved lymph node is initially replaced by granulation tissue, which then undergoes subsequent slow conversion to mature fibrotic tissue. Granulation tissue, or "immature fibrosis," has relatively increased signal intensity on T2-weighted images because of its prominent vascularity and interstitial water content. Thus MR signal criteria are of limited value in the characterization of mediastinal masses during the period immediately following completion of a treatment course.[22,33] During this time period, any increase in size of a nodal mass should arouse suspicion of tumor recurrence.

The precise length of time required for a lymph node or other mass to undergo complete conversion to mature fibrotic tissue has not been determined. Many variables may influence this process, including the type and duration of therapy, any concomitant treatment that the patient has undergone, and patient age and general health status. In addition, the ability to visualize this transition in lymph node signal intensity may also be influenced by the field strength at which imaging is performed, other features of the MR imaging system, and the particular set of imaging parameters used. Because of the variability in time course for observation of such signal changes, serial examinations at regular intervals are recommended following the completion of therapy. It is also important to obtain a baseline examination prior to therapy, so that subsequent subtle signal intensity alterations can be appreciated. Signal alterations caused by inflammatory tissue that simulate active tumor are uncommon when imaging is performed more than 6 months after treatment.[70]

It has been generally accepted that observation of uniform decreased signal intensity on adequately T2-weighted images reliably indicates the presence of mature fibrotic tissue. However, some controversy has involved observation of paradoxic increased signal intensity in association with mature fibrotic tissue on T2-weighted MR images.[57,65] One should also be aware that some tumors, particularly desmoplastic tumors or those associated with calcification and/or hemorrhage, can demonstrate decreased signal intensity on T2-weighted sequences. This can lead to misinterpretation of active tumor sites for mature fibrosis. Furthermore, microscopic tumor foci can be present, even when a mass appears uniformly hypointense on T2-weighted images.[70]

Retained secretions within paramediastinal lung tissue following radiation therapy can cause hyperintensity on T2-weighted images that simulates active tumor.[70] Another cause for false positive diagnoses is foci of medi-

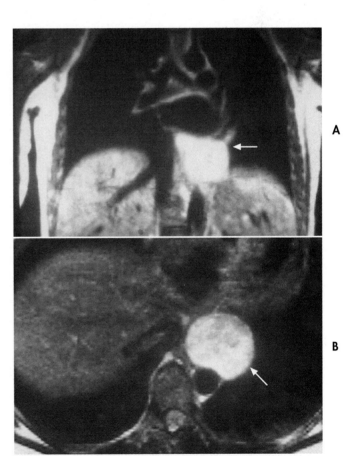

A

B

Fig. 1-6. T1-weighted coronal **(A)** and transaxial **(B)** images demonstrate a rounded hyperintense mass *(arrow)* within the posterior mediastinum representing a bronchogenic cyst. Hyperintensity is due to proteinaceous contents within the cyst.

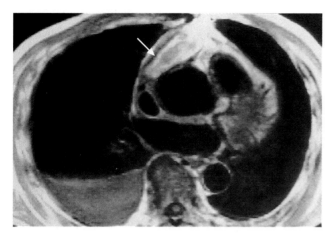

Fig. 1-7. An oval focus of increased signal intensity is demonstrated within the anterior mediastinum *(arrow)* on this transaxial T1-weighted image. This represents a pericardial hematoma in a patient who underwent recent coronary bypass surgery. Also note moderate sized right pleural effusion with some hyperintensity indicating hemothorax.

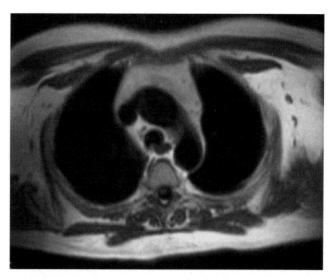

Fig. 1-8. Abundant fat throughout the anterior mediastinum is demonstrated on this transaxial T1-weighted image (TR 740, TE 12, 4 Nex).

astinal fat located within or adjacent to mature fibrotic tissue.[70] Fat-suppressed T2-weighted images will allow the latter entity to be distinguished from active tumor.

Mediastinal lesions in asymptomatic subjects

Some mediastinal masses can be incidentally discovered in asymptomatic subjects. These may include bronchogenic and foregut duplication cysts (Figs. 1-6, *A* and *B*). These cysts can appear hyperintense on T1-weighted images, because of their proteinaceous contents, and occasionally demonstrate fluid-fluid levels.[59] Lymphangioma is another mediastinal mass that can demonstrate T1 shortening on the same basis. Mediastinal edema and hematoma formation can be observed following surgery such as coronary artery bypass grafting (Fig. 1-7).

Mediastinal Fat

Abundant mediastinal fat can be present in obese patients, patients with Cushing disease, or those receiving exogenous steroid therapy (Figs. 1-8 and 1-9). While lipomatosis results in masslike enlargement of the mediastinum, the signal intensity characteristics of fat allow this entity to be easily recognized. Prominent collections of fat can be observed in the posterior mediastinum, particularly in patients with diaphragmatic defects or hernias (Fig. 1-10). Although usually unnecessary, fat suppressed sequences allow for definitive characterization of lipomatous tissue in equivocal cases.

The relatively high signal intensity of mediastinal fat on T1-weighted images is relied on for visualization of subtle mediastinal invasion by pulmonary neoplasms.

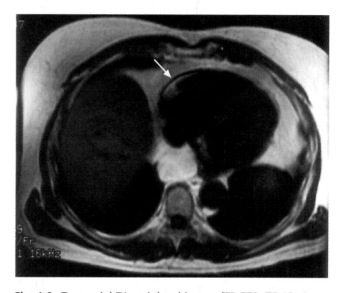

Fig. 1-9. Transaxial T1-weighted image (TR 770, TE 12, 4 Nex) demonstrates abundant fat throughout the posterior mediastinum in 59-year-old slightly male. Also note that the pericardium appears to be thickened or contain fluid *(arrow)* due to shear effects between the pericardial layers.

Therefore, tumor staging can be difficult in regions of the mediastinum containing relatively little fat, such as along the course of the aortic arch and descending thoracic aorta.

Thymus Gland

The thymus gland appears as a soft tissue structure within the anterior mediastinum, where it can simulate a mass lesion.[7,19] The thymus typically demonstrates sig-

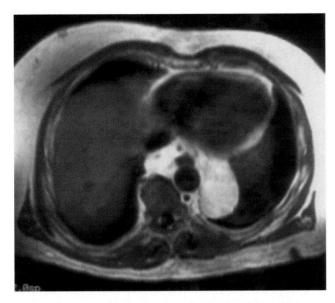

Fig. 1-10. Transaxial T1-weighted image (TR 500, TE 12, 4 Nex) demonstrates extensive posterior mediastinal fat, which extends up from the abdomen through a diaphragmatic defect. Also note small lesion in hepatic dome.

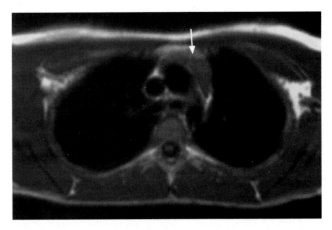

Fig. 1-11. Residual thymic tissue *(arrow)* is present in this 14-year-old male on transaxial T1-weighted image (TR 600, TE 12, 4 Nex). Note asymmetric prominence of the left thymic lobe.

nal intensity characteristics that are intermediate between those of muscle and fat on both T1- and T2-weighted images. However, thymic signal intensity is somewhat variable.

The thymus is prominent in infants and children and undergoes regression and fatty replacement during adolescence and early adulthood[7,75] (Fig. 1-11). However, the timing of thymic regression is somewhat variable, and residual thymic tissue can be frequently observed in young adults. The presence of residual thymic tissue can lead to misinterpretation as mediastinal lymphadenopathy, thymoma, or other forms of neoplastic or inflammatory mediastinal lesions.

Residual thymic tissue demonstrates several features that usually allow it to be distinguished from other masses. For example, residual thymic tissue frequently has a triangular or bilobed configuration, which is atypical for other mediastinal masses.[62] While the thymic lobes are usually symmetric, asymmetric prominence of one thymic lobe (usually the left lobe) is not uncommon and does not necessarily indicate pathology[62] (Fig. 1-11). The lateral margins of the thymus are usually straight or concave, though some degree of convexity can also be encountered as a normal variation in children.[62] The thymus can also have a quadrilateral configuration in some subjects.

The thymus is typically located within the anterior compartment of the mediastinum. However, ectopic descent of the thymus can occur, with thymic tissue extending into the superior and/or posterior medias-

tinum.[3,14,62] Within the posterior mediastinum, the thymus may become interposed between the superior vena cava and the trachea. The presence of ectopic thymic tissue increases the likelihood of confusion for a neoplasm, enlarged lymph nodes, or other mass. Correct identification is based on continuity of the apparent mass with the remainder of the thymus and isointensity between the apparent mass and thymus on all pulse sequences.[71]

Diffuse thymic enlargement can occur secondary to neoplastic involvement, such as lymphoma or thymoma. Neoplastic thymic enlargement can be difficult to distinguish from benign thymic hyperplasia. The latter entity may occur in patients with hyperparathyroidism or red cell aplasia.[62] Another cause for diffuse thymic enlargement is the "thymic rebound" phenomenon,[7,12,51] observed in patients undergoing chemotherapy. In such patients, benign thymic enlargement occurs on the basis of hyperplasia during or after chemotherapy.

Thymic cysts may be congenital or acquired and can simulate cystic or necrotic thymic neoplasms.[7,62] Cysts are recognized by uniform signal intensity characteristics that closely follow those of fluid on all pulse sequences, absence of soft tissue nodularity, septations or a thickened wall, and lack of enhancement when intravenous contrast material is administered. An unusual cause for apparent thymic cyst or mass is the presence of anomalous parathyroid tissue contained within the thymus.[4a]

Posterior Mediastinum

A number of masses arise in the posterior mediastinum. Of these, benign and malignant neurogenic tumors are most common. Many entities can simulate the appearance of posterior mediastinal masses. Such pseudomasses are often related to the gastrointestinal tract. The normal collapsed esophagus, for example, can appear to represent a mass. The potential for such confusion is increased when esophageal dilatation is present, which may be secondary to distal esophageal stricture, achalasia, scleroderma, or other causes (Fig. 1-12). Sliding or paraesophageal hiatal hernias and large esophageal diverticula can result in similar findings (Fig. 1-13). Pseudomasses may be related to previous esophageal surgical procedures, including colonic interposition or gastric pull-through procedure in patients who have undergone esophagectomy (Fig. 1-14).

Signal characteristics are usually not helpful in distinguishing the above entities from other mediastinal masses because gastrointestinal tract structures can have variable signal intensity, ranging from marked hyperintensity caused by fluid to marked hypointensity resulting from air. Heterogeneity within these structures caused by retained food debris represents another confounding factor, and it can simulate soft tissue nodularity within an apparent cystic lesion.

Distinction is therefore based on continuity of the apparent lesion and the gastrointestinal tract. Clinical information is also essential, particularly when previous surgery has been performed. In problematic cases, oral contrast material may be administered to mark the gastrointestinal tract. For example, a high-viscosity barium paste can be combined with a dilute solution of gadopentetate dimeglumine for this purpose.[66] This contrast material can facilitate identification of the esophagus on thoracic MR images, while at the same time improving distinction of the esophageal lumen from its wall. The latter feature can be instrumental in improving recognition of esophageal wall thickening and ulceration, which are otherwise difficult to appreciate on MR images.

Following intravenous contrast material administration, the normal esophagus can demonstrate a target-like appearance that can potentially simulate a necrotic lymph node or other mass (Fig. 1-15).

The azygoesophageal recess of the mediastinum is usually concave in normal individuals. When convexity of this recess is observed, the presence of pathology, including lymphadenopathy, should be suspected. However, convexity of the azygoesophageal recess can also represent an anatomic variant.[27] Retrocrural lymph nodes may also be simulated by osteophytes projecting anteriorly from the thoracic vertebral bodies or by partial volume averaging of the proximal ribs with adjacent fat (Figs. 1-16, *A* and *B*). Relatively slow flow within a dilated azygos or hemiazygos vein can lead to increased signal intensity and appear to represent an enlarged retrocrural lymph node. Ectopic pulmonary tissue may occasionally be found within the retrocrural space as an anatomic variation. This is unlikely, however, to simulate a mass lesion unless there is associated consolidation.

Extramedullary hematopoiesis can occur in the thoracic paravertebral regions in patients with chronic

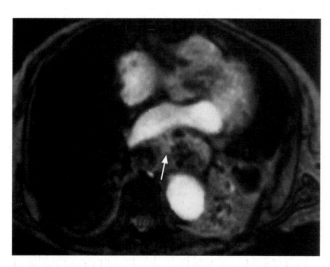

Fig. 1-12. Transaxial spoiled gradient echo image (TR 200, TE 12, 60-degree flip angle, 2 Nex) depicts apparent posterior mediastinal mass *(arrow)*, which impresses on the posterior wall of the left atrium. The mass represents a massively dilated esophagus, caused by distal esophageal stricture. Air-containing debris is recognized as foci of marked decreased signal intensity. Also note large left pleural effusion that appears hyperintense because of fluid motion.

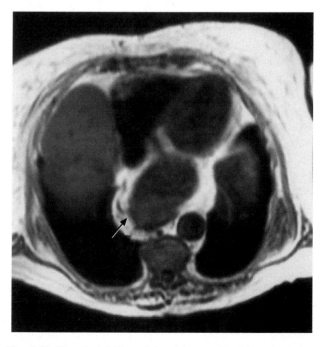

Fig. 1-13. Transaxial T1-weighted image (TR 500, TE 11, 4 Nex) of lower thorax demonstrates large moderate to low signal intensity structure within the posterior mediastinum, representing a hiatal hernia *(arrow)*.

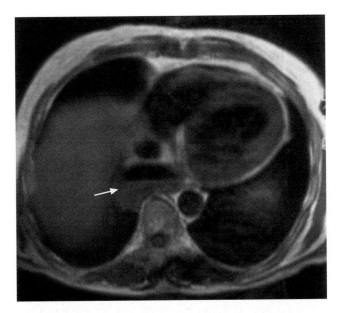

Fig. 1-14. T1-weighted image (TR 500, TE 12, 4 Nex) in 64-year-old male who underwent previous resection of esophageal carcinoma and gastric pull-through procedure. A posterior mediastinal structure containing a large air-fluid level is observed, representing the neoesophagus *(arrow).*

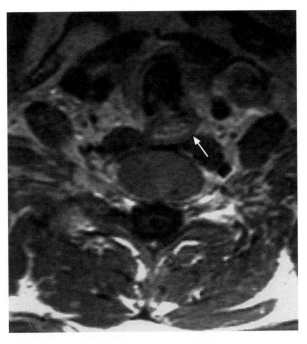

Fig. 1-15. Gadolinium chelate enhanced transaxial T1-weighted image (TR 400, TE 14, 2 Nex) demonstrates concentric ring–like enhancement pattern of normal esophagus *(arrow).* A large syrinx cavity is also noted within the cervical spinal cord.

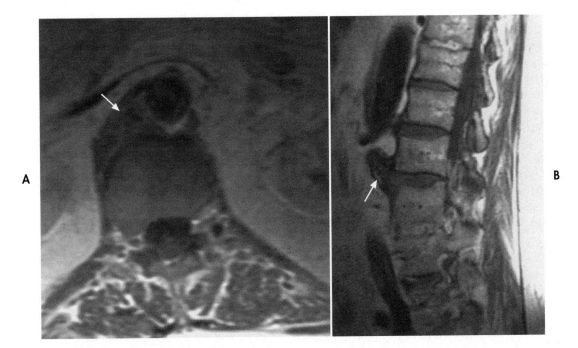

Fig. 1-16. A, Retrocrural lymphadenopathy is suggested on transaxial T1-weighted gadopentetate enhanced image (TR 500, TE 15, 4 Nex) *(arrow).* **B,** The apparent enlarged retrocrural lymph nodes actually represent osteophytes projecting from the anterior vertebral bodies, as demonstrated on sagittal T1-weighted image (TR 500, TE 12, 2 Nex) *(arrow).*

hemiglobinopathy and anemia, where it may simulate a posterior mediastinal neoplasm.[73] The presence of prominent reconverted hematopoietic marrow throughout the skeleton and the appropriate clinical history should alert one to this possibility.

Vasculature

A wide spectrum of congenital variation can affect the mediastinal vessels. A comprehensive review of these anomalies is beyond the scope of this chapter. Among the most frequent variations to affect the thoracic aorta and its major branches are right aortic arch, aberrant origin of the right subclavian artery, aortic coarctation, patent ductus arteriosus, truncus arteriosus, and aortic ring. The branching order of the great vessels from the aortic arch can be variable. Variations from the typical branching pattern are estimated to occur in approximately 20% of subjects.[4a] For example, the brachiocephalic and left common carotid arteries share a common origin in approximately 11% of subjects.[4a] A number of accessory arteries can also arise from the thoracic aorta.

The mediastinal veins similarly demonstrate considerable variation. A persistent left superior vena cava can exist that communicates with the coronary sinus, left atrium, left innominate vein, or right superior vena cava.[4a] The superior vena cava may be duplicated or absent, with the brachiocephalic veins opening directly into the right atrium. The azygos vein can empty into the right atrium, right brachiocephalic vein, or subclavian vein rather than into the superior vena cava.[4a]

The pulmonary arteries may originate from the thoracic aorta and rarely are duplicated. The left pulmonary artery may take an anomalous course through the mediastinum (pulmonary sling). The pulmonary veins are subject to variation in their number and size. Instead of communicating with the left atrium, they may occasionally enter the right atrium, inferior vena cava, or superior vena cava.[4a]

The thoracic duct usually terminates near the junction of the superior vena cava and left internal jugular vein. However, the duct can communicate with any of the major mediastinal veins.[4a]

LUNGS
Anatomic Variations

Many variations are seen in the pattern of pulmonary lobar division. The interlobar fissures can be absent, or various accessory fissures may be present; these may be complete or incomplete. The size and configuration of the trachea are variable, and the carina can be located anywhere between the T5 and T7 vertebral levels.[4a] A sabre sheath trachea is a common variant and can be ob-

served in patients with obstructive lung disease. There is also considerable variability in the organization of bronchopulmonary segments and in the branching pattern of lobar bronchi.[4a] These variations are usually not evident on MR images.

An "azygos lobe" is present in approximately 0.5% of subjects, and an accessory inferior lobe is also not infrequently present[4a] (Figs. 1-17, *A* and *B*). The lungs may be asymmetric in size on the basis of hypoplasia, and occasionally agenetic or aplastic lungs are encountered. Sequestered lung tissue can be located in various sites, though the most common is the lower left hemithorax.

Pulmonary Nodules

Conventional MR imaging has demonstrated limited ability to depict pulmonary nodules.[88] This is particularly true for relatively small nodules. The poor sensitivity of MR is attributable to several factors, the most significant of which is the effect of respiratory motion. Periodic motion of the chest wall, lungs, and diaphragm during the respiratory cycle results in artifactual bands of increased signal intensity that propagate along the phase encoding direction of the image. These "ghosting artifacts" appear as complete or incomplete representations of the moving structure, with their prominence directly related to the signal intensity of the moving structure. Because of its relatively high signal intensity, fat within the chest wall is the primary contributor to such artifacts. In addition to these structured phase encode errors, respiratory motion also leads to generalized blurring throughout the image. Both of these factors combine to obscure small pulmonary nodules.

During the respiratory cycle, lung nodules also undergo significant periodic motion, resulting in phase shifts that decrease the conspicuousness of such nodules. As these nodules move into and out of a particular section, partial volume averaging of the lesion with adjacent lung tissue will also occur, further decreasing their visibility.

A number of methods have been developed to reduce the impact of respiratory motion for thoracic MR imaging. An overview of these methods has been provided by Haacke and Patrick.[40] The performance of multiple data acquisitions (excitations) results in improved signal-to-noise ratio and proportional reduction in severity of respiratory motion phase encoding artifacts. However, image acquisition time increases in direct proportion to the number of excitations, and this method does not alleviate blurring.

With respiratory gating, data acquisition occurs only during specific points in the respiratory cycle. This method substantially prolongs imaging time and limits the operator's choice of repetition time (TR), since this parameter is determined by the length of the respiratory cycle. For these reasons, respiratory gating is seldom

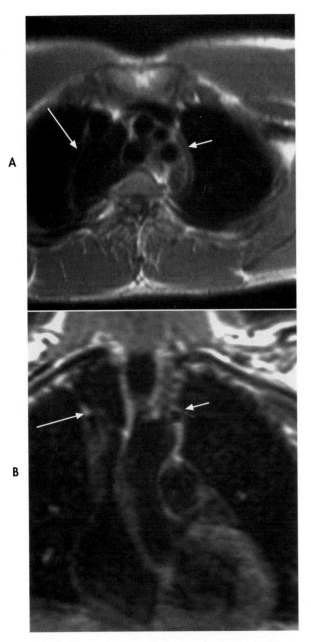

METHODS FOR SUPPRESSING RESPIRATORY MOTION ARTIFACTS

- Respiratory gating
- Respiratory pseudogating
- Respiratory ordered phase encoding
- Spatial presaturation pulses
- Gradient moment nulling
- Binder
- Multiple excitations
- Breathhold imaging

Fig. 1-17. A, Transaxial (TR 900, TE 11, 4 Nex) and **B,** coronal (TR 640, TE 10, 4 Nex) T1-weighted images in 24-year-old male. The azygos arch *(arrow)* encompasses a portion of pulmonary tissue in the right apical region, forming an "azygos lobe". In addition, the left superior intercostal vein is shown forming an "aortic nipple" *(small arrow).*

a bellows device placed around the patient's chest. This simulates the effect of a long slow expiration and reduces respiratory motion artifact without significantly increasing imaging time.

Spatial presaturation radiofrequency pulses are most commonly used to decrease vascular pulsation artifacts. However, such pulses can be applied within the field-of-view, so as to overlap the chest wall. This will decrease the signal intensity of fat within the chest wall, and thus related motion artifacts can be proportionally diminished. In prescribing such presaturation bands, the operator must be careful to avoid overlap with the mediastinum and anterior lung fields, since unintended presaturation in these locations could obscure lesions.

Gradient moment nulling (flow compensation) uses gradient lobes, usually along the slice-select and readout directions, to reestablish phase coherence among moving spins at the time of echo collection.[13] The implementation of this method requires a relatively long echo time, and it is therefore most often used for acquisition of T2-weighted images. Gradient moment nulling is also capable of decreasing blurring artifacts, which many of the other techniques do not address.

While each of the preceding methods can reduce the severity of respiratory related artifacts, none is capable of completely eliminating them. The only way such artifacts can be eliminated is by imaging during suspended respiration. This requires image acquisition times substantially shorter than those allowed by conventional sequences. Gradient echo sequences are the most widely used method for performing rapid imaging. Gradient echo sequences are poorly suited to pulmonary imaging, however, because of their sensitivity to susceptibility artifacts. Rapid spin echo pulse sequences can be performed during suspended respiration, though the limitations of such sequences include their limited signal-to-noise ratio and vulnerability to vascular pulsation artifacts.

In addition to the effects of respiratory motion, a second major factor has limited ability of MR to depict

used at the present time. Respiratory pseudogating refers to prescription of the TR to approximate the duration of the patient's respiratory cycle. The technique is of limited effectiveness because of variability in the length of the respiratory cycle during image acquisition.

Respiratory ordered phase encoding involves retrospective reordering of phase encoding steps with reference to the respiratory cycle, which is monitored using pulmonary nodules. The lungs are comprised primarily of air, with parenchymal tissue accounting for relatively little of their total volume. This creates a problem on MR images, where air contributes to artifactual signal void. This signal void often extends beyond the actual location of such air, and it can reduce the signal intensity of neighboring tissues. Such artifacts reflect marked differences in the magnetization properties of air and soft tissues and are generally referred to as "susceptibility effects." Susceptibility artifacts increase in prominence according to the echo time (TE) used; therefore, T2-weighted images are affected more severely than T1-weighted images. They are also accentuated on gradient echo images, because of the absence of a 180-degree radiofrequency refocusing pulse.[16] Susceptibility artifacts limit visualization of peripheral pulmonary vessels as well as pulmonary nodules on MR images.

Because of these considerations, short TR and TE (i.e., T1-weighted) spin echo sequences generally provide the best depiction of pulmonary nodules as well as pulmonary infiltrates and other abnormalities. While reduced echo time is advantageous in reducing susceptibility effect, it also leads to relative increased intravascular signal intensity. This increased signal intensity can reduce distinction between mediastinal/hilar lymph nodes and blood vessels. Specific pulse sequences have been investigated that may reduce susceptibility effects for pulmonary MR imaging.[4]

A number of pulmonary lesions have low signal intensity on spin echo pulse sequences. Among these entities are calcified pulmonary nodules, arteriovenous malformations, and lesions containing acute or chronic hemorrhagic breakdown products. Such hypointense lesions may be particularly difficult to visualize on conventional spin echo sequences because of the lack of contrast between the lesions and surrounding low signal intensity pulmonary tissue. The visibility of some of these lesions—including pulmonary nodules—is often improved with the use of intravenous contrast material.

Because of their similar appearance, some low signal intensity pulmonary lesions are also difficult to characterize. For example, calcified lesions can simulate flow void in vessels or vascular lesions. One report describes a similar low signal intensity appearance of pulmonary arteriovenous malformation and chronic hematoma, with signal characteristics attributable to rapid blood flow and hemoglobin breakdown products, respectively.[6] While conventional spin echo images may not allow for differentiation of these entities, other techniques such as phase reconstructions and flow sensitive gradient echo images can often assist in this process. On spin echo images, the low signal intensity of

air-containing bronchi can appear similar to pulmonary vessels, particularly in the hilar regions (Fig. 1-1). Gradient echo images are again useful in distinguishing these structures.

Many entities are capable of simulating the appearance of pulmonary nodules; some of these are familiar from CT. For example, partial volume averaging of the first rib can result in an apparent nodule in the anterior chest. Callus associated with healed rib fractures may lead to similar findings, usually along the lateral chest wall. The air-filled esophagus may appear to represent a dilated and thick walled left lower lobe bronchus, or it can be confused for a cavitary pulmonary nodule. Plugs of mucous within the airways can simulate a pulmonary nodule. Mediastinal fat extending into the interlobar fissures, inferior pulmonary ligament, or accessory pulmonary fissures can appear nodular or can be volume averaged with adjacent lung tissue, again simulating a pulmonary nodule.[26] Thickening of the interlobar fissures caused by previous inflammation or the presence of pleural fluid within these fissures are additional causes of pulmonary pseudotumors.

Pulmonary vessels can have intermediate to high intraluminal signal intensity because of relatively slow blood flow, entry phenomenon, or the use of gradient moment nulling. Such vessels may appear to represent pulmonary nodules, particularly when they are relatively prominent and/or asymmetric. Pulmonary vessels within the dependent portions of the lungs are generally of relatively increased caliber. A generalized increased signal intensity can also be observed within the dependent aspect of the lungs (Fig. 1-18). The azygos vein can also mimic a pulmonary nodule, particularly when an acces-

---

SIMULATION OF PULMONARY NODULES

- Partial volume averaging of first rib
- Healed rib fractures
- Esophagus
- Mucous plugs
- Mediastinal fat
- Thickening or fluid in interlobar fissures
- Pulmonary vessels
- Azygos/superior intercostal veins
- Rounded atelectasis
- Collapsed/consolidated lung
- Pulmonary infarct/organizing pneumonia
- Atrial appendages
- Partial volume averaging of diaphragm
- Aliasing of humeral head
- Postoperative/radiation changes
- Atypical pleural fluid collections/masses

sory azygos lobe is present (Figs. 1-17, *A* and *B*, 1-19, *A* and *B*, and 1-20, *A* and *B*). Similarly, the left superior intercostal vein can simulate a pulmonary nodule when it creates a so-called aortic nipple (Fig. 1-17).

Rounded atelectasis usually occurs in association with pleural disease, such as that related to asbestos exposure, and can simulate a peripheral pulmonary nodule.[60,84] Curvilinear low signal intensity may be observed within rounded atelectasis, representing thickened pleural indentations.[84] Collapsed or consolidated lung tissue often enhances prominently when contrast material is administered, further contributing to diagnostic difficulties in some patients. Simple atelectasis can appear similar to postobstructive collapse cause by a mass. Simple (i.e., nonobstructive) atelectasis usually demonstrates decreased signal intensity on T2-weighted images, whereas increased signal intensity is often seen in patients with postobstructive atelectasis.[43]

Pulmonary infarct and focal organizing pneumonia are other entities that can lead to confusion for a mass lesion.[53] The atrial appendages can simulate a lung mass when they undergo partial volume averaging with adjacent pulmonary parenchyma (Figs. 1-21, *A* and *B*). Partial volume averaging of the diaphragm with lung tissue can lead to similar findings in the lung bases; this is most likely to occur when there is diaphragmatic eventration or herniation.

Central or diffuse calcification within a pulmonary nodule on plain radiographs or CT usually signifies a healed granuloma. MR is limited in its ability to depict calcification, and thus distinction between granulomatous and neoplastic nodules is more difficult.[76,81] This is an important limitation of MR in the evaluation of pulmonary nodules, because of the high prevalence of patients with old granulomatous disease.

Aliasing (i.e., wraparound) artifacts occur when there is excitation of tissue located outside the prescribed field-of-view. This results in mismapping of the signal intensity corresponding to such tissue into the field-of-view, where it has the potential to simulate or obscure lesions. In the chest, aliasing of the humeral heads into the upper lung fields can occur on either coronal or transaxial

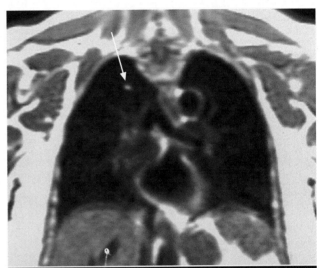

A

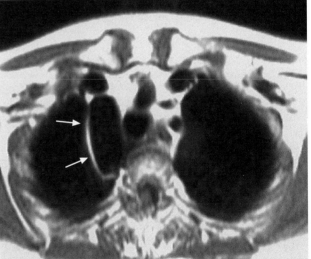

B

Fig. 1-19. A, Coronal T1-weighted image (TR 500, TE 11, 4 Nex) demonstrates an apparent right upper lobe pulmonary nodule *(arrow)*. **B,** This represents the azygos vein in a patient with an "azygos lobe" (TR 500, TR 11, 4 Nex) *(small arrows)*. Increased intravascular signal intensity is related to slow blood flow.

Fig. 1-18. Relative increased signal intensity is observed within the dependent aspect of both lungs *(arrows)* on this transaxial T1-weighted image (TR 970, TE 11, 4 Nex) in patient with right pulmonary mass *(arrowhead)*.

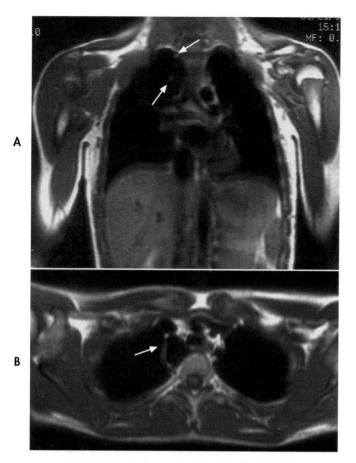

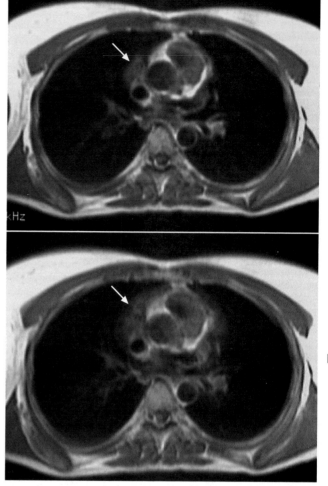

Fig. 1-20. A, Coronal T1-weighted image (TR 620, TE 12, 4 Nex) depicts two apparent nodules *(arrows)* in the right pulmonary apex. **B,** These represent the azygos vein, which is arched forward to form an azygos lobe, as documented on transaxial T1-weighted image (TR 600, TE 12, 4 Nex) *(arrow).*

Fig. 1-21. T1-weighted transaxial image **(A)** (TR 1030, TE 12, 4 Nex) demonstrates apparent mass or infiltrate in the right middle lobe *(arrow).* This is due to partial volume averaging of lung with the right atrial appendage, which is seen on more caudal image **(B)** *(arrow).*

images and can simulate the appearance of unilateral or bilateral apical pulmonary masses (Figs. 1-22, *A* and *B*). Aliasing can be avoided with the use of algorithms such as "nophase wrap," which provide oversampling and effective extension of the field-of-view along the phase encoding direction. An alternative approach is to suppress the signal intensity of tissue extending beyond the field-of-view with the use of radiofrequency presaturation pulses or external shielding with a material such as aluminum foil. The phase and frequency encode gradients may be reoriented, which will redirect aliasing artifacts into another portion of the image. The use of some filters will also assist in reducing aliasing artifacts. The prescribed field-of-view, of course, can simply be enlarged to accommodate tissue that extends beyond the field-of-view, thereby preventing aliasing at the expense of decreased spatial resolution.

The presence of a retained surgical sponge following thoracic surgery can simulate a mass lesion.[48] An unusual

cause for a thoracic mass is the presence of an intrathoracic spleen.[24] In the latter situation, the "mass" demonstrates signal intensity characteristics similar to those of normal splenic tissue. Abnormal contrast enhancement of lung parenchyma can be observed following radiation therapy; these findings should not be interpreted as evidence of malignant involvement.[89] In patients who have undergone pneumonectomy, the postpneumonectomy space often contains fluid and manifests heterogeneous signal intensity because of hemorrhagic and fibrotic material; these features can simulate recurrent neoplasm[55,56] (Fig. 1-23). The presence of calcifications within the postpneumonectomy space, as elsewhere, is poorly depicted on MR images.[55,56] The location of surgical clips following pneumonectomy may not be apparent on MR images, which can create difficulty in the planning of

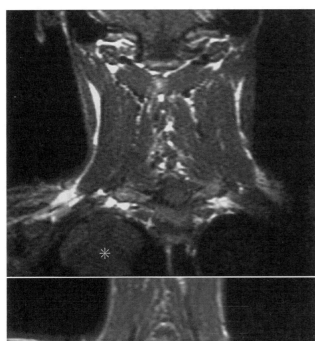

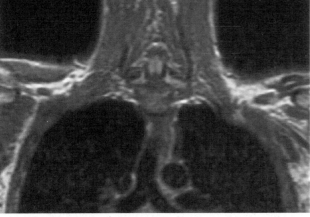

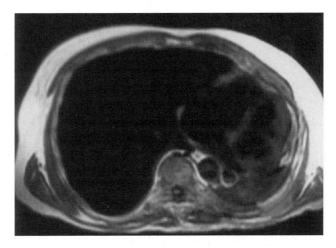

Fig. 1-23. Transaxial T1-weighted image (TR 700, TE 12, 4 Nex) in 68-year-old male who has undergone previous left pneumonectomy. The mediastinal and cardiac structures are shifted into the left hemithorax. Fluid containing some high signal intensity hemorrhage products fills the postpneumonectomy space.

Fig. 1-22. A, There is an apparent rounded mass lesion *(asterisk)* involving the right pulmonary apex (Pancoast tumor) on this coronal T1-weighted image (TR 300, TE 16, 0.5 Nex). This image was acquired using a cervical spine coil and a 24 cm field-of-view. **B,** Subsequent coronal image acquired using body coil and 34 cm field-of-view (TR 2000, TE 30, 2 Nex) reveals no mass to be present. The apparent mass in **A** represents the humeral head that has undergone aliasing because of the restricted field-of-view.

subsequent radiotherapy.[55,56] Heterogeneous masslike thickening may be observed in the hilar region in patients who have undergone previous lung transplantation. This represents gastrocolic omentum that has been used to encourage healing of the bronchial anastomosis.[32] Signal intensity characteristics of this omental flap reflect the predominant presence of fat and vascular structures.

Pulmonary hemorrhage results in a variety of signal intensity patterns, depending on the oxygenation state of the blood breakdown products. Following acute hemorrhage, deoxyhemoglobin leads to markedly reduced (signal) intensity on T2-weighted images, which can be indistinguishable from adjacent pulmonary air.[47] The for-

mation of methemoglobin is marked by increased signal intensity on T1-weighted images. Subacute pulmonary hemorrhage can therefore have an appearance similar to lipoid pneumonia.[8,9]

PLEURAL SPACE

A small amount of pleural fluid can be observed on T2-weighted images in normal subjects.[63] Atypical pleural fluid collections can be difficult to distinguish from pulmonary or mediastinal masses. Pleural fluid may collect along the diaphragmatic pleural surface in a so-called subpulmonic location. Such collections redistribute with alteration in patient position, indicating that they are not loculated. Pleural fluid may collect within the interlobar fissures, where it can again simulate a pulmonary mass or a loculated fluid collection.[63] The location of the collection, its lenticular morphology, and its isointensity with fluid on all sequences allow for recognition.

Pleural effusion can be difficult to distinguish from abdominal fluid (i.e., ascites) in some patients. Distinction between these entities is based on four observations.[63] First, the diaphragm is located peripheral to abdominal structures, whereas it is central with reference to the lungs and pleura. Second, the interface between the liver and ascitic fluid is sharp, whereas its interface with pleural fluid is not. Third, the diaphragmatic crus may be displaced anteriorly by pleural effusion, but not by ascites. Finally, ascitic fluid is not able to extend behind the bare area of the liver.

Although these signs are helpful in distinguishing pleural effusion from ascites, several pitfalls can be encountered.[63] For example, pleural fluid can appear to be located central to the diaphragm when the latter structure is inverted as a result of a large pleural fluid collection. In this situation, ascites can be simulated. Basilar pulmonary atelectasis can appear to represent the hemidiaphragm, also leading to an erroneous diagnosis of ascites.

Pleural fluid usually has signal intensity similar to that of other fluids, though aberrant signal characteristics can be observed. For example, proteinaceous or hemorrhagic material related to exudative pleural effusions can lead to relative increased signal intensity on T1-weighted images and decreased signal intensity on T2-weighted images. These findings can occur in association with infection (empyema), tumor, trauma (hemothorax), or lymphatic obstruction or disruption (chylothorax).[61] Complicated exudative effusions such as those caused by malignancy or infection often appear more intense than simple exudates, which are in turn more intense than transudative effusions on T2-weighted images.[18]

Atypical signal intensity characteristics can be observed even when a simple transudate is present, related to movement of such fluid during the respiratory cycle. Pleural fluid may display relative increased signal intensity on T1-weighted spin echo images because of entry phenomenon or slow flow. Conversely, relative decreased intensity on T2-weighted spin echo images can be caused by phase shifts related to rapid or turbulent motion. Movement of pleural fluid can result in high signal intensity on gradient echo images[87] (Figs. 1-12 and 1-24). Therefore, high signal intensity pleural fluid on T1-weighted gradient echo images does not necessarily indicate hemothorax or chylothorax. Motion of pleural fluid causes phase encoding errors that are manifested as alternating high and low signal intensity ghost artifacts (Fig. 1-2). These artifacts can simulate or obscure pleural or pulmonary lesions.

Diffuse or localized pleural thickening can result from neoplastic involvement. However, these findings may also be caused by inflammation or infection or occur after radiotherapy, thoracotomy, or administration of sclerosing agents. Nodular areas of benign pleural thickening can simulate a pleural-based pulmonary mass, pleural metastasis, or a primary pleural neoplasm such as mesothelioma. Pulmonary volume loss can occur in association with both benign and malignant pleural disease.[63] Circumferential pleural thickening and involvement of the mediastinal pleural surfaces are more frequently due to mesothelioma than other causes.[63] Inflammatory pleural thickening usually does not involve the mediastinal pleura, although tuberculosis can be an exception.[63] Pleural thickening caused by old granulomatous disease is frequent in the apical regions, where it can simulate a superior sulcus carcinoma. Small pleural effusions can be difficult to distinguish from pleural thickening, though

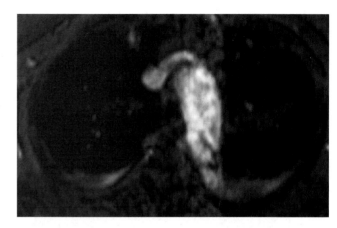

Fig. 1-24. Relative T1-weighted spoiled gradient echo image (TR 50, TE 13, 60-degree flip angle, 2 Nex) demonstrates bilateral hyperintense pleural fluid collections suggestive of hemorrhagic collections. However, these findings represent bland pleural effusions in a patient with congestive heart failure. Hyperintensity is related to motion of fluid within the pleural space.

the former entity usually appears more intense on T2-weighted images.

Pleural calcification may result from asbestos exposure, tuberculosis, or previous hemothorax or empyema. The presence of such calcification is poorly visualized on MR images. Pleural calcification can also be caused by mesothelioma.[63] When extensive pleural calcification is present, a curvilinear signal intensity void may be seen. The signal void of calcified pleura can simulate an extrapleural air collection (i.e., pneumothorax) (Figs. 1-25, A-C).

Fat is normally present in the extrapleural space. Such fat can be prominent in some patients, such as those receiving exogenous steroid therapy. Extrapleural fat collections can simulate pleural thickening or fluid, though signal intensity characteristics usually allow for distinction. Fat suppression methods may be used in problematic cases. Prominent costal fat can simulate pleural plaques and can thicken because of scarring within the adjacent lung parenchyma.[26] Costal fat can also extend into the pleural space along the path of a thoracostomy drainage tube.[26]

BREAST
Carcinoma

The use of MR to evaluate breast pathology is gaining considerable attention. This attention results from recent studies indicating that MR can be used to stage patients with documented breast carcinoma prior to surgery, to detect radiographically occult breast carcinoma in women with dense fibroparenchymal changes, and to

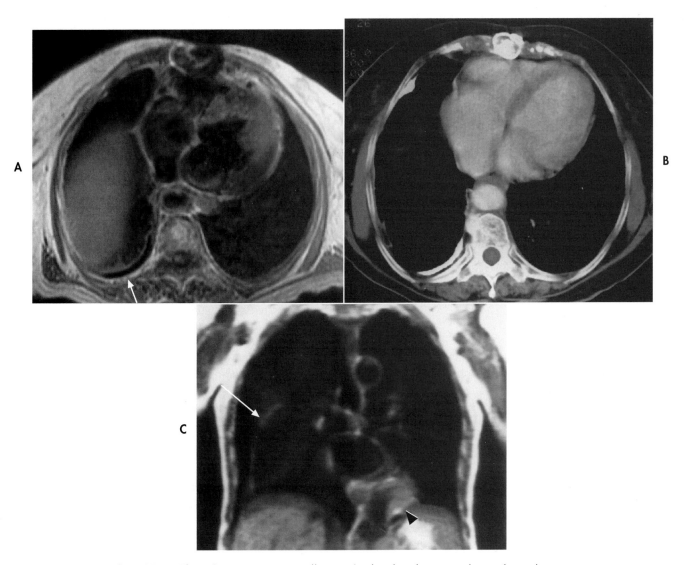

Fig. 1-25. A, There is an apparent small posterior loculated pneumothorax *(arrow)* on transaxial proton density–weighted image (TR 1430, TE 11, 4 Nex). This appearance is due to a calcified pleural plaque as confirmed on CT image **B**. A second calcified plaque, located along the anterior pleural surface, is not visualized on MR because of its poor sensitivity for calcium. **C,** Findings in **A** can be compared with actual pneumothorax *(arrow)* in another patient with left lower lobe lung carcinoma *(arrowhead)* (TR 780, TE 12, 4 Nex). Note artifact secondary to metallic sternal suture wires in **A**.

characterize lesions that have an indeterminate appearance on mammography.

Parenchymal breast tissue can be distinguished from surrounding fatty components of the breast on conventional T1-weighted or T2-weighted MR images. However, such images generally do not allow for distinction between tumor and normal or hyperplastic breast parenchyma. Conventional MR imaging, therefore, has relatively poor sensitivity for breast cancer detection as well as limited ability to stage its extent.[1]

Focal prominence or asymmetry of breast tissue is not a reliable indicator of neoplasm. Breast tissue is frequently bilaterally asymmetric in normal individuals, with the right breast usually larger than the left.[4a] Supernumerary breasts can occur. Parenchymal tissue within the axillary portion of the breast can simulate a mass lesion. Focal areas of prominent tissue are frequently due to fibrocystic changes rather than neoplasm.[54] Fibrocystic changes of the breast fluctuate in prominence throughout the menstrual cycle and may also vary in response to hormonal therapy or dietary substances. Physiologic prominence of breast parenchyma and associated hyperintensity on T2-weighted images also occur during pregnancy and lactation (Fig. 1-26).

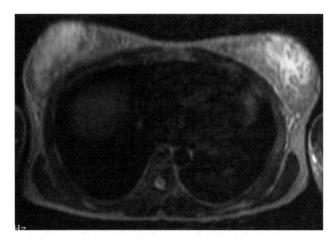

Fig. 1-26. Transaxial T2-weighted image (TR 3400, TE 80, 2 Nex) demonstrates symmetric prominence and hyperintensity of glandular breast tissue in woman imaged during first trimester of pregnancy.

All of the above anatomic and physiologic variations limit the usefulness of observed prominence of breast tissue as a means for diagnosing malignancy.

Because of these limitations, initial attempts to use MR to evaluate breast carcinoma generated disappointing results. Renewed efforts have centered on use of paramagnetic contrast agents for improving the depiction of breast malignancy as well as for determining its extent. Breast carcinoma undergoes significant enhancement when an agent such as gadopentetate dimeglumine is administered intravenously,[45,50,68,79] while normal breast tissue does not.

Enhancing breast lesions can be difficult to discern on standard T1-weighted spin echo images because enhancing lesions can be isointense with adjacent high signal intensity fatty tissues. Consequently, the use of fat suppression techniques has been critical to improve demonstration of pathologic contrast enhancement in the breast.[72] In order to detect small lesions and offer precise staging information, high spatial resolution methods are also required. Therefore, the prescribed section thickness and field-of-view should be small and the data acquisition matrix relatively large. Three-dimensional Fourier transform (i.e., volume) fat suppressed T1-weighted gradient echo sequences have been used to provide thin contiguous images in reasonable acquisition times.

Surface coils help to compensate for reduced signal-to-noise ratio that otherwise occurs on high-resolution images. A variety of unilateral and bilateral breast coils are now available. Significant artifacts related to coil motion with respiration can degrade image quality, particularly when the patient is imaged in the supine position. Improved image quality is achieved with prone patient

positioning, with the breast extending downward into the coil.[36]

Focal areas of contrast material enhancement within the breast are associated with malignancy. However, enhancement can also occur as a result of many benign entities. Enhancement normally occurs in the retroareolar region and within the vascular structures of the breast.[68] Enhancement of the normal nipple can preclude determination of nipple involvement by carcinoma.[42] Benign breast lesions such as proliferative and nonproliferative fibroparenchymal tissue, fibroadenoma, sclerosing adenosis, and atypical hyperplasia can all undergo enhancement, simulating carcinoma.[42,45,50,68,79] Prominent contrast enhancement can also occur in patients with fat necrosis caused by associated inflammation.[30] Evaluation of lesion morphology is useful in distinguishing these benign entities from neoplasm, with a spiculated appearance suggestive of malignancy. However, in one study of 30 breasts, MR demonstrated a specificity of only 37% for diagnosing carcinoma, despite a sensitivity of 94%.[42]

Physiologic variations in contrast enhancement of breast tissue also occur during the menstrual cycle.[50] Use of dynamic contrast enhanced imaging can allow for improved distinction between benign and malignant breast lesions as compared with routine contrast enhanced images. Breast carcinoma tends to enhance faster and more intensely than benign lesions using this technique.[30]

Previous intervention can result in morphologic and signal intensity alterations within the breast. Air-fluid levels in patients who have undergone recent excision of breast lesions can suggest abscess (Fig. 1-27). Focal or diffuse edema may be related to recent surgery or radiation therapy. T2-weighted images do not allow for distinction between postradiation fibrosis and recurrent tumor.[17] However, using dynamic contrast enhanced imaging, early enhancement (i.e., before 3 minutes) usually indicates tumor recurrence, whereas fibrosis tends to enhance later and less prominently.[17]

BREAST ENHANCEMENT THAT MAY SIMULATE CARCINOMA

- Normal retroareolar region/nipple
- Normal vascular structures
- Menstrual related changes
- Fibroparenchymal tissue
- Fibroadenoma
- Sclerosing adenosis
- Atypical hyperplasia
- Fat necrosis

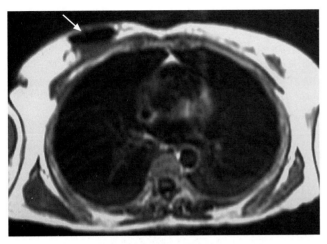

Fig. 1-27. Transaxial T1-weighted image demonstrates an air-fluid level within the right breast *(arrow)*. While this finding could represent abscess, this is due to recent biopsy and lumpectomy for breast carcinoma performed 2 days earlier.

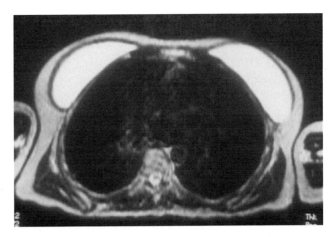

Fig. 1-28. Transaxial T2-weighted image demonstrates uniformly hyperintense breast prostheses bilaterally.

Breast Prostheses

Another application of MR is the evaluation of patients with breast implants for possible implant rupture or other complications. Breast prostheses display signal characteristics of fluid (Fig. 1-28) and can demonstrate some deformity in the absence of disruption. The prosthesis is normally surrounded by a thin fibrous capsule. Radial folds may be observed within an intact implant on MR images and do not imply that rupture or leakage has occurred.[36,64] Rather, these are normal infoldings of the elastomer shell. When intracapsular rupture has occurred, curvilinear areas of decreased signal intensity are observed, representing the implant shell floating within silicone gel; this has been termed the "linguine sign."[64]

Silicone within breast implants demonstrates signal intensity features similar to those of fluid on T1- and T2-weighted images.[36] Consequently, the presence of small amounts of silicone leakage outside of the prosthesis capsule can be difficult to discern. Specialized pulse sequences employing radiofrequency presaturation at the resonant frequency of silicone, as well as other techniques, have been developed to improve identification of silicone leakage and to distinguish it from related inflammatory changes.[20,74] More widely available water saturation T2-weighted images can also be used to distinguish inflammatory changes from extracapsular silicone collections. Microscopic leakage of silicone can occur through the implant shell and is poorly visualized on MR images.[64]

Postoperative scarring in patients with prostheses can simulate the appearance of breast carcinoma.[44] While mature scar does not undergo significant contrast enhancement, variable enhancement ranging from absent to intense has been observed during the first 6 months following surgery.[44]

CHEST WALL AND DIAPHRAGM
Anatomic Variations
Chest wall

The sternum appears concave or convex in patients with pectus excavatum or carinatum deformity, respectively. The sternum can also be cleft, and suprasternal ossicles can be observed.[4a] The xiphoid process is highly variable in size and shape. The ribs and related abnormalities are usually poorly visualized on MR images because of their small size and their motion during the respiratory cycle.[2,58] There is considerable variation in the number of ribs, and the ribs may be bifid or fused. Cervical ribs are present in up to 1% of the population[4a] and can simulate a supraclavicular mass lesion[28]; lumbar ribs may also occur. Hypertrophy, calcification, or ossification at the costochondral junctions can result in a heterogeneous masslike appearance.[23] A distorted appearance of the chest wall is seen in patients with severe kyphoscoliosis. The number of internal mammary vessels is variable.[31] Absence of the internal mammary artery may be related to previous harvesting for coronary bypass grafting.

Diaphragm

The muscular diaphragm is of variable thickness and can be congenitally deficient.[10] The crura may appear nodular or redundant, simulating a mass lesion.[10] The thickness of the diaphragmatic crura varies during the respiratory cycle.[91] Partial volume averaging of the hepatic dome can simulate a diaphragmatic mass.

Artifacts that Simulate or Obscure Chest Wall Abnormalities

Foci of abnormal signal intensity along the chest wall can arise from silver chloride electrocardiographic (ECG) leads[83] (Figs. 1-29, *A* and *B*). These artifacts appear as foci of hypointensity with surrounding curvilinear hyperintensity. Susceptibility effects from ECG leads can also result in focal fat suppression failure artifacts when fat saturation is used (Figs. 1-29, *A* and *B*

and 1-30, *A* and *B*). A series of signal voids within the sternum usually indicates metallic sutures related to previous median sternotomy (Fig. 1-31). Susceptibility artifacts caused by ECG leads and sternal wires are markedly accentuated on gradient echo images, where they can obscure abnormalities involving the chest wall and anterior mediastinum (Figs. 1-31, *A* and *B*).

A rounded signal void within the anterior chest wall can result from an implanted drug infusion port[85] (Fig. 1-32). Following removal of Hickman or other related

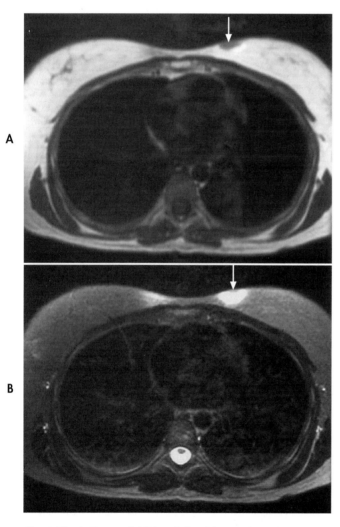

Fig. 1-29. A, Transaxial T1-weighted image (TR 360, TE 12, 4 Nex) depicts focus of artifactual signal void with surrounding hyperintensity in the left anterior chest wall *(arrow)*. These findings are due to the presence of an ECG electrode. **B,** Corresponding fat saturation fast spin echo T2-weighted image (TR 5300, effective TE 104, 4 Nex, 16 echo train) demonstrates failure to suppress fat signal in vicinity of electrode caused by local alterations in magnetic field *(arrow)*.

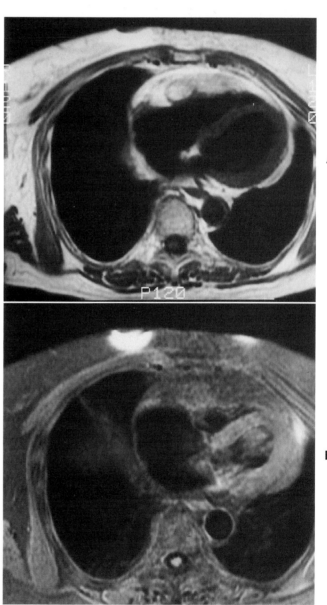

Fig. 1-30. Transaxial T1-weighted images (TR 970, TE 11, 4 Nex) obtained **A,** without and **B,** with fat saturation in patient with extensive epicardial fat and fatty infiltration of the right ventricular free wall. Note increased prominence of susceptibility artifacts related to ECG leads on fat saturation image.

venous catheters, a chest wall "pseudonodule" may result.[25] Another cause of chest wall "pseudotumor" is an elastofibroma, which occurs in the periscapular region and can simulate malignancy.[5,37] Lymph nodes can be present within the interpectoral region, where they may be mistaken for other masses.[46] The pectoral muscles may be absent in patients who have undergone previous radical mastectomy.

Coronal gradient echo images frequently demonstrate "zebra stripe" artifacts along the periphery of the thorax (Fig. 1-33). These artifacts result from phase cancellation and are accentuated where there is aliasing, or wraparound, of tissue into the image. Therefore, they can often be reduced or eliminated when a larger field-of-view is prescribed. Chemical shift phase cancellation artifacts are manifested as hypointense lines at fat-water interfaces, such as along the fascial planes of the chest wall, and are observed on gradient echo images acquired us-

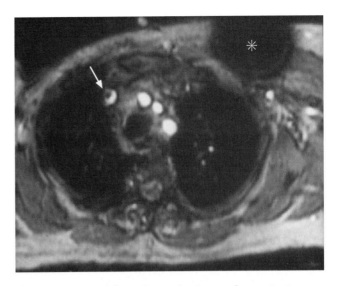

Fig. 1-32. Transaxial gradient echo image demonstrates signal void within the left anterior chest wall *(asterisk)* caused by drug infusion port. Also note defect in superior vena cava caused by catheter *(arrow)*, which can simulate thrombus.

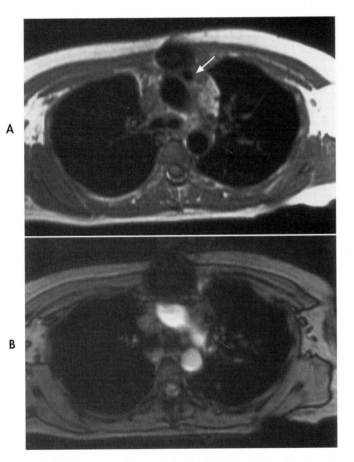

Fig. 1-31. A, Transaxial T1-weighted spin echo image (TR 790, TE 20, 2 Nex) in patient with graft *(arrow)* extending from left innominate vein to right atrial appendage. **B,** Metallic artifact related to previous median sternotomy is markedly accentuated on corresponding gradient echo image (TR 200, TE 12, 50-degree flip angle, 2 Nex), which obscures the graft.

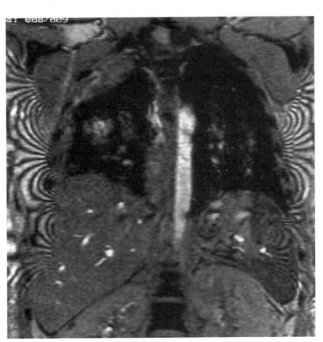

Fig. 1-33. Coronal steady state gradient echo image (TR 50, TE 15, 30-degree flip angle, 1 Nex) demonstrates "zebra stripe" banding artifact along the periphery of the thorax and upper abdomen, with artifacts extending into lateral aspect of body. These artifacts are due to phase cancellation and are accentuated by aliasing related to a relatively small field-of-view.

ing an echo time at which fat and water protons are of opposed phase.

NECK
Thyroid Gland

The thyroid gland usually consists of two relatively symmetric lateral lobes united by a narrow isthmus. Many variations in the configuration of the thyroid gland can occur. Among the most frequent is the presence of

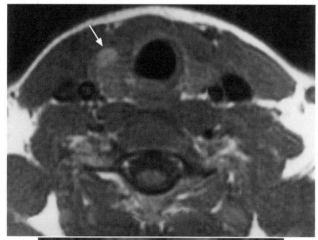

A

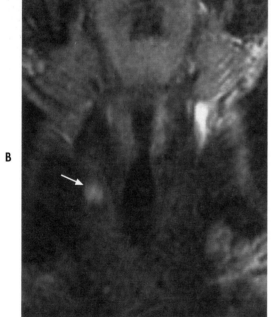

B

Fig. 1-34. Small focus of relative increased signal intensity *(arrows)* is noted on **A,** transaxial T1-weighted (TR 600, TE 12, 2 Nex) and **B,** coronal T2-weighted (TR 2400, TE 80, 1 Nex) images within the thyroid gland. This was an incidental finding in a 28-year-old female, representing a presumed colloid cyst.

a pyramidal lobe, an extension of thyroid tissue that rises superiorly from the isthmus. The pyramidal lobe can also originate from either of the lateral lobes and may be partially composed of fibrous tissue.[4a] The lateral thyroid lobes are frequently asymmetric in size, and the isthmus can be of variable prominence. Absence or hypoplasia of either lateral lobe or of the isthmus can occur. Thyroid tissue may be located in an ectopic position, such as in the tongue (lingual thyroid) or in the mediastinum.

Funari et al identified asymptomatic thyroid nodules in 46% of patients undergoing MR imaging for evaluation of suspected parathyroid adenomas[29] (Figs. 1-34, *A* and *B*). These nodules can appear either hyperintense or, less commonly, hypointense on T2-weighted images and may represent colloid cysts, adenomas, or other relatively common entities. The high prevalence of incidental thyroid signal abnormalities presents a limitation for the detection of thyroid carcinoma and other thyroid lesions.

Parathyroid Glands

The parathyroid glands can vary in number between two and six.[4a] These glands are usually located along the posteroinferior aspect of the thyroid gland but may be found in a variety of other locations, including anterior or inferior to the thyroid. In addition, they may be located in the mediastinum, thymus gland, posterior mediastinum, or epicardial region.[4a]

Parathyroid adenomas are typically hyperintense on T2-weighted images, allowing for their distinction from lymph nodes. However, the signal intensity of parathyroid adenomas is variable, and some may demonstrate only mild or moderate intensity. In this situation, they may simulate cervical lymph nodes or can be difficult to detect because of isointensity with surrounding fat on T2-weighted images.[67,78] Marked decreased signal intensity on T2-weighted images can occur when parathyroid adenomas are calcified. When contrast material enhanced images are obtained, parathyroid adenomas can also be difficult to identify because of their isointensity with fat. This can be remedied with use of fat suppressed T1-weighted images.

Parathyroid adenomas may simulate colloid cysts, adenomas, or other lesions arising from the thyroid gland when a tissue plane between the adenoma and the thyroid is not evident. Parathyroid adenomas can occasionally be located within the thyroid gland, where they are difficult to distinguish from colloid cysts and other benign or malignant high signal intensity thyroid lesions.[80]

Approximately 20% of parathyroid adenomas are located in an ectopic site such as the thymus, paraesophageal, or other regions.[49] Therefore, images of the mediastinum should be routinely acquired in patients with suspected parathyroid adenoma.

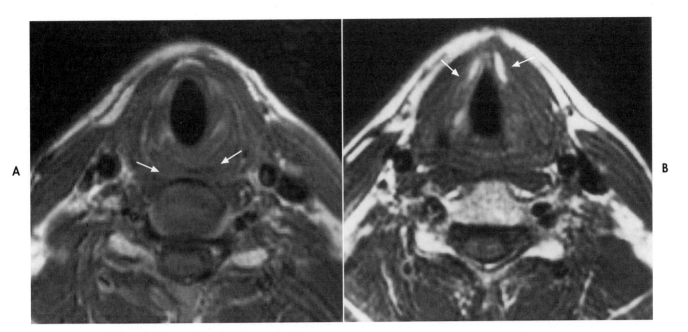

Fig. 1-35. T1-weighted images (TR 500, TE 12, 2 Nex) demonstrate heterogeneous signal intensity within the cricoid **A,** and **B,** thyroid cartilages *(arrows)*. These findings are due to irregular foci of ossification within these cartilages. This heterogeneous appearance may simulate or obscure tumor involvement.

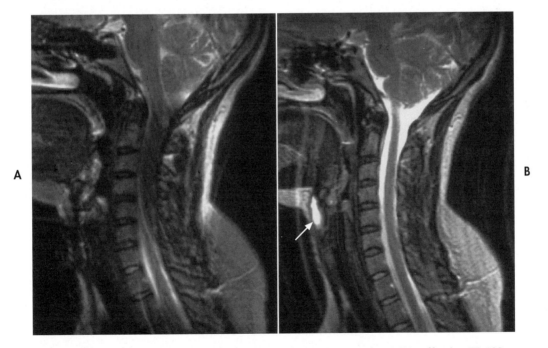

Fig. 1-36. A, Initial sagittal fast spin echo T2-weighted image (TR 3400, effective TE 102, 4 Nex, 16 echo train) is limited by phase encode artifacts related to patient swallowing. These artifacts obscure visualization of a thyroglossal duct cyst within the anterior neck. **B,** Repeat imaging using similar parameters clearly demonstrates the lesion *(arrow)*.

Neck

The thyroid and cricoid cartilages can appear highly heterogeneous on MR images (Figs. 1-35, *A* and *B*). Foci of relative increased signal intensity, particularly on T1-weighted images, represent marrow fat resulting from ossification of these structures. This heterogeneous appearance can simulate tumor involvement or can render tumor involvement difficult to discern.[11,15] Fat within these cartilages, which is juxtaposed to soft tissues, can give rise to chemical shift misregistration artifacts, which may obscure subtle tumor invasion.

The configuration of the vocal cords changes considerably during phonation. The piriform sinuses and valleculae may be collapsed and poorly visualized; performance of Valsalva or other maneuvers during rapid imaging can show them distended and allow for better evaluation.

Necrosis of cervical lymph nodes is a reliable sign of malignant involvement. Such necrosis is usually best visualized on contrast material enhanced T1-weighted images, particularly when fat suppression is used. The target appearance of necrotic lymph node can simulate a thrombosed vessel. Use of gradient echo sequences allows for improved visualization of cervical vessels and their distinction from nodes and other structures. Large necrotic lymph nodes can also simulate an abscess. A small focus of relative increased signal intensity can be observed with normal lymph nodes; this represents fat within the nodal hilum. Cervical lymph nodes may be simulated by prominent or asymmetric cervical muscles, such as the sternocleidomastoid or scalene muscle.

Artifacts resulting from patient swallowing are a major source of image degradation in the neck. This is manifested as generalized image blurring, as well as structured ghosting artifacts that extend across the phase encoding direction of the image. These artifacts can simulate or obscure cervical lesions (Figs. 1-36, *A* and *B*).

REFERENCES

1. Adachi Y, Kanasugi K, Mizuno H et al: MRI of the breast: spectral presaturation with inversion recovery (SPIR), SMRM Book of Abstracts 3205, 1992.
2. Axel L, Summers RM, Kressel HY et al: Respiratory effects in two-dimensional fourier transform MR imaging, Radiology 160:795-801, 1986.
3. Bach AM, Hilfer CL, Holgersen LO: Left-sided posterior mediastinal thymus—MRI findings, Pediatr Radiol 21:440-441, 1991.
4. Bergin CJ, Noll DC, Pauly JM et al: MR imaging of lung parenchyma: a solution to susceptiblity, Radiology 183:673-676, 1992.
4a. Bergman RA, Thompson SA, Afifi AK et al: Compendium of human anatomic variation: text, atlas, and world literature, Baltimore, 1988, Urban & Schwarzenberg.
5. Berthoty DP, Shulman HS, Miller HAB: Elastofibroma: chest wall pseudotumor, Radiology 160:341-342, 1986.
6. Brown JJ, Gilbert T, Gamsu G et al: MR imaging of low signal intensity pulmonary lesions using flow-sensitive techniques, J Comput Assist Tomogr 12:560-564, 1988.
7. Brown LR, Augenhabugh GL: Masses of the anterior mediastinum: CT and MR imaging, Am J Roentgenol 157:1171-1180, 1991.
8. Carette MF, Grivaux M, Monod BB et al: MR findings in lipoid pneumonia, Am J Roentgenol 153:1097-1098, 1989.
9. Carrillon Y, Tixier E, Revel D et al: MR diagnosis of lipoid pneumonia, J Comput Assist Tomogr 12:876-877, 1988.
10. Caskey CI, Zerhouni EA, Fishman EK et al: Aging of the diaphragm: a CT study, Radiology 171:385-389, 1989.
11. Castelijns JA, Gerritsen GJ, Kaiser MC et al: Invasion of laryngeal cartilage by cancer: comparison of CT and MR imaging, Radiology 167:199-206, 1988.
12. Choyke PL, Zeman RK, Gootenberg JE et al: Thymic atrophy and regrowth in response to chemotherapy: CT evaluation, Am J Roentgenol 149:269-272, 1987.
13. Colletti PM, Raval JK, Benson RC et al: The motion artifact suppression technqiue (MAST) in magnetic resonance imaging: clinical results, Magn Reson Imaging 6:293-299, 1988.
14. Cory DA, Cohen MD, Smith JA: Thymus in the superior mediastinum simulating adenopathy: appearance on CT, Radiology 162:457-459, 1987.
15. Curtin HD: Imaging of the larynx: current concepts, Radiology 173:1-11, 1989.
16. Czervionke LF, Daniels DL, Wehrli FW et al: Magnetic susceptibility artifacts in gradient-recalled echo MR imaging, Am J Neuroradiol 9:1149-1155, 1988.
17. Dao TH, Rhahumouni A, Campana F et al: Tumor recurrence versus fibrosis in the irradiated breast: differentiation with dynamic gadolinium-enhanced MR imaging, Radiology 187: 751-755, 1993.
18. Davis SD, Henschke CI, Yankelevitz DF et al: MR imaging of pleural effusions, J Comput Assist Tomogr 14:192-198, 1990.
19. de Geer G, Webb WR, Gamsu G: Normal thymus: assessment with MR and CT, Radiology 158:313-317, 1986.
20. Derby KA, Frankel SD, Kaufman L et al: Differentiation of silicone gel from water and fat in MR phase imaging of protons at 0.064 T, Radiology 189:617-620, 1993.
21. Duvernoy O, Larsson SG, Thuren J et al: Epicardial fat causing pitfalls in CT and MR imaging of the pericardium, Acta Radiol 33:1-5, 1992.
22. Ebner F, Kressel HY, Mintz MC et al: Tumor recurrence versus fibrosis in the female pelvis: differentiation with MR imaging at 1.5 T, Radiology 166:333-340, 1988.
23. Ehara S, Sugisawa M, Matsuda M: MR imaging of the anterior chest wall by using a flat coil (letter), Am J Roentgenol 156:1110-1111, 1991.
24. Fairhurst JJ, Christensen SL, Kuhn JP et al: Isolated intrathoracic spleen presenting as an enlarging chest mass: CT and MRI findings, Pediatr Radiol 22:305-306, 1992.
25. Fernandez G, Coblentz CL, Cooper C et al: Hickman nodule: a mimick of metastatic disease, Radiology 171:401-402, 1989.
26. Fisher ER, Godwin JD: Extrapleural fat collections: pseudotumors and other confusing manifestations, Am J Roentgenol 161:47-52, 1993.

27. Fitzgerald SW, Donaldson JS: Azygoesophageal recess: normal CT appearance in children, Am J Roentegenol 158:1101-1104, 1992.

28. Flemming MC, Kellman GM, Haggar AM: Cervical rib: a cause of supraclavicular mass on MR imaging, Am J Roentgenol 153:1102-1103, 1989.

29. Funari M, Campos Z, Gooding GA et al: MRI and ultrasound detection of asymptomatic thyroid nodules in hyperparathyroidism, J Comput Assist Tomogr 16L:615-619, 1992.

30. Gilles R, Guinebretiere J-M, Shapeero LG et al: Assessment of breast cancer recurrence with contrast-enhanced subtraction MR imaging: preliminary results in 26 patients, Radiology 188:473-478, 1993.

31. Glassberg RM, Sussman SK, Glickstein MF: CT anatomy of the internal mammary vessels: importance in planning percutaneous transthoracic procedures, Am J Roentgenol 155:397-400, 1990.

32. Glazer HS, Anderson DJ, Cooper JD et al: Omental flap in lung transplanation, Radiology 185:395-400, 1992.

33. Glazer HS, Niemeyer JH, Balfe DM et al: Neck neoplasms: MR imaging. Part I. Initial evaluation, Radiology 160:343-348, 1986.

34. Glazer GM, Orringer MB, Chenevert TL et al: Mediastinal lymph nodes: relaxation time/pathologic correlation and implications in staging of lung cancer with MR imaging, Radiology 168:429-431, 1988.

35. Goei R, Tjwa MKT: Leutic aneurysm of the innominate artery mimicking a mass in the right side of the anterior mediastinum: MR appearance (letter), Am J Roentgenol 159:1343, 1992.

36. Gorczyca DP, Sinha S, Ahn CY et al: Silicone breast implants in vivo: MR imaging, Radiology 185:407-410, 1992.

37. Gould ES, Javors BR, Morrison J et al: MR appearance of bilateral periscapular elastofibromas, J Comput Assist Tomogr 13:701-703, 1989.

38. Gronemeyer SA, Langston JW, Hanna SL et al: MR imaging detection of calcified intracranial lesions and differentiation from iron-laden lesions, J Magn Reson Imaging 2:271-276, 1992.

39. Gross BH, Glazer GM, Orringer MB et al: Bronchogenic carcinoma metastatic to normal-sized lymph nodes: frequency and significance, Radiology 166:71-74, 1988.

40. Haacke EM, Patrick JL. Reducing motion artifacts in two-dimensional Fourier transform imaging, Magn Reson Imaging 4:359-376, 1986.

41. Hackney DB, Grossman RI, Zimmerman RA et al: Low sensitivity of clinical MR imaging to small changes in the concentration of nonparamagnetic protein, Am J Neuroradiol 8:1003-1008, 1987.

42. Harms SE, Flamig DP, Hesley KL, et al: MR imaging of the breast with rotating delivery of excitation off resonance: clinical experience with pathologic correlation, Radiology 187:493-501, 1993.

43. Herold CJ, Kuhlman JE, Zerhouni EA: Pulmonary atelectasis: signal patterns with MR imaging, Radiology 178:715-720, 1991.

44. Heywang SH, Hilbertz T, Beck R et al: Gd-DTPA enhanced MR imaging of the breast in patients with postoperative scarring and silicone implants, J Comput Assist Tomogr 14:348-356, 1990.

45. Heywang SH, Wold A, Pruss E et al: MR imaging of the breast with Gd-DTPA: use and limitations, Radiology 171:95-103, 1989.

46. Holbert BL, Holbert JM, Libshitz HI: CT of interpectoral lymph nodes, Am J Roentgenol 149:687-688, 1987.

47. Hsu BY, Edwards DK III, Trambert MA: Pulmonary hemorrhage complicating systemic lupus erythematosus: role of MR imaging in diagnosis, Am J Roentgenol 158:519-520, 1992.

48. Ishii K, Maeda K: MR appearance of a retained surgical sponge (letter), Am J Roentgenol 158:460, 1992.

49. Kang YS, Rosen K, Clark OH et al: Localization of abnormal parathyroid glands of the mediastinum with MR imaging, Radiology 189:137-141, 1993.

50. Kelcz F, Santyr G, Fairbanks EJ: Characterization of breast masses using gadolinium enhanced, fat suppressed rapid MR imaging and colorflow duplex Doppler ultrasound, SMRM Book of Abstracts 3206, 1992.

51. Kisslin CM, Husband JE, Nicholas D et al: Benign thymic enlargement in adults after chemotherapy: CT demonstration, Radiology 163:67-70, 1987.

52. Kiyono K, Sone S, Sakai F et al: The number and size of normal mediastinal lymph nodes: a postmortem study, Am J Roentgenol 150:771-776, 1988.

53. Kohno N, Ikezoe J, Johkoh T et al: Focal organizing pneumonia: CT appearance, Radiology 189:119-123, 1993.

54. Kopans DB, Swann CA, White G et al: Asymmetric breast tissue, Radiology 171:639-643, 1989.

55. Laissy JP, Rebibo G, Iba-Zizen MT et al: MR appearance of the normal chest after pneumonectomy, J Comput Assist Tomogr 13:248-252, 1989.

56. Laissy JP, Rebibo G, Tortot PM et al: Postpneumonectomy evaluation of the chest: a prospective comparative study of MRI with CT, Magn Reson Imaging 7:55-60, 1989.

57. Lee JKT, Glazer HS: Controversy in the MR imaging appearance of fibrosis, Radiology 177:21-22, 1990.

58. Lewis CE, Prato FS, Drost DJ et al: Comparison of respiratory triggering and gating techniques for the removal of respiratory artifacts in MR imaging, Radiology 160:803-810, 1986.

59. Lyon RD, McAdams HP: Mediastinal bronchogenic cyst: demonstration of a fluid-fluid level at MR imaging, Radiology 186:427-428, 1993.

60. McHugh K, Blaquiere RM: CT features of rounded atelectasis, Am J Roentgenol 153:257-260, 1989.

61. McLoud TC, Flower CDR: Imaging the pleura: sonography, CT, and MR imaging, Am J Roentgenol 156:1145-1153, 1991.

62. Molina PL, Siegel MJ, Glazer HS: Thymic masses on MR imaging, Am J Roentgenol 155:495-500, 1990.

63. Muller NL: Imaging of the pleura, Radiology 186:297-309, 1993.

64. Mund DF, Farria DM, Gorczyca DP et al: MR imaging of the breast in patients with silicone-gel implants: spectrum of findings, Am J Roentgenol 161:773-778, 1993.

65. Negendank WG, Al-Katib Am, Karanes C et al: Lymphomas: MR imaging contrast characteristics with clinical-pathologic correlations, Radiology 177:209-216, 1990.

66. Pavone P, Cardone G-P, Cisternino S et al: Gadopentetate dimeglumine-barium paste for opacification of the esophageal lumen on MR images, Am J Roentgenol 159:762-764, 1992.

67. Peck WW, Higgins CB, Fisher MR et al: Hyperparathyroid-

ism: comparison of MR imaging with radionuclide scanning, Radiology 163:415-420, 1987.

68. Pierce WB, Harms SE, Flamig DP et al: Three-dimensional gadolinium-enhanced MR imaging of the breast: pulse sequence with fat suppression and magnetization transfer contrast, (work in progress), Radiology 181:757-763, 1991.

69. Poon PY, Bronskill MJ, Henkelman RM et al: Mediastinal lymph node metastases from bronchogenic carcinoma: detection with MR imaging at CT, Radiology 162:651-656, 1987.

70. Rahmouni A, Tempany C, Jones R et al: Lymphoma: monitoring tumor size and signal intensity with MR imaging, Radiology 188:445-451, 1993.

71. Rollins NK, Currarino G: MR imaging of posterior mediastinal thymus, J Comput Assist Tomogr 12:518-520, 1988.

72. Rubens D, Totterman S, Chacko AK et al: Gadopentetate dimeglumine-enhanced chemical-shift MR imaging of the breast, Am J Roentgenol 157:267-270, 1991.

73. Savader SJ, Otero RR, Savader BL: MR imaging of intrathoracic extramedullary hematopoiesis, J Comput Assist Tomogr 12:878-880, 1988.

74. Schneider E, Chan TW: Selective MR imaging of silicone with the three-point Dixon technique, Radiology 187:89-93, 1993.

75. Siegel MJ, Glazer HS, Wiener JI et al: Normal and abnormal thymus in childhood: MR imaging, Radiology 172:367-371, 1989.

76. Siegel MJ, Nadel SN, Glazer HS et al: Mediastinal lesions in children: comparison of CT and MR, Radiology 160:241-244, 1986.

77. Som PM: Detection of metastasis in cervical lymph nodes: CT and MR criteria and differential diagnosis, Am J Roentgenol 158:961-969, 1992.

78. Spritzer CE, Gefter WB, Hamilton R et al: Abnormal parathyroid glands: high-resolution MR imaging, Radiology 162:487-491, 1987.

79. Stack JP, Redmond OM, Codd MB et al: Breast disease: tissue characterization with Gd-DTPA enhancement profiles, Radiology 174:491-494, 1990.

80. Stevens SK, Chang J-M, Clark OH et al: Detection of abnormal parathyroid glands in postoperative patients with recurrent hyperparathyroidism: sensitivity of MR imaging, Am J Roentgenol 160:607-612, 1993.

81. Tsuruda JS, Bradley WG: MR detection of intracranial calcification: a phantom study, Am J Neuroradiol 8:1049-1055, 1987.

82. van den Brekel MW, Castelijns JA, Stel HV et al: Detection and characterization of metastatic cervical adenopathy by MR imaging: comparison of different MR techniques, J Comput Assist Tomogr 14:581-589, 1990.

83. van Genderingen HR, Sprenger M, de Ridder RW et al: Carbon-fiber electrodes and leads for electrocardiography during MR imaging, Radiology 171:872, 1989.

84. Verschakelen JA, Demaerel P, Coolen J et al: Rounded atelectasis of the lung: MR appearance, Am J Roentgenol 152:965-966, 1989.

85. von Roemeling R, Lanning RM, Eames FA: MR imaging of patients with implanted drug infusion pumps, J Magn Reson Imaging 1:77-81, 1991.

86. Wagle WA: Technique for RF isolation of a pulse oximeter in a 1.5-T MR unit (letter), Am J Neuroradiol 10:208, 1989.

87. Wallner B, Edelman RR, Finn JP et al: Bright pleural effusion and ascites on gradient-echo MR images: a potential source of confusion in vascular MR studies, Am J Roentgenol 155:1237-1240, 1990.

88. Webb WR, Sostman HD: MR imaging of thoracic disease: clinical uses, Radiology 182:621-630, 1992.

89. Werthmuller WC, Schiebler ML, Whaley RA et al: Gadolinium-DTPA enhancement of lung radiation fibrosis, J Comput Assist Tomogr 13:946-948, 1989.

90. Wiener JI, Chako AC, Merten CW et al: Breast and axillary tissue MR imaging: correlation of signal intensities and relaxation times with pathologic findings, Radiology 160:299-305, 1986.

91. Williamson BRJ, Gouse JC, Rohrer DG et al: Variation in the thickness of the diaphragmatic crura with respiration, Radiology 163:683-684, 1987.

92. Winer-Muram HT, Gold RE: Effusion in the superior pericardial recess simulating a mediastinal mass, Am J Roentgenol 154:69-71, 1990.

2

Vasculature

ANATOMIC VARIATIONS

The vascular system demonstrates significant variation in vessel branching patterns and anatomic course, presence of accessory vessels, and related anomalies. Only the most frequent of these variations will be mentioned. The aortic arch may be located on the right side, possibly with an associated anomalous left subclavian artery that courses behind the esophagus.[18,26] An aberrant right subclavian artery can occur in patients with a left-sided aortic arch.[17,26,41] The anomalous vessel may arise from a diverticulum of Kommerell, which can simulate a subclavian artery aneurysm.[29,59] The number, order of origination, and branching pattern of the great vessels are highly variable. The mediastinal arteries are frequently tortuous or ectatic in older individuals.

Variations of the thoracic venous system include anomalous left brachiocephalic vein, persistence of the left superior vena cava, and anomalous right superior vena cava that drains into the left atrium.[17,26] The inferior vena cava can be absent, with venous return from the lower body provided by dilated azygos and hemiazygos veins. The pulmonary arteries and veins can vary in number and anatomic course.[17,22] MR findings have been described in patients with aberrant left pulmonary artery (pulmonary artery sling),[32] congenital absence of the pulmonary artery,[9] various forms of anomalous pulmonary venous return,[55] and corrected transposition of the aortic root and pulmonary artery.[38] Significant variations involving the vasculature of the abdomen, pelvis, and extremities are also frequent. Bilateral veins are frequently asymmetric in size in normal individuals (Fig. 2-1).

VASCULAR THROMBOSIS

Appearance of Flowing Blood

Spin echo images

MR has developed an important role in the noninvasive evaluation for suspected vascular thrombosis. A recent overview of MR principles of blood flow has been provided by Stahlberg et al.[49] Flowing blood is usually depicted as a "flow void" on both T1- and T2-weighted spin echo images. This flow void refers to absence of intraluminal signal intensity, which results from time-of-flight as well as spin phase effects. Signal intensity on spin echo images requires that spins be exposed to slice selective 90- and 180-degree radiofrequency pulses. Whereas stationary protons experience both pulses, flowing spins may escape the section prior to experiencing both pulses and hence do not effectively generate signal. Signal loss on this basis is most prominent in the presence of high-velocity blood flow. In addition, flowing spins rapidly gain and lose phase relative to one another, particularly under nonlaminar flow conditions. These phase cancellation effects also contribute to intraluminal signal loss.[6,58]

Gradient echo images

In contrast to spin echo images, gradient echo images typically depict flowing blood as hyperintense relative to stationary tissues. Several factors contribute to this "flow enhancement" phenomenon. First, the use of relatively short echo times provides less opportunity for flowing spins to escape a given section prior to receiving radiofrequency excitation. In addition, gradient echo images employ only a single radiofrequency pulse. Because of these factors, time-of-flight signal loss is minimized on gradient echo sequences. Because gradient echo images are often acquired as consecutive single slices, rather than as a multislice acquisition, there is continuous entry of fully magnetized (i.e., unsaturated) spins into the section. Such unsaturated spins are capable of generating relatively higher signal intensity than stationary spins that have been exposed to repeated radiofrequency pulses. Finally, flow-compensating gradient pulses (i.e., gradient moment nulling) are often used with gradient echo sequences. This leads to rephasing of flowing spins at the time of echo collection and minimizes signal loss on the basis of spin phase cancellation.

Intravascular thrombus appears as increased intraluminal signal intensity on spin echo images or decreased signal intensity on gradient echo images relative to flowing blood. There are many pitfalls in the evaluation for vascular thrombosis. These entities are described according to whether they are observed primarily on spin echo or gradient echo images. Pitfalls relating specifically to MR angiography are discussed in Chapter 4.

Pitfalls in Diagnosing Thrombosis on Spin Echo Images

Slow blood flow

When there is reduced flow velocity, the expected flow void on spin echo images may not be observed (Figs. 2-2, *A* to 2-4, *B*). Slowly flowing spins remain within the imaging section for a relatively long time, allowing them to experience both 90- and 180-degree radiofrequency pulses. The precise flow velocity necessary to cause a flow void appearance depends on many variables, including the echo time and slice thickness used. Both very short echo times and increased slice thickness will contribute to relative increased intraluminal signal intensity on spin echo images (Figs. 2-5, *A-C*).

Increased intraluminal signal intensity resulting from slow flow is more frequently observed in venous rather than arterial vessels. However, slow arterial flow can occur distal to a site of severe stenosis, within the lumen of large aneurysms, and on images acquired during ventricular diastole. Images may be intentionally acquired during diastole with the use of ECG triggering. However,

the prescribed repetition time (TR) may coincide with the patient's heart rate on nontriggered sequences, resulting in "diastolic pseudogating."[6,58] This can also result in increased intraluminal signal intensity. In order to distinguish diastolic pseudogating from actual thrombosis, the sequence can be repeated using a different TR or with cardiac gated image acquisition targeted to ventricular systole.

Relatively slow flow can occur along the periphery of the vessel lumen under laminar flow conditions. Another cause for slow flow is increased vascular resistance. This can occur, for example, within the pulmo-

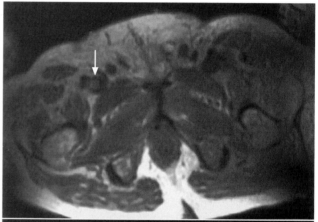

A

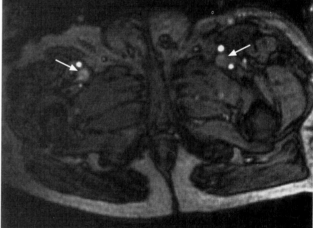

B

Fig. 2-2. A, Transaxial T1-weighted image (TR 500, TE 12, 4 Nex) in 74-year-old male with lower extremity swelling. There is apparent enlargement and increased intraluminal signal intensity involving the right common femoral vein *(arrow)*. **B,** The corresponding flow-compensated spoiled gradient echo image (TR 50, TE 12, 60-degree flip angle, 2 Nex) shows relative decreased signal intensity involving both femoral veins *(arrows)*. Whereas findings on both spin echo and gradient echo images are suggestive of thrombosis, these findings are due to slow blood flow in this patient who underwent a subsequent normal venogram.

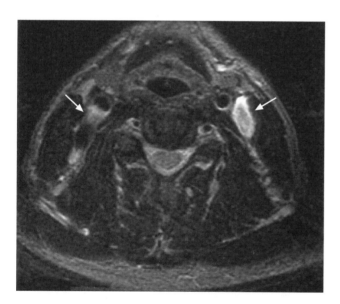

Fig. 2-1. Transaxial flow compensated T2-weighted image (TR 3200, TE 80, 1 Nex) shows increased signal intensity within the jugular veins *(arrows)*. Note that signal void is present within the carotid arteries, which are located anteromedial to the jugular veins. Asymmetric prominence of the left jugular vein is also noted as a normal variant.

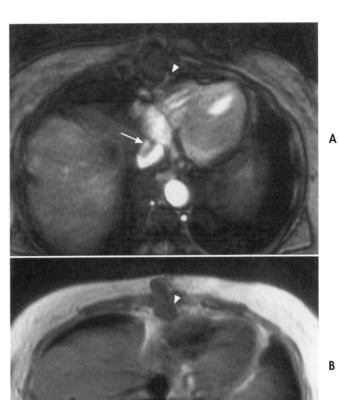

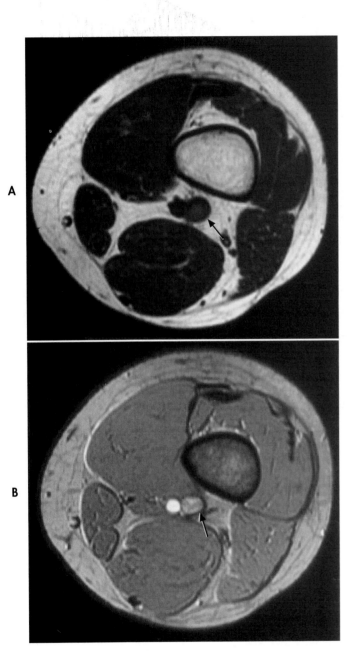

Fig. 2-3. A, T1-weighted image (TR 350, TE 25, 2 Nex) demonstrates absence of expected flow void within popliteal vein *(arrow).* **B,** The corresponding gradient echo image (TR 200, TE 15, 40-degree flip angle, 2 Nex) shows relative decreased signal intensity in similar location *(arrow).* While these findings suggest venous thrombosis, a venogram performed later the same day was normal. Findings on MR images are explained by relatively slow blood flow.

Fig. 2-4. A, Flow-compensated spoiled gradient echo image (TR 46, TE 12, 25-degree flip angle, 2 Nex) demonstrates a defect in the proximal inferior vena cava that appears to represent thrombus *(arrow).* However, these findings are due to turbulent blood flow, as verified on corresponding T1-weighted spin echo image **(B)** (TR 500, TE 12, 4 Nex). A cystic mass is located anterior to the right ventricle on the spin echo image *(arrowhead).* The gradient echo image suffers from susceptibility artifacts caused by sternal sutures that obscure portions of the mass. However, the visualized portion of the mass demonstrates high signal intensity on gradient image, suggestive of flow. At surgery, the mass was found to represent a loculated cyst without a vascular component. Findings on gradient echo image are due to transmitted cardiac pulsations resulting in fluid motion within this cyst. Note that the descending thoracic aorta demonstrates increased intraluminal signal intensity on spin echo image as a result of slow flow. The corresponding gradient echo image confirms absence of thrombus in this location.

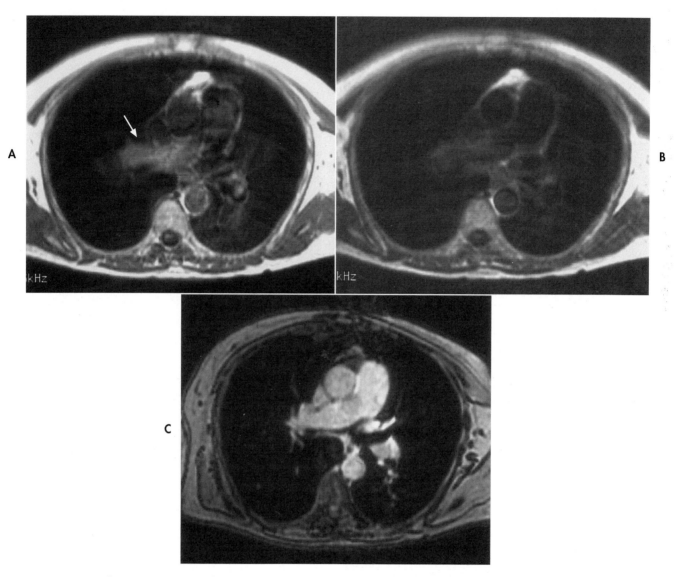

Fig. 2-5. A, Transaxial T1-weighted image (TR 730, TE 11, 4 Nex) demonstrates extensive signal intensity within the right pulmonary artery *(arrow)* in a patient with suspected pulmonary embolism. **B,** T1-weighted image acquired using a longer echo time (TR 770, TE 18, 4 Nex) demonstrates the pulmonary vessels to be patent, which is also indicated on a bolus contrast material enhanced rapid gradient echo image **(C)** (TR 19, TE 2.7, 60-degree flip angle, 1 Nex).

nary arteries in patients with pulmonary hypertension (Figs. 2-6 and 2-7). In this situation, slow flow in the pulmonary arteries produces increased signal intensity that can simulate thrombus. While increased pulmonary arterial signal intensity on a systolic image is an ancillary sign of pulmonary hypertension, these findings can be observed on diastolic images in normal subjects (Fig. 2-8).

In-plane flow

In addition to the echo time (TE) and slice thickness, the plane of image acquisition also affects intravascular signal intensity. Flow void is most prominent on images acquired perpendicular to the primary direction of blood flow. When images are acquired parallel to the direction of flow, spins remain within the imaging section for longer periods of time. Such spins are able to generate

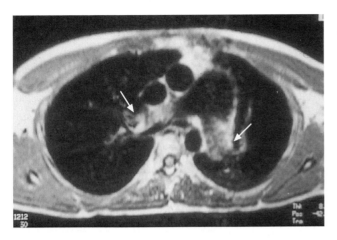

Fig. 2-6. Dilatation of the pulmonary arteries is seen on this transaxial T1-weighted image in patient with pulmonary hypertension. Note relative increased signal intensity within both the right and left central pulmonary arteries *(arrows)*.

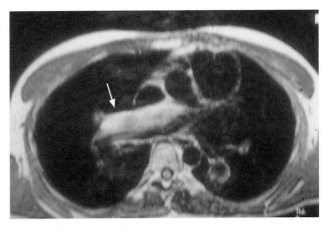

Fig. 2-7. There is markedly increased intensity noted on this transaxial T1-weighted image within the right pulmonary artery in patient with pulmonary hypertension *(arrow)*.

PITFALLS IN DETECTION OF THROMBUS: SPIN ECHO IMAGES

- Slow blood flow
- Diastolic pseudogating
- In-plane flow
- Phase shifts caused by nonvascular motion
- Phase shifts caused by mobile thrombus
- Partial volume averaging of vessels with fat/soft tissue
- Entry phenomenon
- Even echo rephasing
- Gradient moment nulling
- Asymmetric vascular signal patterns
- Hemorrhagic thrombus
- Motion artifacts

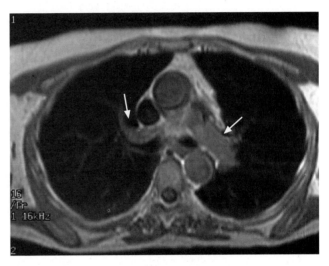

Fig. 2-8. Transaxial T1-weighted spin echo image (TR 1000, TE 11, 4 Nex) demonstrates diffuse signal intensity throughout the central pulmonary arteries bilaterally *(arrows)*. These findings are due to relatively slow blood flow occurring during diastole and simulate slow pulmonary arterial flow secondary to pulmonary hypertension.

relatively greater signal intensity. Thus to maximize flow void in the abdominal aorta, images should be acquired in the transaxial plane. However, to optimally evaluate the horizontally oriented renal veins, sagittal images are preferred.

Radiofrequency presaturation pulses

Spatial presaturation is another method that assists in distinguishing between slow blood flow and thrombus. This technique involves application of spatially selective radiofrequency pulses prior to the 90-degree excitation pulse. The objective of this prepulse is to saturate the signal intensity of tissue to which it is exposed.[14] When presaturation pulses are applied superior and inferior to the imaging section, they reduce the signal intensity of protons that enter and/or exit that section. In the abdomen, for example, presaturation pulses applied cephalad to a group of imaging sections will reduce the signal intensity of spins within the abdominal aorta, whereas caudal presaturation pulses will saturate spins within the inferior vena cava. Spatial presaturation can be implemented on either T1- or T2-weighted spin echo sequences. Its limitations include increased radiofrequency power deposition to the patient and reduced number of imaging slices that can be obtained for a given TR.

Phase images

Phase map images can also be used to distinguish between slow blood flow and thrombus. Phase information is routinely collected during imaging but is discarded and only magnitude data displayed. When vascular MR studies are performed, phase data should be saved, since they can provide important information without increasing imaging time. There is a slight delay in image reconstruction time when phase images are generated. Phase images depict moving spins as either high or low signal intensity, contrasted against a background of intermediate signal intensity representing stationary tissue. Visualization of phase shifts within a vessel lumen suggests that the vessel is patent, although flow may be very slow.

While phase images can be valuable, they are subject to their own set of pitfalls. Observation of phase shifts is not specific for blood flow but can result from any type of motion (Figs. 2-9, *A* and *B*). Therefore respiration, gastrointestinal peristalsis, or gross patient movement can also generate phase shifts that can simulate blood flow.[37,44,57] Intraluminal thrombus may be mobile; its motion can also result in phase shifts simulating vessel patency.[37,44,57,62] On the other hand, phase shifts are not always evident within patent vessels. When flow is very slow or stagnant, significant phase shifts may not result.[37,52,61] For example, slow flow on images acquired during cardiac diastole may not produce apparent phase shifts and can simulate thrombosis.

Aliasing of phase information can occur; very rapid flow may generate phase shifts similar to those of very slow flow. Protons with large phase shifts (i.e., 360 degrees) can have a similar appearance as those with no phase shift, and rapidly flowing blood can thereby simulate thrombus.[37,57,61,62]

Some types of stationary tissue can produce apparent phase shifts. For example, susceptibility effects related to iron within hemorrhagic breakdown products can generate apparent phase shifts.[57,62] Consequently, thrombus that contains hemorrhagic products can simulate flowing blood. Spurious phase shifts can also be caused by calcification.[65]

Partial volume averaging

Other causes for artifactual intraluminal signal intensity on spin echo images, in addition to slow flow, are found. Partial volume averaging of vessels with adjacent

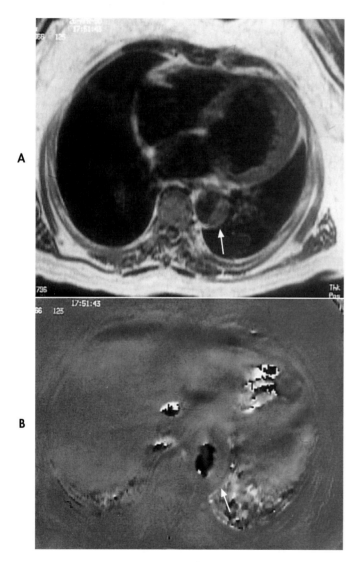

Fig. 2-9. A, Transaxial T1-weighted image in patient with Type B aortic dissection. There is relative increased signal intensity noted within the false lumen of the aorta *(arrow)*, which may represent slow blood flow or thrombosis. **B,** Corresponding phase reconstruction demonstrates absence of phase shift within the false lumen *(arrow)*, confirming thrombosis. Note that phase shifts are not only present within vascular structures but also within the lung fields.

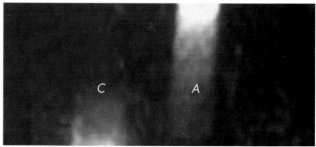

Fig. 2-10. Coronal projection from three-dimensional rapid gradient echo acquisition in the abdomen (TR 11.5, TE 2.7, 30-degree flip angle, 1 Nex). Increased intraluminal signal intensity is present within the upper abdominal aorta *(A)* and lower inferior vena cava *(C)*. These findings are due to entry of relatively unsaturated spins in these loci. Progressive loss of signal intensity is due to saturation of spins as they flow through the imaging volume.

fat or other soft tissues can result in apparent increased intraluminal signal intensity compatible with thrombosis.

Entry phenomenon

Vessels can display increased intraluminal signal intensity on peripheral images acquired as part of a multi-slice sequence (Figs. 2-10 to 2-12, *B*). This "entry phenomenon" reflects the ability of unsaturated spins flowing into the imaging section to generate relatively greater signal intensity as compared with saturated stationary tissue. As spins traverse the imaging volume, they experience repeated radiofrequency excitation and thus become saturated and less intense.

When entry phenomenon is suspected as the cause for increased intraluminal signal intensity, one must consider the direction of flow and the relative ordering of imaging slices. For example, an abdominal T1-weighted sequence can provide 10 imaging slices. The most cranial image in the series will have increased signal intensity

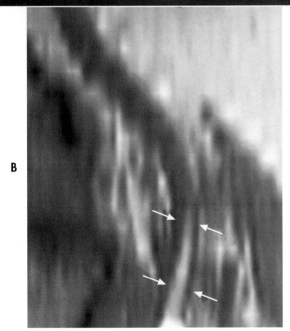

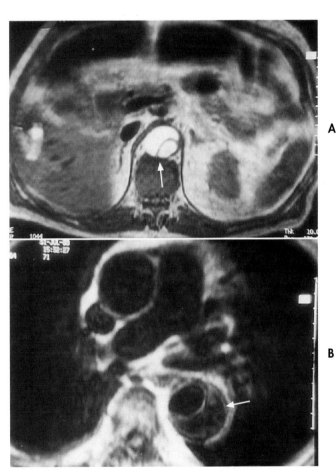

Fig. 2-11. **A,** A series of transaxial T1-weighted gradient echo images (TR 400, TE 5, 90-degree flip angle, 2 Nex) demonstrates high signal intensity throughout the popliteal vein *(arrow)*. This is due to entry of relatively unsaturated spins. Progressive reduction in signal intensity on successive images results from saturation effects. **B,** The parabolic flow profile resulting from these effects can be visualized on a sagittal reformation of images from the above series *(arrows).*

Fig. 2-12. **A,** Transaxial T1-weighted image obtained as initial image of multisection series. There is marked increased signal intensity within both the true and false lumina of a dissected abdominal aorta *(arrow)*. While these findings simulate vascular thrombosis, they were due to entry of unsaturated spins, as verified on additional images that documented patency of the aorta. **B,** Image obtained at slightly higher level in same patient verifies patency of the true and false lumina, with relative increased signal intensity within the false lumen *(arrow),* resulting from slow flow.

within the aorta. Increased intensity within the inferior vena cava does not occur, since its spins have already traversed the entire imaging volume and therefore have been saturated by repeated radiofrequency exposure. On the most caudal slice, however, increased signal intensity will be present within the inferior vena cava, where unsaturated venous spins first enter the imaging volume. Increased signal intensity within the inferior vena cava on a mid to cranial imaging slice could not be explained by entry phenomenon, and the possibility of thrombosis or an alternate flow effect should be considered.

Observation of entry phenomenon is not limited to just a single imaging section. Rather, relatively unsaturated flowing spins can penetrate variable distances into the group of imaging sections before they become fully saturated. Therefore the initial several images often demonstrate intraluminal signal intensity. A parabolic flow profile frequently exists, where high-velocity flow occurs in the center of the vessel lumen and slower flow occurs along the vessel wall. Central rapidly flowing spins are able to extend farther into the imaging volume before becoming saturated; therefore a target appearance with central intraluminal signal intensity and peripheral hypointensity can be observed. In some cases, entry phenomenon appears asymmetric when bilateral vessels are imaged.[34] Differences in depiction of cocurrent versus countercurrent flow patterns can also be observed.[63]

Several methods can be used to distinguish entry phenomenon from thrombosis. Spatial presaturation pulses, described previously, reduce intraluminal signal intensity caused by entry phenomenon. When entry phenomenon is being considered as the cause for intravascular signal intensity, one can repeat the sequence, placing the section(s) in question in the middle of the imaging volume. If intraluminal signal intensity persists, entry phenomenon is unlikely to be a causative factor. Images can also be acquired in an alternate plane, since entry phenomenon is most prominent on images acquired perpendicular to the direction of blood flow.

Entry phenomenon contributes to the flow enhancement that occurs on gradient echo images. Absence of increased intraluminal signal intensity on gradient echo images is supportive of thrombus rather than entry phenomenon. Phase images are also useful for determining the cause of intravascular signal intensity, since flowing spins generate phase shifts whereas thrombus material usually does not.

Even echo rephasing

Loss of phase coherence among flowing spins is maximal on the first echo and subsequent odd numbered echoes of a multiecho sequence (odd echo dephasing).[6,58] Conversely, phase coherence is partially restored on even echo images (even echo rephasing). As a result, intraluminal signal intensity can be in-

creased on even echo images of a multiecho pulse sequence (Figs. 2-13, *A* and *B*). Even echo rephasing is maximal when symmetric echoes (e.g., TE 40 and 80 msec) are used. However, asymmetric echoes (e.g., TE 20 and 90 msec) can also give rise to this effect. Even echo rephasing is most prominent when there is relatively slow laminar blood flow. Distinction of even echo rephasing from thrombosis is based on inspection of the corresponding odd echo image. If the odd echo

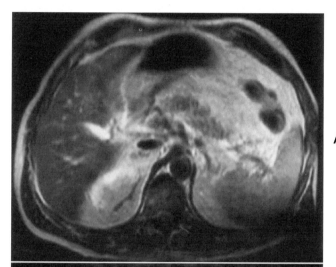

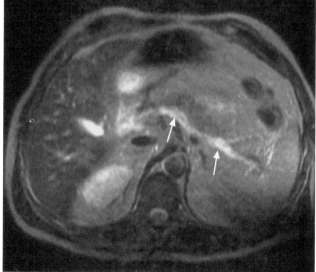

Fig. 2-13. **A,** The first echo image of a dual echo sequence (TR 3400, TE 40, 2 Nex) demonstrates the splenic vein to have similar signal intensity to surrounding mesenteric fat. This results in poor visualization of the splenic vein. **B,** The corresponding second echo image (TR 3400, TE 80, 2 Nex) shows the splenic vein to be markedly hyperintense *(arrows).* These findings are attributable to use of gradient moment nulling as well as to inherent even echo rephasing.

image also demonstrates intraluminal signal intensity, then thrombosis should be considered. T1-weighted spin echo, gradient echo, and phase images can also be used as problem solving tools. Observation of even echo rephasing can be useful for verifying vessel patency with slow flow rather than thrombosis when intraluminal signal intensity is observed on T1-weighted or other images.[24]

Gradient moment nulling

Gradient moment nulling (i.e., flow compensation) is used to reduce motion artifacts, including those related to vascular pulsation and respiratory motion.[14] This technique involves use of additional gradient lobes to rephase moving spins; it is therefore analogous to even echo rephasing. Several levels of flow compensation can be used, with each successive level correcting for more complex flow. First, second, and third order flow compensation corrects for phase shifts related to laminar flow, turbulent flow, and acceleration, respectively. In most clinical settings, first order flow compensation is used. When flow compensation is prescribed, increased intraluminal signal intensity occurs, particularly within veins that typically have slow laminar flow. Use of flow compensation gradient pulses can lengthen the minimum TE for a given sequence. Thus flow compensation is usually reserved for use on T2-weighted sequences.

Spatial presaturation and flow compensation are often used together to maximize motion artifact suppression. These techniques have counteracting effects on intraluminal signal intensity. Their combined use creates intermediate intraluminal signal intensity, which can simulate thrombus. Fat suppression techniques can also contribute to increased intraluminal signal intensity on spin echo images. This is related to alteration of the dynamic range for tissue contrast display.

Asymmetric signal intensity patterns

Bilateral vessels can demonstrate asymmetric signal intensity characteristics on MR images. Fujita et al. observed this phenomenon in the vertebral arteries and attributed it to motion-induced intraluminal phase shifts.[20] These phase shifts are related to the angle formed by flowing spins and the readout and slice select gradients. Normal vessels with asymmetric signal intensity can simulate abnormalities including vascular stenosis, occlusion, dissection, or unusually slow flow.

Misregistration of oblique flow

Signal intensity corresponding to flow within vessels oriented oblique to the plane of imaging can undergo spatial misregistration on both spin echo and gradient echo images. This is due to the time that elapses between application of the phase and frequency encoding gradients.[27] This is manifested as a line or rounded focus of high signal intensity adjacent to the vessel and is more prominent on images acquired using a long echo time.

Effect of hemorrhagic products on visualization of thrombus

Thrombus material usually displays intermediate signal intensity on both T1- and T2-weighted spin echo images. However, various signal characteristics can be observed and can contribute to diagnostic difficulty. For example, either hyperintensity or hypointensity can result from hemorrhagic breakdown products, which are frequently present within thrombus. Deoxyhemoglobin and/or intracellular methemoglobin that occur in acute or early subacute hemorrhagic thrombus appear hypointense on T2-weighted images. In this situation, the thrombus may not be visualized, and vascular patency will be simulated.[1,4] Correlation with T1-weighted spin echo and gradient echo sequences will allow the correct diagnosis to be made.

Gradient echo images depict thrombus with intermediate to low signal intensity; this contrasts with the high signal intensity of flowing blood. Methemoglobin within subacute thrombus produces T1 shortening effects that can simulate flowing blood on T1- or proton density–weighted gradient echo images[2,67] (Figs. 2-14, *A* and *B*). In this situation, thrombus material will be obscured. To avoid this pitfall, gradient echo images should be closely correlated with T1-weighted spin echo images, which depict hemorrhagic thrombus as hyperintense as opposed to the signal void of flowing blood. The proximal and distal aspects of thrombus can have disparate signal characteristics; this could lead to underestimation of the actual extent of such thrombus.[56]

Effect of contrast material

Paramagnetic contrast agents, such as gadopentetate dimeglumine, are often used to detect and characterize visceral lesions. Atypical intravascular signal patterns can be observed following contrast material administration. When flow is rapid, high-velocity signal loss overwhelms the T1 shortening effects of the contrast agent and a signal void appearance is observed. However, when there is slow flow, significant intraluminal signal intensity can result on contrast enhanced images. Heterogeneous signal patterns can result from regional variations in flow velocity within the vessel lumen. For example, high signal intensity may be observed along the vessel periphery, where flow is slower, with flow void within the central lumen. Intraluminal thrombus can be difficult to detect on some contrast enhanced images.

Differences in the contrast enhancement pattern of bland and tumor thrombus can assist in their distinction. Tumor thrombus, which consists of vascularized tissue, enhances following contrast material administration.[21] Bland thrombus, which is avascular, usually does not en-

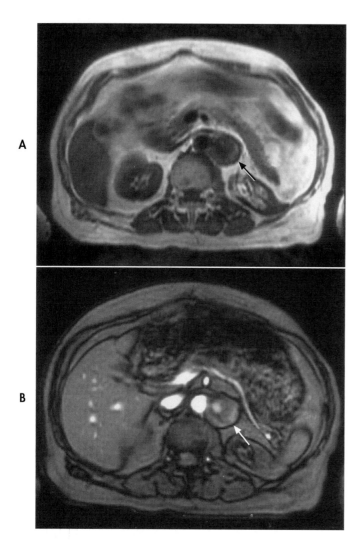

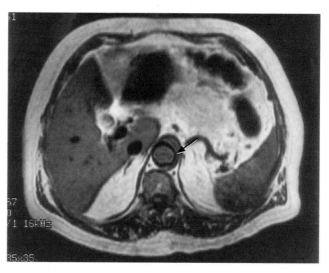

Fig. 2-15. T1-weighted image (TR 970, TE 20, 2 Nex) demonstrates intermediate signal intensity throughout aortic lumen caused by slow flow. In addition, a concentric ring of marked decreased signal intensity parallels the aortic wall resulting from shear effects *(arrow)*.

Fig. 2-14. A, Transaxial T1-weighted spin echo image (TR 500, TE 20, 4 Nex) depicts saccular abdominal aortic aneurysm *(arrow)*, with relative increased signal intensity along its periphery consistent with mural thrombus. **B,** Corresponding gradient echo image (TR 50, TE 12, 30-degree flip angle, 2 Nex) demonstrates peripheral thrombus to be relatively hyperintense *(arrow)*, because of T1 shortening effects of methemoglobin. Distinction between patent and thrombosed portions of the aneurysm is significantly improved on the gradient echo image.

hance. However, chronic bland thrombus can become organized with ingrowth of vascular supply and thus may occasionally demonstrate contrast enhancement.[46]

Flow separation effects

Shearing or flow separation effects occurring at the interface between endothelium and flowing blood also result in regional differences in signal intensity within the vessel lumen. These are manifested as a ring of low

signal intensity that outlines the interior of the vessel wall (Figs. 2-15 and 2-16, *A* and *B*). A layer of slowly flowing spins along the periphery of the vessel lumen can result in relative increased signal intensity.[45]

Motion artifacts

Motion of vessels during image acquisition results in phase encode errors (i.e., ghosting artifacts) that project across the image. It also contributes to blurring of the vessel, which can restrict its evaluation. Although ECG triggering is not routinely used for imaging of extrathoracic vessels, it can be useful for improving vessel clarity in selected situations where greater anatomic detail is required (Figs. 2-17, *A* and *B*).

Pitfalls in Diagnosis of Thrombus on Gradient Echo Images

Slow blood flow

Gradient echo imaging presents a number of additional pitfalls in the evaluation for vascular thrombosis. Slow blood flow can appear relatively hypointense on gradient echo images, simulating thrombus.[1,13,48] Use

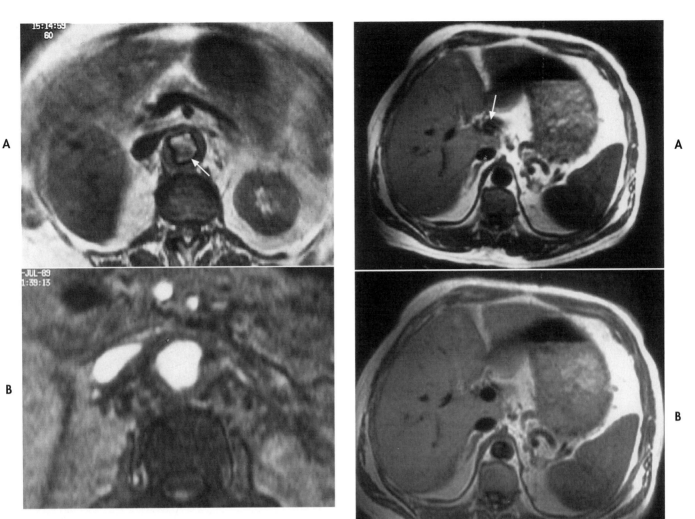

Fig. 2-16. A, T1-weighted transaxial image demonstrates relative increased signal intensity within the aortic lumen, caused by slow blood flow on a diastolic image. **B,** Corresponding gradient echo image demonstrates flow-related enhancement within the aorta, confirming its patency. Also note black ring along inside of aortic lumen on spin echo image *(arrow),* caused by shear effects.

Fig. 2-17. A, T1-weighted image (TR 625, TE 12, 4 Nex) demonstrates the portal vein to be poorly defined and contains intraluminal signal intensity, probably resulting from slow flow *(arrow).* **B,** The portal vein is of increased clarity and without intraluminal signal on corresponding image acquired using peripheral gating (TR 500, TE 12, 4 Nex).

PITFALLS IN DETECTION OF THROMBUS: GRADIENT ECHO IMAGES

- Slow blood flow
- Long TE, large flip angle images
- Eddy currents
- Thick sections
- High-velocity/turbulent flow
- In-plane flow
- Intravascular/juxtavascular metal
- Vascular catheters
- Hemorrhagic thrombus

---

of a relatively long echo time or large flip angle also contributes to decreased intraluminal signal intensity on the basis of increased spin dephasing or saturation effects, respectively. The signal intensity of flowing blood as compared with stationary tissues is generally maximized when a short TR, short TE, and small to intermediate flip angle are used. Gradient moment nulling or flow compensation also helps to maximize the signal intensity of

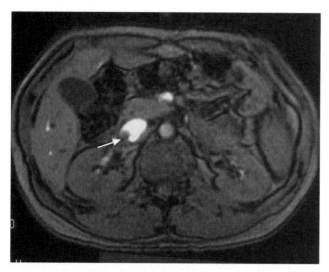

Fig. 2-18. An apparent filling defect is evident within the inferior vena cava on this rapid spoiled gradient echo image (TR 118, TE 3, 90-degree flip angle, 1 Nex) *(arrow)*. This finding is caused by turbulent flow resulting from wash-in of blood from the right renal vein.

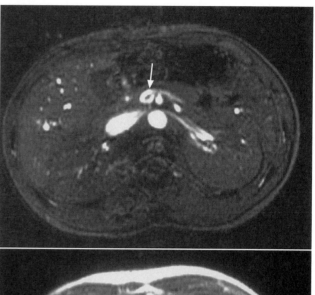

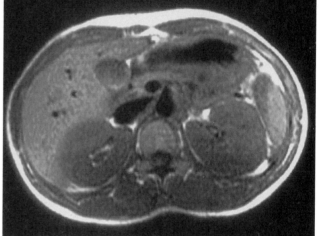

Fig. 2-19. A, Transaxial gradient echo image (TR 50, TE 13, 60-degree flip angle, 2 Nex) depicts low signal intensity defect within the superior mesenteric vein *(arrow)* due to turbulent flow. **B,** Corresponding T1-weighted spin echo image (TR 550, TE 10, 4 Nex) demonstrates this vessel to be patent.

flowing blood, though it may require a somewhat longer TE to be used, which can be counterproductive. Flow-compensating gradient pulses are usually applied along the slice-select and readout directions.[12] Eddy currents can distort these gradient profiles, diminishing the benefits of gradient moment nulling.[12] The use of a relatively large section thickness contributes to saturation of flowing spins and decreased intraluminal signal intensity. Therefore flowing blood is best depicted on gradient echo images that have a small to moderate section thickness.

Turbulent flow

Intravascular signal intensity is maximal on gradient echo images when flow is laminar. High-velocity or turbulent blood flow leads to phase cancellation effects; these are manifested as areas of decreased intraluminal signal intensity that can simulate thrombosis.[2,15] Disruption of laminar flow patterns can occur in normal subjects at vessel bifurcations and curves and at sites of venous washin[16] (Figs. 2-4, *A* and *B*, 2-18, and 2-19, *A* and *B*). Foci of decreased intraluminal signal intensity can occur in these locations, which can again simulate thrombus. Similar findings can occur adjacent to venous valves or sites of atherosclerotic plaque and within the lumen of aneurysms.

In-plane flow

Vascular thrombosis can also be simulated by flow parallel to the plane of image acquisition on gradient echo images. Time-of-flight flow enhancement is maximal on images acquired perpendicular to the direction of flow. Spins that remain within an imaging section for an extended time become saturated and are thus capable of generating less signal. Therefore artifactual decreased intraluminal signal intensity can be observed within transversely oriented vessels such as the renal veins when transaxial gradient echo images are acquired. In-plane flow can also result in a striated appearance of the vessel.[23]

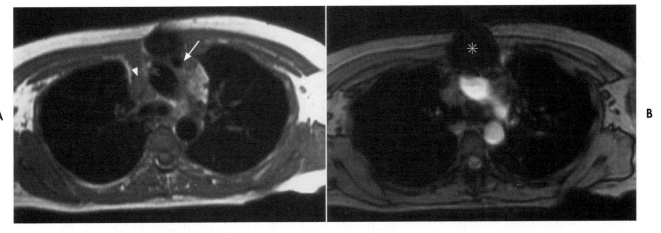

Fig. 2-20. A, Transaxial T1-weighted spin echo image (TR 790, TE 20, 2 Nex) in patient with fibrosing mediastinitis. A graft *(arrow)* has been placed from the left innominate vein to the right atrial appendage, as a result of previous occlusion of the superior vena cava. Multiple enlarged mediastinal lymph nodes are noted *(arrowhead)*, as well as artifact caused by metallic sutures from previous sternotomy. **B,** Metallic artifact is markedly accentuated on corresponding gradient echo image (TR 200, TE 12, 50-degree flip angle, 2 Nex) *(asterisk)*, obscuring the graft.

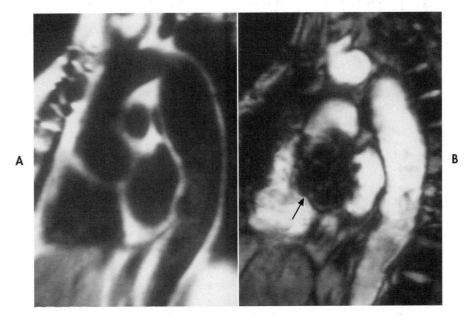

Fig. 2-21. A, Sagittal oblique T1-weighted spin echo and **B,** gradient echo images in patient with prosthetic aortic valve. There is marked accentuation of signal void caused by susceptibility artifact arising from the prosthetic valve on the gradient echo image *(arrow)*, obscuring portions of cardiac anatomy.

Susceptibility effects

Because susceptibility artifacts are accentuated on gradient echo images, the presence of vascular clips and other metallic items can obscure visualization of vessels in their vicinity and simulate thrombosis of such vessels (Figs. 2-20, *A* and *B* and 2-21, *A* and *B*). Intravascular devices such as stents, filters, or coils can also cause prominent intraluminal signal loss on gradient echo images.[30,33,53,54,60] Susceptibility artifacts can preclude vascular evaluation and can potentially simulate thrombosis or cause morphologic distortion of a vessel that simulates aneurysm (Figs. 2-22, *A* and *B*).

Intravenous or intraarterial catheters appear as a rounded focus of decreased intraluminal signal intensity on gradient echo images; these findings can simulate thrombus (Fig. 2-23).

AORTIC DISSECTION

MR is frequently used to evaluate patients with suspected aortic dissection. It offers the ability to sensitively determine the presence and extent of aortic dissections noninvasively and without the need for intravenous contrast material. Both T1-weighted spin echo and flow-compensated gradient echo images are usually acquired in patients with suspected aortic dissection. Phase data from the spin echo sequence can also provide additional useful information.

Diagnosis of aortic dissection is based on observation of a linear region of relative increased (spin echo) or decreased (gradient echo) signal intensity within the aortic lumen. This represents the intimal flap, which divides the aorta into true and false lumina. Clinically important data that should be sought include determination of the proximal and distal extent of the dissection, involvement of major aortic branch vessels, and whether the false lumen is patent or thrombosed.

Chemical Shift Misregistration

A number of entities can simulate the appearance of an intimal flap. The interface between the aortic wall and

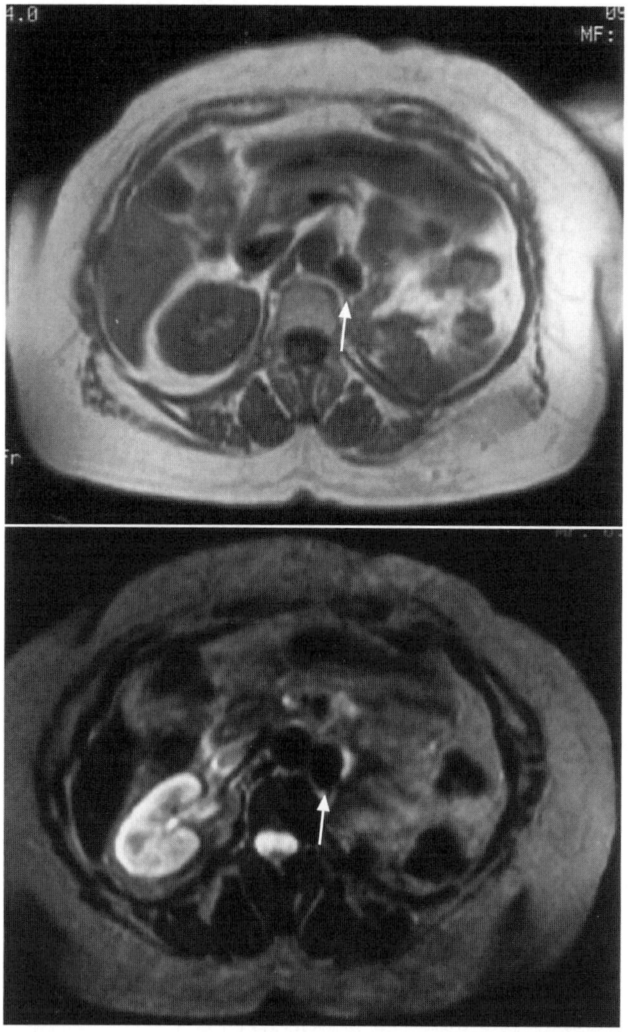

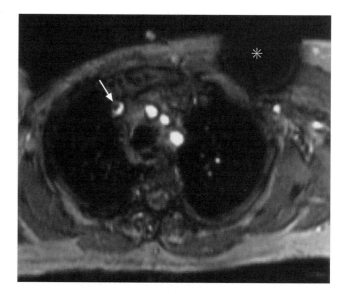

Fig. 2-22. A, Transaxial T1-weighted (TR 500, TE 12, 4 Nex) and **B,** T2-weighted (TR 3400, TE 80, 2 Nex) images depict spherical area of signal void that is contiguous with lateral aspect of abdominal aorta, suggestive of a saccular aortic aneurysm *(arrows)*. This signal void, however, is due to susceptibility artifact related to a surgical clip placed at the time of a left nephrectomy.

Fig. 2-23. Transaxial gradient echo image (TR 50, TE 15, 40-degree flip angle, 2 Nex) demonstrates filling defect suggestive of thrombus within the superior vena cava *(arrow)*. The apparent defect represents an infusion catheter. A large area of signal void along the anterior chest wall is seen corresponding to a metallic port *(asterisk)*.

adjacent periaortic fat gives rise to chemical shift misregistration artifacts. These artifacts propagate along the frequency encode direction of the image, causing curvilinear signal intensity to be shifted over the aortic lumen[31,47] (Fig. 2-24). Chemical shift misregistration is more prominent with use of high field strength systems, reduced receiver bandwidth sequences, and large voxel sizes. With reorientation of the phase and frequency encode gradients, chemical shift artifacts are aligned along the anterior-posterior axis of the aorta. This allows the artifactual nature of these findings to be confirmed and to be distinguished from aortic dissection.

Motion Artifacts

Aortic pulsation artifacts appear as a series of replications of the aortic wall that propagate along the phase encode direction of the image. When they overlie the aortic lumen, such ghosting artifacts can simulate or obscure an intimal flap[47] (Figs. 2-25 and 2-26). Techniques such as spatial presaturation, averaging of multiple data excitations, and ECG triggering can decrease vascular pulsation artifacts. Respiratory motion of the chest wall also generates phase encode artifacts and generalized blurring, which can obscure the aorta.[47] Respiratory ordered phase encoding can be helpful in reducing these artifacts, in addition to the methods mentioned above.

Truncation Artifacts

Truncation artifacts are manifested as a series of alternating high and low signal intensity bands; they are evident on images acquired using a relatively low resolution (e.g., 128 × 256) matrix. Truncation artifacts are usually observed along the phase encode direction. When they overlie the aortic lumen, truncation artifacts can

simulate an intimal flap.[39] Gradient reorientation can again be useful as a problem solving technique in difficult cases. Sequences employing filtration algorithms and a higher resolution imaging matrix can also be used to reduce these artifacts.

Complex Flow Patterns

Complex intraluminal signal intensity patterns can be observed within the aorta, as discussed in the previous section. Regions of aberrant increased and/or decreased signal intensity on spin echo or gradient echo images can contribute to difficulty in the diagnosis of aortic dissection.[25]

Neighboring Structures

Structures that border the aorta can also create a spurious appearance of aortic dissection. The juxtaposed walls of the aorta and neighboring structure appear to represent an intimal flap, with the aortic lumen and the adjacent structure simulating the true and false lumina, respectively. Both the superior pericardial recess, located posterior to the aortic root, and the preaortic recess, located anterior to the aortic arch, can contain a small amount of fluid in normal individuals. Both structures can simulate the appearance of aortic dissection[35,47] (Figs. 2-27 to 2-29). Simulation for aortic dissection can also occur on gradient echo images, where fluid within the pericardial recesses can demonstrate high signal intensity because of transmitted pulsatile motion.[5]

SIMULATION OF AORTIC DISSECTION

- Chemical shift misregistration artifact
- Motion artifacts
- Truncation artifact
- Complex flow patterns
- Pericardial recesses
- Left brachiocephalic vein
- Proximal great vessels
- Left superior intercostal vein
- Trachea/proximal bronchi
- Azygos vein
- Diaphragmatic crus
- Periaortic atelectasis
- Atherosclerotic plaque/mural thrombus
- Fibrosing mediastinitis/retroperitoneal fibrosis
- Postoperative changes
- Penetrating aortic ulcer

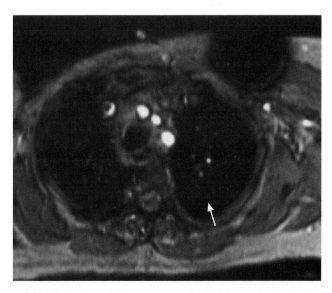

Fig. 2-24. Transaxial fast spin echo T2-weighted image (TR 4000, effective TE 117, 4 Nex, 16 echo train) shows curvilinear increased signal intensity projecting across the descending thoracic aorta *(small arrow),* suggestive of dissection. This apparent intimal flap is due to chemical shift misregistration artifact.

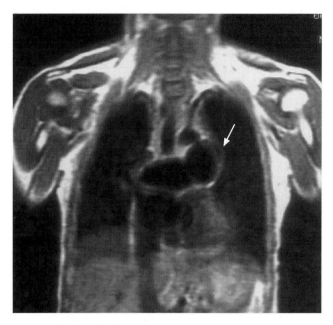

Fig. 2-25. Coronal T1-weighted image (TR 730, TE 11, 4 Nex) demonstrates apparent dissection of main pulmonary artery *(arrow),* which is aneurysmally dilated as a result of long-standing pulmonary stenosis and pulmonary hypertension. The apparent intimal flap is related to motion artifact, as verified on repeat imaging and subsequent pulmonary arteriography that demonstrated no corresponding abnormality.

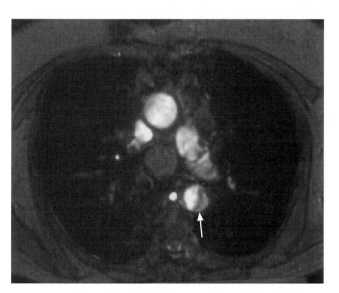

Fig. 2-26. Motion artifact results in apparent dissection of the descending thoracic aorta *(arrow)* on this transaxial spoiled gradient echo image (TR 50, TE 13, 60-degree flip angle, 2 Nex). Corresponding spin echo images demonstrated a normal appearance of the aorta.

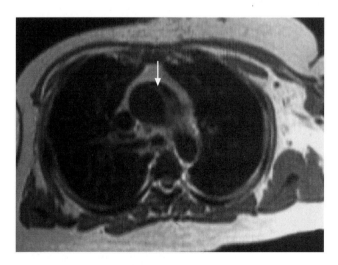

Fig. 2-27. The anterolateral wall of the ascending aorta appears to represent an intimal flap *(arrow)* on this T1-weighted image (TR 800, TE 20, 2 Nex), as it intervenes between the signal void of the aortic lumen and that of fluid within the anterior pericardial recess.

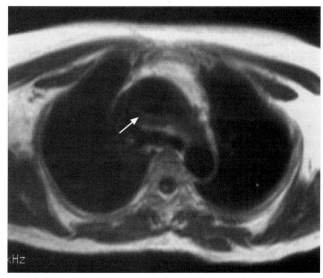

Fig. 2-28. Transaxial T1-weighted image (TR 550, TE 12, 4 Nex) demonstrates apparent dissection of the ascending aorta *(arrow)* in a patient with fluid within the superior pericardial recess.

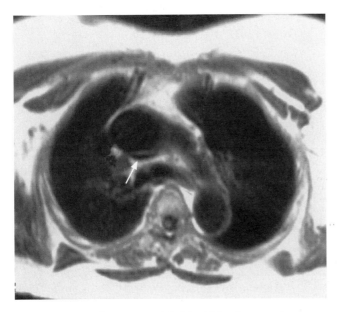

Fig. 2-29. A small amount of fluid within the superior pericardial recess *(arrow)* contributes to the appearance of an intimal flap involving the posterior wall of the ascending aorta on this transaxial T1-weighted image (TR 860, TE 11, 4 Nex).

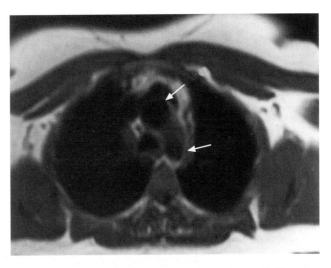

Fig. 2-30. The medial walls of the left brachiocephalic vein and left superior intercostal vein simulate an intimal flap *(arrows)*, where these vessels are closely applied to the aorta on this T1-weighted image (TR 500, TE 12, 4 Nex).

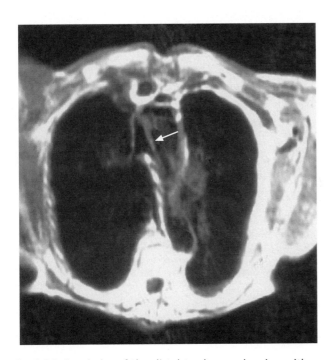

Fig. 2-31. Proximity of the distal trachea and carina with the ascending aorta simulates the appearance of an aortic dissection *(arrow)* on this transaxial T1-weighted image (TR 800, TE 12, 4 Nex) in a patient with severe kyphosis.

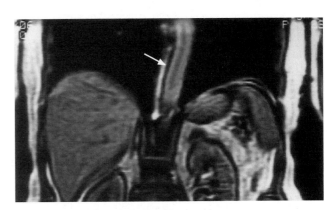

Fig. 2-32. Coronal spoiled gradient echo image (TR 120, TE 3, 90-degree flip angle, 1 Nex) demonstrates apparent dissection of the descending thoracic aorta *(arrow)* caused by the adjacent azygos vein. The apparent intimal flap is composed of the juxtaposed walls of the azygos vein and aorta, as well as to chemical shift phase cancellation artifact on this image acquired using an opposed phase echo time.

The left brachicephalic vein, which courses obliquely across the superior mediastinum, borders the aortic arch, where it can mimic dissection[47] (Fig. 2-30). The proximal aspects of the great vessels, as they arise from the aortic arch, can present a similar pitfall.[47] The left superior intercostal vein can simulate dissection involving the proximal descending thoracic aorta[47] (Fig. 2-30). The walls of the trachea and proximal bronchi can appear to represent an intimal flap, where these structures are contiguous with the aorta (Fig. 2-31). The azygos vein can simulate dissection of the distal descending thoracic and

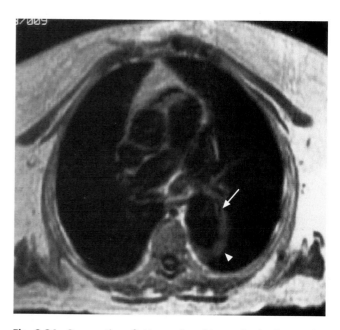

Fig. 2-34. Crescentic soft tissue signal intensity is observed along the lateral aspect of descending thoracic aorta *(arrowhead)* on this T1-weighted image (TR 860, TE 35, 2 Nex). This finding is suggestive of slow flow or thrombus within the false lumen of an aortic dissection. However, this soft tissue mass represents periaortic atelectasis, as confirmed by visualization of a bronchus entering the apparent false channel *(arrow)*. The patient did not have clinical evidence of aortic dissection.

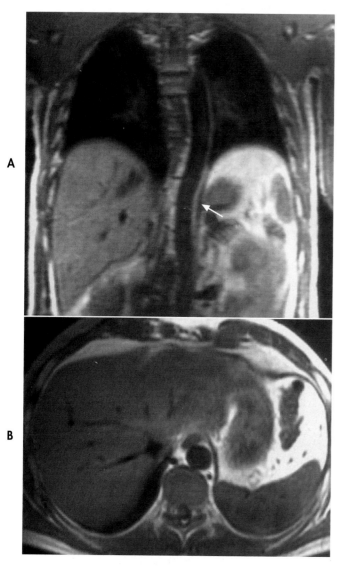

Fig. 2-33. A, Coronal T1-weighted image (TR 950, TE 11, 4 Nex) demonstrates linear increased signal intensity along the lateral aspect of the thoracic aorta *(arrow)*, simulating aortic dissection. This represents fat interposed between the aorta and diaphragmatic crus, as verified on transaxial T1-weighted image **(B)** (TR 920, TE 12, 4 Nex).

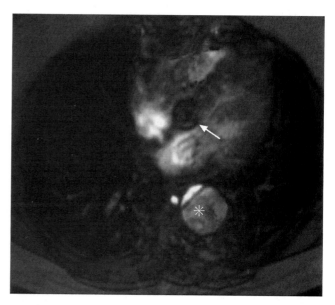

Fig. 2-35. Transaxial spoiled gradient echo image (TR 50, TE 12, 60-degree flip angle, 2 Nex) in patient with Marfan disease and dissection of descending thoracic aorta. Reduced signal intensity is noted throughout the false lumen *(asterisk)* as a result of relative slow blood flow. Also note signal void related to prosthetic St. Jude aortic valve *(arrow)* and phase encode artifact related to cardiac motion.

abdominal aorta[47] (Fig. 2-32). The fat plane located between the lateral wall of the aorta and the diaphragmatic crus can simulate an intimal flap on coronal images (Figs. 2-33, *A* and *B*). Atelectatic lung located adjacent to the lateral wall of the descending thoracic aorta can also simulate dissection (Fig. 2-34). Close inspection of the apparent false lumen may reveal evidence of an entering bronchus, verifying that it actually represents lung tissue.

Determination of False Lumen Patency

The false lumen of a dissected aorta frequently contains slowly flowing blood. This can result in increased signal intensity that makes it difficult to distinguish patency versus thrombosis of the false lumen (Figs. 2-9, *A* and *B* and 2-16, *A* and *B*). Display of phase data and use of gradient echo images can be useful in this distinction[11,25,52,57,61,62] (Fig. 2-35). Cine MR can be per-

formed using velocity mapping techniques, allowing for estimation of flow rates within the true and false lumina.[7] Flow velocity in the false lumen is usually significantly slower than in the true lumen. Retrograde flow is also found within the false lumen in some patients. A patent false lumen can be simulated by hyperintensity related to subacute hemorrhagic thrombus on gradient echo images.[47,67]

Atherosclerotic plaque along the aortic wall can simulate slow flow or thrombus within a false lumen.[47,66] Mural thrombus located along the wall of aortic aneurysms can result in similar findings.[25]

Difficulty in Visualizing Intimal Flap

Dissection involving smaller vessels, such as the carotid and vertebral arteries, can be difficult to detect.[51] Because an intimal flap may not be directly visualized, ancillary findings should be sought. These findings include increased perivascular signal intensity with associated luminal narowing, increased intravascular signal intensity, and poor visualization of the involved vessel.[51] Because of the limited ability of MR to demonstrate dissection of smaller vessels, angiography may be required to evaluate the status of the coronary arteries in patients with dissections involving the ascending thoracic aorta.[8]

The medial layer of the aortic wall can tear without associated intimal rupture.[64,66] This unusual form of dissection can be difficult to detect; it is manifested as concentric thickening of the aortic wall, without an intimal

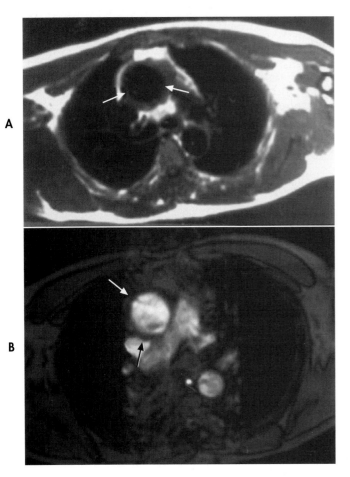

A

B

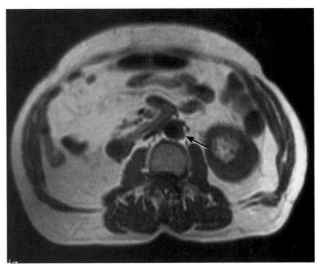

Fig. 2-36. A, Concentric thickening of the ascending aorta *(arrows)* is noted on transaxial T1-weighted spin echo image (TR 500, TE 12, 4 Nex). However, a discrete flap or flowing blood within a false lumen is not visualized on this or on corresponding spoiled gradient echo image **(B)** (TR 50, TE 12, 60-degree flip angle, 2 Nex). This represents surgically proven aortic dissection into the vessel media, in the absence of an intimal tear.

Fig. 2-37. Transaxial T1-weighted image (TR 400, TE 15, 4 Nex) depicts crescentic rim of soft tissue signal intensity lateral to the abdominal aorta *(arrow)*. This finding raises suspicion for aortic dissection, with slow flow or thrombus within the false lumen. However, these findings are due to known retroperitoneal fibrosis, which has resulted in ureteral obstruction, in a patient with no symptoms or clinical findings to suggest aortic dissection.

flap[64] (Figs. 2-36, *A* and *B*). Fibrosing mediastinitis can also result in concentric thickening of the aortic root,[47] and retroperitoneal fibrosis can cause thickening of the abdominal aorta (Fig. 2-37). Additional causes for peri-aortic soft tissue thickening include previous vascular surgery or complications of surgery such as graft infection. All of the above entities can simulate aortic dissection. Penetrating aortic ulcerations can also simulate aortic dissection.[68]

Although dissections usually involve the aorta and its branches, the pulmonary artery can rarely undergo dissection. In one reported case, spin echo MR images failed to demonstrate an intimal flap in a patient with pulmonary artery dissection, though differential signal intensity between the true and false lumina was apparent on cine gradient echo images.[50]

AORTIC COARCTATION

MR is useful for demonstrating coarctation of the aorta, particularly in older children or adolescents in whom echocardiographic visualization of the aortic arch is limited. Focal narrowing of the aortic isthmus may be difficult to visualize on standard orthogonal images. Sagittal oblique images allow for improved depiction of the coarctation site. Partial volume averaging of the aorta with adjacent lung can occur on sagittal oblique images, particularly when thick sections are used. These partial volume effects can simulate aortic coarctation on both spin echo and gradient echo images[36] (Figs. 2-38 and 2-39). In addition to demonstrating apparent narrowing of the aortic isthmus, cine gradient echo images can also depict an apparent signal void in the aortic isthmus. This signal void simulates turbulent flow that frequently occurs distal to the coarctation site. This latter finding is due to out-of-plane motion of the aorta during image acquisition, again resulting in partial volume averaging with adjacent pulmonary air. In one study, these findings of "pseudocoarctation" were observed in eight of 20 normal subjects (40%).[36] In patients with actual coarctation, partial volume effects can cause the severity of narrowing or of poststenotic turbulent flow to be overestimated.

There is, of course, a distinct entity known as pseudocoarctation of the aorta, in which elongation and kinking of the aorta simulate coarctation. There is no pressure gradient across the site of apparent stenosis in patients with pseudocoarctation, and no mediastinal collateral vessels are present.[28] Pseudocoarctation is associated with congenital defects involving the heart and other organs.

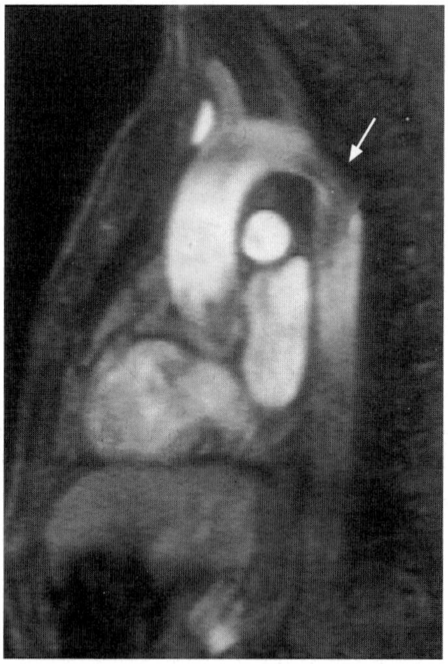

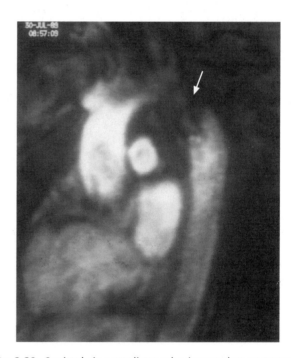

Fig. 2-38. Sagittal cine gradient echo image demonstrates apparent narrowing in the region of the aortic isthmus *(arrow),* suggestive of aortic coarctation. In addition, there is a suggestion of abnormal decreased signal intensity in this vicinity, potentially representing turbulent blood flow distal to an area of stenosis. However, these findings are due to partial volume averaging with adjacent lung in a normal subject.

Fig. 2-39. Sagittal cine gradient echo image demonstrates apparent narrowing and abnormal decreased signal intensity in the region of aortic isthmus *(arrow),* suggestive of aortic coarctation with associated turbulent flow. However, these findings are due to partial volume averaging with adjacent pulmonary air in a normal subject.

POSTOPERATIVE CHANGES

MR is also used to follow patients with aortic coarctation who have undergone intervention.[40] In such patients, continued evidence of turbulent flow has been observed on gradient echo images, even in the absence of a significant residual pressure gradient.[42]

A variety of complications can be observed on MR images in patients who have undergone aortic surgery. These include graft occlusion, graft infection, aneurysmal graft dilatation, pseudoaneurysm formation, hemorrhage adjacent to the graft, and aortoenteric fistula.[3] Hematoma is routinely observed adjacent to the graft site in patients who have undergone recent vascular bypass surgery. The hematoma initially displays high signal intensity on T2-weighted images, with progressive reduction in signal intensity after approximately 3 months. Six months following surgery, it is replaced by a fibrotic mass with low signal intensity on all pulse sequences.[10] Soft tissue thickening is frequently observed surrounding an aortic graft on MR images.[43]

REFERENCES

1. Arrive L, Menu Y, Dessarts I et al: Diagnosis of abdominal venous thrombosis by means of spin-echo and gradient-echo MR imaging: analysis with receiver operating characteristic curves, Radiology 181:661-668, 1991.
2. Atlas SW, Mark AS, Fram EK et al: Vascular intracranial lesions: applications of gradient-echo MR imaging, Radiology 169:455-461, 1988.
3. Auffermann W, Olofsson P, Stoney R et al: MR imaging of complications of aortic surgery, J Comput Assist Tomogr 11:982-989, 1987.
4. Augustyn GT, D'Amour PG, Scott JA et al: Thrombus simulating flow void: a pitfall in diagnosing aqueductal patency by high-field MR imaging, Am J Neuroradiol 8:1139-1141, 1987.
5. Black CM, Hedges LK, Javitt MC: The superior pericardial sinus: normal appearance on gradient-echo MR images, Am J Roentgenol 160:749-751, 1993.
6. Bradley WG Jr: Flow phenomena in MR imaging, Am J Roentgenol 150:983-994, 1988.
7. Chang JM, Friese K, Caputo GR et al: MR measurement of blood flow in the true and false channel in chronic aortic dissection, J Comput Assist Tomogr 15:418-423, 1991.
8. Cigarroa JE, Isselbacher EM, DeSanctis RW et al: Medical progress. Diagnostic imaging in the evaluation of suspected aortic dissection: old standards and new directions, Am J Roentgenol 161:485-493, 1993.
9. Debatin JF, Moon RE, Spritzer CE et al: MRI of absent left pulmonary artery, J Comput Assist Tomogr 16:641-645, 1992.
10. Di Cesare E, Di Renzi P, Pavone P et al: Evaluation of hematoma by MRI in follow-up of aortofemoral bypass, Magn Reson Imaging 9:247-253, 1991.
11. Dinsmore RE, Wedeen V, Rosen B et al: Phase-offset technique to distinguish slow blood flow and thrombus on MR images, Am J Roentgenol 148:634-636, 1987.
12. Duerk JL, Pattany PM: Analysis of imaging axes significance in motion artifact suppression technique (MAST): MRI of turbulent flow and motion, Magn Reson Imaging 7:251-263, 1989.
13. Edelman RR, Zhao B, Liu C et al: MR angiography and dynamic flow evaluation of the portal venous system, Am J Roentgenol 153:755-760, 1989.
14. Ehman RL, Felmlee JP: Flow artifact reduction in MRI: a review of the roles of gradient moment nulling and spatial presaturation, Magn Reson Med 14:293-307, 1990.
15. Evans AJ, Hedlund LW, Herfkens RJ et al: Evaluation of steady and pulsatile flow with dynamic MRI using limited flip angles and gradient refocused echoes, Magn Reson Imaging 5:475-482, 1987.
16. Evans AJ, Sostman HD, Knelson MK et al: Detection of deep venous thrombosis: prospective comparison of MR imaging with contrast venography, Am J Roentgenol 161:131-139, 1993.
17. Fletcher BD, Jacobstein MD: MRI of congenital abnormalities of the great arteries, Am J Roentgenol 146:941-948, 1986.
18. Fletcher BD, Jacobstein MD, Abramowsky CR et al: Right atrioventricular valve atresia: anatomic evaluation with MR imaging, Am J Roentgenol 148:671-674, 1987.
19. Fujimoto K, Abe T, Kumabe T et al: Anomalous left brachiocephalic (innominate) vein: MR demonstration, Am J Roentgenol 159:479-480, 1992.
20. Fujita N, Harada K, Hirabuki N et al: Asymmetric appearance of intracranial vessels on routine spin-echo MR images: a pulse sequence-dependent phenomenon, Am J Neuroradiol 13:1153-1159, 1992.
21. Gehl HB, Bohndorf K, Klose KC: Inferior vena cava tumor thrombus: demonstration by Gd-DTPA enhanced MR, J Comput Assist Tomogr 14:479-481, 1990.
22. Greene R, Miller SW: Cross-sectional imaging of silent pulmonary venous anomalies, Radiology 159:279-281, 1986.
23. Henkelman RM, McVeigh ER, Crawley AP et al: Very slow in-plane flow with gradient echo imaging, Magn Reson Imaging 7:383-393, 1989.
24. Jaspan T, Wilson M, O'Donnell H et al: Magnetic resonance imaging with even-echo rephasing sequences in the assessment and management of giant intracranial aneurysms, Br J Radiol 61:351-357, 1988.
25. Kersting-Sommerhoff BA, Higgins CB, White RD et al: Aortic dissection: sensitivity and specificity of MR imaging, Radiology 166:651-655, 1988.
26. Kersting-Sommerhoff BA, Sechtem UP, Fisher MR et al: MR imaging of congenital anomalies of the aortic arch, Am J Roentgenol 149:9-13, 1987.
27. Larson TC III, Kelly WM, Ehman RL et al: Spatial misregistration of vascular flow during MR imaging of the CNS: cause and clinical significance, Am J Neuroradiol 11:1041-1048, 1990.
28. LePage JR, Szechenyi E, Ross-Duggan JW: Pseudocoarctation of the aorta, Magn Reson Imaging 6:65-68, 1988.
29. Levine E: Kommerell diverticulum or subclavian aneurysm? [letter], Am J Roentgenol 150:695, 1988.
30. Liebman CE, Messersmith RN, Levin DN et al: MR imaging of inferior vena caval filters: safety and artifacts, Am J Roentgenol 150:1174-1176, 1988.
31. Lotan CS, Cranney GB, Doyle M et al: Fat-shift artifact simulating aortic dissection on MR images, Am J Roentgenol 152:385-386, 1989.

32. Malmgren N, Laurin S, Lundstrom NR: Pulmonary artery sling. Diagnosis by magnetic resonance imaging, Acta Radiol 29:7-9, 1988.

33. Matsumoto AH, Teitelbaum GP, Barth KH et al: Tantalum vascular stents: in vivo evaluation with MR imaging, Radiology 170:753-755, 1989.

34. Mayo J, McVeigh ER, Hoffman N et al: Disappearing iliac vessels: an MR phase cancellation phenomenon, Radiology 164:555-557, 1987.

35. McMurdo KK, Webb WR, von Schultess GK et al: Magnetic resonance imaging of the superior pericardial recesses, Am J Roentgenol 145:985-988, 1985.

36. Mirowitz SA, Lee JKT, Gutierrez FR et al: "Pseudocoarctation" of the aorta: pitfall on cine MR imaging, J Comput Assist Tomogr 14:753-755, 1990.

37. Nadel L, Braun IF, Kraft KA et al: Intracranial vascular abnormalities: value of MR phase imaging to distinguish thrombus from flowing blood, Am J Roentgenol 156:373-380, 1991.

38. Park JH, Man CH, Kim CW: MR imaging of congenitally corrected transposition of the great vessels in adults, Am J Roentgenol 153:491-494, 1989.

39. Petasnick JP: Radiologic evaluation of aortic dissection, Radiology 180:297-305, 1990.

40. Pinzon JL, Burrows PE, Benson LN et al: Repair of coarctation of the aorta in children: postoperative morphology, Radiology 180:199-203, 1991.

41. Proto AV, Cuthbert NW, Raider L: Aberrant right subclavian artery: further observations, Am J Roentgenol 148:253-257, 1987.

42. Rees S, Somerville J, Ward C et al: Coarctation of the aorta: MR imaging in late postoperative assessment, Radiology 173:499-502, 1989.

43. Rofsky NM, Weinreb JC, Grossi EA et al: Aortic aneurysm and dissection: normal MR imaging and CT findings after surgical repair with the continuous-suture graft-inclusion technique, Radiology 186:195-201, 1993.

44. Rumancik WM, Naidich DP, Chandra R et al: Cardiovascular disease: evaluation with MR phase imaging, Radiology 166:63-68, 1988.

45. Schiebler ML, Listerud J: Common artifacts encountered in thoracic magnetic resonance imaging: recognition, derivation, and solutions, Magn Resonan Q 4:1-17, 1992.

46. Semelka RC, Hricak H, Stevens SK et al: Combined gadolinium-enhanced and fat-saturation MR imaging of renal masses, Radiology 178:803-809, 1991.

47. Solomon SL, Brown JJ, Glazer HS et al: Thoracic aortic dissection: pitfalls and artifacts in MR imaging, Radiology 177:223-228, 1990.

48. Spritzer CE, Sussman SK, Blinder RA et al: Deep venous thrombosis evaluation with limited-flip-angle, gradient-refocused MR imaging: preliminary experience, Radiology 166:371-375, 1988.

49. Stahlberg F, Ericsson A, Nordell B et al: MR imaging, flow and motion, Acta Radiol 33:179-200, 1992.

50. Stern EJ, Graham C, Gamsu G et al: Pulmonary artery dissection: MR findings, J Comput Assist Tomogr 16:481-483, 1992.

51. Sue DE, Brant-Zawadzki MN, Chance J: Dissection of cranial arteries in the neck: correlation of MRI and arteriography, Neuroradiology 34:273-278, 1992.

52. Tavares NJ, Auffermann W, Brown JJ et al: Detection of thrombus by using phase-image MR scans: ROC curve analysis, Am J Roentgenol 153:173-178, 1989.

53. Teitelbaum GP, Bradley WG, Klein BD: MR imaging artifacts, ferromagnetism, and magnetic torque of intravascular filters, stents, and coils, Radiology 166:657-664, 1988.

54. Teitelbaum GP, Ortega H, Vinitski S et al: Low-artifact intravascular devices: MR imaging evaluation, Radiology 168:713-719, 1988.

55. Thorsen MK, Erickson SJ, Mewissen MW et al: CT and MR imaging of partial anomalous pulmonary venous return to the azygos vein, J Comput Assist Tomogr 14:1007-1009, 1990.

56. Totterman S, Francis CW, Foster TH et al: Diagnosis of femoropopliteal venous thrombosis with MR imaging: a comparison of four MR pulse sequences, Am J Roentgenol 154:175-178, 1990.

57. von Schultess GK, Augustiny N: Calculation of T2 values versus phase imaging for the distinction between flow and thrombus in MR imaging, Radiology 164:549-554, 1987.

58. von Schultess GK, Higgins CB: Blood flow imaging with MR: spin-phase phenomena, Radiology 157:687-696, 1985.

59. Walker TG, Geller SC: Aberrant right subclavian artery with a large diverticulum of Kommerell: a potential for misdiagnosis, Am J Roentgenol 149:477-478, 1987.

60. Watanabe AT, Teitelbaum GP, Gomes AS et al: MR imaging of the bird's nest filter, Radiology 177:578-579, 1990.

61. White EM, Edelman RR, Wedeen VJ et al: Intravascular signal in MR imaging: use of phase display for differentiation of blood-flow signal from intraluminal disease, Radiology 161:245-249, 1986.

62. White RD, Ullyot DJ, Higgins CB: MR imaging of the aorta after surgery for aortic dissection, Am J Roentgenol 150:87-92, 1988.

63. Whittemore AR, Bradley WG, Jinkins JR: Comparison of cocurrent and countercurrent flow-related enhancement in MR imaging, Radiology 170:265-271, 1989.

64. Wolff KA, Herold CJ, Tempany CM et al: Aortic dissection: atypical patterns seen at MR imaging, Radiology 181:489-495, 1991.

65. Yamada N, Imakita S, Kaminaga T et al: Potential of gradient echo phase image to depict intracranial calcification, SMRM Book of Abstracts 1992, p 1718.

66. Yamada T, Tada S, Harada J: Aortic dissection without intimal rupture: diagnosis with MR imaging and CT, Radiology 168:347-352, 1988.

67. Yousem DM, Balakrishnan J, Debrun GM et al: Hyperintense thrombus on GRASS MR images: potential pitfall in flow evaluation, Am J Neuroradiol 11:51-58, 1990.

68. Yucel EK, Steinberg FL, Egglin TK et al: Penetrating aortic ulcers: diagnosis with MR imaging, Radiology 177:779-781, 1990.

3

Heart

PERICARDIAL/EPICARDIAL SPACES
Fat Collections

Prominent collections of epicardial and/or pericardial fat may occur as a normal variation[9,23,29] (Figs. 3-1, *A* and *B*). These fat collections can extend into the atrioventricular grooves (particularly on the right side), and may surround the aortic root.[12,23] Discrete epicardial lipomas can also be incidentally discovered in asymptomatic patients.[22]

Pericardial Defects

The pericardium may be partially or completely absent on a congenital basis.[42] Acquired pericardial defects may relate to a pericardial window created for treatment of cardiac tamponade or in association with previous coronary artery bypass grafting.[42]

Pericardial Recesses

The pericardial recesses can be of variable prominence.[4,19,24] These include the superior, transverse, oblique, left pulmonic, postcaval, and pulmonary venous recesses. When these recesses contain pericardial fluid, they can undergo volume averaging with adjacent mediastinal fat, simulating the appearance of mediastinal lymph nodes or other lesions.

Pericardial Cysts

Pericardial cysts can be encountered in asymptomatic individuals; their most frequent location is the right cardiophrenic angle. They are typically unilocular and have fluid-like signal characteristics on all sequences.[47] Pericardial cysts can simulate other cystic mediastinal masses including teratomas and bronchogenic cysts, among others.[47]

Misdiagnosis is more likely to occur when pericardial cysts display atypical signal characteristics. For example, they can appear relatively hyperintense on T1-weighted images because of proteinaceous fluid contents, thus simulating a solid mass, a cystic hemorrhagic lesion, or perhaps melanoma. Heavily T2-weighted sequences can be helpful in confirming the cystic nature of such le-

sions.[47] However, pericardial cysts can also appear heterogeneous with foci of decreased signal intensity on T2-weighted images as a result of the dephasing effects of transmitted cardiac pulsations. This can also contribute to simulation of a solid mass or cystic mass with solid components (Figs. 3-2, *A* and *B*). The use of cardiac gating is important for reducing the impact of such transmitted cardiac pulsations.

Pericardial Fluid

A small amount of fluid is present within the pericardial sac under physiologic conditions.[19,35,36] However, the apparent volume of pericardial effusion is often overrepresented on MR images (Fig. 3-3) because of shear effects between the parietal and visceral pericardial layers resulting from cardiac motion.[36,37] These shear effects lead to spin dephasing with subsequent artifactual signal loss.

Movement of pericardial fluid may also cause simple transudative pericardial effusions to appear hyperintense on gradient echo images[37] (Fig. 3-4). This appearance can suggest the presence of hemopericardium, particularly when T1-weighted gradient echo images are acquired.

Documentation of pericardial calcification is important, particularly in the setting of constrictive pericarditis. However, such calcification is usually poorly depicted on MR images. Cardiac gated (cine) gradient echo imaging may be useful for improving visualization of pericardial calcifications.

It may be difficult to distinguish between a small amount of pericardial fluid and pericardial thickening (Figs. 3-5, *A* and *B*). Thickening of the pericardium can be observed following cardiac surgery, though these findings usually remit after several weeks.[18] Partial volume averaging with the diaphragm or with a high left hepatic lobe can simulate a pericardial mass.

Bypass Grafts

MR imaging has been used to evaluate coronary bypass grafts for patency.[15,50] Susceptibility effects related to adjacent hemostatic clips, graft calcification, and adjacent mediastinal fibrosis may each lead to artifactual signal loss, which can simulate patency of a thrombosed graft on spin echo images.[50,51]

Chemical shift phase cancellation effects may be seen in the epicardial tissues. These artifacts occur on gradient echo images acquired using an echo time at which the phase of fat and water protons is opposed. They result in signal void at fat-water interfaces, such as in the region of the coronary arteries (Fig. 3-5).

Coronary Arteries

There are many variations in the branching pattern of the coronary arteries, coronary veins, and coronary sinus. These findings are usually not apparent on standard MR images, which display limited detail regarding the coronary vessels.

MYOCARDIUM
Motion Artifacts

The heart undergoes a continuous cycle of expansion, contraction, and complex rotational motion, which can

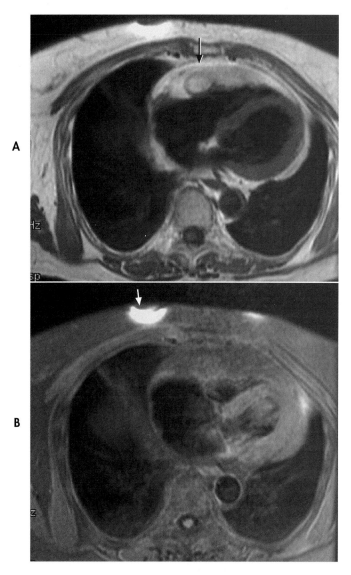

Fig. 3-1. A, Transaxial T1-weighted image (TR 970, TE 11, 4 Nex) demonstrates extensive epicardial fat, which extends into the right atrioventricular groove, with associated fatty infiltration of the right ventricular free wall (*arrow*). **B,** The presence of fat is confirmed by a decrease in signal intensity on corresponding fat saturation T1-weighted image (TR 1030, TE 11, 4 Nex). Increased prominence of susceptibility artifacts related to ECG lead is noted on fat saturation image (*arrow*).

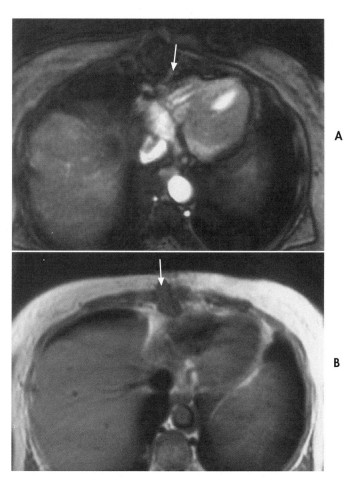

Fig. 3-2. A, Transaxial flow-compensated spoiled gradient echo image (TR 46, TE 12, 25-degree flip angle, 2 Nex) demonstrates partial visualization of a high signal intensity mass (*arrow*) subjacent to the anterior chest wall, suggestive of a vascular lesion. The mass is partially obscured by susceptibility artifact arising from sternal sutures. **B,** Corresponding T1-weighted spin echo image (TR 900, TE 12, 4 Nex) demonstrates the lesion to better advantage (*arrow*). The mass was found to represent a loculated cyst at surgery, with findings on gradient echo image resulting from transmitted cardiac pulsations.

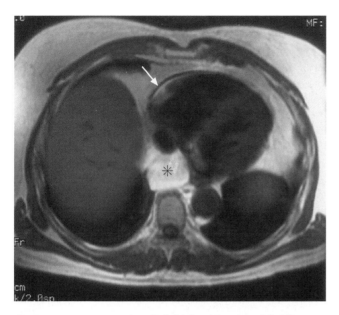

Fig. 3-3. Apparent pericardial thickening and/or fluid (*arrow*) on this transaxial T1-weighted image (TR 770, TE 12, 4 Nex) results from shear effects between the two pericardial layers. Abundant posterior mediastinal fat is also noted on this image (*asterisk*).

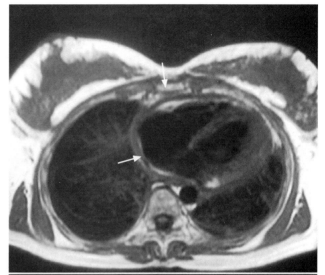

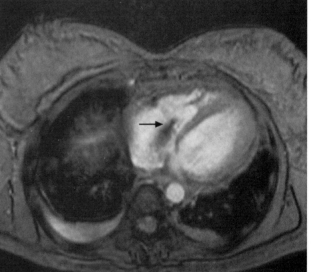

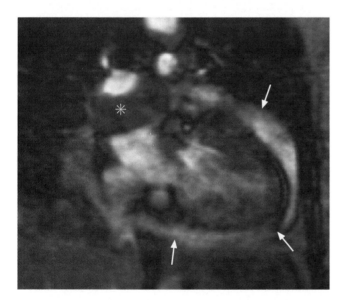

Fig. 3-4. A large pericardial effusion (*arrows*), which is of relative increased signal intensity, as seen on this coronal steady state gradient echo image (TR 50, TE 12, 45-degree flip angle, 2 Nex). Although hyperintensity is suggestive of hemopericardium, the corresponding T1-weighted spin echo images showed pericardial fluid to be markedly hypointense, indicating simple fluid. Hyperintensity on this image is due to motion of pericardial fluid. Note also mass situated above the left atrium (*asterisk*), representing metastatic ovarian carcinoma.

Fig. 3-5. Transaxial T1-weighted spin echo **(A)** (TR 670, TE 12, 4 Nex) and spoiled gradient echo **(B)** (TR 80, TE 13, 30-degree flip angle, 2 Nex) images. Thickening of the pericardium results in decreased signal intensity on T1-weighted image (*arrows*), though it is difficult to determine whether this is due to pericardial fluid or thickening. Note small jet of decreased signal intensity proximal to the tricuspidal valve on gradient echo image (*arrow*), representing physiologic tricuspidal regurgitation. There are also bilateral pulmonary infiltrates and bilateral pleural effusions that appear hyperintense because of motion on gradient echo image. Curvilinear areas of decreased signal intensity, representing chemical shift phase cancellation artifact, are noted on gradient echo image as well.

have devastating effects on the ability to depict cardiac anatomy on MR images. Artifacts related to cardiac motion are manifested as severe blurring, artifactual signal loss, and structured ghost artifacts along the phase encode direction. They are also affected by respiratory-induced variations in heart rate.[32] These artifacts can obscure or simulate cardiac/juxtacardiac masses,[52] myocardial infarcts,[11] or other abnormalities.

The solution to these problems has been to reference data acquisition to specific points in the cardiac cycle, thereby minimizing the effects of cardiac motion[49] (Figs. 3-6, *A* and *B* and 3-7, *A* and *B*). Electrocardiographic chest leads are used to monitor the cardiac cycle. While peripheral plethysmographic sensors are more easily applied, standard chest electrodes provide a more accurate tracing and are recommended for cardiac imaging.

Cardiac Gating

Difficulties may be encountered in attempting to perform effective cardiac gating, which can severely affect image quality and diagnostic efficacy. Since the R wave is used to trigger data acquisition, an effective tracing displays recognizable R wave peaks, which are substantially higher than all other components of the tracing. The placement of electrodes on the chest wall has consider-

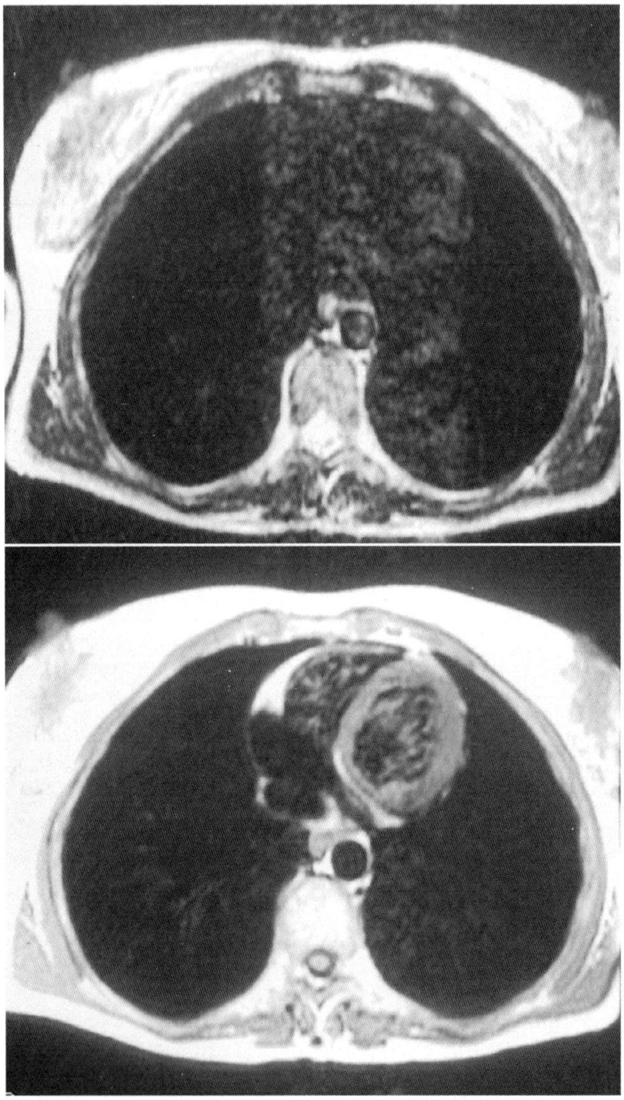

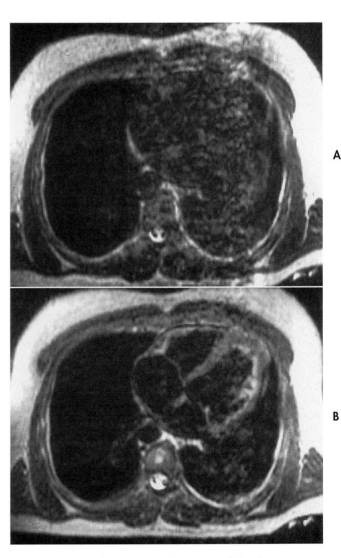

Fig. 3-6. A, T2-weighted image (TR 2200, TE 80, 2 Nex) demonstrates extremely poor visualization of cardiac anatomy, attributable to absence of ECG gating. A band of phase encode artifact is observed in the region of the heart. **B,** Corresponding ECG gated transaxial T1-weighted image (TR 660, TE 12, 4 Nex) demonstrates high-quality depiction of cardiac anatomy.

Fig. 3-7. Transaxial T2-weighted images of the chest obtained without **(A)** and with **(B)** ECG gating. Cardiac structures are poorly defined on the nongated image, with marked improvement with use of ECG gating.

able impact on the quality of the resultant electrocardiographic tracing. Often the electrodes must be positioned several times to optimize the tracing. These electrodes are more frequently positioned on the anterior chest wall, though in this location they undergo significant motion as a result of respiration. In patients with pulmonary hyperinflation, such as that resulting from chronic obstructive lung disease, electrodes may be relatively distant from the heart and thus the electrical tracing is not sensitively recorded.

Some electrodes, particularly those containing silver chloride, can generate artifacts that can obscure visualization of adjacent structures including the heart (see Figs. 3-1, *A* and *B*). In addition, anterior leads can cause image distortion and signal loss affecting the cardiac apex. For all of these reasons, positioning of electrocardiographic leads on the patient's back rather than anterior chest wall may sometimes be useful.

Suboptimal tracings may be achieved in particularly large patients and in patients with reduced cardiac electrical potential resulting from previous myocardial infarction, cardiomyopathy, or other factors. When a poor tracing is obtained, other factors that should be considered include the possibility of defective leads or inadequate lead contact. Cardiac gating may be ineffective in patients with severe cardiac dysrhythmias. The impact of isolated dysrythmic events can be reduced with the use of filters that cause aberrant impulses to be rejected. Retrospective cardiac gating techniques can also be used to correct for dysrhythmic events.

The MR system itself may be responsible for undesirable alterations in the electrocardiographic tracing. The presence of blood flow within the strong static magnetic field leads to artifactual heightening of the T waves of the ECG tracing (magnetohemodynamic effect). This effect remits when the patient is removed from the magnet and imposes no safety risks to the patient. However, it may be detrimental to effective gating of cardiac MR images because the height of the T wave can exceed that of the R wave, causing aberrant triggering. The switching gradient magnetic fields may also alter the ECG pattern, producing less distinct and recognizable peaks that likewise reduce the effectiveness of cardiac gating.

MYOCARDIAL SIGNAL INTENSITY VARIATIONS

- Motion artifacts (cardiac, respiratory)
- Partial volume averaging with epicardial fat
- Left ventricular hypertrophy
- Myocardial ischemia/infarction
- Fatty infiltration
- Regional variations

Signal Variations

The signal intensity of the myocardium should be relatively homogeneous in normal individuals, with foci of heterogeneous increased/decreased signal intensity usually representing pathology. However, inhomogeneous myocardial signal intensity may also be caused by ghosting artifacts from respiratory or cardiac motion. Partial volume averaging of myocardium with epicardial fat is another artifactual cause of abnormal myocardial signal intensity. The heterogeneous high signal intensity that results from these entities can simulate the appearance of myocardial infarction.[11]

Heterogeneous myocardial signal intensity has also been noted in patients with left ventricular hypertrophy in the absence of infarction.[53] Signal alterations in these patients may result from fibrosis or other alterations within the myocardium. The prominence of these signal intensity changes does not correspond directly with myocardial wall thickness.

Foci of increased myocardial signal intensity can be observed on T2-weighted images caused by ongoing myocardial ischemia as well as completed infarction. Unfortunately, signal characteristics provide no distinction between these two entities.[1] Consequently, patients with unstable angina may demonstrate signal patterns simulating myocardial infarcts. Signal intensity alterations on T2-weighted images resulting from myocardial infarction remain evident for several months following the acute event. There is, however, a progressive decline in conspicuousness of these signal alterations with a concomitant localization of such signal abnormalities to the subendocardial region.[44] When an increase in myocardial signal intensity is visualized during this time period, ongoing ischemia or reinfarction should be suggested.

Relaxation times of myocardium have been found to vary according to location. The right ventricle exhibits significantly longer T1 relaxation than does the left atrium, and the left ventricle has shorter T2 relaxation than all other chambers.[33] Alterations in T1 relaxation correspond to myocardial water content, and changes in myocardial hydroxyproline (collagen) contribute to variations in both T1 and T2 relaxation. Myocardial signal alterations involving the free wall of the right ventricle may result from infiltration by fat[23] (see Figs. 3-1, *A* and *B*). Fatty infiltration of the right ventricular free wall can occur with associated dysplasia and may be associated with dysrhythmias and contractile abnormalities.[2,18]

Wall Thickening

Partial volume averaging of the cardiac chambers or walls with epicardial fat can simulate cardiac mass lesions or myocardial wall thickening.[11] The thickness of the myocardium varies considerably during the cardiac cycle.[30] The appearance of normal wall thickening as depicted on a systolic image would be considered distinctly

---

SIMULATION OF CARDIAC MASSES

- Motion artifacts
- Partial volume averaging
- Prominent papillary muscles
- Slow blood flow
- Atrial appendages
- Lipomatous infiltration
- Crista terminalis
- Eustachian
- Thebesian valves
- Chiari network
- Thrombus
- Combination of gradient moment nulling and spatial presaturation

---

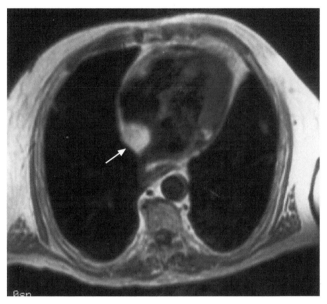

Fig. 3-9. Transaxial T1-weighted image (TR 860, TE 25, 4 Nex) at level of atrioventricular valves demonstrates lipomatous infiltration of the atrial septum (*arrow*), which was discovered as an incidental finding in a 75-year-old male.

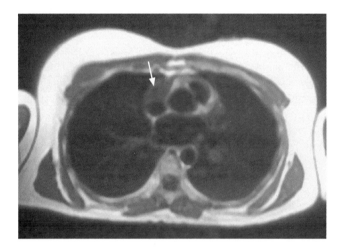

Fig. 3-8. Transaxial T1-weighted image (TR 600, TE 11, 4 Nex) depicts intermediate signal intensity that could relate to a mass or thrombus (*arrow*) in the region of a normal right atrial appendage.

abnormal on an image acquired during diastole. Thus evaluation of myocardial wall thickness should be correlated with the phase of the cardiac cycle during which an image was acquired. This can be determined by the position of the atrioventricular valves on the image or, more reliably, by image annotation when available.

Cardiac Masses

Motion artifacts and partial volume effects have already been mentioned as possible causes for simulation of cardiac masses. Prominent papillary muscles represent another cause for false diagnosis of an intraventricular mass lesion.[14] Slow blood flow within the ventricular or atrial chambers can result in focal increased signal

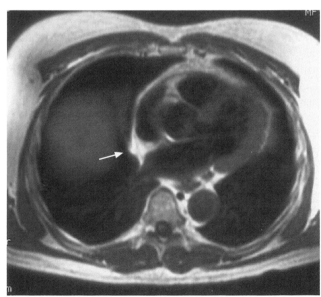

Fig. 3-10. Lipomatous infiltration of the interatrial septum (*arrow*) is demonstrated on this transaxial T1-weighted image (TR 770, TE 12, 4 Nex).

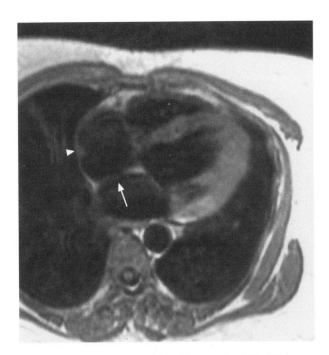

Fig. 3-11. Transaxial T1-weighted image (TR 720, TE 11, 4 Nex) demonstrates nodular tissue along the posterior right atrial wall, corresponding to the normal crista terminalis (*arrowhead*). Thinning of the interatrial septum is also noted in the region of the fossa ovalis (*arrow*).

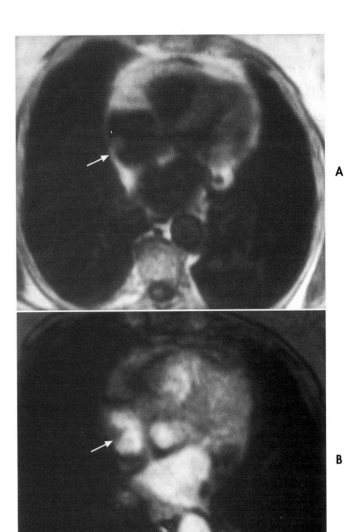

Fig. 3-12. Transaxial T1-weighted spin echo **(A)** and cine gradient echo **(B)** images demonstrate nodular structure along posterior wall of right atrium (*arrows*) representing a prominent crista terminalis. (From Mirowitz SA, Gutierrez FR: Radiology 182:231-233, 1992.)

intensity that can simulate a mass lesion.[52] Signal abnormalities related to slow blood flow are usually not consistently present on various pulse sequences, and cine gradient echo imaging can be used to verify the absence of a mass. The prominent trabeculae of the atrial appendages can also appear to represent a soft tissue mass (Fig. 3-8). Masslike enlargement of the atrial septum can result from benign lipomatous infiltration[21,23] (Figs. 3-9 and 3-10), and lipomas may also involve the atrial walls.[27] Such lipomas are usually not clinically significant.[17] However, atrial septal lipomas have been associated with dysrhythmias in some patients, and some lipomas can lead to distortion of the coronary arteries.[17]

The appearance of a small nodular mass is frequent within the right atrium, related to prominence of normal fibromuscular structures.[25] The crista terminalis is a fibromuscular ridge extending longitudinally from the orifice of the superior vena cava to the orifice of the inferior vena cava. This structure separates the smooth-walled and trabeculated portions of the right atrium. When the crista terminalis is prominent, it may appear to represent a nodular soft tissue mass along the posterior wall of the right atrium (Figs. 3-11, 3-12, *A* and *B*, and 3-13).

The crista terminalis merges inferiorly with the valves for the inferior vena cava (eustachian valve) and coronary sinus (thebesian valve). A series of strandlike fibrous structures can be observed traversing the caudal portion of the right atrial chamber, representing the Chiari network (Figs. 3-14, *A* and *B*). Each of these structures can contribute to the appearance of a right atrial mass on spin echo or cine gradient echo MR images.

The distinction between thrombus and tumor can be difficult on standard spin echo images. Bland thrombus

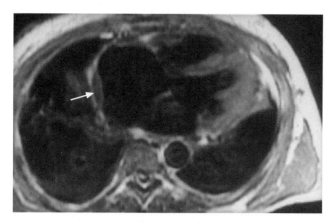

Fig. 3-13. Transaxial T1-weighted image (TR 625, TE 15, 2 Nex) demonstrates thrombus along the posterior right atrial wall (*arrow*). This appears larger and less discrete than normal fibromuscular structures of the right atrium. Also note bilateral pulmonary infiltrates.

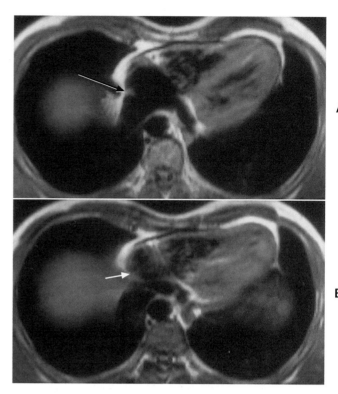

Fig. 3-14. A and **B,** Transaxial T1-weighted images at two consecutive levels (TR 1075, TE 25, 4 Nex) in 18-year-old male. A nodular structure (*arrow*) is seen along the posterior right atrial wall, representing a prominent crista terminalis **(A).** At a more caudal level, a series of radiating structures is seen coursing across the right atrial chamber (*small arrow*), near the entrance of the inferior vena cava. These structures represent components of the Chiari network. (From Mirowitz SA, Gutierrez FR: Radiology 182:231-233, 1992.)

is frequently hypointense whereas tumor is often hyperintense relative to skeletal muscle on cine gradient echo images.[38] However, certain tumors such as atrial myxoma may contain iron, which can also result in hypointensity on gradient echo images,[38,39] and subacute thrombus may have high signal intensity.[18] Intravenous paramagnetic contrast material can be used to distinguish enhancing cardiac tumors from nonenhancing thrombus material.[39]

Cardiac masses can be poorly depicted on spin echo images, even when cardiac gating is used, because of signal loss caused by motion of the mass throughout the cardiac cycle. In addition, low signal intensity masses may be isointense with the cardiac blood pool. In such cases, cine gradient echo images usually demonstrate the mass.[18] The ability to detect as well as to stage cardiac masses on conventional spin echo images may be limited because of the isointensity between tumor and normal adjacent myocardial tissue. This limitation can also be obviated with the use of intravenous contrast material, which frequently results in differential enhancement of lesions as compared with myocardium.[13] However, the prominence of contrast material enhancement of cardiac tumors is highly variable.[39]

Heterogeneous signal intensity can be observed within the cardiac chambers when gradient moment nulling and spatial presaturation are used in combination (Fig. 3-15). This results from the counteracting effects of these artifact reduction techniques on the signal intensity of flowing blood and can simulate a mass or thrombus. Partial volume averaging of the ventricular chambers with inferior wall myocardium can also simulate a mass lesion (Fig. 3-16). Slow venous flow, such as in the left atrium,

can result in increased signal intensity on the basis of even echo rephasing.

Contrast Material

Contrast material has also been useful for evaluating patients with myocardial infarcts. Myocardial infarcts have variable contrast enhancement, depending on the age of the infarct.[46] Acute and subacute infarcts generally undergo prominent enhancement, whereas chronic infarcts usually do not.[5,28,46] Prominent myocardial enhancement is not diagnostic of myocardial infarction, since similar findings may also result from myocarditis. Mild heterogeneous myocardial contrast enhancement may also be observed in normal individuals.[46] Enhancement of normal myocardium can appear relatively prominent, particularly when fat suppressed T1-weighted images are acquired (Figs. 3-17, *A* and *B*).

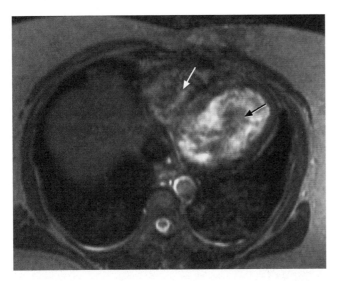

Fig. 3-15. Heterogeneous signal intensity (*arrows*) is noted within the cardiac chambers on this transaxial T2-weighted image (TR 2300, TE 80, 2 Nex). High signal intensity is related to use of flow compensation, with lower signal intensity components attributable to saturation effects and turbulence. The low signal intensity areas can potentially simulate thrombus or tumor. A physiologic volume of fluid can be seen in both pleural spaces.

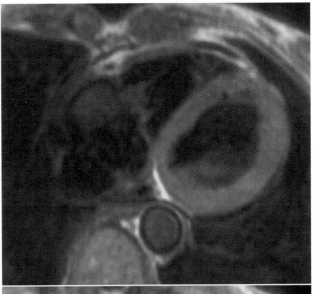

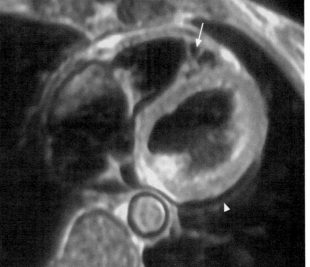

Fig. 3-17. Transaxial T1-weighted images (TR 845, TE 11, 4 Nex) acquired before **(A)** and after **(B)** intravenous gadoteridol administration. Prominent enhancement throughout the myocardium is noted on **B**. Also observed is depiction of the moderator band (*arrow*) and a small pericardial effusion (*arrowhead*).

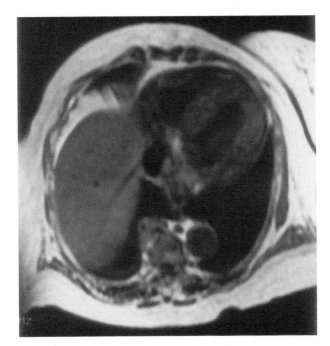

Fig. 3-16. Partial volume averaging with hypertrophic inferior wall of left ventricle simulates an intraventricular mass on this T1-weighted transaxial image. Note that the apparent mass maintains isointensity with remaining myocardium.

Septal Defects

Congenital defects of the atrial or ventricular septa are well demonstrated on MR images. The foramen ovale can be patent in otherwise normal individuals, with probe patency present in approximately 25% of the adult population.[3] MR images frequently demonstrate an apparent defect in the atrial septum where none exists anatomically. This is due to extreme thinning of the atrial septum in the region of the fossa ovalis and the presence of

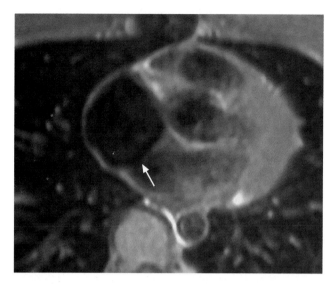

Fig. 3-18. A focus of apparent signal loss within the midportion of the interatrial septum (*arrow*) is demonstrated on this transaxial T1-weighted image (TR 1150, TE 11, 4 Nex). This represents normal thinning of the septum in the region of the fossa ovalis and may simulate an atrial septal defect.

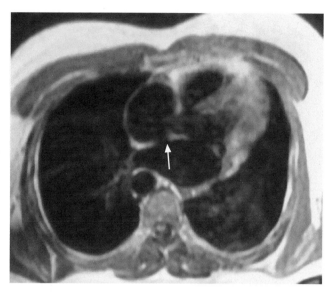

Fig. 3-19. T1-weighted transaxial image (TR 760, TE 25, 2 Nex) demonstrates apparent interruption of the interatrial septum (*arrow*), suggestive of an atrial septal defect. This is due to normal thinning of the atrial septum in the region of the fossa ovalis. Also note that the thoracic aorta descends on the patient's right side.

low signal intensity fibrous tissue in this location.[6-8] These features result in focal signal dropout, which simulates a septal defect (Figs. 3-11, 3-18, and 3-19). A true atrial septal defect usually demonstrates angular rather than blunted margins, as well as associated enlargement of the cardiac chambers and pulmonary vessels.

CARDIAC CHAMBERS/VALVES
Congenital Variations

The cardiac valves can have a variable number of cusps; a bicuspid aortic valve is the most common variation. The coronary sinus may be absent or can terminate in the left atrium rather than the right atrium.[3] The coronary arteries demonstrate many variations in their number, size, and branching patterns.

Cine MR

Cine MR imaging is used to determine the presence and severity of valvular regurgitation and stenosis as well as for evaluation of cardiac wall motion and other abnormalities. Between 12 and 16 flow-compensated gradient echo images are acquired at a single anatomic level, each representing a different point in the cardiac cycle. These images are then presented as a repeating movie loop.

Normal blood flow is usually depicted with uniform high signal intensity on cine MR images. Shear effects resulting in phase dispersion of flowing spins can result in a thin zone of decreased signal intensity along the endocardial surfaces.[10] In the presence of valvular stenosis or insufficiency, the resultant pressure gradient creates high velocity and/or turbulent flow patterns. Similar pressure gradients also result from cardiac shunts, such as ventricular septal defects.[34] In either situation, dephasing of flowing spins occurs and is reflected as marked decrease in intraluminal signal intensity, usually in a perivalvular jetlike configuration.

The size, extent, and duration of the dephasing jet indicate the severity of the underlying valvular lesion. However, the underlying pressure gradient is not the only factor that affects the appearance of such signal intensity alterations. The imaging parameters prescribed can affect the sensitivity of cine MR images to depiction of spin dephasing.[41] Generally a short to moderate TR, short TE, moderate flip angle, and gradient moment nulling are utilized. Overaccentuation of spin dephasing occurs when relatively large echo times and/or flip angles are used and when gradient moment nulling is not implemented. These imaging parameters also influence distinction between the blood pool and endocardial surfaces on cine MR images; this is important for accurate determination of myocardial wall function. Image display settings also affect the appearance of perivalvular jets on

---

NORMAL CARDIAC CINE MR SIGNAL VARIATIONS

- Right atrium: entrance of coronary sinus, proximal to tricuspid valve, near entrance of superior vena cava
- Left atrium: between mitral valve leaflets
- Atrial appendages
- Left ventricle: caudal chamber, along papillary muscles, proximal to aortic valve leaflets, along mitral valve leaflets
- Left ventricular outflow tract
- Aortic root: lateral wall, posterior wall
- Sinuses of Valsalva
- Descending thoracic aorta
- Inferior vena cava: near entrance into right atrium
- Main pulmonary artery: inferiorly
- Pulmonary veins: proximally

SIGNAL VOID ON CINE (GRADIENT ECHO) IMAGES

- Calcification
- Metal artifact
- Chemical shift phase cancellation artifact
- Shear effects
- High-velocity/turbulent flow
- Imaging parameters: TR, TE, flip angle
- Image display factors: window width, level
- Partial volume averaging with adjacent air
- Slow flow
- Catheters, other intravascular devices

---

cine MR images.[41] The size and extent of spin dephasing can appear quite different when the display window width and level settings are altered.

Signal variations on cine MR

Foci of decreased signal intensity are frequently observed on cine MR studies in the juxtavalvular regions in normal individuals.[26,34,45] These findings are due to physiologic flow turbulence from high-velocity flow through normal cardiac chambers or across nondiseased cardiac valves. The appearance of these flow patterns is relatively consistent, though some variation may be related to factors such as patient age, heart rate, and preload and afterload conditions. Awareness of these normal cardiac flow patterns is important so that such findings are not confused with pathology. These normal cardiac flow patterns will be described according to the imaging plane in which they are most frequently observed. These patterns are also summarized in schematic format (Figs. 3-20, A-H).

Transaxial cine MR images at the level of the coronary sinus demonstrate an early systolic triangular signal void proximal to the tricuspid valve leaflets. This finding is due to physiologic tricuspid regurgitation, which frequently occurs in normal subjects (see Figs. 3-5, A and B). This signal void is confined to the juxtavalvular region, unlike significant tricuspid regurgitation, which produces a larger signal void extending farther into the right atrial chamber. Near the inferior aspect of the left ventricular chamber, a globular signal void caused by rapid ventricular filling is seen during early diastole. A linear signal void is often present within the coronary sinus or near its entrance in the right atrium (Fig. 3-21). During systole, a rounded signal void is ob-

served in the inferior vena cava that may reflect transient flow reversal.

On the next higher imaging section, some of the phenomena described above continue to be observed. Additional observations at this level include a linear signal void extending along the anterior leaflet of the mitral valve during its opening in early diastole (Figs. 3-22 and 3-23). This finding can simulate diastolic signal void that results from aortic regurgitation. The latter condition, however, usually results in a pandiastolic signal void and does not have a linear configuration. Following mitral leaflet closure in early systole, a small circular signal void can be observed between or slightly proximal to these leaflets. This reflects trivial mitral regurgitation, which is known by Doppler echocardiography to occur frequently in normal individuals. Distinction from significant mitral regurgitation is again made by the limited duration and extent of the normal signal void region.

At the next higher level, central or peripheral linear foci of signal void are observed during early systole within the left ventricular outflow tract (Fig. 3-24). Small rounded foci are seen within the proximal pulmonary veins throughout the cardiac cycle, and the previously described findings relating to the mitral valve leaflets are again observed.

At the level of the aortic root, early systolic signal void is observed along the left lateral wall of the aortic root as a result of high velocity blood flow (Fig. 3-25). The poststenotic jet associated with aortic stenosis is more central in location and of considerably greater duration and extent during mid-systole. A small rounded signal void may be present in the descending thoracic aorta. Diffuse signal loss can occur in the left atrial appendage because of relative slow flow and/or out-of-plane motion of this structure resulting in partial volume averaging with adjacent pulmonary air.

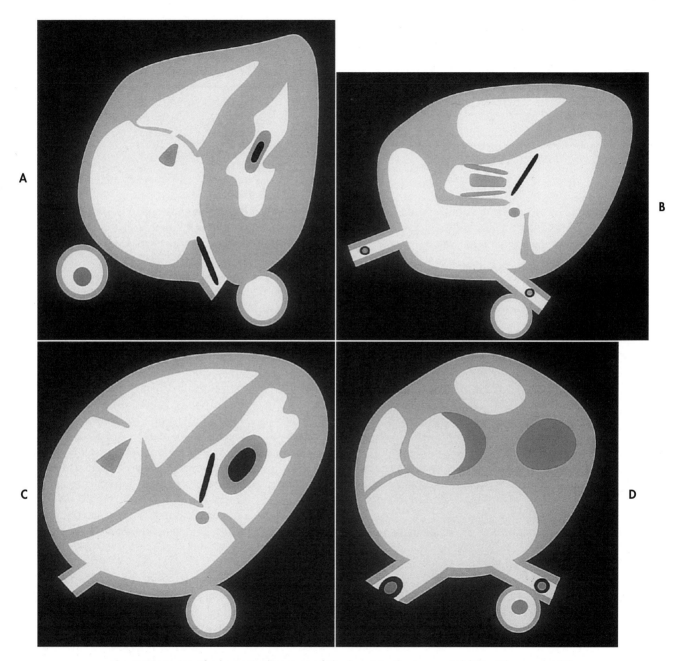

Fig. 3-20. Series of schematic diagrams of the heart in the transaxial (**A** to **D**), coronal (**E**), sagittal oblique (**F**), horizontal long axis (**G**), and short axis (**H**) views. These illustrations depict areas of signal void observed in normal subjects on cardiac cine MR imaging. Signal void areas occurring during ventricular systole are depicted in light gray, whereas those occurring in diastole are shown in darker gray. (Reprinted from Mirowitz SA, Lee JKT, Guterriez FR et al: Radiology 176:49-55, 1990.)

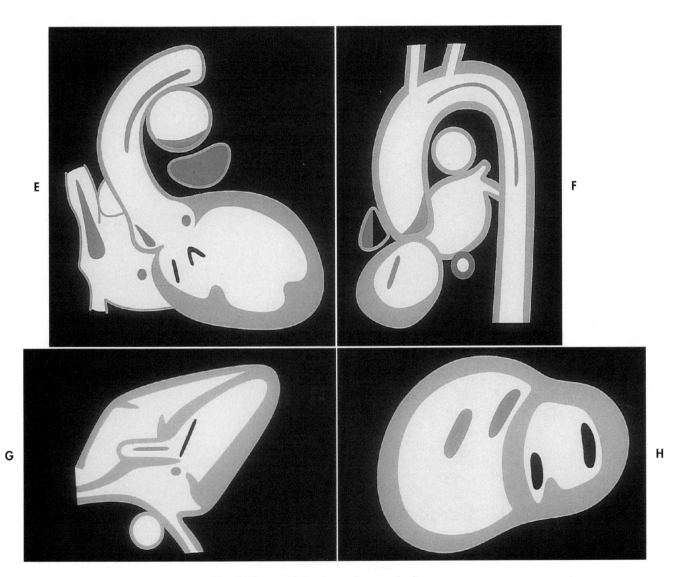

E

F

G

H

Fig. 3-20, cont'd For legend see opposite page.

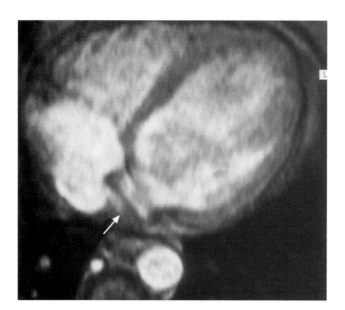

Fig. 3-21. Transaxial cine gradient echo image obtained during diastole demonstrates linear focus of signal void (*arrow*) within the coronary sinus.

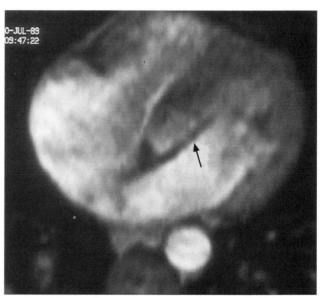

Fig. 3-22. Transaxial cine gradient echo image obtained during diastole demonstrates signal void along the anterior mitral valve leaflet (*arrow*).

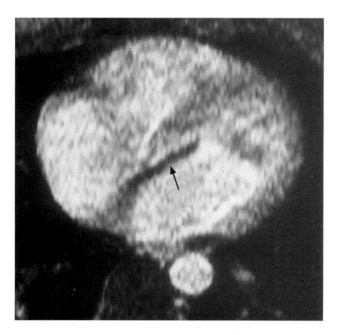

Fig. 3-23. Transaxial cine gradient echo image obtained during diastole demonstrates linear signal void (*arrow*) along the opening anterior leaflet of the mitral valve.

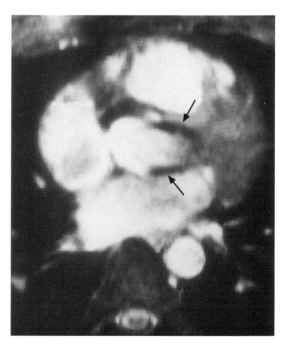

Fig. 3-24. Transaxial cine gradient echo image obtained during systole demonstrates two linear foci of signal void within the left ventricular outflow tract (*arrows*). (From Mirowitz SA, Lee JKT, Guterriez FR et al: Radiology 176:49-55, 1990.)

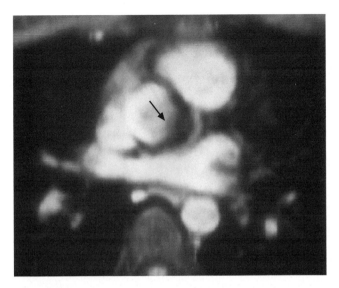

Fig. 3-25. Curvilinear signal void (*arrow*) is seen along the medial wall of the ascending aorta on this systolic transaxial cine gradient echo image.

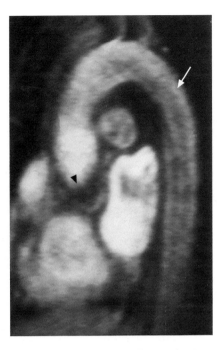

Fig. 3-26. Sagittal oblique cine gradient echo image demonstrates signal void within the aortic root (*arrowhead*). Some linear foci of signal void are also seen within the descending thoracic aorta (*arrow*).

Coronal cine MR images often reveal an oval-shaped focus of signal loss extending from the distal superior vena cava into the right atrium during systole. Signal loss along the septal aspect of the right atrium during early systole corresponds to physiologic tricuspid regurgitation. During systole, signal void is also observed along the inferior aspect of the main pulmonary artery, probably because of high-velocity flow. The left atrial appendage can demonstrate diffuse reduced signal intensity throughout the cardiac cycle, possibly related to slow flow and/or flow alterations resulting from its highly trabeculated architecture. A signal void that resembles an inverted V is often present proximal to the aortic valve during early systole. Small rounded foci can also be seen at this time within the sinuses of Valsalva and are often followed by a curvilinear signal void extending along the ascending aorta and aortic arch. A focus of signal void is noted within the left ventricle during early diastole, corresponding to flow disturbances along the opening mitral valve leaflets.

Sagittal oblique cine MR studies demonstrate early systolic signal void along the posterior wall of the aortic root, which may relate to physiologic flow reversal (Fig. 3-26). Slightly later in systole, a curvilinear signal void extends across the aortic arch into the proximal descending thoracic aorta. Systolic linear signal void within the right atrium and continuous diffuse signal loss within the right atrial appendage are again visualized.

The short axis view demonstrates diastolic signal void along the papillary muscles of the left ventricle. Curvilinear signal void is present within the left ventricular chamber during systole and in the right ventricle during diastole.

Slow Blood Flow

Intraluminal signal loss on cine gradient echo images usually reflects turbulent and/or high-velocity blood flow. However, slow flow may also lead to reduced signal intensity on cine studies, while also producing relatively increased signal intensity within the cardiac chambers on T1-weighted spin echo images. Slow blood flow can occur adjacent to sites of myocardial infarction or within large cardiac (pseudo)aneurysms. Signal alterations resulting from slow flow can simulate thrombus material or neoplasm.[14,20] The use of spatial presaturation radiofrequency pulses assists in reducing the signal intensity of flowing blood on spin echo images but is often incompletely successful. The use of a very short TE (e.g., less than 10 msec) contributes to signal generation from slowly flowing blood, and a TE on the order of 20 msec or more is often preferable. Cine MR images can serve a problem-solving role in such cases, since they are generally less severely affected by signal alterations related to slow flow. Phase images can also be used in an effort to distinguish between slow flow and soft tissue masses. However, marked phase shifts may be generated by myocardial motion that can obscure visualization of underlying lesions.[43,48]

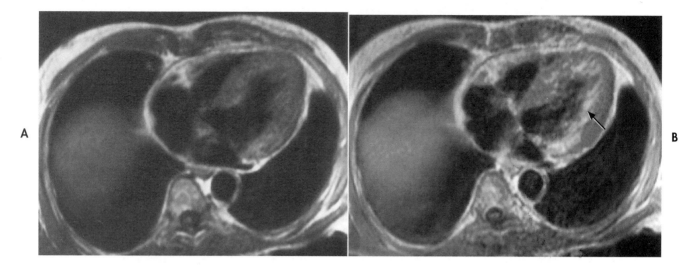

Fig. 3-27. Transaxial T1-weighted images (TR 1270, TE 11, 4 Nex) obtained before **(A)** and after **(B)** gadolinium chelate administration. Increased signal intensity is observed along the endocardial surfaces of the left ventricular chamber following contrast material administration (*arrow*). This represents T1 shortening caused by contrast material within areas of blood flow stasis.

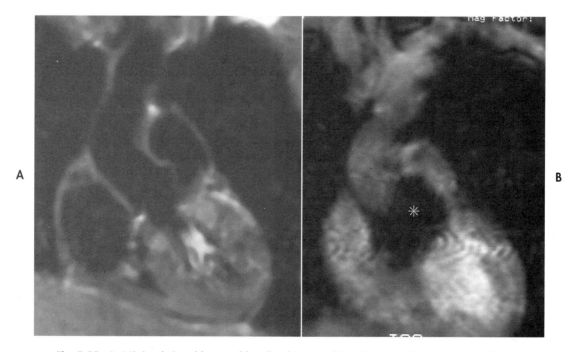

Fig. 3-28. A, Minimal signal loss and localized image distortion is evident on coronal T1-weighted image (TR 620, TE 20, 2 Nex) in patient with Marfan disease who has undergone previous aortic valve replacement and ascending aortic graft. **B,** Marked signal void resulting from the metallic prosthetic aortic valve is observed on the corresponding coronal gradient echo image (TR 130, TE 12, 30-degree flip angle, 2 Nex) (*asterisk*).

Slow flow can indicate that the overlying myocardium is poorly functioning, usually because of a previous myocardial infarction. However, relatively slow flow is often present under physiologic conditions along the endocardial surfaces of the heart, particularly on images acquired during ventricular diastole.[11] Marked increased signal intensity can be observed in these locations following contrast material administration (Figs. 3-27, *A* and *B*).

Relatively slow blood flow can lead to increased signal intensity in the juxtavalvular areas on spin echo images. These findings can simulate thickening of the valve leaflets from endocarditis.

Metal Artifacts

Foci of decreased signal intensity on spin echo and gradient echo images may reflect the presence of cardiac or juxtacardiac metallic objects. For example, valvular prostheses generate profound signal loss, particularly on gradient echo images, which can obscure large portions of cardiac anatomy (Figs. 3-28, *A* and *B* and 3-29). These artifactual signal void foci can affect the ventricular septum, simulating the appearance of a septal defect.[40] Catheters and other devices that traverse the heart can also result in signal void foci, particularly on gradient echo images.

Calcifications

Calcification of cardiac valvular leaflets or annulus can lead to susceptibility artifacts, though they are usually less extensive than those associated with ferromagnetic items. Intracardiac calcifications may also be related to the coronary arteries, calcific pericarditis, calcified thrombus, mural calcification, tumors, and other entities. The presence of such calcifications is usually not detectable on conventional spin echo images, though profound signal void regions often render them apparent on gradient echo images.[16,31] Confusion of normal or pathologic flow void regions for sites of intracardiac calcification on cine gradient echo imaging represents a potential pitfall.

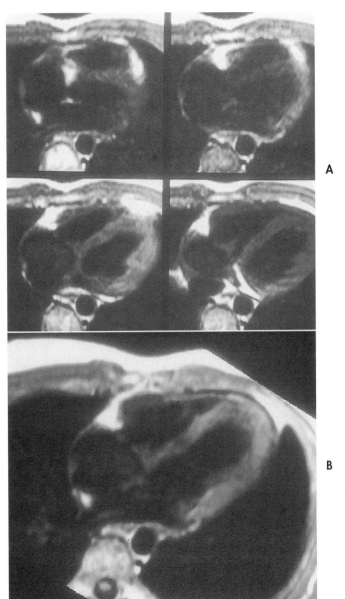

Fig. 3-30. A, Series of consecutive T1-weighted transaxial images of the heart. **B,** Retrospective reformatting of the data using a tricubic interpolation method provides orientation of image along the long axis of the heart, parallel to the interventricular septum.

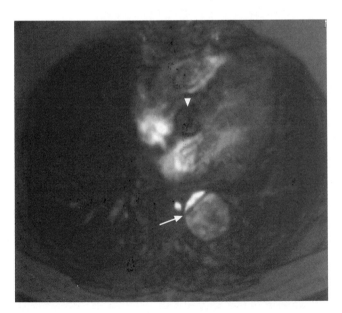

Fig. 3-29. Transaxial spoiled gradient echo image (TR 50, TE 12, 60-degree flip angle, 2 Nex) in patient with Marfan disease. A signal void results from a prosthetic St. Jude aortic valve (*arrowhead*). Also noted is dissection of the descending thoracic aorta (*arrow*).

Imaging Axes

The axis of the heart is oblique with reference to that of the thorax. Consequently, images acquired orthogonal to the thorax intersect the heart at an oblique angle, resulting in suboptimal depiction of cardiac anatomy. These images can present a distorted appearance of the true contour and size of the cardiac chambers and result in foreshortening of the atrial/ventricular septae and myocardium (Figs. 3-30, *A* and *B*). Therefore cardiac analysis is best performed when images are acquired orthogonal to the heart, such as long axis and short axis views.

REFERENCES

1. Ahmad M, Johnson RF Jr, Fawcett HD et al: Magnetic resonance imaging in patients with unstable angina: comparison with acute myocardial infarction and normals, Magn Reson Imaging 6:527-534, 1988.
2. Auffermann W, Wichter T, Breithardt G et al: Arrythmogenic right ventricular disease: MR imaging vs angiography, Am J Roentgenol 161:549-555, 1993.
3. Bergman RA, Thompson SA, Afifi AK et al: Compendium of human anatomic variation: text, atlas and world literature, Baltimore, 1988, Urban & Schwarzenberg.
4. Choe YH, Im JG, Park JH et al: The anatomy of the pericardal space: a study in cadavers and patients, Am J Roentgenol 149:693-697, 1987.
5. de Roos A, Doornbos J, van der Wall EE et al: MR imaging of acute myocardial infarction: value of Gd-DTPA, Am J Roentgenol 150:531-534, 1988.
6. Didier D, Higgins CB, Fisher MR et al: Congenital heart disease: gated MR imaging in 72 patients, Radiology 158:227-235, 1986.
7. Diethelm L, Dery R, Lipton MJ et al: Atrial-level shunts: sensitivity and specificity of MR in diagnosis, Radiology 162:181-186, 1987.
8. Dinsmore RE, Wismore GL, Guyer D et al: Magnetic resonance imaging of the interatrial septum and atrial septal defects, Am J Roentgenol 145:697-703, 1985.
9. Duvernoy O, Larsson SG, Thuren J et al: Epicardial fat causing pitfalls in CT and MR imaging of the pericardium, Acta Radiol 33:1-5, 1992.
10. Edelman RR, Thompson R, Kantor H et al: Cardiac function: evaluation with fast-echo MR imaging, Radiology 162:611-615, 1987.
11. Fisher MR, McNamara MT, Higgins CB: Acute myocardial function: MR evaluation in 29 patients, Am J Roentgenol 148:247-251, 1987.
12. Fletcher BD, Jacobstein MD, Abramowsky CR et al: Right atrioventricular valve atresia: anatomic evaluation with MR imaging, Am J Roentgenol 148:671-674, 1987.
13. Funari M, Fujita N, Peck WW et al: Cardiac tumors: assessment with Gd-DTPA enhanced MR imaging, J Comput Assist Tomogr 15:953-958, 1991.
14. Gomes AS, Lois JF, Child JS et al: Cardiac tumors and thrombus: evaluation with MR imaging, Am J Roentgenol 149:895-899, 1987.
15. Gomes AS, Lois JF, Drinkwater DC et al: Coronary artery by-pass grafts: visualization with MR imaging, Radiology 162:175-179, 1987.
16. Hammersmith SM, Colletti PM, Norris SL et al: Cardiac calcifications: difficult MRI diagnosis, Magn Reson Imaging 9:195-200, 1991.
17. Hananouchi GI, Goff WB 2d: Cardiac lipoma: six-year follow-up with MRI characteristics, and a review of the literature, Magn Reson Imaging 8:825-828, 1990.
18. Higgins CB, Caputo GR: Role of MR imaging in acquired and congenital cardiovascular disease, Am J Roentgenol 161:13-22, 1993.
19. Im J-G, Rosen A, Webb WR et al: MR imaging of the transverse sinus of the pericardium, Am J Roentgenol 150:79-84, 1988.
20. Jungehuslihng M, Sechtem U, Theissen P et al: Left ventricular thrombi: evaluation with spin-echo and gradient-echo MR imaging, Radiology 182:225-229, 1992.
21. Kaplan KR, Rifkin MD: MR diagnosis of lipomatous infiltration of the interatrial septum, Am J Roentgenol 153:495-496, 1989.
22. King SJ, Smallhorn JF, Burrows PE: Epicardial lipoma: imaging findings, Am J Roentgenol 160:261-262, 1993.
23. Krieghauser JS, Julsrud PR, Lund JT: MR imaging of fat in and around the heart, Am J Roentgenol 155:271-274, 1990.
24. McMurdo KK, Webb WR, von Schultess GK et al: Magnetic resonance imaging of the superior pericardial recesses, Am J Roentgenol 145:985-988, 1985.
25. Mirowitz SA, Gutierrez FR: Fibromuscular elements of the right atrium: pseudomass at MR imaging, Radiology 182:231-233, 1992.
26. Mirowitz SA, Lee JKT, Gutierrez FR et al: Normal signal-void patterns in cardiac cine MR images, Radiology 176:49-55, 1990.
27. Mousseaux E, Idy-Peretti I, Bittoun J et al: MR tissue characterization of a right atrial mass: diagnosis of a lipoma, J Comput Assist Tomogr 16:148-151, 1992.
28. Nishimura T, Kobayashi H, Ohara Y et al: Serial assessment of myocardial infarction by using gated MR imaging and Gd-DTPA, Am J Roentgenol 153:715-720, 1989.
29. Paling MR, Williamson BRJ: Epipericardial fat pad: CT findings, Radiology 165:335-339, 1987.
30. Pflugfelder PW, Sechtem UP, White RD et al: Quantification of regional myocardial function by rapid cine MR imaging, Am J Roentgenol 150:523-529, 1988.
31. Pucillo AL, Schechter AG, Kay RH et al: Identification of calcified intracardiac lesions using gradient echo MR imaging, J Comput Assist Tomogr 14:743-747, 1990.
32. Rogers WJ, Shapiro EP: Effect of RR interval variation on image quality in gated, two-dimensional, Fourier MR imaging, Radiology 186:883-887, 1993.
33. Scholz TD, Fleagle SR, Burns TL et al: Nuclear magnetic resonance relaxometry of the normal heart: relationship between collagen content and relaxation times of the four chambers, Magn Reson Imaging 7:643-648, 1989.
34. Sechtem U, Pflugfelder P, Cassidy MC et al: Ventricular septal defect: visualization of shunt flow and determination of shunt size by cine MR imaging, Am J Roentgenol 149:689-692, 1987.
35. Sechtem U, Pflugfelder PW, White RD et al: Cine MR imag-

ing: potential for the evaluation of cardiovascular function, Am J Roentgenol 148:239-246, 1987.

36. Sechtem U, Tscholakoff D, Higgins CB: MRI of the abnormal pericardium, Am J Roentgenol 147:245-252, 1986.

37. Sechtem U, Tscholakoff D, Higgins CB: MRI of the normal pericardium, Am J Roentgenol 147:239-244, 1986.

38. Seelos KC, Caputo GR, Carrol CL et al: Cine gradient refocused echo (GRE) imaging of intravascular masses: differentiation between tumor and nontumor thrombus, J Comput Assist Tomogr 16:169-175, 1992.

39. Semelka RC, Shoenut JP, Wilson ME et al: Cardiac masses: signal intensity features on spin-echo, gradient-echo, gadolinium-enhanced spin-echo, and TurboFLASH images, J Magn Reson Imaging 2:415-420, 1992.

40. Soulen RL, Fishman EK, Pyeritz RE et al: Marfan syndrome: evaluation with MR imaging versus CT, Radiology 165:697-701, 1987.

41. Suzuki J, Caputo GR, Kondo C et al: Cine MR imaging of valvular heart disease: display and imaging parameters affect the size of the signal void caused by valvular regurgitation, Am J Roentgenol 155:723-727, 1990.

42. Takasugi JE, Godwin JD: Surgical defects of the pericardium: radiographic findings, Am J Roentgenol 152:951-954, 1989.

43. Tavares NJ, Auffermann W, Brown JJ et al: Detection of thrombus by using phase-image MR scans: ROC curve analysis, Am J Roentgenol 153:173-178, 1989.

44. Thompson RC, Liu P, Brady TJ et al: Serial magnetic resonance imaging in patients following acute myocardial infarction, Magn Reson Imaging 9:155-158, 1991.

45. Utz JA, Herfkens RJ, Heinsimer JA et al: Valvular regurgitation: dynamic MR imaging, Radiology 168:91-94, 1988.

46. van Dijkman PRM, van der Wall EE, de Roos A et al: Acute, subacute, and chronic myocardial infarction: quantitative analysis of gadolinium-enhanced MR images, Radiology 180:147-151, 1991.

47. Vinee P, Stover B, Sigmund G et al: MR imaging of the pericardial cyst, J Magn Reson Imaging 2:593-596, 1992.

48. von Schultess GK, Augustiny N: Calculation of T2 values versus phase imaging for the distinction between flow and thrombus in MR imaging, Radiology 164:549-554, 1987.

49. Wendt RE III, Rokey R, Vick GW III et al: Electrocardiographic gating and monitoring in NMR imaging, Magn Reson Imaging 6:89-95, 1988.

50. White RD, Caputo GR, Mark AS et al: Coronary artery bypass graft patency: noninvasive evaluation with MR imaging, Radiology 164:681-686, 1987.

51. White RD, Pflugfelder PW, Lipton MJ et al: Coronary artery bypass grafts: evaluation of patency with cine MR imaging, Am J Roentgenol 150:1271-1274, 1988.

52. Winkler M, Higgins CB: Suspected intracardiac masses: evaluation with MR imaging, Radiology 165:117-122, 1987.

53. Zahler R, Chelmow D, Gore J et al: Heterogeneous signal intensity in magnetic resonance images of hypertrophied left ventricular myocardium, Magn Reson Imaging 7:517-528, 1989.

4

MR Angiography

MR angiography is usually based on flow-compensated gradient echo images. Following their acquisition, images are postprocessed using a software algorithm (e.g., maximum intensity projection, MIP) that removes the signal intensity of background soft tissues and renders an image resembling a conventional angiogram. "Time-of-flight" MR angiograms are performed utilizing two- or three-dimensional Fourier transform sequences. Less frequently used MR angiography techniques include phase contrast and "black blood" methods.

Evaluation of the carotid arteries and vertebrobasilar circulation has been the most frequent application for MR angiography thus far. MR angiography has been principally used for noninvasive screening for atherosclerotic disease involving these vessels. However, MR angiography has also been used to evaluate cerebral aneurysms and vascular malformations and to depict vascular supply to neoplasms. MR angiography has had more limited application outside of the head and neck, mostly because of difficulties related to physiologic motion. However, promising results are now being achieved using MR angiography for evaluating the thoracoabdominal aorta, renal arteries, lower extremity vasculature, portal vein, renal veins, and peripheral venous system.

TURBULENT FLOW

Normal laminar flow patterns often become disrupted distal to a site of vascular stenosis; flow in this region can become frankly turbulent. Turbulence leads to spin dephasing, which is reflected as intraluminal signal loss on gradient echo images.[47] Signal loss resulting from poststenotic turbulent flow can cause significant overestimation of the length and severity of vascular stenosis on MR angiograms*; (Figs. 4-1 and 4-2, *A* and *B*). It can also cause high-grade stenotic lesions to simulate vessel occlusion[2,14,17,28] (Fig. 4-3). Complete absence of signal intensity within a segment of the affected vessel is observed with high-grade stenoses as well as occlu-

*References 2, 14, 17, 23, 26, 41, 46.

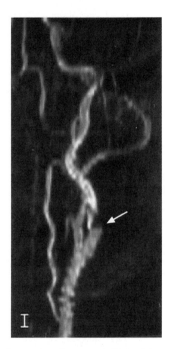

Fig. 4-1. Two-dimensional time-of-flight MR angiogram (TR 45, TE 8, 60-degree flip angle, 1 Nex) in 67-year-old female demonstrates high-grade stenosis involving origin of left internal carotid artery *(arrow)*. MR angiography significantly overestimated the severity of this lesion. Also noted is pulsatility artifact involving the left common carotid artery, which is without correlate on a conventional angiogram.

CAUSES OF SIGNAL LOSS ON MR ANGIOGRAPHY IMAGES

- Disordered/turbulent flow
- Slow/absent flow
- In-plane flow
- Large voxel size/section thickness/volume
- Inappropriate imaging parameters (TR, TE, flip angle)
- Susceptibility effects (air, metal, calcium, iron)
- Motion artifacts
- Unintended radiofrequency presaturation
- Postprocessing artifacts

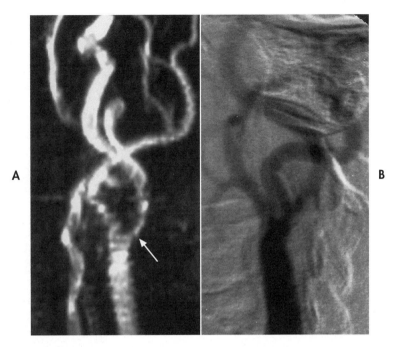

Fig. 4-2. A, Sagittal oblique projection from two-dimensional time-of-flight MR angiogram (TR 45, TE 9, 60-degree flip angle, 1 Nex) demonstrates apparent severe narrowing involving the origin of the left internal carotid artery *(arrow)*. **B,** Subsequent intraarterial digital subtraction angiogram documents that actual luminal narrowing is less severe than indicated by MRA.

sions. However, "reconstitution" of intraluminal signal intensity immediately distal to the focus of signal void usually indicates that there is severe, though subtotal, luminal narrowing.[39] It is conceivable that this appearance could also occur in patients with an occluded vessel that is immediately reconstituted by collateral flow. However, this is an unusual situation, and both entities would require surgical treatment.[39]

When the internal carotid artery is occluded at its origin, branches of the external carotid artery can simulate a patent carotid bifurcation and continuation of the internal carotid artery (Fig. 4-4).

The length of signal loss distal to a stenosis on MR angiography correlates with the severity of the stenosis and with flow rate within the vessel.[20,23] Poststenotic signal intensity loss is usually not observed in association with hemodynamically insignificant lesions (i.e., <50% luminal narrowing).[23] Imaging parameters also affect the appearance of poststenotic signal voids. In general, signal voids are less prominent when shorter echo times and smaller voxels are prescribed.[23,26]

Alternate techniques such as phase contrast MR angiography can be useful when the nature of poststenotic signal voids remains problematic. "Black blood" MR angiography offers another means for elucidating these findings.[7] Black blood images can be obtained using spin echo sequences; however, these are subject to ghosting artifacts caused by pulsatile flow. Gradient echo sequences can be used to generate black blood images. However, even when presaturation pulses are used, intraluminal signal intensity is usually not effectively eliminated. One method for eliminating intraluminal signal intensity on gradient echo images is use of magnetization preparation prepulses.[7] Other limitations of black blood MR angiography include difficulty in accurate depiction of vessels as they pass through bony canals and vessels containing calcific plaque.[14]

Turbulence is not limited to vessels affected by severe vascular stenosis. Aneurysms are also predisposed to turbulent flow; resultant signal loss can cause the size of the aneurysm to be underestimated.[13] Signal loss foci within aneurysms can also simulate mural thrombus.

Disordered flow patterns can also occur in some normal vessels. For example, laminar flow is disrupted in the carotid bulb of normal subjects, where flow reversal and creation of vortex flow patterns occur[2,17,34] (Figs. 4-5, *A* and *B*). This leads to signal loss, which can simulate luminal narrowing. Physiologic flow reversal also occurs in the aortic root (Fig. 4-6). Phase contrast images, which are sensitive to flow direction, can be used to verify flow reversal.

Disruption of laminar flow patterns can occur at sites of arterial bifurcations or venous confluences in normal subjects and in tortuous vessels[3,29,31,32] (Fig. 4-7). Flow

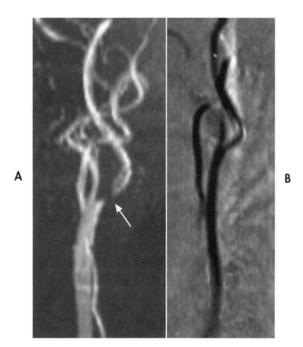

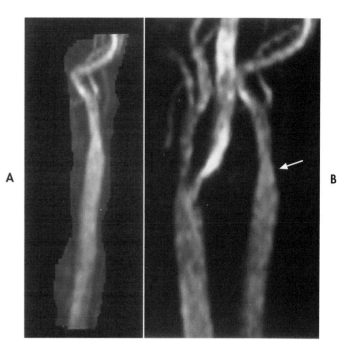

Fig. 4-3. A, Two-dimensional time-of-flight MRA image (TR 45, TE 8, 60-degree flip angle, 1 Nex) indicates a short segment of discontinuity involving the proximal left internal carotid artery *(arrow)*. This appearance suggests vascular occlusion with subsequent reconstitution. **B,** Corresponding two-dimensional phase contrast MRA (TR 31, TE 7, 20-degree flip angle, 12 Nex) indicates continuity of the vessel throughout this segment. Findings on time-of-flight MRA are due to turbulent flow distal to a site of significant vascular stenosis.

Fig. 4-4. A, Two-dimensional time-of-flight MR angiogram (TR 45, TE 9, 60-degree flip angle, 1 Nex) of left carotid artery. The image was initially interpreted as demonstrating stenosis of the distal common carotid artery, with patent internal and external carotids. **B,** Oblique projection of both carotid arteries demonstrates left internal carotid artery to be occluded at its origin *(arrow)*. The apparent carotid bifurcation on **A** actually represents two branches of the external carotid artery.

separation can occur along the walls of a vessel. This also leads to intravascular signal loss, which may cause the vessel to appear diffusely narrowed or can simulate mural thrombus.[2]

SLOW FLOW/SATURATION EFFECTS

Inflow of unsaturated spins—those not subjected to multiple previous radiofrequency excitations—into the section of interest is a major contributor to the flow enhancement effect demonstrated on gradient echo images. After experiencing repetitive radiofrequency pulses, flowing spins become saturated and generate reduced signal intensity, similar to stationary tissue. When blood flow is particularly slow, spins remain within the imaging slice for an extended period of time and become saturated. Slow arterial flow can occur distal to occlusions, within aneurysms or other vascular abnormalities, or be caused by systemic factors such as poor cardiac output (Figs. 4-8, *A-C* and 4-9, *A-D*). Venous flow is typically relatively slow, and veins may be poorly visualized on some time-of-flight MR angiograms on this basis.[6]

Segments of vessels that are distal to a site of proximal occlusion may also appear to be occluded on MR angiograms. For example, flow within the carotid siphons may not be evident in patients with occlusion of the internal carotid artery at its origin because of slow blood flow (Figs. 4-10, *A-C*).

The appropriate choice of imaging parameters can help to minimize saturation effects related to slow flow. One approach is to reduce the section thickness. This requires flowing spins to traverse a shorter distance before becoming saturated. Thin slices and smaller voxel sizes also contribute to reduced signal from stationary soft tissues and to improved spatial resolution. Intravenous administration of paramagnetic contrast material can also be used to increase the signal intensity of slowly flowing spins[6,30] (Figs. 4-11, *A* and *B*). This can improve visualization of small and peripheral vessels. However, when such contrast agents are given, enhancement of soft tissues also occurs, which can render vascular structures less conspicuous.[6,29] Improved results may be obtained with contrast agents that remain confined to the intravascular space, such as those bound to macromolecules.

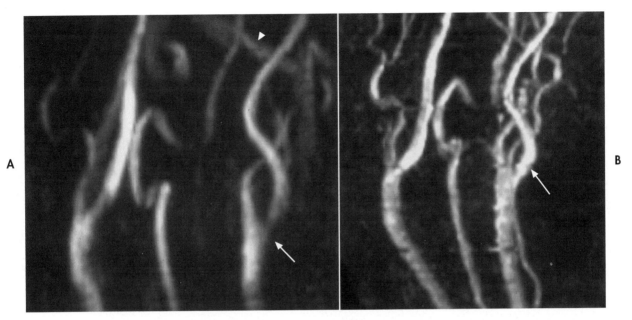

Fig. 4-5. **A,** There is apparent stenosis involving the left internal carotid artery *(arrow)* on three-dimensional phase contrast MRA image (TR 35, TE 8, 20-degree flip angle, 1 Nex) in which the designated flow encoding direction was superior-inferior. This appearance is related to flow reversal and turbulence in the carotid bulb. **B,** This region is shown to be normal on the corresponding two-dimensional time-of-flight MRA (TR 45, TE 9, 60-degree flip angle, 1 Nex) *(arrow)*. Other differences between time-of-flight and phase contrast MRA are also noted, including improved suppression of stationary tissues, increased venous signal intensity *(arrowhead),* and decreased pulsatility artifact on phase contrast images.

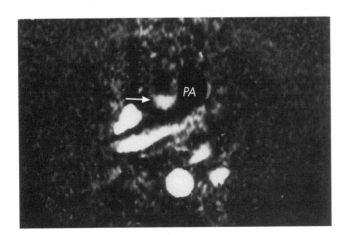

Fig. 4-6. Transaxial image from cine phase contrast MRA (TR 66, TE 10, 30-degree flip angle, 4 Nex). Flow in the caudal direction is designated as white, whereas cephalad flow is black. There is evidence of physiologic retrograde flow within the posterior aortic root *(arrow)*. In addition, a complex flow pattern is observed within the main and right pulmonary arteries *(PA)*.

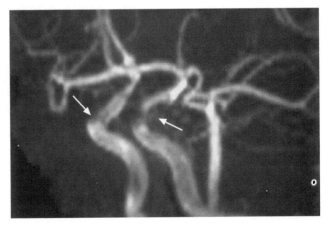

Fig. 4-7. Sagittal oblique projection from three-dimensional time-of-flight MR angiogram (TR 48, TE 5, 25-degree flip angle, 1 Nex) demonstrates symmetric foci of relative decreased signal intensity within the supraclinoid segments of the internal carotid arteries *(arrows)*. These artifactual foci are due to turbulent flow within this tortuous vascular segment.

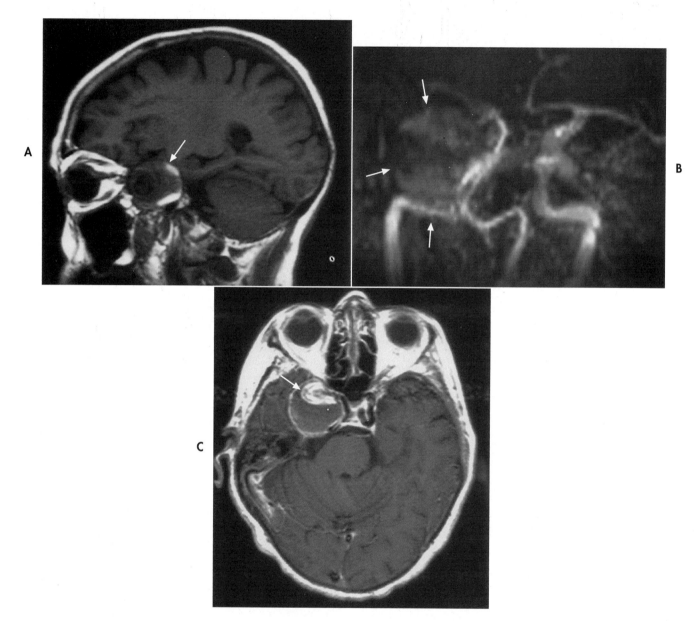

Fig. 4-8. A, Intermediate signal intensity on T1-weighted sagittal image (TR 433, TE 11, 2 Nex) indicates relatively slow blood flow within the lumen of a giant right internal carotid artery aneurysm *(arrow)*. Hyperintensity along the periphery of the aneurysm is related to methemoglobin within mural thrombus. **B,** The corresponding three-dimensional time-of-flight MRA (TR 48, TE 5, 25-degree flip angle, 1 Nex) shows relatively little flow-related enhancement within the aneurysm *(arrows)*, due to slow flow. Peripheral hyperintensity simulating active flow is observed, as a result of the T1 shortening effects of methemoglobin. **C,** Contrast enhanced T1-weighted image (TR 500, TE 11, 2 Nex) accurately depicts the patent central lumen of the aneurysm *(arrow)* and distinguishes it from peripheral thrombus material.

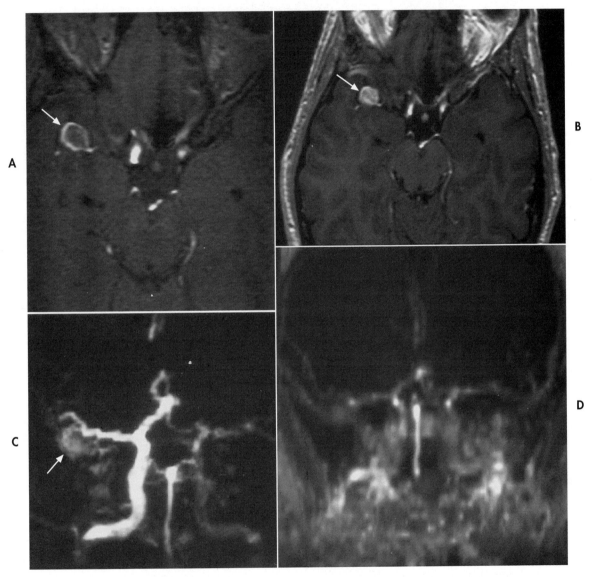

Fig. 4-9. A, Transaxial image from three-dimensional time-of-flight MRA (TR 48, TE 5, 25-degree flip angle, 1 Nex) depicts right middle cerebral artery aneurysm *(arrow)*. There is absence of flow-related enhancement within the central aspect of the aneurysm suggestive of thrombosis. These findings are likely due to turbulent flow and are eliminated on corresponding image obtained following gadopentetate administration **(B)**. **C,** The projection image from the unenhanced MRA data set depicts the aneurysm *(arrow)*. However, additional apparent aneurysms are spuriously indicated, because of poor suppression of background soft tissues. **D,** Projection image from the contrast-enhanced MRA data set demonstrates very poor background tissue suppression related to enhancement of extracranial soft tissues.

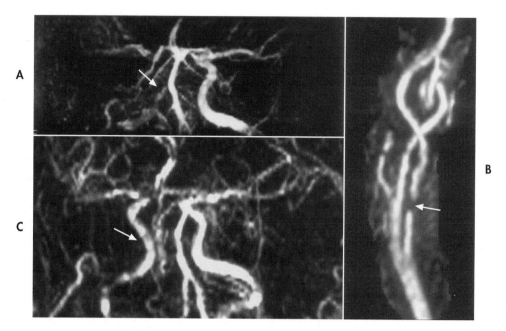

Fig. 4-10. A, Coronal projection from three-dimensional time-of-flight MRA (TR 48, TE 5, 25-degree flip angle, 1 Nex) demonstrates apparent occlusion of the right internal carotid artery siphon *(arrow)*. The patient had a high-grade stenosis of the proximal right internal carotid artery, as demonstrated on two-dimensional time-of-flight MRA **(B)** (TR 45, TE 9, 60-degree flip angle, 1 Nex) *(arrow)*. **C,** Repeat evaluation of the intracranial circulation using two-dimensional time-of-flight MRA (TR 45, TE 9, 60-degree flip angle, 1 Nex) reveals the right internal carotid artery siphon to be patent *(arrow)*. Apparent occlusion on the three-dimensional time-of-flight sequence was due to relative slow blood flow occurring distal to the area of stenosis. These images also illustrate the decreased sensitivity to depiction of slow blood flow on three-dimensional as compared with two-dimensional time-of-flight MRA.

THREE-DIMENSIONAL MRA

Three-dimensional Fourier transform (i.e., volume) data acquisition has many features favorable for MR angiography. Advantages relative to two-dimensional acquisitions include ability to achieve reduced slice thickness and hence improved spatial resolution, increased signal-to-noise ratio, and reduced echo times to minimize dephasing effects.

On three-dimensional time-of-flight MR angiograms, flowing spins become saturated when a large imaging volume is prescribed* (Fig. 4-12). As moving spins traverse the volume, they are exposed to repetitive radio-frequency excitations, which causes them to progressively lose signal intensity. As a result, flow within smaller arterial vessels and venous structures may not be evident on these images.

Saturation of spins flowing through the imaging volume can be reduced by acquiring multiple contiguous or overlapping small volumes, which are then processed as a single composite image. One implementation of this

*References 13, 24, 25, 29, 31, 33.

technique has been termed "multiple overlapping thin slab acquisition" (MOTSA).[38] Patient motion can result in misregistration between adjacent volumes, which can simulate vascular narrowing or ulceration.[17] The signal intensity of flowing blood can vary within each slab as a result of saturation effects. This can result in the "Venetian blind artifact."[12]

FLIP ANGLE

Optimization of the excitation flip angle is important for performance of MR angiography. A very low flip angle can lead to reduction of the signal-to-noise ratio, whereas a large flip angle can result in excess signal intensity arising from the soft tissues and increased saturation of flowing spins (Fig. 4-12). Therefore a moderate flip angle is generally recommended for most MR angiography applications. However, the flip angle should be chosen with consideration to the specific TR, TE, slice thickness, and type of gradient echo sequence used.

The flip angle can be varied in magnitude across a three-dimensional imaging volume, resulting in improved depiction of flowing spins.[6,43] With this method,

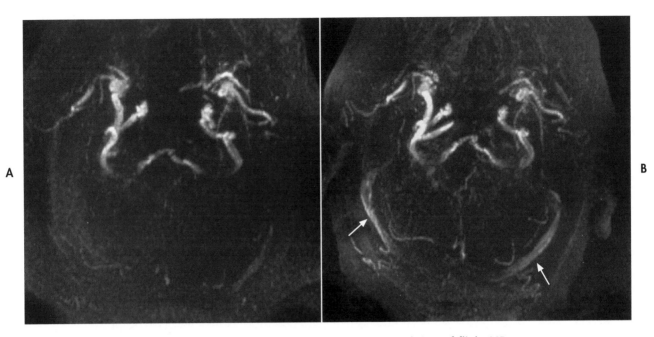

Fig. 4-11. Transaxial projection images from two-dimensional time-of-flight MR angiogram (TR 45, TE 9, 60-degree flip angle, 1 Nex) performed before **(A)** and after **(B)** gadolinium chelate administration. On the contrast-enhanced image, there is relative increased signal intensity within the venous structures *(arrows),* despite the use of superior presaturation bands on both images. The cervical soft tissues are also higher signal intensity than on the unenhanced images.

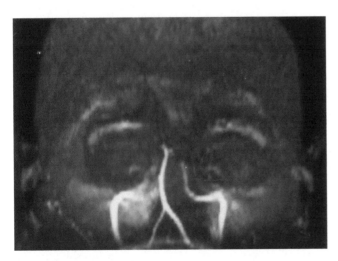

Fig. 4-12. Projection image from three-dimensional time-of-flight MR angiogram (TR 38, TE 5, 45-degree flip angle, 1 Nex) obtained using 13 cm thick slab. There is decreasing visualization of intravascular signal intensity progressing from caudal to cranial within the imaging volume. This is attributable to use of excessively large volume thickness, leading to intravascular saturation effects. In addition, poor suppression of background stationary soft tissues are attributable to use of relatively large flip angle.

a relatively large flip angle is used for acquisition of initial slices, with progressive reduction in flip angle on subsequent slices. This allows for decreased saturation of flowing spins as they traverse the imaging volume.

REPETITION TIME

A moderate repetition time (TR) is also usually optimal for MR angiography. Use of a long TR results in increased signal intensity of soft tissues, whereas a very short TR will reduce the signal intensity of slowly flowing spins.[29] Very short repetition times also lead to a reduced signal-to-noise ratio, which is manifested as image graininess and can impair visualization of small vessels.[26] The signal-to-noise ratio can be improved with use of local coils, particularly those using quadrature or phased array technology.

ECHO TIME

The shortest available echo time (TE) should generally be used for MR angiography. As noted previously, increased echo time leads to greater dephasing of flowing spins and artifactual intraluminal signal loss.[6,46]

Gradient moment nulling (i.e., flow compensation) prolongs the minimum echo time that can be used. However, use of gradient moment nulling is usually justified, because it provides improved intraluminal signal intensity as a result of rephasing of flowing spins at the time of echo collection. Asymmetric (i.e., fractional) echo sampling is often used to reduce echo times. Because only a portion of the echo is sampled, this technique results in increased truncation artifacts, which can reduce vessel edge definition.[24]

VOXEL SIZE

Signal loss resulting from dephasing of flowing spins is also accentuated with relatively large voxel sizes.[4,13] Therefore smaller voxel sizes contribute to improved depiction of flowing spins and improved spatial resolution. Disadvantages of small voxel sizes include increased image acquisition time and decreased signal-to-noise ratio.[26] Because of their ability to provide smaller voxel sizes with adequate signal-to-noise ratio, as well as their ability to provide shorter echo times, three-dimensional (volume) acquisitions generally display less dephasing effects than two-dimensional sequences.

IN-PLANE FLOW

Saturation of flowing spins can occur when images are acquired parallel to the direction of blood flow. This can simulate vascular stenosis or occlusion (Figs. 4-13, A and B). The plane of image acquisition should be oriented perpendicular to the primary direction of flow for maximal flow-related enhancement. Thus cervical internal carotid arteries are usually best evaluated using transaxial images. However, transaxial images demonstrate artifactual signal loss within horizontal segments of the inter nal carotid arteries because of in-plane flow.[39] Artifactual signal loss can also occur when vessels are oriented oblique to the plane of image acquisition.[36]

SUSCEPTIBILITY EFFECTS

Gradient echo images are highly sensitive to local variations in magnetic field homogeneity because they lack a 180-degree refocusing pulse. Such field inhomogeneities can occur in the vicinity of metal, air, iron, or calcium and result in artifactual foci of signal void. These susceptibility artifacts can obscure vessels or cause them to appear artifactually narrowed on MR angiograms. For example, the cavernous and supraclinoid segments of the

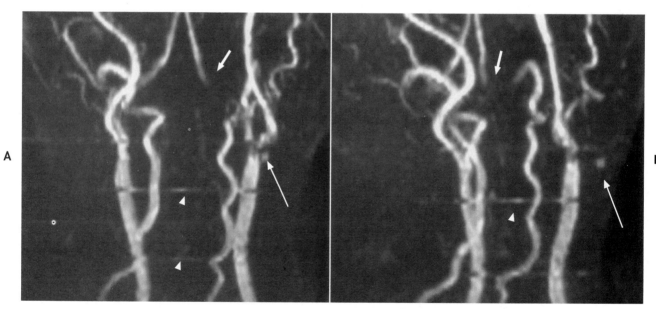

Fig. 4-13. A, Projection image from two-dimensional time-of-flight MR angiogram (TR 45, TE 9, 60-degree flip angle, 1 Nex) demonstrates narrowing of the left internal carotid artery with apparent ulceration near its origin *(arrow)*. The apparent ulcer represents a focus of artifactual signal intensity and can be separated from the carotid artery on oblique projection image, **B** *(arrow)*. Also note linear vascular pulsation artifacts extending horizontally across the image *(arrowheads)*. Artifactual loss of signal intensity resulting from in-plane flow is noted involving the horizontal segments of the vertebral arteries *(thick arrows)*.

internal carotid arteries can appear artifactually narrowed because of air in the sphenoid sinuses.[18,21] Vessels can also appear to have poorly defined edges when they are in proximity to the paranasal sinuses (Figs. 4-14, *A* and *B*). This effect is due to reduction in signal-to-noise ratio caused by susceptibility effects.[26] Another manifestation of this phenomenon is apparent narrowing or occlusion of the petrous segment of the internal carotid artery as it extends through the skull base[18,40] (Figs. 4-15 to 4-17, *B*). Vessels located adjacent to surgical clips or orthopedic prostheses can also appear to be narrowed or occluded[3,15,22,37,42] (Figs. 4-18, *A* and *B*). In the abdomen and pelvis, bowel gas can also result in susceptibility artifacts that obscure nearby vessels.

Highly ferromagnetic items, such as some clamps used in patients with intracranial aneurysms, can lead to anatomic distortion and extensive signal loss.[49] These ar-tifacts are considerably less prominent when nonferrous tantalum clamps are used. When metallic objects are suspected as the cause of apparent vascular occlusion, spin echo images should be inspected for a localized signal void, possibly with peripheral hyperintensity.

Intraluminal thrombus or atheromatous plaque can contain hemorrhagic or calcific components, which can also generate susceptibility artifacts and lead to overestimation of vascular stenosis.[28] Apparent carotid artery stenosis has been noted in patients who have undergone endarterectomy, probably from related causes.[41] In patients who have undergone previous vein grafting, apparent vascular dilatation may be seen (Fig. 4-19). Susceptibility artifacts are minimized on gradient echo images when a short echo time, small voxel sizes, and three-dimensional rather than two-dimensional image acquisitions are used.

MOTION ARTIFACTS

Motion is another cause for artifactual decreased intravascular signal intensity on MR angiograms. This is of particular concern in the chest and abdomen, where respiratory motion can contribute to poor visualization of small vessels.[25,53]

IMAGE DISTORTION

Gradient nonlinearities and eddy currents may lead to spatial distortion on MR angiograms; these alterations can be significant when such images are used for radio-

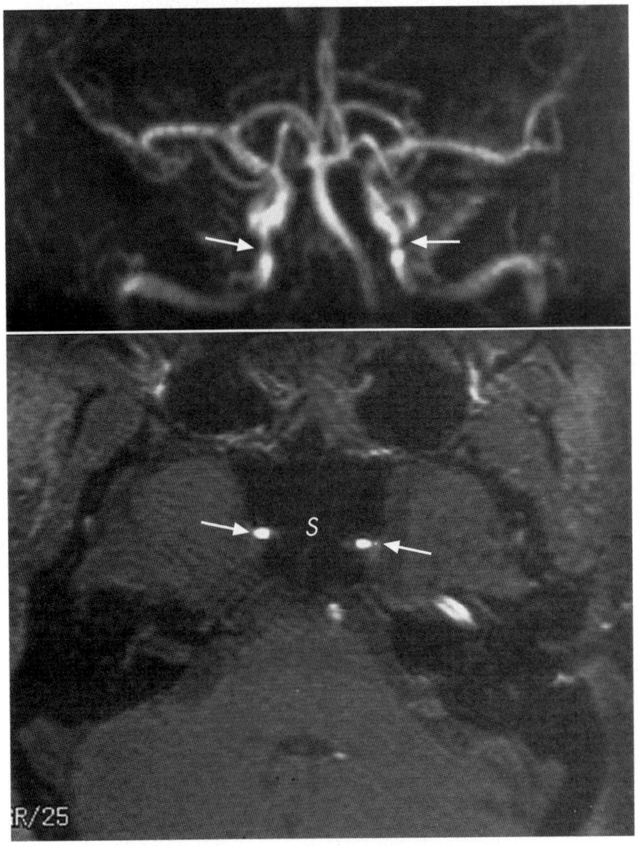

Fig. 4-14. A, Coronal projection image from three-dimensional time-of-flight MRA (TR 48, TE 5, 25-degree flip angle, 1 Nex) demonstrates apparent narrowing involving the cavernous segments of both internal carotid arteries *(arrows)*. This appearance is due to signal void (i.e., susceptibility artifact) arising from air in the adjacent sphenoid sinuses *(S)*, as seen on transaxial partition image **(B).**

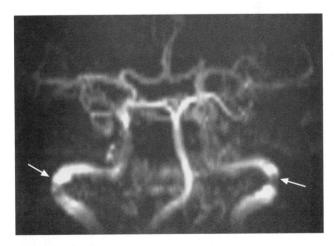

Fig. 4-15. Apparent stenosis of both internal carotid arteries is demonstrated on three-dimensional time-of-flight MRA (TR 48, TE 5, 25-degree flip angle, 1 Nex) *(arrows)*. This appearance is due to susceptibility artifacts encountered as the carotid arteries enter the skull base.

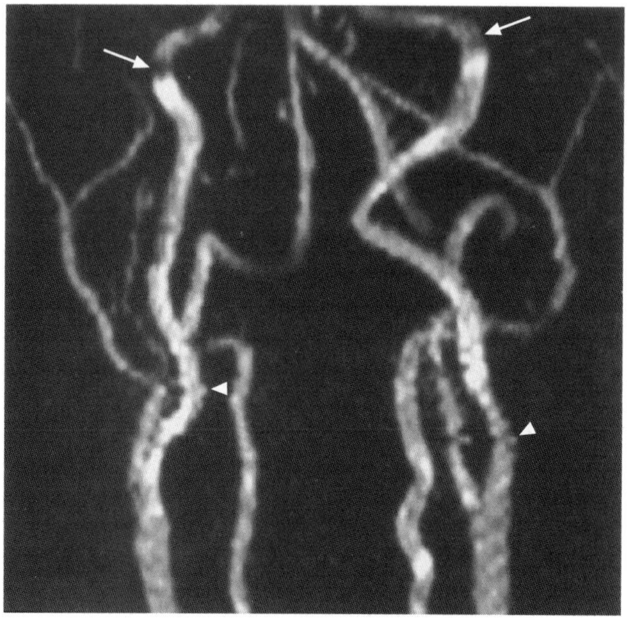

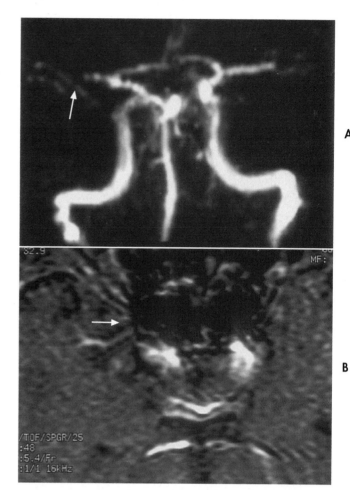

Fig. 4-16. Two-dimensional time-of-flight MR angiogram image (TR 45, TE 9, 60-degree flip angle, 1 Nex) demonstrates symmetric regions of signal loss involving the internal carotid arteries bilaterally *(arrows)*. These findings are due to susceptibility effects as the vessel enters the skull base. Misregistration artifact caused by vascular pulsation is also noted, simulating ulceration of the vessel *(arrowheads)*.

surgical planning.[44] Such distortions can be corrected on the basis of data acquired during phantom experiments.

SPATIAL PRESATURATION

Overlap between arterial and venous structures can lead to diagnostic difficulties on MR angiograms. Spatial presaturation radiofrequency pulses can be used to address this problem. Presaturation pulses are applied to eliminate signal intensity from venous spins when arterial imaging is being performed, and vice versa.[22] For example, when the cervical carotid arteries are being evaluated, a presaturation band placed cephalad to each section saturates spins within the jugular veins, rendering them unable to generate significant signal intensity.

While presaturation is usually successful, it has some limitations. First, the effectiveness of presaturation pulses diminishes as their distance from the imaging section increases. Spins are maximally saturated immediately after encountering the presaturation band; these spins regain magnetization rapidly. Consequently, unwanted venous signal intensity may appear on images that are relatively remote from the presaturation band and result in diagnostic difficulties. Presaturation bands that

Fig. 4-17. A, Coronal projection from three-dimensional time-of-flight MR angiogram (TR 48, TE 5, 25-degree flip angle, 1 Nex) demonstrates apparent stenosis involving the proximal aspect of the right middle cerebral artery *(arrow)*. This finding is due to susceptibility artifact arising from pneumatized bone *(arrow)* as demonstrated on the transaxial partition acquired at the level of apparent stenosis **(B)**.

move with the imaging slice result in improved effectiveness throughout the imaging volume.[15,22] Banding artifacts can occur when the presaturation band is located close to the imaging section.[5] Contrast agents such as gadopentetate dimeglumine are useful for some applications of MR angiography, as noted already. The effectiveness of spatial presaturation is reduced on contrast-enhanced images because of the T1 shortening effects of the agent.

Caution is required to avoid inadvertent presaturation of vessels being evaluated. For example, in a looping vessel, flow within the descending limb of the loop can be saturated when a presaturation band is prescribed superior to the imaging section. This can simulate stenosis

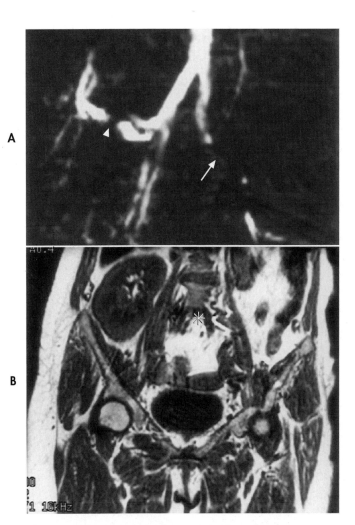

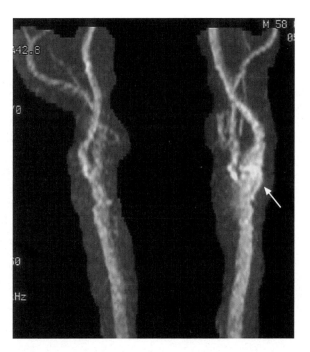

Fig. 4-19. Coronal projection from two-dimensional time-of-flight MR angiogram (TR 45, TE 9, 60-degree flip angle, 1 Nex) in patient who underwent previous left carotid endarterectomy. There is marked asymmetric dilatation of the left carotid bulb related to a vein graft *(arrow).*

Fig. 4-18. A, Coronal projection from two-dimensional time-of-flight MR angiogram (TR 45, TE 7, 60-degree flip angle, 1 Nex) in patient with renal transplant. There is apparent occlusion of the left common iliac artery *(arrow)* as well as the artery supplying the renal graft *(arrowhead).* These findings are due to susceptibility artifacts arising from surgical clips in the vicinity of the graft *(asterisk),* as verified on coronal T1-weighted image **(B)** (TR 400, TE 12, 2 Nex), which also depicts the transplant kidney.

or occlusion of this vessel. Vascular loops can also simulate the appearance of an aneurysm on MR angiogram images (Figs. 4-20, *A* and *B*). High signal intensity within the jugular veins can be observed despite the use of superior presaturation bands. This can occur in patients with retrograde venous flow resulting from right heart failure or tricuspid regurgitation (Figs. 4-21, *A* and *B*). Triphasic flow patterns occur normally in the extremities. This can result in artifactual decreased signal intensity in the popliteal artery, as flowing spins encounter the saturation band placed inferior to the imaging sec-

tion to eliminate venous signal intensity and reenter the section.[53] This can result in apparent vessel occlusion or dark stripes across the vessel.[37] Increasing the distance between the inferior presaturation band and the imaging section will eliminate this artifact.

Presaturation bands are most frequently used to reduce intravascular signal intensity. However, they can also be used to suppress the signal intensity of peripheral soft tissues, so as to increase the conspicuousness of vessels.[19] For example, presaturation bands prescribed along the periphery of the cranium can reduce the high signal intensity of fat within the scalp and orbits. It is important that these presaturation bands not intersect any portion of the vessel(s) being evaluated. Even when the presaturation band is located close to a vessel, its imperfect slice profile can lead to inadvertent presaturation of flowing spins, which can simulate vascular occlusion. When the peripheral presaturation technique is used for cranial MR angiography, lateral presaturation bands can approach the lateral aspect of the petrous segment of the internal carotid arteries, saturating flowing spins in this vessel[35] (Figs. 4-22, *A-F* and 4-23, *A* and *B*). Another method for decreasing the signal intensity of background soft tissues is sequences that use magnetization transfer contrast.[12,27] This refers to delivery of off-resonance radio-

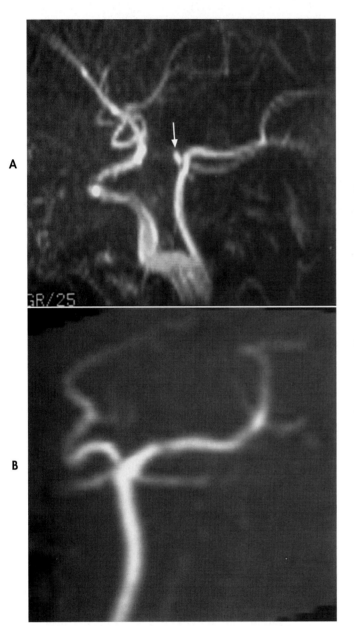

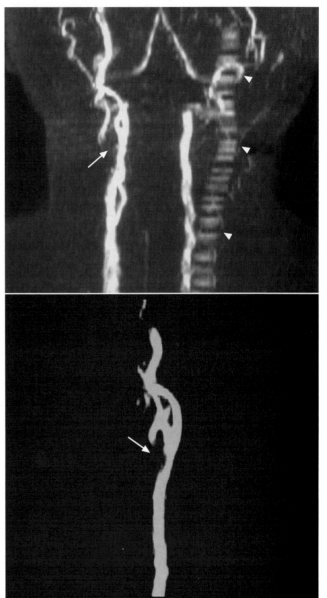

Fig. 4-20. **A,** Lateral projection image from three-dimensional time-of-flight MR angiogram (TR 48, TE 5, 25-degree flip angle, 1 Nex) suggests possible small aneurysm arising from the posterior circulation (*arrow).* **B,** Targeted projection image, obtained from same data set, indicates that no aneurysm is present. Findings on the previous image are attributable to tortuous posterior cerebral artery with vascular loop simulating aneurysm.

Fig. 4-21. **A,** Coronal projection image from two-dimensional time-of-flight MR angiogram (TR 45, TE 8, 60-degree flip angle, 1 Nex) demonstrates a large tubular structure in the left side of the neck *(arrowheads).* This represents the internal jugular vein, which demonstrates signal intensity despite the use of superior presaturation bands. This is due to retrograde flow within the internal jugular vein, caused by tricuspid regurgitation. There is also a segment of absent signal intensity, suggestive of occlusion, involving the right external carotid artery on the standard projection image *(arrow).* **B,** Projection of a limited portion of the original data set demonstrates this segment to be continuous though there is evidence of stenosis.

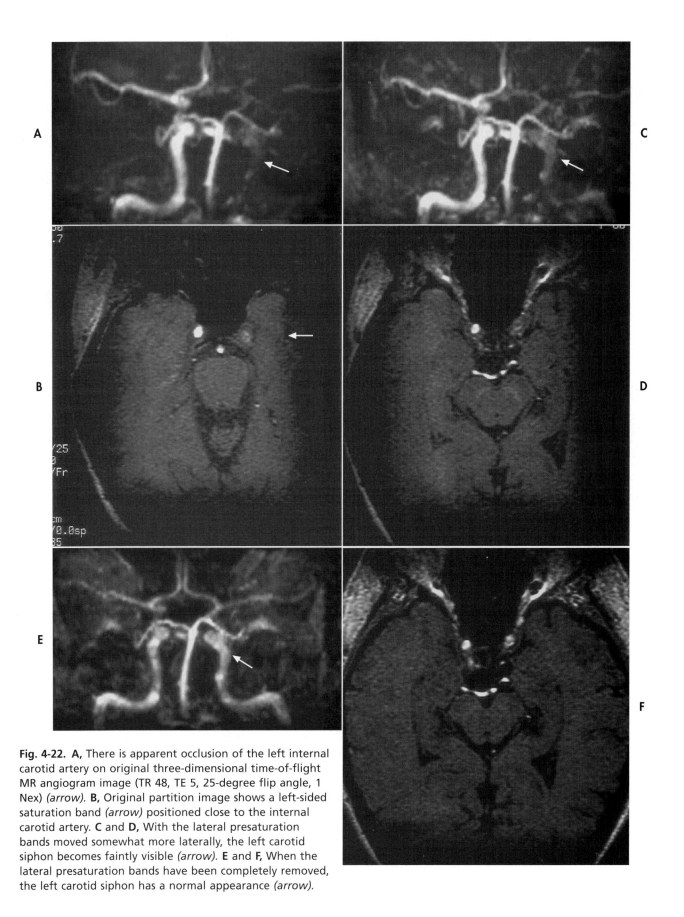

Fig. 4-22. A, There is apparent occlusion of the left internal carotid artery on original three-dimensional time-of-flight MR angiogram image (TR 48, TE 5, 25-degree flip angle, 1 Nex) *(arrow).* **B,** Original partition image shows a left-sided saturation band *(arrow)* positioned close to the internal carotid artery. **C** and **D,** With the lateral presaturation bands moved somewhat more laterally, the left carotid siphon becomes faintly visible *(arrow).* **E** and **F,** When the lateral presaturation bands have been completely removed, the left carotid siphon has a normal appearance *(arrow).*

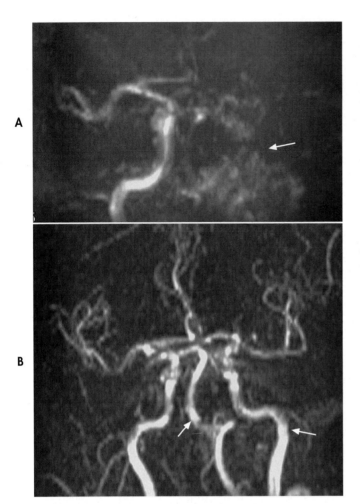

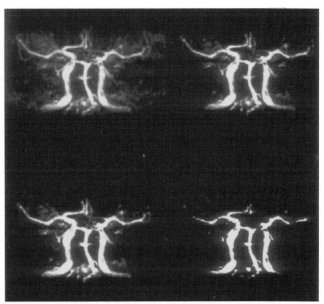

Fig. 4-24. Coronal projections from three-dimensional time-of-flight MR angiogram (TR 48, TE 5, 25-degree flip angle, 1 Nex) were obtained using progressively increased threshold values. As the threshold value is increased, there is corresponding improvement in suppression of background signal intensity. At the same time, there is progressive artifactual narrowing of vessels and decreased ability to visualize small vessels.

Fig. 4-23. A, Three-dimensional time-of-flight MR angiogram (TR 48, TE 5, 25-degree flip angle, 1 Nex) depicts apparent occlusion of the left internal carotid artery *(arrow)*. The basilar artery is also not visualized on this image. **B,** Repeat performance of identical pulse sequence, but with left-sided presaturation band displaced further laterally, demonstrates the left internal carotid artery *(arrow)* as well as the basilar artery *(arrowhead)* to be normal.

frequency irradiation, which decreases the signal intensity of brain parenchyma while maintaining the high signal intensity of flowing blood. Magnetization transfer pulses do not, however, suppress the signal intensity of fat.

POSTPROCESSING

All of the artifacts discussed thus far affect MR angiograms at the level of gradient echo image acquisition. However, even when image acquisition is optimized, artifacts can be introduced during the postprocessing of such images. A maximum intensity projection (MIP) algorithm is most commonly used, wherein multiple rays are directed through the image set at various angles. Pixels with the highest signal intensity along the course of the ray are retained, whereas all other pixels are eliminated. This provides a means for eliminating the signal intensity of soft tissues and rendering a projection image resembling a conventional angiogram. However, significant information can be lost during postprocessing of gradient echo images, and erroneous data can also be generated. Therefore individual images should be inspected, particularly when any aberrant findings are suspected.[24]

The MIP algorithm must be performed using appropriate threshold settings (Fig. 4-24). An inappropriately high threshold value can cause intravascular signal intensity to be excluded from the projection image, simulating vessel stenosis or occlusion. Conversely, a threshold value that is too low will allow extraneous signal that does not correspond to flowing spins to be incorporated into the projection image. This will reduce the conspicuousness of vessels. In addition, extraneous signal can simulate vascular malformations or ulcerations when located adjacent to a vessel.

When nonvascular foci of high signal intensity become incorporated into the projection image, they can also lead to a spurious appearance of vascular stenosis

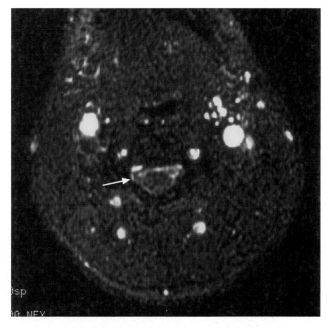

Fig. 4-26. Transaxial image acquired as a part of a two-dimensional time-of-flight MR angiogram (TR 45, TE 9, 60-degree flip angle, 1 Nex) demonstrates hyperintensity caused by CSF flow within the thecal sac *(arrow)*. This can lead to visualization of the thecal sac on resultant projection image.

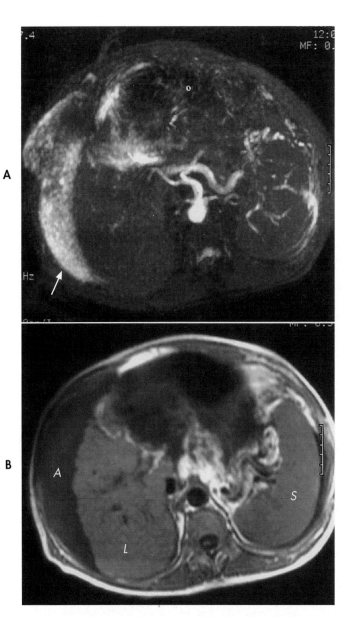

Fig. 4-25. A, Projection image from two-dimensional time-of-flight MR angiogram (TR 45, TE 8, 45-degree flip angle, 2 Nex) demonstrates high signal intensity within the lateral abdomen *(arrow)*. This is due to motion of ascitic fluid. **B,** The presence of ascites (*A*), as well as a small nodular liver (*L*) and splenomegaly (*S*), is demonstrated on transaxial T1-weighted image (TR 500, TE 12, 4 Nex) in patient with hepatic cirrhosis and portal hypertension.

POSTPROCESSING ARTIFACTS ON MR ANGIOGRAPHY

- Inappropriate threshold settings
- Nonvascular sources of high signal intensity (hemorrhage, contrast enhancement, other lesions/structures, motion artifact, fat, noise)
- Exclusion of portion of vessel
- Partial volume averaging of small vessels
- Misregistration caused by vessel motion

---

or occlusion. When the ray tracing algorithm encounters such high signal intensity foci, it can disregard the relatively less intense signal corresponding to flowing spins. Extravascular foci of high signal intensity can result from random noise and motion, among other causes.[2,6,14] Fluid collections such as pleural and pericardial effusions, ascites, cerebrospinal fluid, and some cystic lesions can appear hyperintense on gradient echo images

because of fluid motion[51] (Figs. 4-25, *A* and *B* and 4-26). Hemorrhagic or proteinaceous fluid collections or fatty tissues can also appear bright on proton density– or T1-weighted gradient echo images. For example, in one reported case, a thyroid cyst containing hemorrhagic and/or proteinaceous contents appeared hyperintense and simulated a carotid artery pseudoaneurysm at MR angiography.[1] The posterior pituitary gland normally has a high signal intensity on T1-weighted images. This structure can simulate an aneurysm arising from the circle of Willis on cranial MR angiograms (Figs. 4-27, *A-D* and 4-28, *A-C*). Following contrast material administration, significant enhancement of stationary soft tissues occurs, which

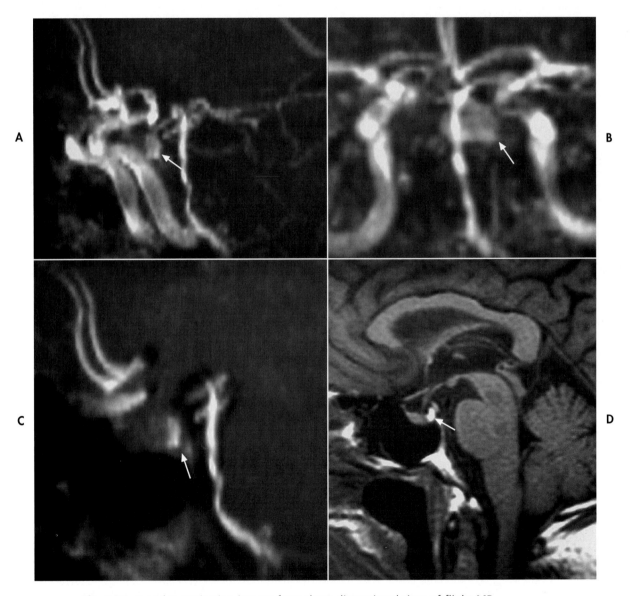

Fig. 4-27. A and **B,** Projection images from three-dimensional time-of-flight MR angiogram (TR 48, TE 5, 25-degree flip angle, 1 Nex) demonstrate an apparent aneurysm arising from the circle of Willis *(arrow)*. This focus of hyperintensity represents the posterior pituitary gland and not a vascular structure. This is evidenced by the lateral limited projection image **(C),** as well as the corresponding T1-weighted midsagittal image **(D)** (TR 430, TE 11, 2 Nex), which depict the posterior pituitary *(arrow).*

can interfere with depiction of vascular anatomy on projection images[8,13] (Figs. 4-9 and 4-11). Enhancing lesions within the brain can also appear on projection images and simulate vascular abnormalities (Figs. 4-29, *A* and *B*).

Thrombus can contain subacute hemorrhagic products (i.e., methemoglobin); its high signal intensity on proton density– or T1-weighted gradient echo images can simulate flowing blood. This can cause the severity of vessel narrowing to be underestimated[21,29,33] and cause thrombosed vessels to appear patent.[52] Similarly, when methemoglobin is present within hematomas or hemorrhagic tumors, abnormal blood vessels can be simulated on projection images (Figs. 4-30, *A* and *B*). Similarly, mural thrombus in an aneurysm can lead to underestimation of the size of the aneurysm lumen[50] (Fig. 4-8). Careful inspection of the original data set is mandated when a source of extravascular high signal intensity is suspected.

Conventional spin echo images should also be compared when they are available. T1-weighted spin echo images depict subacute hemorrhagic products as hyperintense, whereas flowing blood usually demonstrates a signal void. Other tissues that can appear hyperintense on proton density or T1-weighted images, such as proteinaceous solutions, some forms of calcification, melanin, and paramagnetic contrast material enhancement, can also potentially simulate flowing blood. Fat surrounding vessels, such as the internal carotid or ophthalmic arteries, can also simulate flowing blood on MR angiography.[18,26] The latter situation can be remedied with use of fat suppression. Perivascular fat can also generate chemical shift misregistration artifacts and chemical shift phase cancellation artifacts on opposed phase images. Both of these artifacts can contribute to inaccuracy in the depicted size of the vessel.[26]

Sources of extravascular high signal intensity can be

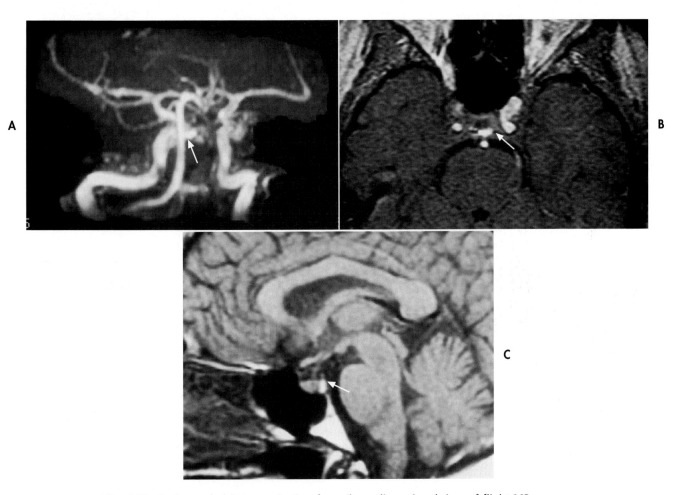

Fig. 4-28. A, Coronal oblique projection from three-dimensional time-of-flight MR angiogram (TR 48, TE 5, 25-degree flip angle, 1 Nex) demonstrates apparent aneurysm arising from the right carotid artery siphon *(arrow).* This focus of high signal intensity represents the normal posterior pituitary gland, as demonstrated on partition image from three-dimensional time-of-flight data set **(B)** and on midsagittal T1-weighted image **(C)** (TR 550, TE 17, 0.5 Nex).

restricted from the data set prior to its postprocessing. A limited or targeted MIP image is performed by manually defining the portion of the data set to be retained with an electronic cursor, excluding sources of aberrant increased signal intensity (Figs. 4-31, *A-C*). Limited MIP projections are useful not only for excluding discrete signal abnormalities that can simulate vascular lesions but also for improving overall quality of MR angiograms. Sources of background signal intensity including fat and random noise are eliminated from the projection image, thus enhancing background tissue suppression and improving the conspicuousness of vessels (Figs. 4-21, 4-32, *A-C*, 4-33, *A* and *B*, 4-34, *A* and *B*, and 4-35, *A* and *B*). Limited MIP images are also useful for selectively displaying a particular vessel of

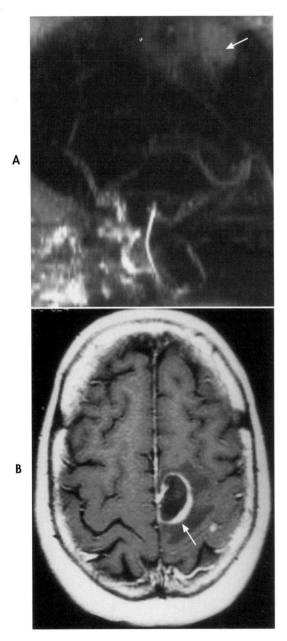

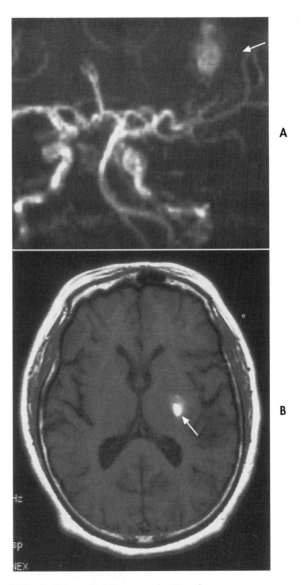

Fig. 4-29. A, Contrast-enhancing metastasis in the left parietal lobe *(arrow)* is evident on three-dimensional time-of-flight MR angiogram image (TR 38, TE 5, 25-degree flip angle, 1 Nex). **B,** The enhancing lesion is demonstrated on transaxial T1-weighted image (TR 500, TE 11, 2 Nex) *(arrow).*

Fig. 4-30. A, Coronal oblique projection from three-dimensional time-of-flight MR angiogram (TR 48, TE 5, 25-degree flip angle, 1 Nex) demonstrates apparent large aneurysm arising from left middle cerebral artery branches *(arrow).* This is due to T1 shortening related to subacute hematoma in lentiform nucleus, as verified on transaxial T1-weighted image **(B)** (TR 500, TE 11, 2 Nex) *(arrow).*

interest. For example, it may be desirable to display the right carotid artery in isolation, so that overlap with the vertebral arteries and left carotid artery do not interfere with interpretation. Overlap between adjacent vessels is frequently present on standard MR angiograms and can lead to significant diagnostic errors.[10]

When a targeted MIP image is being defined, one must be careful not to exclude portions of the vessel(s) being evaluated. This is particularly likely to occur with a tortuous vessel. When a portion of the vessel extends

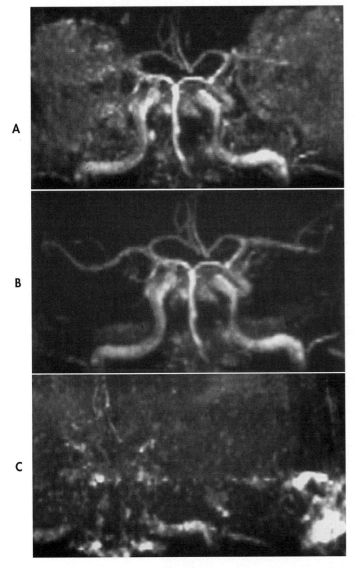

Fig. 4-31. A, Three-dimensional time-of-flight MR angiogram (TR 48, TE 5, 25-degree flip angle, 1 Nex) demonstrates poor vascular detail, attributable to relative increased signal intensity arising from fat within the scalp and orbits. **B,** There is marked improvement in vascular detail demonstrated on limited projection image obtained from the same data set avoiding fat containing areas. **C,** Use of fat saturation leads to suppression of signal intensity from flowing spins.

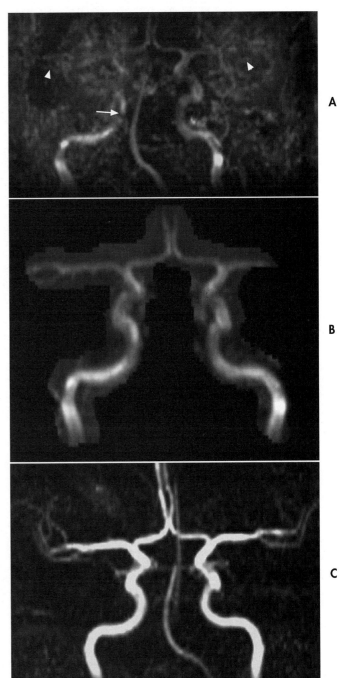

Fig. 4-32. A, The right carotid artery siphon *(arrow)* and both middle cerebral arteries *(arrowheads)* are poorly visualized on original projection from three-dimensional time-of-flight MR angiogram (TR 48, TE 5, 25-degree flip angle, 1 Nex). **B,** Marked improvement in depiction of these vessels is presented on limited projection image, on which subcutaneous and orbital fat have been excluded. **C,** Excellent background soft tissue suppression is also achieved on corresponding three-dimensional phase contrast MR angiogram image (TR 35, TE 10, 20-degree flip angle, 1 Nex).

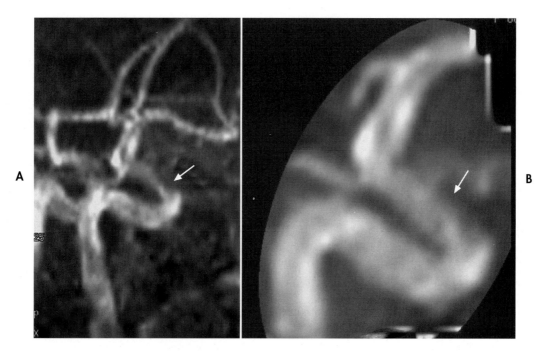

Fig. 4-33. A, Coronal oblique projection from three-dimensional time-of-flight MR angiogram (TR 48, TE 5, 25-degree flip angle, 1 Nex) demonstrates apparent stenosis involving the left carotid artery siphon *(arrow)*. **B,** Selective projection of this vascular segment, excluding extraneous sources of signal intensity, demonstrates it to be of normal caliber *(arrow)*.

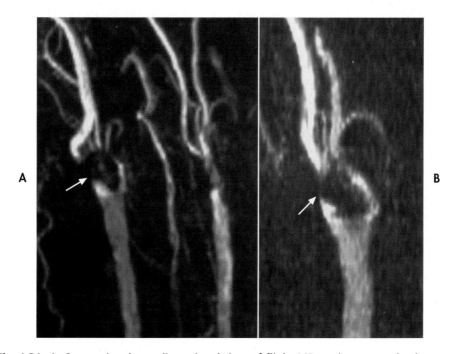

Fig. 4-34. A, Conventional two-dimensional time-of-flight MR angiogram projection image (TR 45, TE 9, 60-degree flip angle, 1 Nex) depicts segment of apparent occlusion involving proximal right internal carotid artery *(arrow)*. **B,** Limited projection of right internal carotid artery demonstrates continuity throughout this portion of the vessel *(arrow)*, which is severely stenotic.

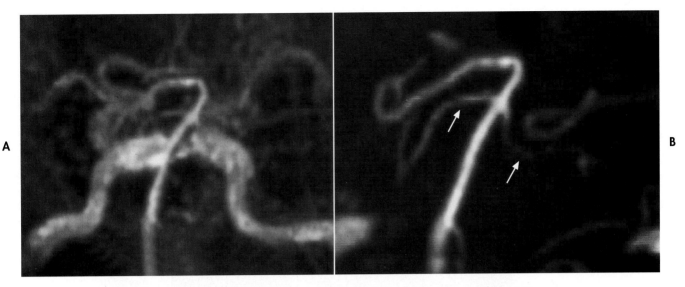

Fig. 4-35. A, Standard projection image from three-dimensional time-of-flight MR angiogram (TR 48, TE 5, 25-degree flip angle, 1 Nex) of Circle of Willis poorly demonstrates superior cerebellar arteries. **B,** Limited projection confined to posterior circulation reveals markedly improved depiction of superior cerebellar arteries *(arrows)* as well as improved suppression of background stationary tissue.

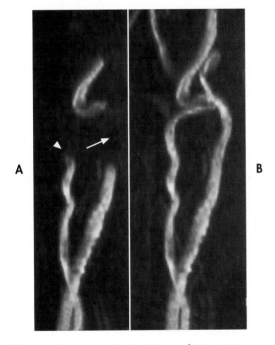

Fig. 4-36. A, Limited projection image from a two-dimensional time-of-flight MR angiogram (TR 45, TE 9, 60-degree flip angle, 1 Nex) demonstrates apparent occlusion of a segment of the left internal carotid artery *(arrow).* The left vertebral artery also appears to be occluded *(arrowhead).* This appearance is due to exclusion of a portion of the image where these vessels are tortuous. **B,** Projection from same data set including larger volume of tissue indicates both vessels are intact.

beyond the confines of the truncated data set, stenosis or occlusion of that vessel can be simulated (Fig. 4-36).

Vessels that are small relative to the voxel sizes used for image acquisition may not be depicted on MR angiograms.[2,26] When such small vessels are visualized, partial volume effects can result in apparent vessel narrowing on projection images.[26] Therefore, individual imaging slices (i.e., partitions) should be inspected carefully.[24] In one study, approximately half of the posterior communicating arteries seen on partition images were not visible following postprocessing.[18]

When a vessel undergoes motion as individual sections are being imaged, its position will vary on successive images. The projection image will demonstrate misregistration artifacts, which are manifested as vascular discontinuity or mural irregularity, which can simulate vessel occlusion, ulceration, or involvement with fibromuscular dysplasia[12,17,25,28] (Figs. 4-1, 4-16, 4-37 to 4-39). Misregistration artifacts can arise from gross patient motion or from vascular pulsation. Misregistration is most frequently observed on two-dimensional time-of-flight acquisitions. Image acquisition can be referenced to the cardiac cycle, so that the effects of pulsatile blood flow can be reduced. This may involve acquiring images during a defined portion of the cardiac cycle or retrospectively reordering phase encode steps with respect to the cardiac cycle.[9] Actual ulcerations are often poorly depicted on MR angiography.[13] This may result from slow flow or retrograde flow within the ulceration.[20] In addi-

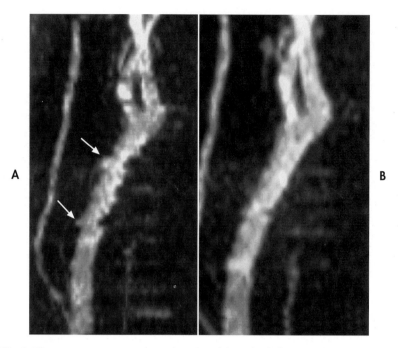

Fig. 4-37. A, There are apparent ulcerations involving the left carotid artery *(arrows)* on two-dimensional time-of-flight MR angiogram image (TR 45, TE 9, 60-degree flip angle). **B,** Repeat evaluation using identical parameters does not corroborate these findings, which are due to misregistration related to vascular pulsation.

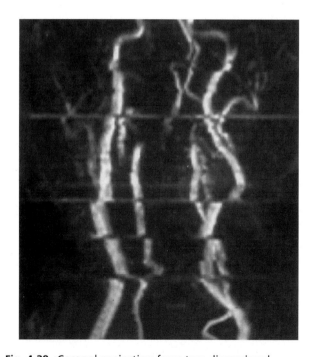

Fig. 4-38. Coronal projection from two-dimensional time-of-flight MR angiogram (TR 45, TE 9, 60-degree flip angle, 1 Nex) demonstrates multiple regions of apparent discontinuity within the carotid and vertebral arteries. These findings are due to misregistration related to gross patient motion occurring during image acquisition.

tion, unsharpness of the vessel margin on projection images can hide the presence of subtle ulceration.[20] Striping artifacts can be observed on projection images, caused by vessels passing obliquely between individual partitions.

Highly tortuous vessels can demonstrate artifactually increased lumen size, because of integration of flow-related signal over the entire section.[26]

It is desirable to quantify the degree of vascular stenosis observed on MR angiogram images. This can also introduce errors. For example, in the carotid arteries, comparison of a stenotic segment with the normally dilated carotid bulb would overemphasize the degree of stenosis present.[16] Consequently, the maximally stenotic lumen should be compared with the internal carotid artery distal to the bulb. When the origin of the internal carotid artery has a straight, rather than bulbous, appearance, 50% reduction of the lumen is usually present.[16]

The relatively limited field-of-view provided by MR angiography can make it difficult and time consuming to interrogate all relevant portions of the vascular anatomy. For example, in patients with suspected carotid artery stenosis, significant abnormalities involving the aortic arch can go undetected when this region is not evaluated.[20]

Although conventional contrast angiography is considered the gold standard for evaluation of the vasculature, occasionally MR angiography provides information that exceeds that of contrast angiography. For example, in the extremities, small vessels can be seen on MR that are often not visible on conventional angiograms.[37] These vessels may be very important in surgical planning for anastomosis of bypass grafts.

PHASE CONTRAST MRA

An alternative to time-of-flight MR angiography is the phase contrast method. Bipolar gradient pulses are used to encode flowing blood and to distinguish it from stationary tissues. Suppression of background soft tissue signal intensity is generally more complete than with time-of-flight methods[40] (Figs. 4-32 and 4-40, *A* and *B*). However, image acquisition and reconstruction times are longer, and phase contrast images are subject to some additional artifacts. The expected flow velocity in the vessel(s) of interest must be specified on phase contrast images (Figs. 4-41, *A* and *B*). When inappropriately high values are prescribed, vessels with slower flow may not be visualized (Figs. 4-42, *A* and *B*).[3] When inappropriately low values are given, aliasing of intravascular signal can occur.[13,21] Difficulties can arise because flow velocity varies during the cardiac cycle. One approach has been to implement variable velocity encoding values during image acquisition that correlate to changes in the cardiac cycle.[48] This has resulted in improved depiction of small vessels.

The direction of flow within the vessel(s) being interrogated must also be specified when phase contrast MR angiograms are acquired. Flow encoding gradients can be used to detect flow in the craniocaudal, left-right, and/or anterior-posterior axes, with increased imaging

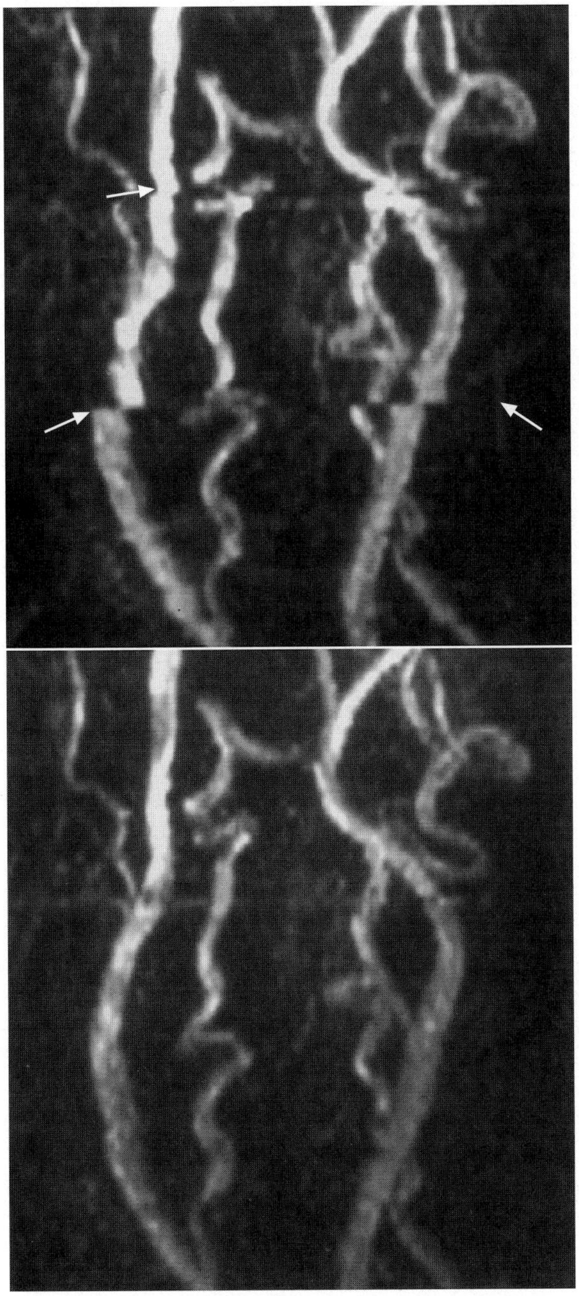

Fig. 4-39. A, There are several areas of apparent vascular discontinuity and stenosis *(arrows)* demonstrated on initial two-dimensional time-of-flight MR angiogram (TR 45, TE 9, 60-degree flip angle, 1 Nex). These findings are due to motion of the neck occurring between acquisition of consecutive images. **B,** Repeat examination using identical parameters reveals the absence of such artifacts, allowing for improved visualization of the vessels.

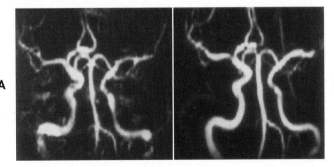

Fig. 4-40. A, Coronal projection images from three-dimensional time-of-flight (TR 48, TE 5, 25-degree flip angle, 1 Nex) and **B,** three-dimensional phase contrast (TR 35, TE 10, 20-degree flip angle 1 Nex) MR angiogram studies. There is greater uniformity of intravascular signal intensity and improved suppression of background soft signal intensity on phase contrast images. Increased signal intensity within the transverse venous sinus is noted on the phase contrast image.

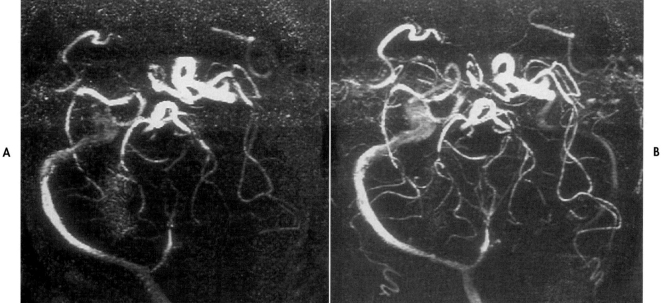

Fig. 4-41. Corresponding images from two different three-dimensional phase contrast MR angiogram examinations (TR 35, TE 10, 60-degree flip angle, 1 Nex). **A** was acquired using a 50 cm/sec velocity encoding value, whereas **B** was acquired using a velocity encoding value of 20 cm/sec. The image acquired using the lower velocity encoding value demonstrates improved depiction of many small vascular structures as well as the right carotid siphon.

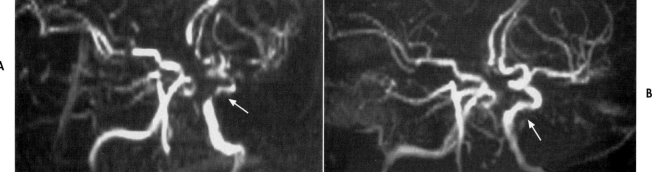

Fig. 4-42. A, Projection image from three-dimensional phase contrast MR angiogram (TR 35, TE 10, 20-degree flip angle, 1 Nex) suggests high-grade stenosis involving the supraclinoid segment of the left internal carotid artery *(arrow).* **B,** The corresponding projection from a three-dimensional time-of-flight acquisition (TR 48, TE 5, 25-degree flip angle, 1 Nex) reveals this segment to be only mildly narrowed *(arrow).*

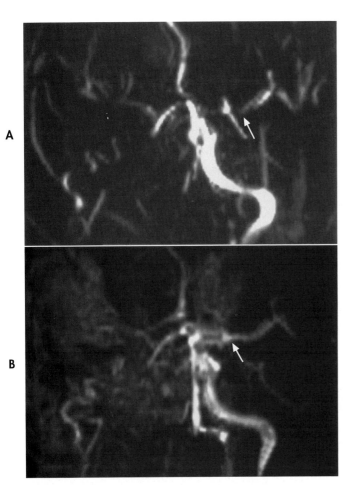

A

B

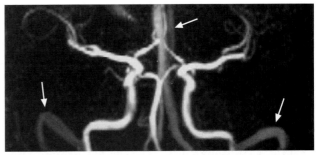

Fig. 4-44. Three-dimensional phase contrast MR angiogram (TR 35, TE 9, 15-degree flip angle, 1 Nex) demonstrates signal intensity within venous structures *(arrows),* including the sagittal and transverse venous sinuses.

Fig. 4-43. A, There is apparent stenosis involving the horizontal segment of the left internal carotid artery *(arrow)* on three-dimensional phase contrast MR angiogram (TR 35, TE 9, 20-degree flip angle, 1 Nex). This is due to flow encoding in the superior-inferior direction only, resulting in insensitivity to flow in the right-left direction. **B,** The corresponding three-dimensional time-of-flight image (TR 48, TE 5, 25-degree flip angle, 1 Nex) demonstrates no evidence of stenosis involving this segment *(arrow).* Patient has an occluded right internal carotid artery. Note improved suppression of background signal intensity on phase contrast image.

Phase shifts can result from sources other than blood flow. These phase shifts can produce artifacts on phase contrast MR angiograms. For example, respiratory motion and peristaltic bowel motion can result in phase shifts,[3] though such artifacts do not severely limit body applications of phase contrast MR angiography.[11] Spurious phase shifts can also result from eddy currents arising within the gradient system.[13]

REFERENCES

1. Anderson CM, Gooding GAW, Lee RE: Thyroid cyst mistaken for carotid pseudoaneurysm by MR angiography: case report, Clin Imaging 16:198-200, 1992.
2. Anderson CM, Saloner D, Tsuruda JS et al: Artifacts in maximum-intensity-projection display of MR angiograms, Am J Roentgenol 154:623-629, 1990.
3. Applegate GR, Talagala SL, Applegate LJ: MR angiography of the head and neck: value of two-dimensional phase-contrast projection technique, Am J Roentgenol 159:369-374, 1992.
4. Brown DG, Riederer SJ, Jack CR et al: MR angiography with oblique gradient-recalled echo technique, Radiology 176:461-466, 1990.
5. Caputo GR, Masui T, Gooding GAW et al: Popliteal and tibioperoneal arteries: feasibility of two-dimensional time-of-flight MR angiography and phase velocity mapping, Radiology 182:387-392, 1992.
6. Chakeres DW, Schmalbrock P, Brogan M et al: Normal venous anatomy of the brain: demonstration with gadopentetate dimeglumine in enhanced 3-D MR angiography, Am J Roentgenol 156:161-172, 1991.
7. Chien D, Goldmann A, Edelman RR: High-speed black blood imaging of vessel stenosis in the presence of pulsatile flow, J Magn Reson Imaging 2:437-441, 1992.
8. Creasy JL, Price RR, Presbrey T et al: Gadolinium-enhanced MR angiography, Radiology 175:280-283, 1990.
9. de Graaf RG, Groen JP: MR angiography with pulsatile flow, Magn Reson Imaging 10:25-34, 1992.
10. Debain JF, Spritzer CE, Grist TM et al: Imaging of the renal arteries: value of MR angiography, Am J Roentgenol 157:981-990, 1991.

and reconstruction time required for each additional direction. When flow direction is inaccurately specified, vascular stenosis or occlusion can be simulated (Figs. 4-43, *A* and *B*). This is most likely to occur in tortuous vessels. For example, artifactual signal loss can occur within a transversely oriented segment of a vessel when only the superior-inferior flow encoding gradient is used.[3]

Phase contrast MR angiograms demonstrate more prominent "bleedthrough" of venous signal intensity on images designed to evaluate the arterial system (Fig. 4-44).

11. Dumoulin CL, Yucel EK, Vock P et al: Two- and three-dimensional phase contrast MR angiography of the abdomen, J Comput Assist Tomogr 14:779-784, 1990.

12. Edelman RR: MR angiography: present and future, Am J Roentgenol 161:1-11, 1993.

13. Edelman RR, Mattle HP, Atkinson DJ et al: MR angiography, Am J Roentgenol 154:937-946, 1990.

14. Edelman RR, Mattle HP, Wallner B et al: Extracranial carotid arteries: evaluation with "black blood" MR angiography, Radiology 177:45-50, 1990.

15. Finn JP, Edelman RR, Jenkins RL et al: Liver transplantation: MR angiography with surgical validation, Radiology 179:265-269, 1991.

16. Fox AJ: How to measure carotid stenosis, Radiology 186:316-318, 1993.

17. Heiserman JE, Drayer BP, Fram EK et al: Carotid artery stenosis: clinical efficacy of two-dimensional time-of-flight MR angiography, Radiology 182:761-768, 1992.

18. Heiserman JE, Drayer BP, Keller PJ et al: Intracranial vascular stenosis and occlusion: evaluation with three-dimensional time-of-flight MR angiography, Radiology 185:667-673, 1992.

19. Hendrix LE, Strandt JA, Daniels DL et al: Three-dimensional time-of-flight MR angiography with a surface coil: evaluation in 12 subjects, Am J Roentgenol 159:103-106, 1992.

20. Huston J III, Lewis BD, Wiebers DO et al: Carotid artery: prospective blinded comparison of two-dimensional time-of-flight MR angiography with conventional angiography and duplex US, Radiology 186:339-344, 1993.

21. Huston J III, Rufenacht DA, Ehman RL et al: Intracranial aneurysms and vascular malformations: comparison of time-of-flight and phase-contrast MR angiography, Radiology 181:721-730, 1991.

22. Kim D, Edelman RR, Kent KC et al: Abdominal aorta and renal artery stenosis: evaluation with MR angiography, Radiology 174:727-731, 1990.

23. Krug B, Kugel H, Friedmann G et al: MR imaging of poststenotic flow phenomena: experimental studies, J Magn Reson Imaging 1:585-591, 1991.

24. Lewin JS, Laub G: Intracranial MR angiography a direct comparison of three time-of-flight techniques, Am J Neuroradiol 12:1133-1139, 1991.

25. Lewin JS, Laub G, Hausmann R: Three-dimensional time-of-flight MR angiography: applications in the abdomen and thorax, Radiology 179:261-264, 1991.

26. Lin W, Haacke EM, Smith AS: Lumen definition in MR angiography, J Magn Reson Imaging 1:327-336, 1991.

27. Lin W, Tkach JA, Haacke EM et al: Intracranial MR angiography: application of magnetization transfer contrast and fat saturation to short gradient-echo, velocity-compensated sequences, Radiology 186:753-761, 1993.

28. Litt AW, Eidelman EM, Pinto RS et al: Diagnosis of carotid artery stenosis: comparison of 2DFT time-of-flight MR angiography with contrast angiography in 50 patients, Am J Neuroradiol 12:149-154, 1991.

29. Marchal G, Bosmans H, Van Fraeyenhoven L et al: Intracranial vascular lesions: optimization and clinical evaluation of three-dimensional time-of-flight MR angiography, Radiology 175:443-448, 1990.

30. Marchal G, Michiels J, Bosmans H et al: Contrast-enhanced MRA of the brain, J Comput Assist Tomogr 16:25-29, 1992.

31. Masaryk TJ, Modic MT, Ross JS et al: Intracranial circulation: preliminary clinical results with three-dimensional (volume) MR angiography, Radiology 171:793-799, 1989.

32. Masaryk TJ, Modic MT, Ruggieri PM et al: Three-dimensional (volume) gradient-echo imaging of the carotid bifurcation: preliminary clinical experience, Radiology 171:801-806, 1989.

33. Mattle HP, Wentz KU, Edelman RR et al: Cerebral venography with MR. Radiology 178:453-458, 1991.

34. Middleton WD, Foley WD, Lawson TL: Flow reversal in the normal carotid bifurcation: color Doppler flow imaging analysis, Radiology 167:207-210, 1988.

35. Mirowitz SA: Apparent vascular occlusion on time-of-flight MR angiography with use of the peripheral presaturation technique, J Comput Assist Tomogr 17:927-931, 1993.

36. Mulligan SA, Matsuda T, Lanzer P et al: Peripheral arterial occlusive disease: prospective comparison of MR angiography and color duplex US with conventional angiography, Radiology 178:695-700, 1991.

37. Owen RS, Baum RA, Carpenter JP et al: Symptomatic peripheral vascular disease: selection of imaging parameters and clinical evaluation with MR angiography, Radiology 187:627-635, 1993.

38. Parker DL, Yuan C, Blatter DD: MR angiography by multiple thin slab 3D acquisition, Magn Reson Med 17:434-451, 1991.

39. Pavone P, Marsili L, Catalano C et al: Carotid arteries: evaluation with low-field-strength MR angiography, Radiology 184:401-404, 1992.

40. Pernicone JR, Siebert JE, Potchen EJ et al: Three-dimensional phase-contrast MR angiography in the head and neck: preliminary report, Am J Roentgenol 155:167-176, 1990.

41. Polak JF, Bajakian RL, O'Leary DH et al: Detection of internal carotid artery stenosis: comparison of MR angiography, color Doppler sonography, and arteriography, Radiology 182:35-40, 1992.

42. Quinn SF, Demlow TA, Hallin RW et al: Femoral MR angiography versus conventional angiography: preliminary results, Radiology 189:181-184, 1993.

43. Ruggieri PM, Laub GA, Masaryk TJ et al: Intracranial circulation: pulse-sequence considerations in three-dimensional (volume) MR angiography, Radiology 171:785-791, 1989.

44. Schad LR, Ehricke HH, Wowra B et al: Correction of spatial distortion in magnetic resonance angiography for radiosurgical treatment planning of cerebral arteriovenous malformations, Magn Reson Imaging 10:609-621, 1992.

45. Schiebler ML, Listerud J: Common artifacts encountered in thoracic magnetic resonance imaging: recognition, derivation, and solutions, Top Magn Reson Imaging 4:1-17, 1992.

46. Schmalbrock P, Yuan C, Chakeres DW et al: Volume MR angiography: methods to achieve very short echo times, Radiology 175:861-865, 1990.

47. Spielmann RP, Schneider O, Thiele F et al: Appearance of poststenotic jets in MRI: dependence on flow velocity and on imaging parameters, Magn Reson Imaging 9:67-72, 1991.

48. Swan JS, Weber DM, Grist TM et al: Peripheral MR angiography with variable velocity encoding: work in progress, Radiology 184:813-817, 1992.

49. Teitelbaum GP, Lin MC, Watanabe AT et al: Ferromagnetism and MR imaging safety of carotid vascular clamps, Am J Neuroradiol 11:267-272, 1990.

50. Tsuruda JS, Sevick RJ, Halbach VV: Three-dimensional time-of-flight MR angiography in the evaluation of intracranial aneurysms treated by endovascular balloon occlusion, Am J Neuroradiol 13:1129-1136, 1992.

51. Wallner B, Edelman RR, Finn JP et al: Bright pleural effusion and ascites on gradient-echo MR images: a potential source of confusion in vascular MR studies, Am J Roentgenol 155:1237-1240, 1990.

52. Yousem DM, Balakrishnan J, Debrun GM et al: Hyperintense thrombus on GRASS MR images: potential pitfall in flow evaluation, Am J Neuroradiol 11:51-58, 1990.

53. Yucel EK, Kaufman JA, Geller SC et al: Atherosclerotic occlusive disease of the lower extremity: prospective evaluation with two-dimensional time-of-flight MR angiography, Radiology 187:637-641, 1993.

Section Two

ABDOMEN

5

Liver and Biliary System

LIVER
Anatomic Variations

The liver is a large organ subject to considerable variation in size, position, and morphology. The liver may be alobar; conversely, accessory hepatic lobes can be present.[6] Accessory liver tissue can be found along the left hepatic lobe, extending into the epiploic foramen, alongside the inferior vena cava (lobus venae cavae), or between the segments of the left lobe (pons hepaticus).[6] Accessory hepatic tissue can also be located in ectopic sites including the gallbladder wall, spleen, ligamentum teres, and omentum.[6]

The left hepatic lobe can have a prominent lateral extension, with its tip located medial to the stomach, interposed between the stomach and spleen, or lateral to the spleen. The medial segment of the left lobe may be very small or, alternatively, masslike prominence of the left lobe can also occur as a normal variation.

A prominent caudal extension of the right hepatic lobe is frequently present, representing the so-called Reidel lobe (Fig. 5-1). Like the left lobe, the right hepatic lobe can also extend into unusual locations, such as a retrorenal position (Fig. 5-2). The right lobe can undergo focal hypertrophy following removal of the right kidney or an insult to the liver. The hypertrophied portion of the liver can fill the right renal fossa and simulate a mass lesion[88] (Figs. 5-3, A-C). In addition, focal enlargement of remaining liver tissue can occur following partial hepatectomy. However, in both situations the apparent mass exhibits signal intensity characteristics identical to those of the remainder of the liver.

The papillary process of the caudate lobe can extend medial and/or posterior to the inferior vena cava[20,49] (Figs. 5-4 and 5-5). This structure can simulate an exophytic hepatic mass or enlarged lymph node in the porta hepatis or retroperitoneum (Figs. 5-6, A and B). The caudate lobe may be focally enlarged in patients with cirrhosis. The appearance of a hepatic mass in this situa-

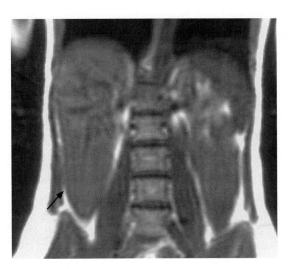

Fig. 5-1. A prominent inferior extension of the right hepatic lobe (Riedel lobe) *(arrow)* is demonstrated on this coronal T1-weighted image (TR 350, TE 12, 4 Nex).

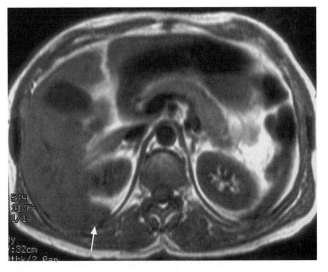

Fig. 5-2. The posterior segment of the right hepatic lobe extends around the posterior aspect of the right kidney (retrorenal liver) *(arrow)* on this transaxial T1-weighted image (TR 550, TE 11, 4 Nex).

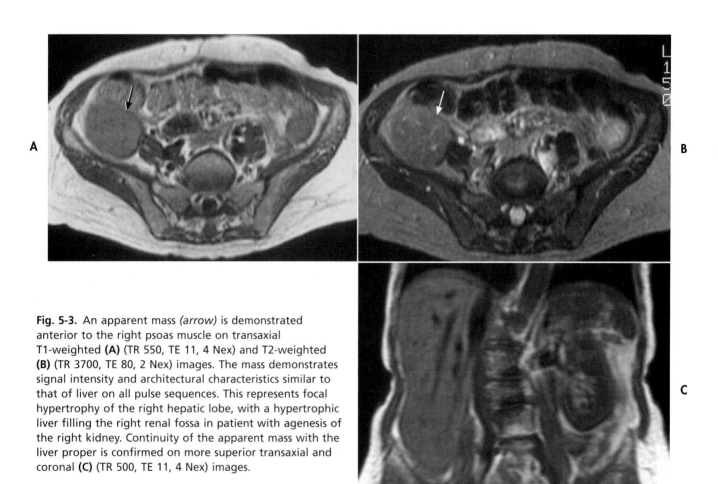

Fig. 5-3. An apparent mass *(arrow)* is demonstrated anterior to the right psoas muscle on transaxial T1-weighted **(A)** (TR 550, TE 11, 4 Nex) and T2-weighted **(B)** (TR 3700, TE 80, 2 Nex) images. The mass demonstrates signal intensity and architectural characteristics similar to that of liver on all pulse sequences. This represents focal hypertrophy of the right hepatic lobe, with a hypertrophic liver filling the right renal fossa in patient with agenesis of the right kidney. Continuity of the apparent mass with the liver proper is confirmed on more superior transaxial and coronal **(C)** (TR 500, TE 11, 4 Nex) images.

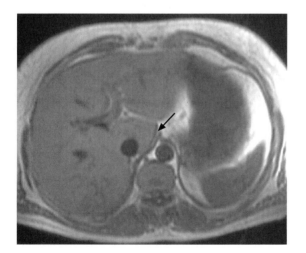

Fig. 5-4. A prominent papillary process of the caudate lobe *(arrow)* is observed extending medial as well as posteromedial to the inferior vena cava on this transaxial T1-weighted image (TR 550, TE 11, 4 Nex).

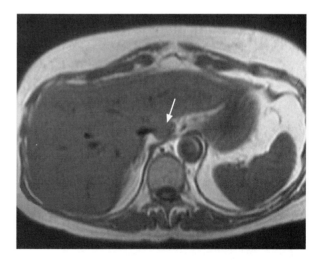

Fig. 5-5. A prominent papillary process of the caudate lobe *(arrow)* projects medial and slightly posterior to the inferior vena cava on this transaxial T1-weighted image (TR 1000, TE 11, 4 Nex), simulating an exophytic hepatic lesion.

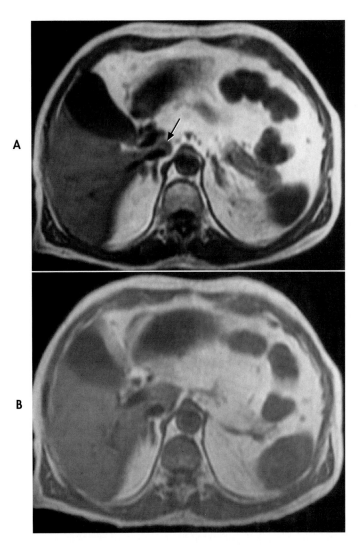

A

B

Fig. 5-6. A, Transaxial T1-weighted image (TR 550, TE 12, 2 Nex) depicts an apparent 1 cm lymph node *(arrow)* in the portacaval region in this 74-year-old male with prostate cancer. **B,** Contiguous image demonstrates continuity with the caudate process, confirming that this represents a papillary process of the caudate lobe.

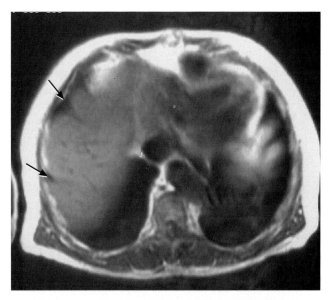

Fig. 5-7. Transaxial T1-weighted image (TR 500, TE 12, 4 Nex) demonstrates multiple clefts along the hepatic dome *(arrow).*

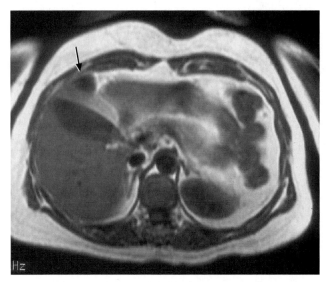

Fig. 5-8. An apparent focal lesion *(arrow)* involving the medial segment of the left hepatic lobe is due to partial volume averaging with subjacent hepatic flexure of the colon on transaxial T1-weighted image (TR 500, TE 11, 4 Nex).

tion is often accentuated as a result of associated atrophy of the right hepatic lobe.

The liver may be malrotated along its anatomic axis. Numerous variations can exist in the lobar division of the liver. The liver can manifest a lobulated rather than smooth contour, and deep clefts within the surface of the liver also occur as normal variants[6] (Fig. 5-7).

Entities That Can Simulate Lesions
Partial volume effects

Partial volume averaging of the colon (usually the hepatic flexure) with adjacent liver parenchyma can lead to the appearance of a focal hepatic lesion (Fig. 5-8). The apparent lesion can manifest variable signal intensity depending on the pulse sequence used and whether the colon contains predominantly air and/or fecal material (low signal intensity on all sequences) or fluid (low signal intensity on T1-weighted images and increased signal intensity on T2-weighted images). Lesions arising from the

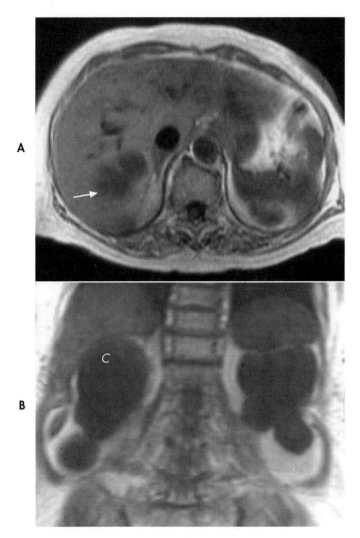

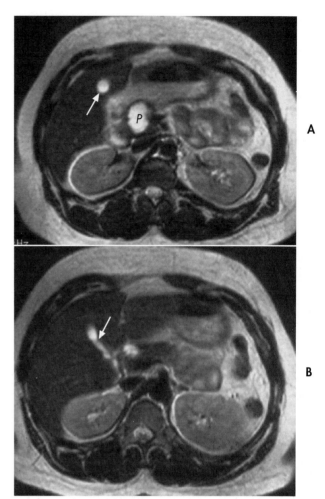

Fig. 5-9. A, An apparent rounded low signal intensity lesion is seen in the right hepatic lobe *(arrow)* on transaxial T1-weighted image (TR 550, TE 11, 4 Nex), caused by partial volume averaging of a right upper pole renal cyst. **B,** This is confirmed on corresponding coronal T1-weighted image (cyst, *C*) (TR 500, TE 12, 4 Nex).

Fig. 5-10. A, An apparent small rounded high signal intensity lesion within the medial segment of the left hepatic lobe *(arrow)* is seen on transaxial fast spin echo T2-weighted image (TR 4000, effective TE 119, 4 Nex, 16 echo train). This represents the gallbladder fundus, as verified by continuity with the remainder of the gallbladder on adjacent image **(B).** Also note cystic mass involving pancreatic head *(P)*.

upper pole of the right kidney or the right adrenal gland may also undergo partial volume averaging with parenchyma of the right hepatic lobe and simulate a liver lesion (Figs. 5-9, *A* and *B*). Close inspection of transaxial images and comparison with coronal or sagittal images will allow for recognition of this entity. In the region of the porta hepatis, the gallbladder may also simulate a hepatic lesion when it projects into the liver or is volume averaged with adjacent liver parenchyma (Figs. 5-10, *A* and *B* and 5-11, *A* and *B*).

The descending portion of the duodenum can appear as an exophytic mass lesion in the region of the porta hepatis. Left lobe lesions can be simulated by volume averaging of the liver with left ventricular myocardium

(Figs. 5-12, *A* and *B*). Deposits of fat may be located within the hepatic fissures or falciform ligament. Such fat can also be volume averaged with the liver, simulating hemorrhagic lesions on both T1- and T2-weighted images. Fat suppression techniques can be useful in problematic cases.

Vascular structures

The hepatic and portal veins are typically hypointense on spin echo images because of the flow void phenomenon. These vessels can simulate focal lesions such as metastases on T1-weighted images[115] (Fig. 5-13). Similar difficulties can be encountered on T2-weighted images when gradient moment nulling is used for artifact

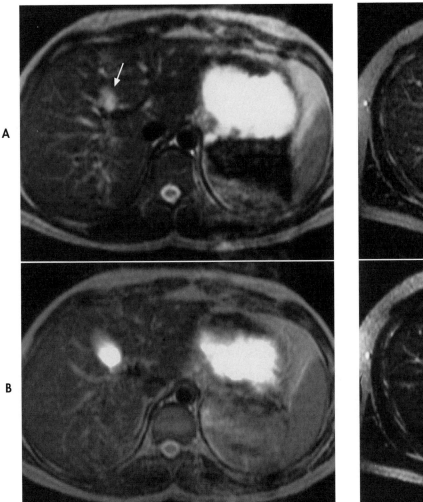

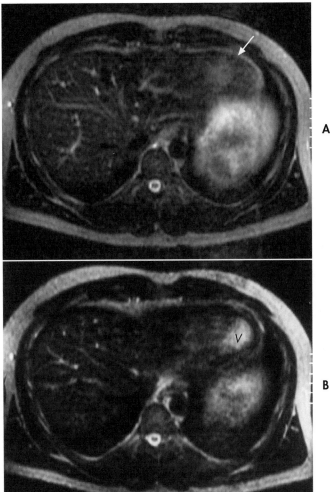

Fig. 5-11. A, Transaxial T2-weighted image (TR 3400, TE 80, 2 Nex) *(arrow)* demonstrates apparent high signal intensity hepatic lesion. This is due to partial volume averaging of hepatic tissue with the gallbladder, as demonstrated on adjacent image **(B).**

Fig. 5-12. A, There is an apparent moderately intense lesion involving the left hepatic lobe *(arrow)* on T2-weighted image (TR 3400, TE 120, 2 Nex). However, this appearance is due to partial volume averaging of blood pool within the inferior left ventricular chamber *(V)*, as depicted on adjacent image **(B).** Blood pool is hyperintense on this flow-compensated image, and the left ventricular myocardium is relatively isointense with hepatic parenchyma.

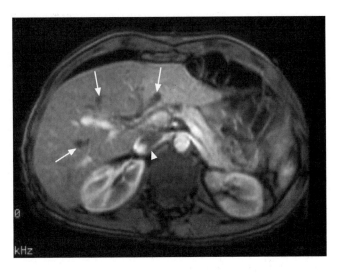

Fig. 5-13. Dynamic gadolinium chelate enhanced rapid gradient echo image (TR 150, TE 2.6, 90-degree flip angle, 1 Nex) demonstrates low signal intensity hepatic foci *(arrows)*, representing unenhanced hepatic veins. These findings may simulate focal hepatic lesions. Also noted is normal cortical enhancement of the kidneys. There is an apparent defect suggestive of thrombus within the inferior vena cava *(arrowhead).* This is related to turbulent flow near the confluence of the renal veins.

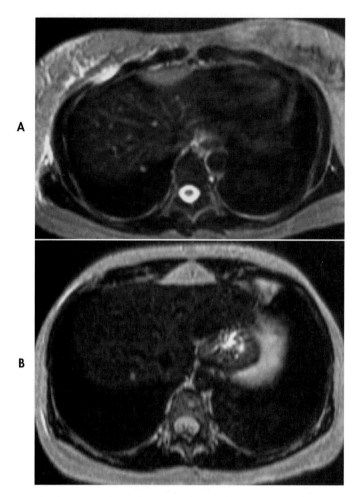

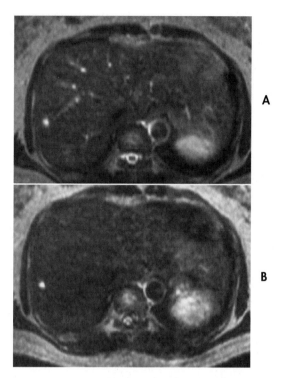

Fig. 5-14. A, There are multiple small hyperintense foci within the hepatic dome on flow-compensated T2-weighted image (TR 3400, TE 120, 2 Nex), which may represent either hepatic vessels or small lesions. **B,** T2-weighted fast spin echo image (TR 2500, effective TE 120, 1 Nex, 16 echo train) obtained without flow compensation reveals that most of the foci in **A** represent normal hepatic vessels. However, persistence of a single small focus is noted, representing a presumed small cyst or cavernous hemangioma.

Fig. 5-15. A, Flow-compensated T2-weighted image (TR 3400, TE 120, 2 Nex) demonstrates multiple small foci of increased intrahepatic signal intensity, which could represent either normal hepatic vessels or hyperintense lesions. **B,** Corresponding image obtained without flow compensation, using identical imaging parameters, demonstrates that most of the foci represent vessels. However, a single focus in the right hepatic lobe represents a small cyst or cavernous hemangioma.

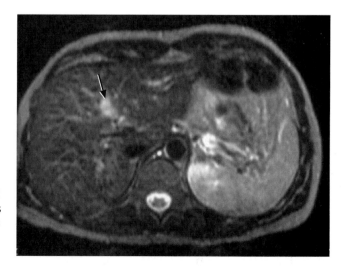

Fig. 5-16. Transaxial T2-weighted image (TR 3400, TE 120, 2 Nex) acquired using gradient moment nulling demonstrates apparent lesion *(arrow)* in left hepatic lobe. This represents a prominent left portal vein, with hyperintensity resulting from rephasing of flowing spins.

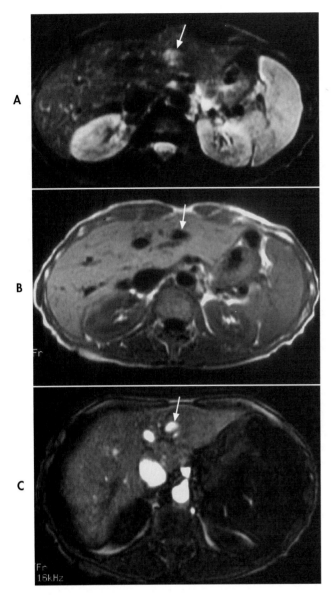

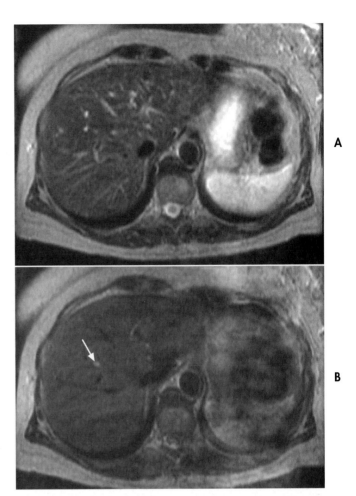

Fig. 5-17. A, Transaxial T2-weighted image (TR 3400, TE 80, 2 Nex) demonstrates high signal intensity lesion in left hepatic lobe *(arrows)*. This represents a prominent left portal vein, as confirmed on corresponding T1-weighted image **(B)** (TR 500, TR 12, 4 Nex) and flow sensitive gradient echo image **(C)** (TR 9, TE 2.6, 30-degree flip angle, 4 Nex). Chemical shift misregistration artifact is present at the margin of the spleen along the frequency-encode direction in A.

Fig. 5-18. Transaxial T2-weighted images (TR 3400, TE 80, 2 Nex) obtained with **(A)** and without **(B)** flow compensation. The flow-compensated image demonstrates reduced respiratory motion artifacts. However, a small high signal intensity cyst *(arrow)*, is difficult to detect because of the high signal intensity of hepatic vessels, whereas it is easily detected without flow compensation.

reduction (Figs. 5-14, *A* to 5-18, *B*). This technique results in hyperintensity of the hepatic vessels that can simulate lesions on T2-weighted images. Vascular structures are recognized by their tubular nature and by their communication with the extrahepatic portal vein or inferior vena cava. When differentiation of vascular structures and lesions remains in doubt, a T1-weighted flow-compensated gradient echo sequence can be performed.

Using this sequence, hepatic vessels will be hyperintense whereas lesions are usually hypointense relative to the surrounding liver.

Pulsation artifacts

Focal hepatic lesions may also be simulated by vascular artifacts of a different type. Vascular pulsations result in an alternating series of high and low signal intensity artifacts that propagate along the phase-encoding direction of the image. Since phase encoding is usually assigned along the anteroposterior axis of the body for abdominal imaging, the artifacts intersect the lateral segment of the left hepatic lobe. In this location, they can appear to represent focal lesions of either increased signal intensity or decreased signal intensity (Figs. 5-17 and 5-19, *A* and *B*).

ENTITIES THAT CAN SIMULATE FOCAL HEPATIC LESIONS

- Partial volume averaging
  Colon (hepatic flexure)
  Right adrenal/kidney lesions
  Gallbladder
  Duodenum
  Left ventricle
  Extrahepatic fat
- Hepatic vessels
- Vascular pulsation artifacts
- Respiratory motion artifacts
- Cardiac pulsations
- Focal fatty infiltration
- Focal sparing of diffuse fatty infiltration
- Heterogeneous contrast enhancement
- Papillary process caudate lobe
- Postoperative changes

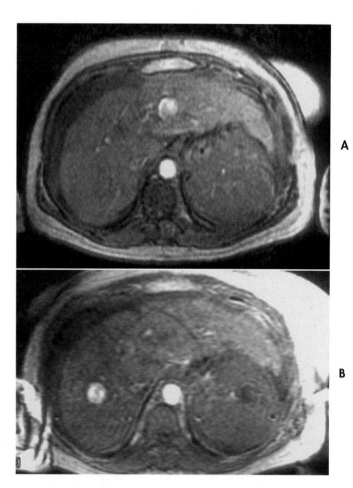

Fig. 5-19. A, Transaxial rapid gradient echo image (TR 120, TE 3, 90-degree flip angle, 1 Nex) demonstrates hyperintense focus in left hepatic lobe as a result of aortic pulsation artifact. **B,** Image obtained following gradient reorientation, using identical imaging parameters, reveals the pseudolesion within the posterior right hepatic lobe.

The intensity of aortic pulsation artifacts is directly proportional to the intensity of flowing blood within the aortic lumen. Spatial presaturation radiofrequency pulses reduce intraluminal signal intensity and therefore the prominence of pulsation artifacts. Because there is increased intraluminal signal intensity on gradient echo images, aortic pulsation artifacts are often accentuated.[125] Pulsation artifacts are particularly prominent on sequences that use high flip angles and long echo times[131] (Figs. 5-20, *A-C*). The combined use of spatial presaturation and gradient moment nulling will reduce but not eliminate pulsation artifacts. The use of gadopentetate dimeglumine and other paramagnetic agents usually accentuate aortic pulsation artifacts because of their T1-shortening effects. However, rapid gradient echo images may demonstrate a paradoxic decrease in such artifacts during bolus injection of contrast material[90] (Figs. 5-21, *A* and *B*).

Pulsation artifacts are recognized by their alignment with the aorta and because the apparent lesion typically resembles the cross-sectional size and shape of the aorta. When distinction between an actual lesion and a pseudolesion based on vascular pulsation remains uncertain, the sequence should be repeated with reorientation of the phase and frequency-encoding gradients. Vascular pulsation artifacts will then propagate along the right-left axis of the body, and the left hepatic lobe can be more accurately evaluated (see Figs. 5-19, *A* and *B*). Persistence of abnormal signal intensity in the left lobe following gradient reorientation indicates that a vascular pulsation artifact is not responsible, and the possibility of a true lesion should be considered.

Motion artifacts

Discrete ghosting artifacts that propagate across the liver along the phase-encoding direction may also arise from motion of high signal intensity lesions in or adjacent to the liver. For example, respiratory related motion of a hepatic cyst or hemangioma may generate a series of such artifacts on T2-weighted images. These artifacts can appear to represent additional hepatic lesions. Since they are usually somewhat less intense than the structure from which they arose, they are most likely to be mistaken for a moderately intense hepatic malignancy (Figs. 5-20, *A-C* and 5-22, *A* and *B*).

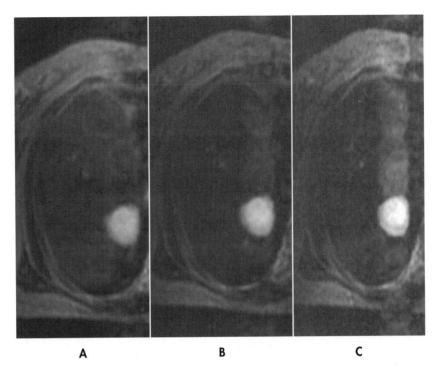

A   B   C

Fig. 5-20. Transaxial T2-weighted images obtained using progressively increased echo times: **A,** TR 3000, TE 80, 2 Nex; **B,** TR 3000, TE 120, 2 Nex; **C,** TR 3000, TE 160, 2 Nex. Ghosting artifacts related to respiratory motion of a hepatic cyst increase in intensity concordant with increasing echo time. These findings are reflective of declining signal-to-noise ratio.

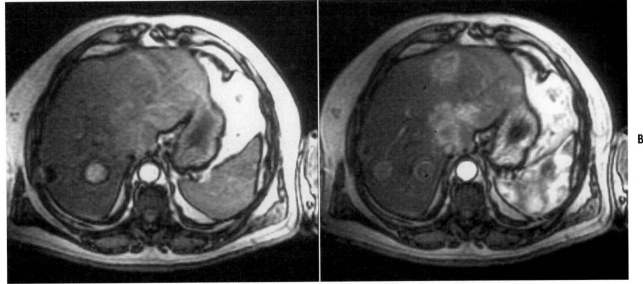

Fig. 5-21. Spoiled gradient echo images (TR 113, TE 2.6, 90-degree flip angle, 1 Nex) obtained before **(A)** and after **(B)** bolus administration of gadolinium chelate contrast material in patient with hepatic metastases. There is paradoxical decreased prominence of aortic pulsation artifacts overlying the right hepatic lobe following contrast material administration as compared with unenhanced image. Heterogeneous contrast enhancement of the spleen is observed in **B.**

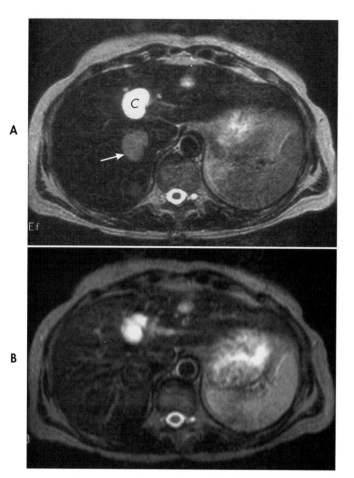

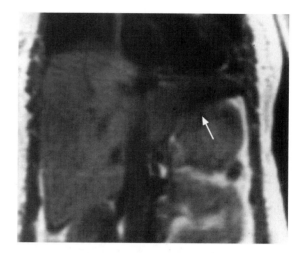

Fig. 5-23. Relative decreased signal intensity is noted throughout the lateral segment of the left hepatic lobe (*arrow*) on coronal T1-weighted image (TR 670, TE 12, 4 Nex). This is due to transmitted pulsations from the overlying heart. Absence of a lesion in this location was verified on additional MR sequences as well as on contrast-enhanced CT images.

Fig. 5-22. A, A markedly hyperintense lesion, representing an hepatic cyst, *(C)* is observed in the medial segment of the left hepatic lobe on transaxial T2-weighted fast spin echo image (TR 4000, effective TE 200, 2 Nex, 16 echo train). There is a moderately intense focus of abnormal signal intensity noted within the right hepatic lobe, simulating a second lesion (*arrow*). However, the latter finding represents a phase-encode artifact due to motion of the previously described cyst. The apparent right lobe lesion is not evident on corresponding T2-weighted conventional spin echo image **(B)** (TR 3400, TE 120, 2 Nex), obtained using shorter echo time as well as gradient moment nulling and respiratory ordered phase encoding. Note the relative hyperintensity of fat on the fast spin echo image as compared to the conventional spin echo image.

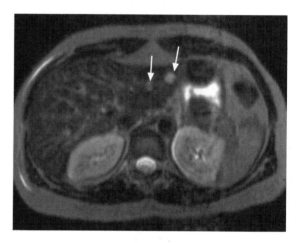

Fig. 5-24. The signal intensity of two cavernous hemangiomas (*arrows*) within the left hepatic lobe is less than expected on this T2-weighted image (TR 3400, TE 120, 2 Nex) related to cardiac pulsation.

Cardiac pulsations

There is yet another cause for vascular related pseudolesions within the left lobe of the liver. The beating heart transmits pulsatile forces to the underlying left hepatic lobe. This results in phase errors that can be manifested as foci of aberrant reduced signal intensity or as more diffuse heterogeneous signal intensity (Figs. 5-23 and 5-24). The use of electrocardiographic (ECG) gating offers a means for reducing such artifacts, since acquisition of specific phase-encoding steps can be referenced to the cardiac cycle. Cardiac gating restricts designation of a specific repetition time (TR), as the TR becomes a function of the patient's heart rate. This may limit the ability to achieve strong T1-weighting, which is desirable for detecting liver lesions, and it can also lengthen examination time. A peripheral plethysmographic sensor can reduce setup time as compared with standard electrocardiographic chest leads. Cardiac gating

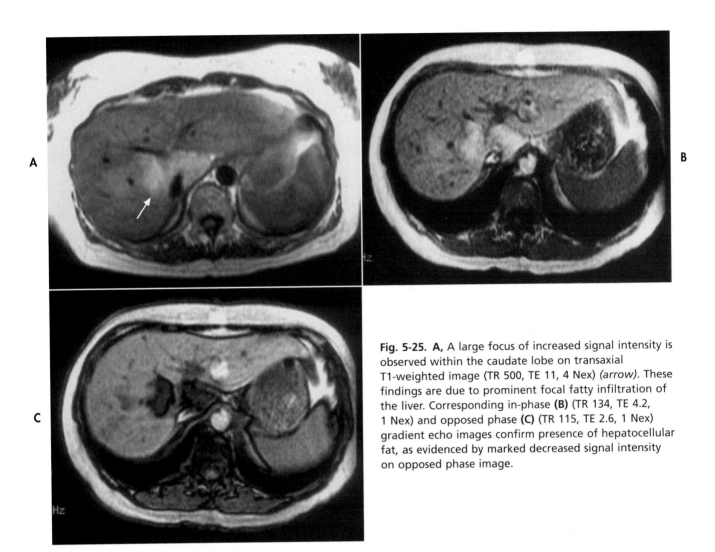

Fig. 5-25. A, A large focus of increased signal intensity is observed within the caudate lobe on transaxial T1-weighted image (TR 500, TE 11, 4 Nex) (arrow). These findings are due to prominent focal fatty infiltration of the liver. Corresponding in-phase **(B)** (TR 134, TE 4.2, 1 Nex) and opposed phase **(C)** (TR 115, TE 2.6, 1 Nex) gradient echo images confirm presence of hepatocellular fat, as evidenced by marked decreased signal intensity on opposed phase image.

should be used when questionable lesions in the left hepatic lobe are observed or when the left lobe is of primary concern based on results of previous studies.

Fatty infiltration

Fatty metamorphosis of the liver occurs relatively frequently; it can be associated with alcoholism, malnutrition, chemotherapy, or other drug administration or can occur on an idiopathic basis. The presence of hepatocellular fat is usually inconspicuous on conventional MR images. However, increased signal intensity on T1-weighted images may be observed in some patients with profound fatty infiltration. Fatty infiltration can simulate hepatic lesions through two mechanisms. First, discrete or patchy foci of abnormal increased signal intensity on T1-weighted images can result from focal fatty infiltration[65,93,119,144,145] (Figs. 5-25, A-C). These findings can simulate hepatic lesions with short T1 relaxation, including some types of hepatocellular carcinoma, hematoma,

and melanoma metastases. Typical locations for focal fat deposition include the left hepatic lobe adjacent to the falciform ligament and adjacent to the intrahepatic segment of the inferior vena cava[94] (Fig. 5-26). Focal fat deposition is often characterized by a wedgelike configuration, absence of mass effect, and visualization of normal vessels coursing through the region of abnormal signal intensity.[93] However, all of these findings are not always present. Furthermore, we have observed several cases in which vascular structures have extended through hepatic neoplasms without apparent distortion.[3]

Lesions can also be simulated when diffuse fatty infiltration spares a limited portion of the liver. This creates the appearance of a focal region of abnormal decreased hepatic signal intensity on T1-weighted images that can simulate a variety of benign or malignant lesions (Figs. 5-27 to 5-29, B). A portion of the left hepatic lobe adjacent to the portal vein is a common site for sparing from diffuse fatty infiltration[93] (Figs. 5-30, A and B). Fo-

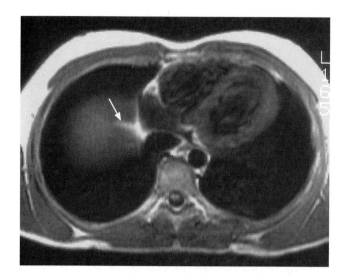

Fig. 5-26. Transaxial T1-weighted image (TR 630, TE 12, 4 Nex) demonstrates focal collection of fat adjacent to the intrahepatic segment of the inferior vena cava *(arrow)*.

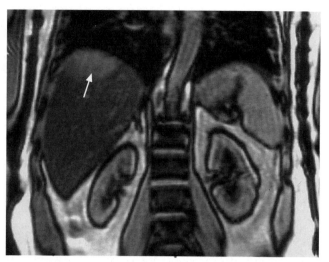

Fig. 5-27. Coronal rapid gradient echo image (TR 113, TE 2.6, 90-degree flip angle, 1 Nex) demonstrates focus of relative increased signal intensity within the hepatic dome *(arrow)*. This is due to focal sparing of diffuse fatty infiltration of the liver on this opposed phase image. The absence of a lesion was confirmed on additional MR pulse sequences as well as CT portography.

cal sparing of diffuse fatty infiltration can also occur distal to an obstructed portal-vein branch.[93]

Several techniques permit identification of fatty infiltration, thereby offering a solution to the diagnostic difficulties mentioned. One method is based on the difference in precessional frequency of fat and water protons. Fat and water protons undergo a cyclic variation by which they are alternately in phase and out of phase with respect to one another, according to the echo time (TE) used. Voxels containing both fat and water protons display reduced signal intensity on opposed phase images (Fig. 5-27). Suppression of signal intensity from either fat or water protons can also be achieved with use of frequency selective radiofrequency pulses followed by gradient spoiling methods (fat or water saturation). Fat saturation is somewhat less sensitive for detection of hepatic fat than is phase contrast imaging.[93] The use of inversion recovery sequences with appropriate choice of inversion time (TI) (short tau inversion recovery; STIR) can also provide suppression of fat signal intensity. Using these methods, fatty changes in the liver can be mapped and focal fat deposition or focal sparing from diffuse fatty infiltration can be recognized. Fatty infiltration of the liver can simulate iron overload on phase contrast or other fat suppression techniques, since both entities produce diffuse hypointensity of the hepatic parenchyma.

Contrast enhancement patterns

An oval focus of prominent enhancement can be observed within the medial segment of the left hepatic lobe during the arterial phase of dynamic contrast-enhanced imaging.[52] This represents a normal variant, provided that no corresponding abnormal signal intensity is observed on conventional T1- or T2-weighted spin echo images or on precontrast or equilibrium phase postcontrast images. This occurs in a location similar to one where localized sparing from diffuse hepatic fatty infiltration is typically seen, and it may reflect a site of more prominent hepatic arterial blood supply and/or more rapid venous drainage.

Adjacent lymph nodes

Enlarged lymph nodes in the porta hepatis and portacaval space usually indicate metastatic disease. However, these findings can also represent Castleman disease, reactive lymphadenopathy caused by an adjacent inflammatory process, or other benign entities. Enlarged lymph nodes can also simulate an hepatic neoplasm.[109]

Lymph nodes in the portocaval space may be larger than other abdominal nodes in normal subjects, with the normal upper limit approximately 1.3 cm in anteroposterior dimension.[51] These nodes may also appear somewhat different than other abdominal nodes, having a flattened rather than rounded configuration. The pancreatic head may extend lateral to the portal vein and appear to represent an enlarged portocaval lymph node.[51] The papillary process of the caudate lobe may be relatively prominent or can extend medial to the inferior vena cava, simulating portocaval lymphadenopathy or an exophytic hepatic lesion (Figs. 5-4 and 5-5).

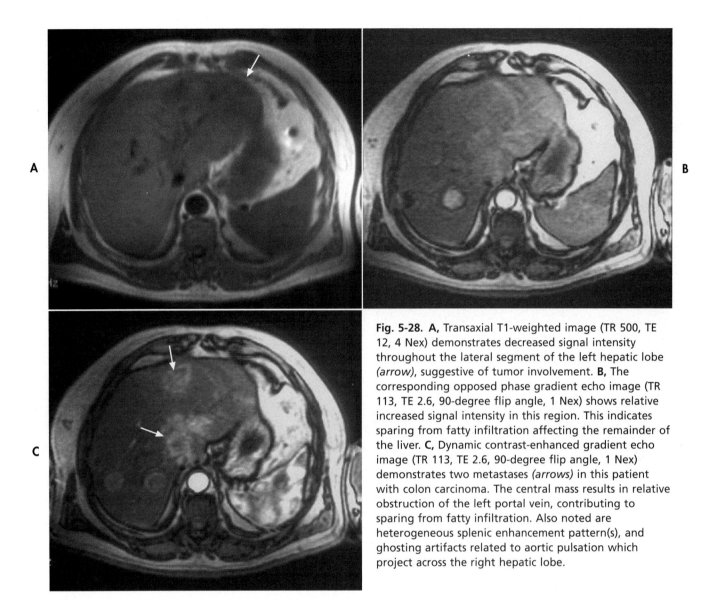

Fig. 5-28. A, Transaxial T1-weighted image (TR 500, TE 12, 4 Nex) demonstrates decreased signal intensity throughout the lateral segment of the left hepatic lobe *(arrow)*, suggestive of tumor involvement. **B,** The corresponding opposed phase gradient echo image (TR 113, TE 2.6, 90-degree flip angle, 1 Nex) shows relative increased signal intensity in this region. This indicates sparing from fatty infiltration affecting the remainder of the liver. **C,** Dynamic contrast-enhanced gradient echo image (TR 113, TE 2.6, 90-degree flip angle, 1 Nex) demonstrates two metastases *(arrows)* in this patient with colon carcinoma. The central mass results in relative obstruction of the left portal vein, contributing to sparing from fatty infiltration. Also noted are heterogeneous splenic enhancement pattern(s), and ghosting artifacts related to aortic pulsation which project across the right hepatic lobe.

Postoperative changes

Alterations in the appearance of the liver can be observed following surgical intervention. For example, in patients who have undergone transplantation of the left hepatic lobe, a collection of blood, bile, lymph, and serous fluid may envelop the graft.[13] The presence of a Roux-en-Y loop adjacent to the liver can simulate a postoperative fluid collection or abscess.[13] Following percutaneous biliary procedures, findings may include collections of fluid and/or blood within the subcutaneous tissues, subcapsular or perihepatic tissues, or intraparenchymal liver as well as free intraperitoneal air.[33]

Following surgery, trauma, infarction, or other insults, the spared portion of the liver can undergo compensatory enlargement, often with an unusual morphologic configuration. These features can simulate a hepatic mass. Focal hepatic hypertrophy can also occur in patients with hepatitis, portal venous or biliary ductal obstruction, sclerosing cholangitis, and other entities.[93] Focal hypertrophied liver can be distinguished from a mass because normal hepatic signal intensity characteristics are maintained in the former entity. Furthermore, hepatic vessels and bile ducts can be observed traversing the hypertrophied segment.[93]

Other causes for focal hepatic alterations

Focal enlargement of the caudate lobe may occur in patients with Budd-Chiari syndrome. The caudate lobe can also demonstrate altered signal intensity and abnormal enhancement pattern, further contributing to confusion for a mass.[93] In patients with cirrhosis, the right hepatic lobe is often atrophic, whereas the caudate and

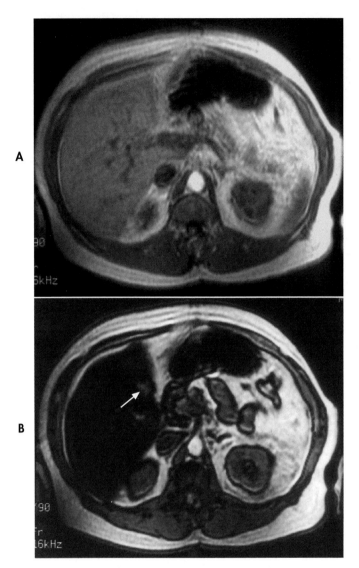

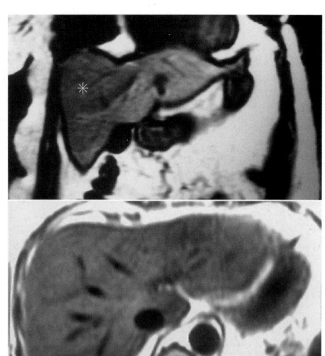

Fig. 5-29. A, Transaxial gradient echo image (TR 133, TE 4.2, 90-degree flip angle, 1 Nex), acquired using an in-phase echo time, demonstrates the liver to have homogeneous signal intensity. **B,** Corresponding opposed phase image (TR 114, TE 2.6, 90-degree flip angle, 1 Nex) reveals marked signal intensity loss throughout the hepatic parenchyma, with nodular focus of relative increased signal intensity observed within the medial segment of the left hepatic lobe (arrow) due to relative sparing from diffuse fatty infiltration. This appearance can simulate tumor involvement.

Fig. 5-30. A, There is relative decreased signal intensity within the right hepatic lobe *(asterisk)* as compared with the left lobe on coronal opposed phase gradient echo image (TR 113, TE 2.6, 90-degree flip angle, 1 Nex). **B,** There is corresponding increased signal intensity within the right lobe of the liver on transaxial T1-weighted spin echo (TR 500, TE 12, 4 Nex). These findings represent fatty infiltration of the liver, with relative sparing of the lateral segment of the left hepatic lobe.

left lobes may be relatively enlarged. The atrophic lobes can have aberrant signal characteristics as compared with the remainder of the liver.[93]

Entities That Can Obscure Lesions
Respiratory motion artifacts

The major source of artifacts on abdominal MR imaging is respiratory motion. Respiratory motion artifacts

---

ENTITIES THAT MAY OBSCURE HEPATIC LESIONS

- Respiratory motion artifacts
- Presaturation of liver
- Inadequate T1-, T2-weighting
- Vascular pulsation artifacts
- Poor tissue contrast
- Gradient echo imaging
- Fast spin echo imaging
- Delayed contrast-enhanced images
- Poor spatial resolution
- Cross-excitation
- Susceptibility artifacts
- Isointense lesions

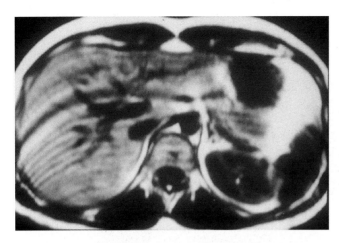

Fig. 5-31. T1-weighted spin echo image demonstrates severe ghosting artifacts resulting from respiratory motion that extend across the phase encode direction of the image.

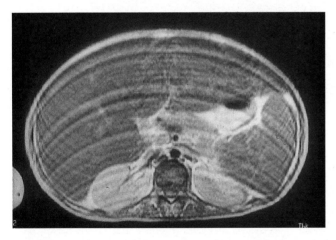

Fig. 5-32. Transaxial proton density–weighted image demonstrates severe ghosting artifacts extending across the phase encode direction of the image.

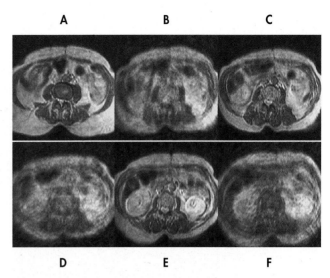

Fig. 5-33. A series of six adjacent transaxial T2-weighted images of the abdomen is displayed. Severe blurring of anatomic structures, in addition to structured ghost artifacts, is present on alternating images **(B, D, F)**, whereas intervening images **(A, C, E)** demonstrate reasonably good image quality. Alternating nature of these motions artifacts is due to use of an interleaved image acquisition, with patient motion occurring during performance of a single data acquisition.

arise as a result of periodic craniocaudal and circumferential motion of the abdominal wall, diaphragm, and abdominal viscera during image acquisition. There are two major effects of respiratory motion on abdominal magnetic resonance (MR) images. First, generalized blurring is created throughout the image. This can result in heterogeneous signal intensity throughout the liver and other organs and general loss of anatomic detail. Second, a series of discrete curvilinear artifacts may be created along the phase-encoding direction of the image (Figs. 5-31 to 5-33, *A-F*). These "ghosting artifacts" are complete or incomplete replications of high signal intensity structures that undergo periodic displacement. The most frequent source of ghost artifacts in the abdomen is fat within the anterior abdominal wall. The number and

spacing of ghost artifacts depend on the respiratory rate.[108] While respiratory motion artifacts may create apparent lesions within the liver, they are even more likely to result in causing actual lesions—particularly small lesions—to be obscured[25,84,142] (Figs. 5-34, *A* to 5-36, *B*).

There are many approaches to reducing respiratory motion artifacts.[118] The use of a simple abdominal binder can be helpful in restricting abdominal motion during respiration.[108] Motion artifacts of all types are of decreased prominence when imaging is performed at low-to-mid field rather than at high field strength. Respiratory gating or pseudogating can be effective in reducing respiratory motion artifacts, though these methods restrict choice of TR and prolong imaging time. Respiratory ordered phase encoding requires a bellows device to be placed around the patient's abdomen for monitoring of the respiratory cycle. Phase-encoding steps are reordered so as to simulate a single slow respiratory cycle, thereby reducing the severity of related artifacts without a significant time penalty. Gradient moment rephasing (nulling) utilizes additional gradient waveforms in order to correct for motion-induced phase shifts. This method cannot be implemented with a short TE and is most frequently used on the second echo of a T2-weighted sequence (Figs. 5-18, 5-37, *A* to 5-38, *B*). Gradient moment rephasing is effective for reducing artifacts related to in-plane or through-plane motion and is usually ap-

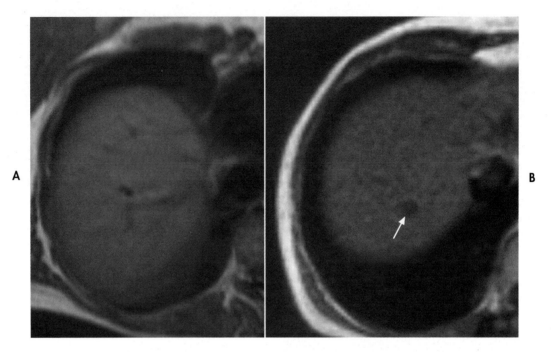

Fig. 5-34. Conventional T1-weighted image **(A)** (TR 500, TE 12, 4 Nex) fails to depict lesion in hepatic dome, which is visualized on breath hold rapid acquisition spin echo image **(B)** (TR 267, TE 11, 0.5 Nex) *(arrow).*

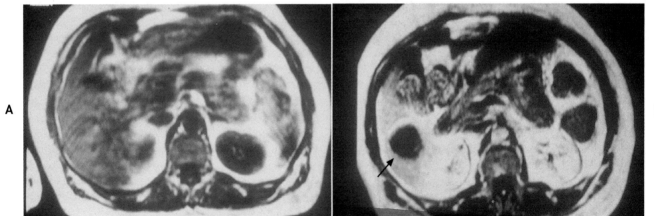

Fig. 5-35. A, Colon cancer metastasis in posterior segment of right hepatic lobe is poorly visualized on conventional transaxial T1-weighted image. **B,** Corresponding dynamic contrast material–enhanced rapid acquisition spin echo image better demonstrates the lesion *(arrow)* because of combined effects of suspended respiration and use of intravenous contrast material. (Reprinted from Mirowitz SA, Lee JKT, Gutierrez E et al: Radiology 179:371-376, 1991.)

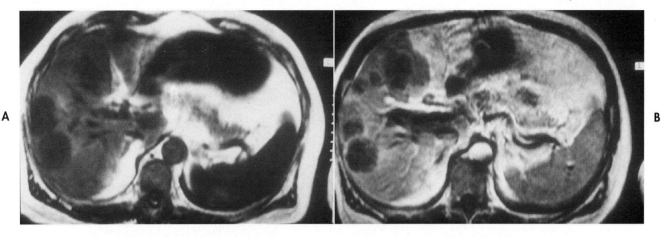

Fig. 5-36. A, Conventional transaxial T1-weighted spin echo image demonstrates three liver metastases in patient with colon cancer. **B,** Bolus contrast material–enhanced rapid acquisition spin echo image acquired at same level reveals a total of five lesions. Improved lesion detection is due to combined effects of suspended respiration and heightened liver-lesion contrast from use of intravenous contrast material. (Reprinted from Mirowitz SA, Lee JKT, Gutierrez E et al: Radiology 179:371-376, 1991.)

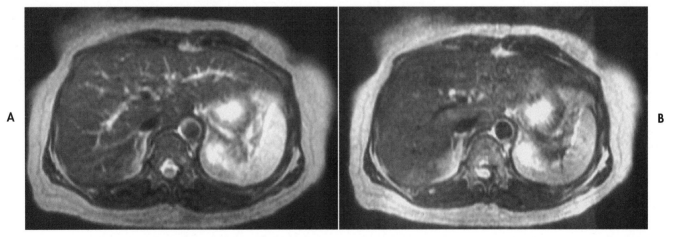

Fig. 5-37. Transaxial T2-weighted images (TR 3400, TE 80, 2 Nex) obtained with **(A)** and without **(B)** use of gradient moment nulling. Reduced respiratory motion artifact is apparent on **A,** as well as relative increased signal intensity of hepatic vessels.

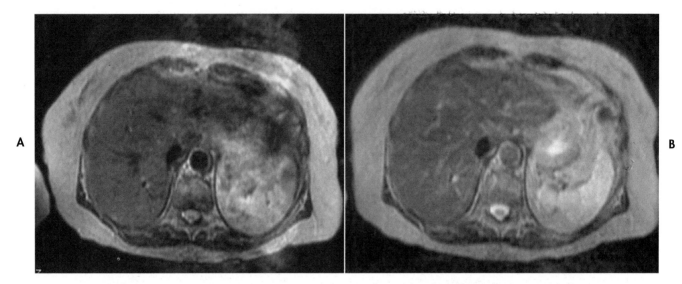

Fig. 5-38. T2-weighted images (TR 3700, TE 80, 2 Nex) obtained without **(A)** and with **(B)** use of gradient moment nulling. Respiratory and vascular motion artifacts result in heterogeneous signal intensity appearance of spleen and left hepatic lobe in **A**. These artifacts are considerably reduced with use of gradient moment nulling. Relative increased signal intensity of hepatic vessels and CSF is also noted on image acquired using gradient moment nulling.

plied on the read out and slice select gradients.[22] Spatial presaturation radiofrequency pulses can be applied along the anterior abdominal wall to reduce the intensity of artifacts arising from motion of this tissue. Care must be taken to avoid unintended presaturation of the subjacent structures. Inadvertent presaturation of the anterior liver can result in artifactual decreased signal intensity and obscured visualization of lesions.

Pulse sequence parameters

The signal-to-noise ratio scales in inverse proportion to echo time; thus long TE images have lower signal-to-noise ratio than short TE images. This is manifested as increased image graininess as well as accentuation of motion related artifacts (Figs. 5-20 and 5-39, *A-D*).

The number of echoes collected during image acquisition also affects image quality. Multiecho sequences generally have less severe motion artifacts because of refocusing of phase shifts.[91] However, multiecho sequences also demonstrate reduced signal intensity of soft tissues relative to that displayed on a single echo sequence because of increased off-resonance radiofrequency generated by the additional 180-degree pulses. More important, the difference in signal intensity between various soft tissues (i.e., tissue contrast) can be reduced on a multiecho sequence. This creates a tradeoff between tissue contrast and motion artifacts. Mitchell et al. found that lesions within the right hepatic lobe were

more conspicuous when a single echo sequence was used, though left lobe lesions were more difficult to identify because of accentuation of motion artifacts.[91]

Delivery of off-resonance irradiation is also accentuated on pulse sequences that provide multiple imaging slices. This results in magnetization transfer effects caused by differences in relaxation of free and bound water protons. Dixon et al. found that the signal intensity of many tissues is reduced by 10% to 20% on multislice sequences as compared with single slice sequences.[19] This phenomenon can also reduce contrast among tissues, potentially obscuring hepatic and other lesions.

Each of the techniques previously discussed is helpful for reducing respiratory motion artifacts. However, none of these methods is completely effective. Superior results are usually achieved when several techniques are used in combination. For example, respiratory ordered phase encoding can be used in conjunction with gradient moment rephasing and spatial presaturation.

Breathhold imaging provides the only means for eliminating rather than ameliorating respiratory motion artifacts. Conventional pulse sequences are, of course, impractical in this regard since they have acquisition times on the order of several minutes. However, several rapid imaging sequences can be performed during a reasonable breathholding interval. Multislice spin echo breathhold imaging can be accomplished using the rapid

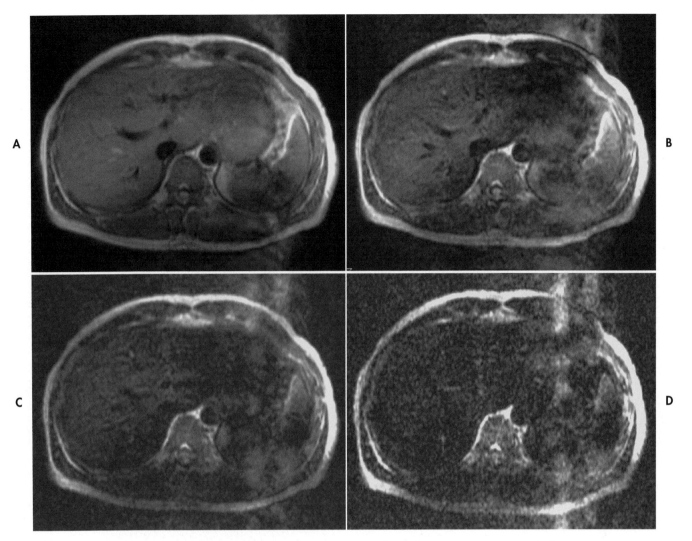

Fig. 5-39. Four images acquired at the same anatomic level are shown at progressively increasing echo times: **A,** TE 30; **B,** TE 60; **C,** TE 90; **D,** TE 120. There is progressive loss of image quality resulting from reduced signal-to-noise ratio, with increasing echo time.

acquisition spin echo (RASE) technique. RASE combines use of short TR and TE, single data excitation, and half-Fourier reconstruction.[83] A number of sequences are based on the gradient echo technique. These include spoiled (e.g., FLASH, spoiled GRASS) and steady state (e.g., GRASS, FISP) gradient echo sequences, as well as rapid (e.g., turbo-FLASH, rapid GRASS) and magnetization prepared rapid (e.g., MP-RAGE) gradient echo techniques.

Vascular pulsation artifacts

Vascular pulsation artifacts can simulate focal hepatic lesions, as previously noted; they can also obscure hepatic lesions. These artifacts can be minimized with spatial presaturation and gradient moment nulling techniques. Similarly, cardiac pulsations transmitted to the left hepatic lobe can mask lesions in this location (Figs. 5-40, *A* and *B*). Cardiac gating can be used to improve visualization of left lobe lesions, though examination time is often prolonged.

Tissue contrast

Detection of liver lesions is highly dependent on the ability of the MR image to sensitively display focal alterations in T1 and T2 relaxation. This is largely determined through selection of appropriate TR and TE; optimization of these imaging parameters is critical to hepatic lesion detection. T1-weighted sequences should generally utilize the minimum echo time available, since considerable T2 weighting may be introduced with even modest prolongation of TE. This results in reduction of signal-to-noise ratio and degrades tissue contrast.[35] Use

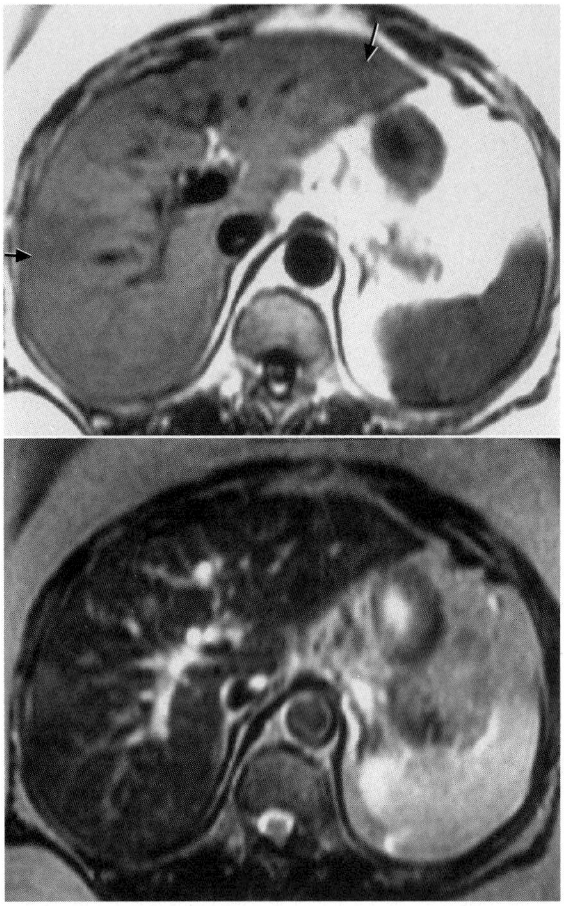

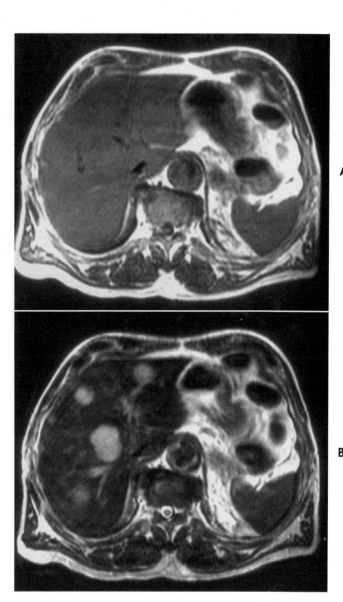

Fig. 5-40. T1-weighted **(A)** (TR 550, TE 12, 4 Nex) and T2-weighted **(B)** (TR 3600, TE 80, 2 Nex) images in patient with colon carcinoma. The T1-weighted image demonstrates two metastatic foci *(arrows)*, one in the anterior segment of the right hepatic lobe and one in the lateral segment of the left lobe. The latter lesion is not visualized on the corresponding T2-weighted image, because of accentuation of artifact related to cardiac pulsations.

Fig. 5-41. A, T1-weighted image (TR 700, TE 11, 4 Nex) in patient with lung carcinoma reveals no evidence of liver metastases. **B,** Corresponding T2-weighted image (TR 4000, TE 68, 4 Nex, 16 echo train) demonstrates multiple metastatic lesions throughout both right and left hepatic lobes.

of an insufficiently short TR and TE on T1-weighted images or use of an insufficiently long TR and TE on T2-weighted images will introduce undesirable proton density weighting characteristics into the image. Consequently, differences between lesions and adjacent normal parenchyma in T1 and T2 relaxation will not be displayed, and lesions may go undetected.[30,46,47,92,107,129] Generally, T1-weighted liver images should be acquired using $TR \leq 500$ msec and $TE \leq 20$ msec, and T2-weighted images should be acquired using $TR \geq 2500$ msec and $TE \geq 80$ msec.

While inadequate T1- and T2-weighting can result from operator error, the ability to achieve heavily T1- and T2-weighted images may also be limited by hardware and software restrictions. For example, very short echo times (≤ 10 msec) on T1-weighted spin echo images cannot be achieved on some systems. On other systems, such short echo times are only provided in conjunction with partial echo sampling, wide receiver bandwidth, or other methods that reduce the signal-to-noise ratio. The use of very long echo times (≥ 120 msec) for performance of heavily T2-weighted images may result in unacceptably low signal-to-noise ratio on low field strength systems.

The strength of the main magnetic field may be influential in detection of hepatic lesions for other reasons. T1 relaxation times increase and undergo convergence

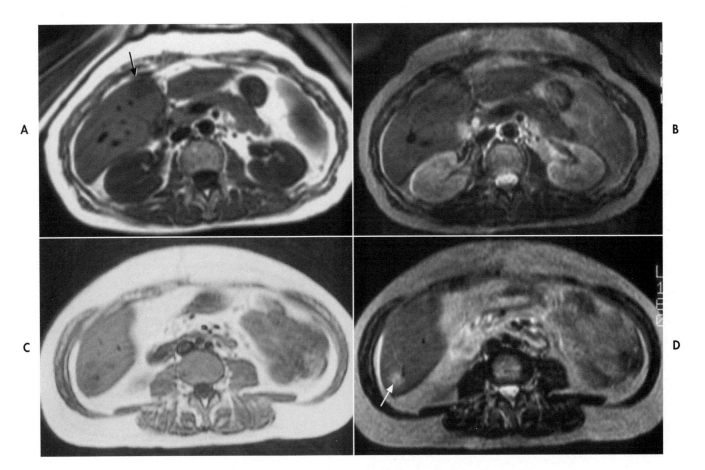

Fig. 5-42. T1-weighted **(A, C)** (TR 450, TE 12, 4 Nex) and T2-weighted **(B, D)** (TR 2500, TE 80, 2 Nex) transaxial images in patient with colon cancer and biopsy proven metastatic liver lesions. A lesion in the medial segment of the left lobe *(arrow)*, is demonstrated on the T1-weighted image **(A)**, though poorly seen on the corresponding T2-weighted image **(B)**. However, at a slightly lower level another lesion *(arrow)* demonstrates an inverse relationship, with greater conspicuousness on T2-weighted **(D)** versus the T1-weighted **(C)** image.

with increasing field strength.[28,30,31,86,110,130] Therefore T1-weighted images acquired at high field strength (1.5 T) may depict focal liver lesions less sensitively than similar images acquired at low field strength. As a result, it has been observed that liver lesions are most sensitively detected using T1-weighted sequences on low-mid-field strength systems and using T2-weighted sequences on high field systems. It is possible that these observations reflect differences among systems that do not relate to field strength alone, such as the availability and effectiveness of artifact reduction methods. Bernardino et al observed that T2 relaxation may also undergo field strength–dependent alterations. They found that the T2 relaxation value of normal hepatic tissue decreased on images acquired at higher field strength.[7] This could contribute to improved liver lesion detection on T2-weighted sequences using high field strength systems.

Tissue contrast between lesions and surrounding liver parenchyma was modeled for several different pulse sequences by Van Lom et al.[136] Their results indicate that T2-weighted spin echo sequences provide higher lesion contrast than T1-weighted sequences at high field strength (1.5 T). However, the tissue contrast provided by inversion recovery images exceeded that of spin echo sequences.

Pulse sequences

Recent experience indicates that, when imaging parameters are optimized and artifact reduction methods used, liver lesions are detected with approximately equal sensitivity using T1- and T2-weighted sequences on high field systems. However, this does not imply that all detected lesions are observed on both sets of images. Lesions are frequently observed on T1-weighted images

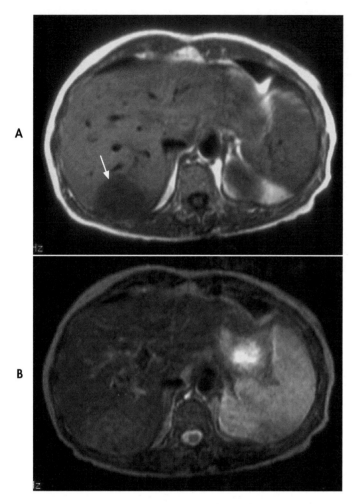

A

B

Fig. 5-43. A, Lymphomatous involvement of the posterior segment of the right hepatic lobe is demonstrated on T1-weighted transaxial image (TR 500, TE 11, 4 Nex) *(arrow).* **B,** The lesion is poorly visualized on the corresponding T2-weighted image (TR 3400, TE 80, 2 Nex).

and not on corresponding T2-weighted images, and vice versa, without apparent explanation[92,130] (Figs. 5-41, *A* to 5-43, *B*). This mandates that both T1- and T2-weighted pulse sequences be performed in all patients to maximize lesion detection.

Gradient echo imaging

The relatively long imaging times associated with conventional spin echo pulse sequences has prompted a search for a more rapid means of evaluating the liver using MR, as noted previously. A number of rapid imaging techniques have been introduced for hepatic imaging. Gradient echo sequences use a short TR and TE, variable flip angle, and substitution of gradient reversal for the 180-degree radiofrequency pulse used in spin echo imaging for echo formation. Tissue contrast on gradient echo images depends on a complex interaction of

the TR, TE, and flip angle prescribed. There is increased opportunity for inappropriate parameter selection to restrict tissue contrast and lead to poor detection of hepatic lesions. For example, a long TR or a very short TR will each contribute undesirable proton density-weighting to gradient echo images. These parameters must be optimized according to the specific type of gradient echo sequence (i.e., steady state, spoiled) used.

Rapid gradient echo sequences use ultrashort TR and TE values, on the order of 10 msec and 3 msec, respectively. These sequences are useful for reducing image acquisition time. However, the use of a very short TR often limits the signal-to-noise ratio and also creates dominantly proton density–weighted tissue contrast (Figs. 5-44, *A-C*). Strong tissue contrast can be achieved on rapid gradient echo sequences, when a magnetization preparation module is carried out prior to the usual excitation pulse. Inversion recovery and driven equilibrium prepulses are used to generate T1- and T2-weighted tissue contrast, respectively. The time that is allowed to elapse between these prepulses and execution of the remainder of the sequence strongly influences the tissue contrast expressed on the image (Figs. 5-45, *A* and *B*). Often the tissue contrast that can be achieved with magnetization prepared rapid gradient echo sequences is more robust than that of conventional spin echo sequences (Figs. 5-48, *A* and *B*), in addition to being considerably more flexible. Through proper choice of these parameters, one may selectively null the signal intensity of fat, flowing blood, spleen, or liver parenchyma. Nulling of spleen and liver tissue would be expected to further improve detection of focal hepatic lesions on relatively T1- and T2-weighted images, respectively.

Phase encoding artifacts may arise as a result of variations in tissue magnetization during data collection.[15] Two methods have been used to address these limitations. Reordering of phase-encoding steps involves initial acquisition of central low order phase encoded data, which is largely responsible for signal-to-noise ratio and tissue contrast. High order phase-encoding steps, which primarily determine spatial resolution, are acquired later. The second method is segmentation of k-space, which involves acquisition of a fraction of phase encoded data lines during a single TR. In a comparative study Chien et al.[16] found that both methods improved tissue contrast on rapid gradient echo images.[15]

Opposed phase images

Opposed phase gradient echo images display relative reduced signal intensity for voxels that contain both fat and water protons. When opposed phase images are obtained using relatively T1-weighted parameters, the low signal intensity of hepatic lesions will therefore be less conspicuous, and such lesions may go undetected in patients with hepatic fatty infiltration.[70]

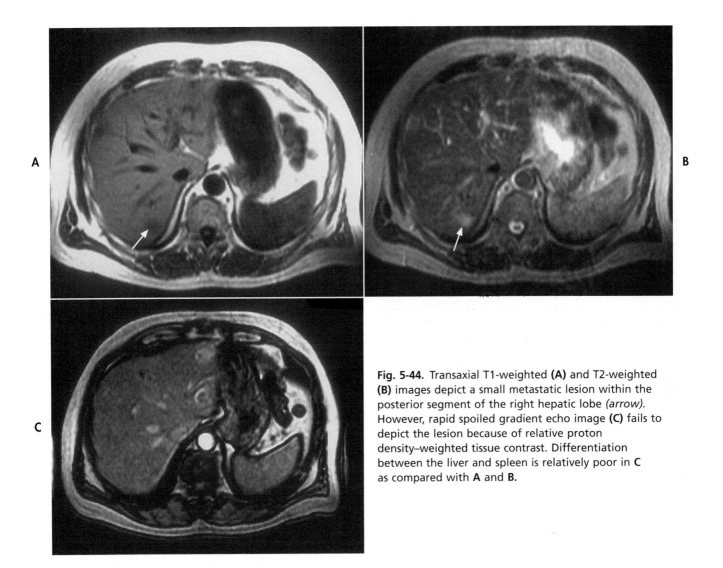

Fig. 5-44. Transaxial T1-weighted **(A)** and T2-weighted **(B)** images depict a small metastatic lesion within the posterior segment of the right hepatic lobe *(arrow)*. However, rapid spoiled gradient echo image **(C)** fails to depict the lesion because of relative proton density–weighted tissue contrast. Differentiation between the liver and spleen is relatively poor in **C** as compared with **A** and **B**.

Vasculature

Hepatic vessels and lesions frequently display similar signal intensity on T1-weighted or flow compensated T2-weighted spin echo pulse sequences. Consequently, a small hepatic lesion can appear to represent a normal vessel and vice versa (Fig. 5-46, *A* and *B*). T2-weighted spin echo sequences acquired without flow compensation or heavily T1-weighted gradient echo sequences can distinguish these entities. Using the former technique, hepatic lesions will be hyperintense while vessels are typically hypointense, whereas with the latter technique the converse relationship will exist.

Fast spin echo imaging

Rapid acquisition relaxation enhanced (RARE) or fast spin echo imaging is another method for reducing image acquisition time. This technique uses a series (i.e., train) of 180-degree radiofrequency pulses to generate multiple data lines per TR, rather than one data line as in conventional imaging. Image acquisition time is reduced proportional to the echo train length, which usually varies between 8 and 16. Early studies indicate that T2-weighted fast spin echo sequences provide tissue contrast equivalent to that of conventional T2-weighted spin echo imaging.[16,56,99] One early study found that T2-weighted fast spin echo images resulted in improved lesion conspicuousness and detection as compared with conventional spin echo counterparts.[71] However, some implementations of fast spin echo can result in suboptimal tissue contrast for detection of solid hepatic lesions[14] (Figs. 5-47, *A* to 5-48, *B*). This may relate to accentuation of magnetization transfer contrast on fast spin echo images or alteration in the dynamic range for tissue contrast display due to the accentuated signal intensity of fat on fast spin echo images. Despite some loss of conspicuousness of solid hepatic lesions, lesions that con-

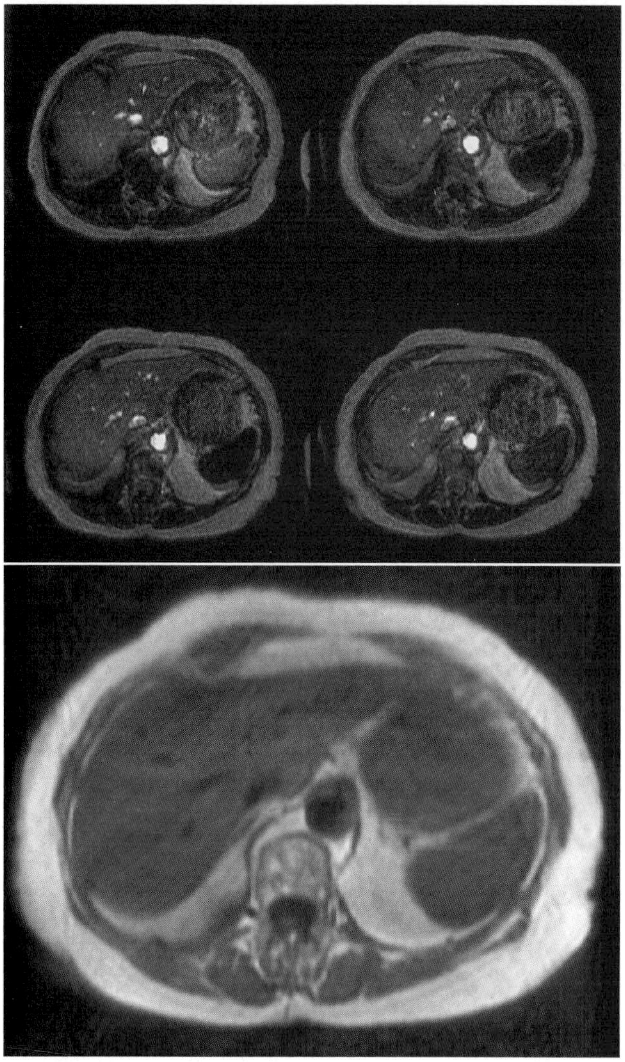

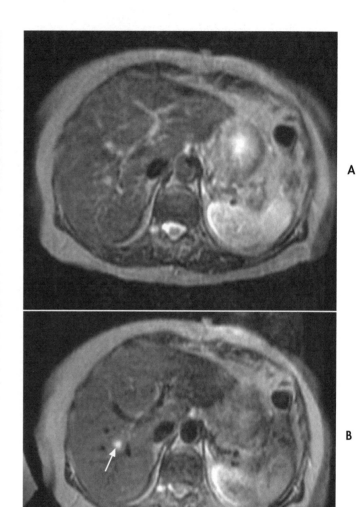

Fig. 5-45. A, Four consecutive images from an inversion recovery prepared rapid gradient echo sequence (TR 10, TE 3, 30-degree flip angle, 2 Nex). There is variable expression of tissue contrast on these images as manifested by varying signal relationship between the liver and spleen. This is due to alterations in the excitation flip angle and inversion time. These images provide considerably greater T1 contrast than does corresponding conventional T1-weighted spin echo image **(B)** (TR 680, TE 11, 4 Nex).

Fig. 5-46. A, Flow compensated T2-weighted image (TR 3700, TE 80, 2 Nex) demonstrates hyperintensity of portal venous branches, without suggestion of focal hepatic lesion. **B,** Image obtained using identical parameters, though without flow compensation, reveals the hepatic vasculature to be hypointense, allowing for clear visualization of a cyst located next to the right portal vein *(arrow).*

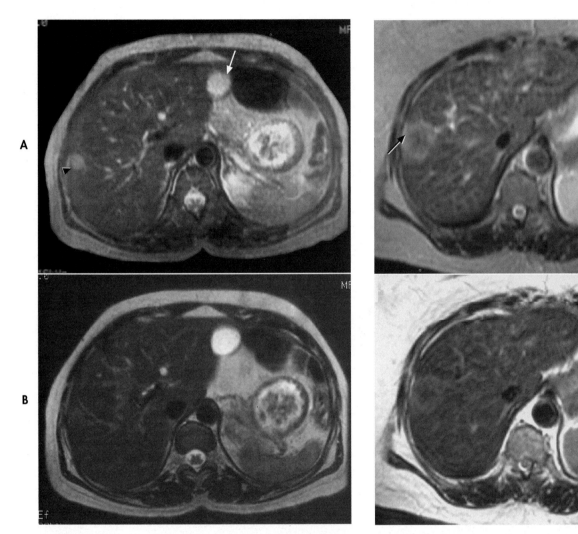

Fig. 5-47. Transaxial T2-weighted images of the liver in patient with colon cancer. Images were obtained using conventional spin echo **(A)** (TR 3400, TE 80, 2 Nex) and **(B)** fast spin echo (TR 4000, effective TE 117, 4 Nex, 16 echo train) techniques. Metastatic lesion in the right hepatic lobe (arrowhead) is less conspicuous on the fast spin echo image as compared with conventional T2-weighted image. However, the left hepatic lobe cyst (arrow) is equally conspicuous on the fast spin echo image. (Reprinted from Catasca JV, Mirowitz SA: Am J Roentgenol 162:61-67, 1994.)

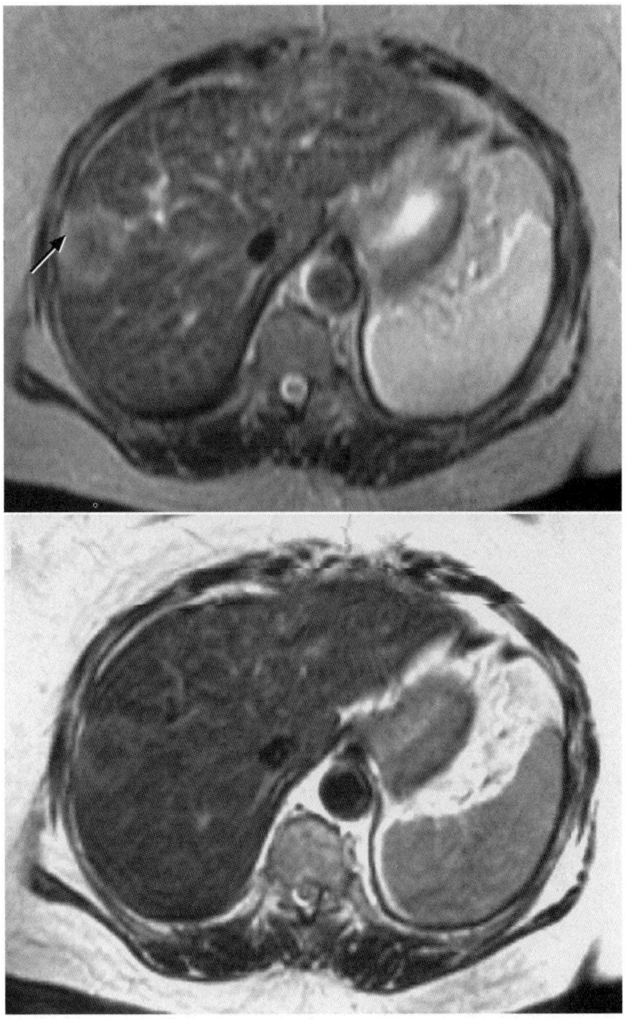

Fig. 5-48. A, Transaxial T2-weighted spin echo image (TR 3600, TE 80, 2 Nex) in patient with colon carcinoma demonstrates metastatic lesion in anterior segment of the right hepatic lobe (arrow). **B,** Corresponding fast spin echo T2-weighted image (TR 4000, effective TE 119, 4 Nex, 16 echo train) demonstrates reduced contrast between the liver and spleen, and the metastatic lesion is poorly visualized. Small foci of intrahepatic hyperintensity noted in **A,** resulting from rephasing of flowing spins on flow compensated image, are not visualized in **B,** since flow compensation was not used.

tain predominantly fluid, such as an hepatic cyst or cavernous hemangioma, are often considerably more conspicuous on fast spin echo as compared with conventional spin echo T2-weighted images (Fig. 5-47, *A* and *B*). This is probably due to the combined effects of (1) reduced signal intensity of the background hepatic parenchyma and (2) greater T2-weighting because of use of longer repetition and echo times on fast spin echo sequences. Fast spin echo images may demonstrate blurring, particularly when short TE or long echo train lengths are used[16,96] (Fig. 5-47, *A* and *B*). The signal intensity of fat is considerably greater on fast spin echo

compared with corresponding conventional spin echo images (Fig. 5-23). This results from decreased J-modulation effects resulting from the repeated refocusing pulses, though other mechanisms may also play a role.[48] As noted previously, the increased signal intensity of fat may degrade the dynamic range for tissue contrast display on fast spin echo images, thereby contributing to decreased lesion conspicuousness. Furthermore, the high signal intensity of fat on T2-weighted fast spin echo images will reduce the conspicuousness of focal hepatic lesions arising in a fatty infiltrated liver.[122] These considerations indicate a role for use of fat suppression in conjunction with fast spin echo imaging of the abdomen (Figs. 5-49, *A* to 5-50, *B*). Difficulty may be en-

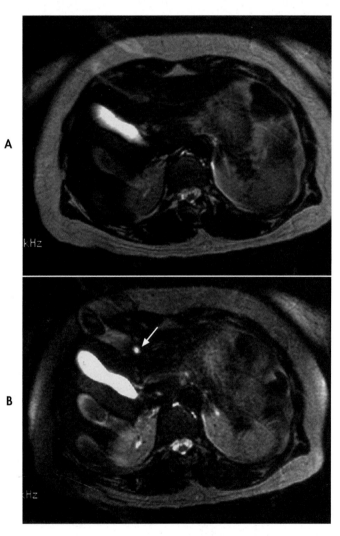

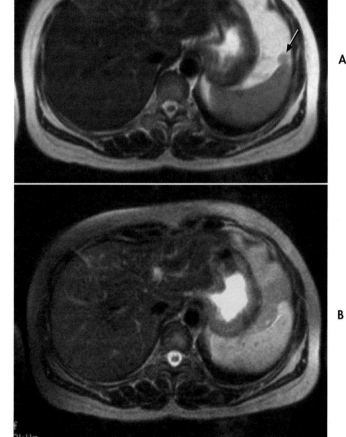

Fig. 5-49. Transaxial fast spin echo T2-weighted images (TR 4000, effective TE 200, 4 Nex, 16 echo train) obtained without **(A)** and with **(B)** use of fat saturation. There is improved conspicuousness of small left hepatic lobe cyst *(arrow)* on fat saturated image. The fat saturated image also demonstrates reduced signal-to-noise ratio as well as uneven fat suppression resulting from inhomogeneity across the field-of-view. Ghosting artifacts related to respiratory motion of the gallbladder can be seen traversing the liver on both images.

Fig. 5-50. T2-weighted fast spin echo images (TR 4000, effective TE 117, 4 Nex, 16 echo train) obtained without **(A)** and with **(B)** fat saturation. There is marked improvement in tissue contrast, as manifested by increased liver-spleen signal intensity difference, on the fat saturation image. A small accessory spleen is seen anterior to the spleen proper *(arrow)*.

countered in achieving uniform fat suppression throughout the relatively large field-of-view used for abdominal imaging when the fat saturation method is used (Fig. 5-49, *A* and *B*). This may be expressed as focal areas of relatively increased signal intensity, which can potentially simulate lesions.

Contrast agents

Paramagnetic contrast agents such as gadopentetate dimeglumine are being used with increasing frequency to assist in detection of hepatic lesions. Bolus injection of contrast material during acquisition of rapid gradient echo or spin echo images has allowed for depiction of lesions that are not observed on conventional unenhanced T1- and T2-weighted images (Figs. 5-35, *A* to

5-36, *B*). This improved lesion conspicuousness with dynamic contrast-enhanced imaging is attributable to two factors. First, images are acquired during suspended respiration, which improves image quality. Second, transient differential contrast enhancement between normal liver parenchyma and liver lesions occurs during the first 2 minutes following contrast material administration, allowing for heightened lesion visibility.[84] It is important to recognize, however, that the conspicuousness of hepatic lesions decreases rapidly with time following contrast material administration. Hepatic lesions can be obscured on images acquired more than 2 minutes following contrast material administration or when contrast material is given as a slow infusion[24,42,84] (Figs. 5-51, *A* to 5-52, *B*). Under these conditions, there is

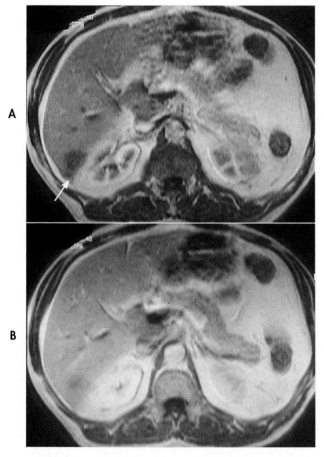

Fig. 5-51. Transaxial T1-weighted rapid acquisition spin echo images obtained during **(A)** and approximately 8 minutes following **(B)** bolus injection of intravenous gadolinium chelate contrast material in patient with melanoma. A metastatic lesion within the posterior segment of the right hepatic lobe *(arrow)* is clearly delineated during the bolus phase of contrast material administration. However, this same lesion is largely obscured on the delayed image. (Reprinted from Mirowitz SA, Lee JKT, Gutierrez E et al: Radiology 179:371-376, 1991.)

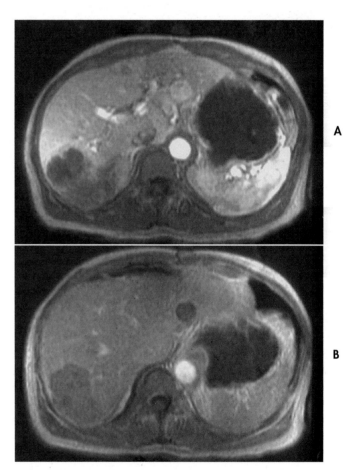

Fig. 5-52. Transaxial gradient echo images (TR 130, TE 4, 90-degree flip angle, 1 Nex) obtained during **(A)** and several minutes following **(B)** bolus injection of gadolinium chelate contrast material. There is diminished conspicuousness of the metastatic lesion in the posterior segment of the right hepatic lobe on the delayed postcontrast image, caused by equilibration of contrast material between the lesion and surrounding hepatic parenchyma.

ample time for contrast material to equilibrate between the intravascular and interstitial tissue compartments; hence liver lesions may become isointense with surrounding normal parenchyma.

Contrast enhancement patterns

Most reports describe the liver as normally undergoing homogeneous contrast enhancement.[41,84,85] However, Semelka et al. reported observing transient areas of relative decreased hepatic enhancement in a segmental or subsegmental distribution.[123] These findings were observed immediately following contrast material administration and converted to a homogeneous pattern within 1 minute. They may reflect regional differences in hepatic perfusion by the portal venous or hepatic arterial systems.

Iron oxide particles

Several new contrast agents are being investigated for use in hepatic MR imaging. Clinical experience with these agents is limited thus far. However, it is already clear that along with their advantageous features, they will present new pitfalls in hepatic lesion detection. For example, superparamagnetic iron oxide particles selectively accumulate in normal liver tissue, where they induce signal loss. Because it does not accumulate in hepatic lesions, this agent is used to heighten the conspicuousness of focal hepatic lesions. However, some liver lesions (e.g., focal nodular hyperplasia and some hepatocellular carcinomas) contain Kupffer cells, which accumulate these particles, thereby potentially obscuring such lesions. Iron oxide particles can also accumulate within the zone of peritumoral signal intensity alteration that frequently surrounds malignant liver lesions, rendering this finding inconspicuous on T2-weighted images.[38]

Manganese-DPDP

Manganese-DPDP is another promising contrast agent, which is designed to provide hepatocellular rather than reticuloendothelial enhancement of normal liver tissue. However, differentiated forms of hepatocellular carcinoma have been found to undergo enhancement when this agent is administered.[113] Other lesions that contain hepatocytes such as focal nodular hyperplasia and regenerative nodules also undergo enhancement with this agent, as does liver that is fatty infiltrated.[113] On delayed images acquired following manganese-DPDP, a hyperintense rim can be observed surrounding some lesions such as metastases and hepatocellular carcinoma.[100] While this finding may indicate tumor infiltration, it may also relate to parenchymal compression and/or proliferation of bile ducts surrounding the lesion.

Spatial resolution

The use of a rectangular matrix (e.g., 128×256) in conjunction with the large fields-of-view required for abdominal imaging (e.g., 38 to 45 cm) results in relatively large pixel sizes. While this is advantageous in terms of improving the signal-to-noise ratio and minimizing image acquisition time, spatial resolution is compromised. Therefore fine anatomic detail and detection of small hepatic and other lesions can be limited. A reasonable compromise between the need for adequate spatial resolution on the one hand and reasonable imaging time and signal-to-noise ratio on the other is to use an intermediate (e.g., 160 to 192×256) imaging matrix. When very small hepatic lesions are suspected, a high resolution (e.g., 256×256) matrix and reduced slice thickness should be considered.

Cross-excitation

Cross-excitation (also known as cross-talk) is due to the imperfections inherent to radiofrequency slice profiles. The radiofrequency pulses used for slice selection are not precisely confined to their intended position, and they produce some inadvertent excitation of adjacent tissues. This reduces the signal-to-noise ratio of these tissues and also limits tissue contrast.[62] Detection of liver lesions may be reduced as a result of both of these effects.[59,121] Cross-excitation can be minimized through several approaches. Image acquisition can be interleaved, so that contiguous images are acquired only after excited tissue has undergone complete relaxation. For example, slice numbers 1, 3, 5, 7, and 9 may be acquired initially, with slices 2, 4, 6, 8, and 10 acquired subsequently. The use of an appropriate interslice gap also reduces the effects of cross-excitation. A gap of 25% to 50% of the slice thickness (e.g., 8 mm slice with $\geq$ 2 mm gap) is desirable. Finally, some vendors offer sequences with specially crafted (i.e., square) radiofrequency pulses that reduce cross-excitation of adjacent tissues.

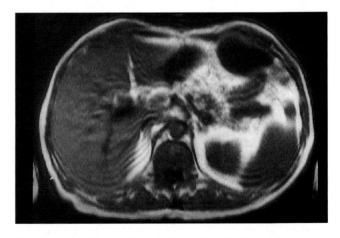

Fig. 5-53. Curvilinear foci of alternating high and low signal intensity are seen along the anterior abdominal wall, liver margin, and stomach, representing truncation artifacts on this transaxial T1-weighted rapid acquisition spin echo image.

Truncation artifacts

Truncation artifacts arise at high tissue contrast interfaces, such as along the anterior abdominal wall or along fat-soft tissue (i.e., viscera) interfaces. They are manifested primarily on images acquired using relatively low-resolution matrixes, such as 128 × 256 images, and are usually obscure on higher resolution images. These artifacts reflect the inability of the Fourier transform to accurately portray sharp transitions in tissue contrast. Truncation artifacts appear as curvilinear foci of alternating increased and decreased signal intensity, which are usually observed along the phase-encoded direction of the image (Figs. 5-53 to 5-54). Use of partial-Fourier reconstruction methods also accentuates truncation artifacts. Although these artifacts have the potential to simulate or obscure hepatic or other lesions, they are rarely of clinical importance in abdominal imaging.

Susceptibility artifacts

Metallic objects located in the vicinity of the liver can obscure hepatic lesions. Examples of extrinsic metal objects that can result in artifacts are keys, paper clips, or other ferromagnetic objects within the patient's pockets or beneath the patient within the magnet bore (Fig. 5-55). Intrinsic metal artifacts can arise from surgical clips, intravascular devices, or embolization coils that have been placed within the liver[8] (Figs. 5-56, A and B). Another source of susceptibility artifacts in abdominal imaging is air within the gastrointestinal tract (Figs. 5-57, A-C).

These entities can result in distortion of local magnetic field gradients and appear as regions of artifactual signal void with possible geometric distortion of anatomic features. In addition to obscuring lesions, susceptibility artifacts can potentially simulate low signal intensity hepatic lesions when they are small and relatively well defined (Figs. 5-57, A-C). Susceptibility artifacts are more severe on gradient echo images compared with spin echo images (Figs. 5-57, A-C) because gradient echo images lack a refocusing 180-degree radiofrequency pulse, which serves to partially correct for local field inhomogeneities caused by metallic objects. Susceptibility artifacts can be made less prominent on both spin echo and gradient echo pulse sequences with the use of a short echo time and small voxel sizes.

Other limitations in lesion detection

For low-contrast lesions, partial volume averaging of lesions with adjacent normal tissue is a dominant cause for poor detection. Therefore, the use of reduced slice thickness is important to detect such lesions. However, detection of high contrast lesions is affected by the thickness of the interslice gap to a greater degree than slice thickness.[10]

Even when imaging parameters are optimized and artifacts effectively controlled, all hepatic lesions are not consistently detected. MR is highly sensitive for detecting focal hepatic lesions, with sensitivities exceeding that of contrast enhanced computed tomography. However, computed tomography performed during arterial portography (CTAP) has demonstrated a greater number of liver lesions than MR in previous studies[45] (Figs. 5-58, A-C). While this relative limitation of MR may be remedied with further technical advances, at this time it is advised that CTAP be considered in addition to MR in patients in whom resection of hepatic metastases is being contemplated and in other exceptional circumstances.

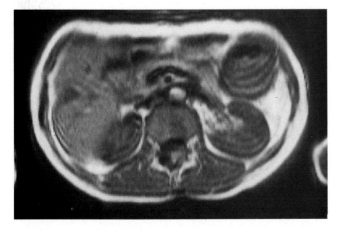

Fig. 5-54. Curvilinear foci of relative increased and decreased signal intensity are seen paralleling the abdominal wall and viscera. These findings represent truncation artifacts related to use of half-Fourier reconstruction.

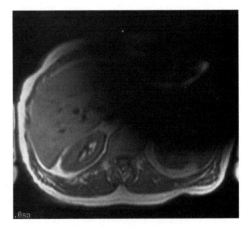

Fig. 5-55. A large signal void artifact obscures portions of the liver, spleen, left adrenal gland, and kidney on this transaxial T1-weighted image (TR 550, TE 12, 2 Nex). This was due to susceptibility artifact related to a metallic key in the patient's pocket.

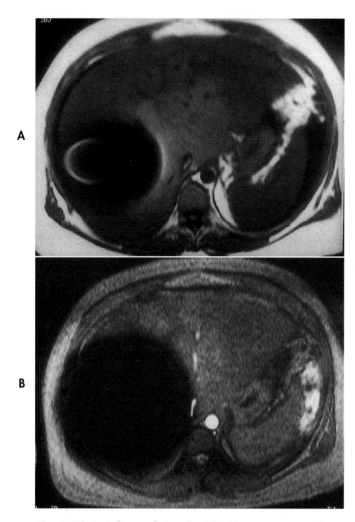

Fig. 5-56. A, A focus of signal void with some surrounding hyperintensity is seen on transaxial T1-weighted image, caused by emobilization coil within liver. Signal void artifact is accentuated on corresponding gradient echo image **(B)** in this patient with Budd-Chiari syndrome.

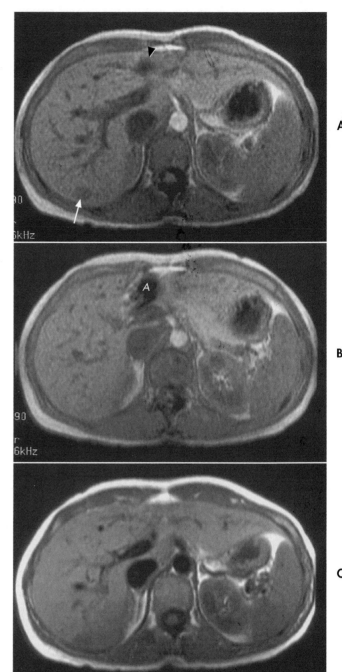

Fig. 5-57. A, Transaxial spoiled gradient echo image (TR 180, TE 4, 90-degree flip angle, 1 Nex) demonstrates lesion in posterior segment of right hepatic lobe *(arrow)*. There is also a second apparent lesion within the left hepatic lobe *(arrowhead)*. However, the latter finding is due to susceptibility artifact from out-of-plane air located within the gastric antrum. **B,** Image obtained 1 cm caudal demonstrates air within the gastric antrum *(A)*. **C,** The T1-weighted spin echo image corresponding to **A** demonstrates no evidence of a lesion in the left hepatic lobe.

Recently, some investigators have attempted to further increase the conspicuousness of hepatic lesions by performing rapid MR imaging during the bolus injection of paramagnetic contrast material into the superior mesenteric artery. This technique, known as MRAP (MR during arterial portography), has demonstrated metastatic lesions that were not evident on conventional spin echo images.[128]

Some hepatic lesions have signal intensity characteristics similar to those of normal liver parenchyma . For example, focal nodular hyperplasia is frequently isointense with surrounding hepatic parenchyma on both T1- and T2-weighted images[29a] (Figs. 5-59, *A* and *B*). As such, it may be difficult to identify focal nodular hyperplasia if a central scar is not evident.[37] Similar signal in-

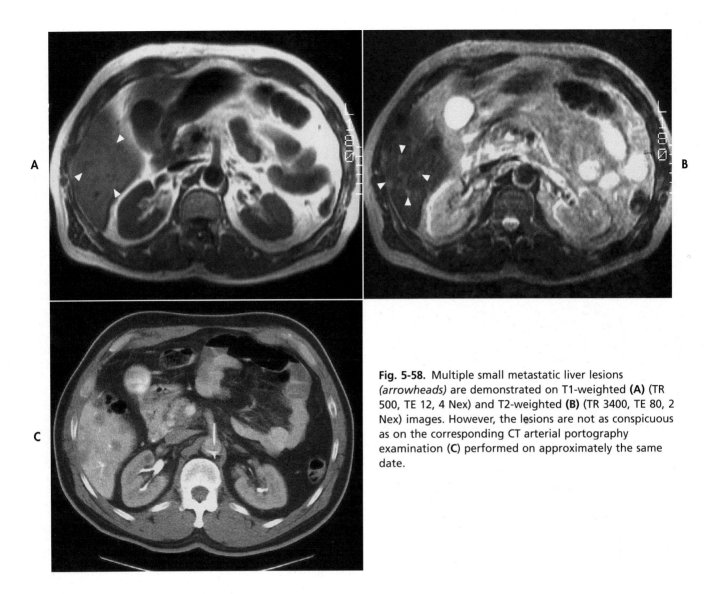

Fig. 5-58. Multiple small metastatic liver lesions *(arrowheads)* are demonstrated on T1-weighted **(A)** (TR 500, TE 12, 4 Nex) and T2-weighted **(B)** (TR 3400, TE 80, 2 Nex) images. However, the lesions are not as conspicuous as on the corresponding CT arterial portography examination **(C)** performed on approximately the same date.

> **CAUSES OF DIFFUSE HETEROGENEOUS HEPATIC SIGNAL INTENSITY**
>
> - Tumor involvement
> - Hepatitis
> - Cirrhosis
> - Infiltrative conditions
> - Passive congestion
> - Portal vein thrombosis
> - Budd-Chiari syndrome
> - Radiation hepatitis
> - Cholestasis
> - Fatty infiltration
> - Iron deposition

tensity characteristics can also be observed with hepatic adenomas.[101]

In patients with sarcoidosis, hepatic involvement can be difficult to visualize, since granulomas may be isointense to slightly hypointense relative to liver parenchyma on T2-weighted images. Hepatic peliosis is another condition that may simulate a mass lesion.[78]

Difficulties Related to Lesion Characterization

In addition to allowing for detection of liver lesions, MR also assists in characterizing some liver lesions based on their signal intensity patterns. These signal patterns are most frequently used to differentiate benign cavernous hemangiomas and cysts from malignancies. There are a number of important pitfalls related to hepatic lesion characterization.

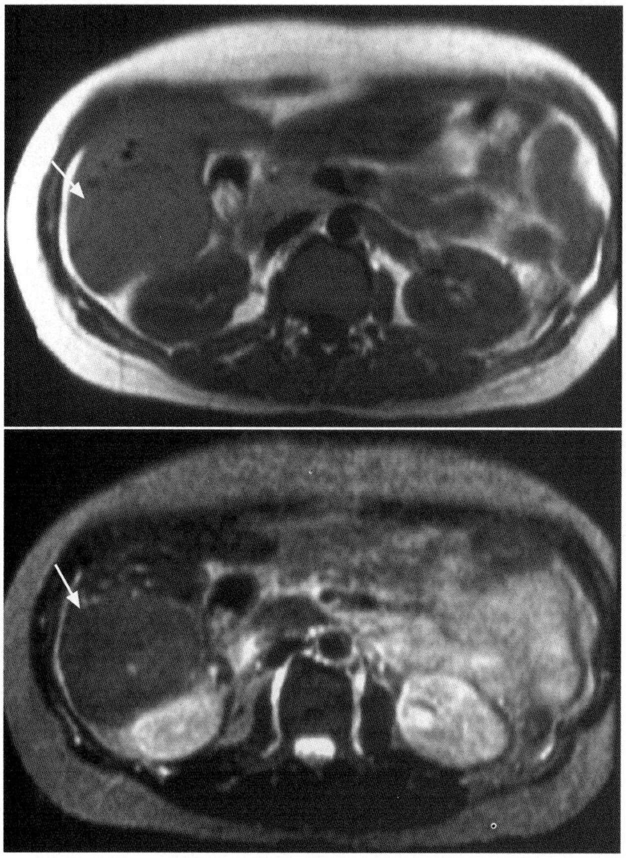

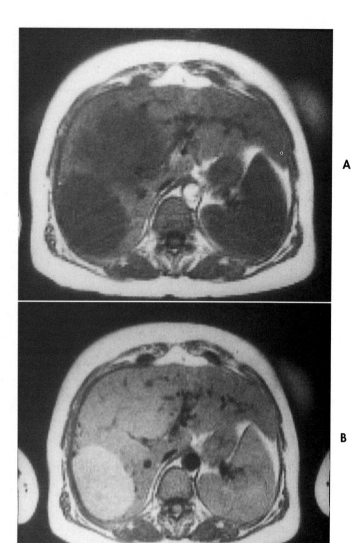

Fig. 5-59. A large lesion within the posterior segment of the right hepatic lobe *(arrow)* is difficult to visualize on transaxial T1-weighted **(A)** (TR 500, TE 12, 4 Nex) and T2-weighted **(B)** (TR 3400, TE 120, 2 Nex) images, because of isointensity with surrounding hepatic parenchyma. This lesion represents focal nodular hyperplasia. A tiny focus of relative increased signal intensity is seen centrally on the T2-weighted image, compatible with central scar.

Fig. 5-60. A, Transaxial T1-weighted image demonstrates two focal hepatic lesions. While the lesions are isointense with one another as well as with splenic parenchyma, the more anterior lesion demonstrates a more irregular contour. **B,** Corresponding proton density–weighted image reveals the anterior lesion to be isointense with surrounding hepatic parenchyma, resulting in difficulty in its visualization. However, the more posterior lesion is considerably hyperintense relative to liver parenchyma and spleen. The more anterior lesion represents a metastasis, whereas the posterior lesion is a cavernous hemangioma.

Pulse sequence parameters

Markedly prolonged T2 relaxation reflects the fluid-like nature of cavernous hemangiomas and cysts and contrasts with the moderately prolonged T2 relaxation that is typical of most metastases. Although T1 relaxation characteristics generally parallel alterations in T2 relaxation, distinction between benign and malignant hepatic lesions is not reliably accomplished using T1-weighted images (Fig. 5-60). Conventional T2-weighted pulse sequences of the abdomen are typically acquired using first and second echo times of approximately 40 and 80 msec, respectively. However, liver lesions cannot be reliably characterized on images acquired with these parameters because these modest echo times do not allow sufficient expression of differences in lesion T2 relaxation.[135] While an echo time of 70 to 90 msec may be suitable for hepatic lesion detection, characterization of hepatic lesions requires prolonged echo times on the order of 120 to 160 msec (Figs. 5-61, *A* and *B*). Cysts/hemangiomas and metastases can have similar signal intensity on a modestly T2-weighted image, whereas a heavily T2-weighted image will depict these benign lesions as mark-

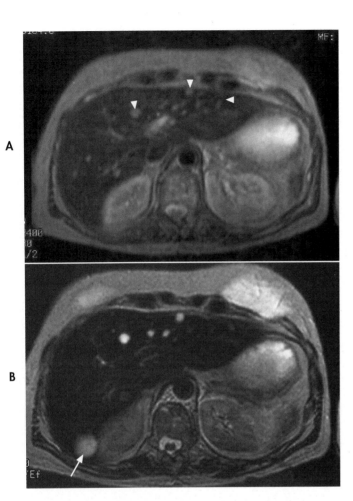

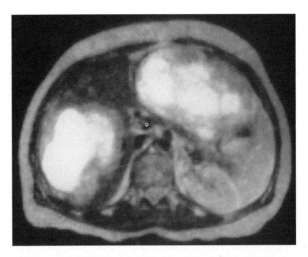

Fig. 5-62. Transaxial T2-weighted image demonstrates two large hepatic lesions, one located in the right lobe and the other in the left lobe. These lesions are markedly hyperintense and relatively well defined, features suggestive of cavernous hemangiomas. However, there is significant heterogeneous signal intensity involving both lesions with apparent soft tissue components along the periphery of the lesions. These lesions represent necrotic vascular metastases secondary to leiomyosarcoma.

Fig. 5-61. A, Several lesions are noted in the left hepatic lobe *(arrowheads)* on transaxial T2-weighted image (TR 3400, TE 80, 2 Nex). The lesions are approximately isointense with renal parenchyma and most suggestive of metastatic foci. **B,** Corresponding heavily T2-weighted fast spin echo image (TR 6000, effective TE 200, 4 Nex, 16 echo train) reveals the lesions to be markedly hyperintense (isointense with fluid), indicating that they represent hepatic cysts. There is a marked discrepancy between the signal intensity of these lesions and that of the kidneys on the prolonged TE image. A larger cyst located in the right hepatic lobe (arrow) demonstrates intermediate signal intensity, suggestive of metastasis, as a result of partial volume averaging with adjacent hepatic parenchyma. All of the lesions were confirmed as cysts by comparison with previous CT examinations.

edly hyperintense relative to most malignant lesions. While heavily T2-weighted images are important for lesion characterization, they have a reduced signal-to-noise ratio that accentuates motion artifacts and limits visualization of many malignant lesions.[25] Thus, acquisition of a moderately T2-weighted image (e.g., TE 70 to 90 msec) remains necessary for complete evaluation of the liver.

Cavernous hemangiomas and cysts can be difficult to differentiate, though such distinction is of limited clinical relevance. The use of a short echo time (e.g., 20 msec) on the first echo of a long TR sequence causes most cysts to be hypointense relative to surrounding liver parenchyma because of their markedly prolonged T1 relaxation values. Conversely, hemangiomas will be hyperintense relative to the liver using these parameters[12,115,141] (Fig. 5-62). Evaluation of contrast material enhancement patterns also allows these entities to be differentiated (discussed below).

Vascular malignancies

Highly vascular and/or necrotic hepatic metastases can demonstrate signal characteristics similar to those of cavernous hemangiomas or cysts[67,69,115,141] (Figs. 5-62 to 5-63, *B*). Representative lesions in this category include metastatic adenocarcinoma of renal, thyroid, or ovarian origin, pancreatic islet cell carcinoma, and melanoma or leiomyosarcoma. Rarely, hepatocellular carcinoma demonstrates markedly long T2 relaxation suggestive of cavernous hemangioma.[102] This can occur with tumors of the pseudoglandular type, with long T2 characteristics due to fluid filled acinar spaces. Conversely, some hepatic cysts or hemangiomas can demonstrate atypical focal or diffuse relative decreased signal intensity which results in confusion for malignancy (Fig. 5-64). These findings may result from proteinaceous

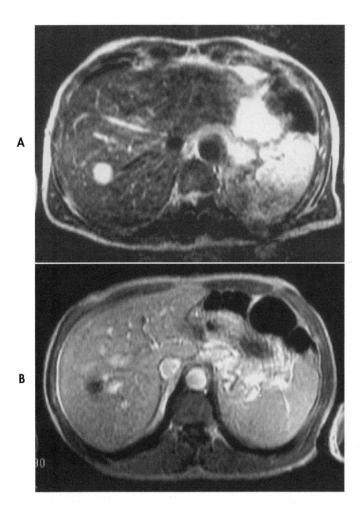

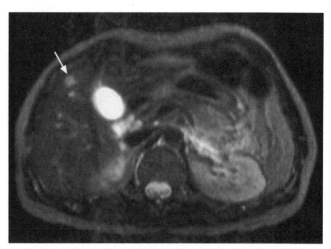

Fig. 5-64. Heavily T2-weighted image (TR 3400, TE 120, 2 Nex) depicts 1 cm lesion in medial segment of left hepatic lobe *(arrow).* The lesion is hypointense relative to fluid within the gallbladder and thecal sac, findings suggestive of malignancy. However, additional breath hold gradient echo images obtained following contrast material administration, as well as corresponding CT images, verified that this represented a hepatic cyst. Atypical signal intensity features on T2-weighted imaging are due to small lesion size leading to partial volume averaging with adjacent liver parenchyma as well as phase shifts related to respiratory motion.

Fig. 5-63. A, Transaxial T2-weighted image (TR 3300, TE 80, 2 Nex) depicts a uniformly hyperintense and relatively well-defined lesion within right hepatic lobe. **B,** Contrast-enhanced gradient echo image (TR 160, TE 4, 90-degree flip angle, 1 Nex) reveals contrast enhancement behavior consistent with necrotic metastasis in patient with recurrent rectal carcinoma.

and/or hemorrhagic contents within the lesion or from signal loss resulting from motion.

Biliary hamartomas

Biliary hamartomas are another type of lesion that demonstrates marked hyperintensity on T2-weighted images because of fluid contained within ductules.[127] These lesions, which are usually rounded and have well-defined margins, may be multiple and can be difficult to distinguish from hepatic cysts and cavernous hemangiomas. Areas of relative decreased signal intensity may represent fibrous stroma.

Image display settings

Image display settings (i.e., window width and level settings) can influence the perceived signal intensity of

hepatic and other lesions. A consistent method for photographing MR images should be established, so that standards of reference for expected signal intensity characteristics of various tissues can be developed.[55]

Alterations in background liver signal intensity

The perceived signal intensity of a liver lesion reflects the signal intensity of the lesion relative to surrounding hepatic parenchyma. This can lead to diagnostic difficulties, since the signal intensity of hepatic parenchyma can be variable. There are biologic variations in hepatic T2 relaxation values that exist among individuals. The liver is also a metabolically active organ that can undergo dramatic alteration in T2 relaxation within a given individual. For example, the signal intensity of hepatic tissue can be markedly reduced on T2-weighted images because of iron deposition. These may be encountered in patients who have received previous transfusions (hemosiderosis) or in patients with hereditary hemochromatosis. In such cases the liver will usually have a signal intensity less than that of skeletal muscle on T2-weighted images.[93]

A number of conditions including hepatitis, hepatic congestion, and fatty infiltration can lead to a diffuse increase in hepatic signal intensity on T2-weighted images.

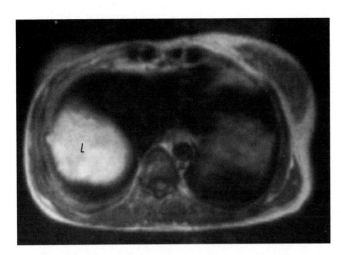

Fig. 5-65. Transaxial T2-weighted image shows well-defined lesion in the hepatic dome (*L*), which appears markedly hyperintense as compared with surrounding liver parenchyma. While these findings suggest cavernous hemangioma, this represents a metastatic lesion. Apparent hyperintensity of the lesion is due to reduced signal intensity of surrounding liver parenchyma secondary to iron overload. (Reprinted from Mirowitz SA, Heiken JP, Lee JKT: J Comput Assist Tomogr 12:323-325, 1988.)

These metabolic alterations in liver signal intensity can influence the apparent signal intensity of focal hepatic lesions. For example, a metastatic lesion arising in a liver affected by iron overload may be misdiagnosed as a benign cyst or hemangioma because it appears markedly hyperintense relative to surrounding hepatic tissue (Fig. 5-65).[36,82] Conversely, high signal intensity benign lesions may be perceived as less intense in a patient with hepatic inflammation or fatty infiltration. Ratios of lesion signal intensity/hepatic signal intensity have been proposed as quantitative indexes for standardizing lesion characterization. Spurious results will also be obtained using such indexes in patients with diffuse hepatic signal alterations.[82] Such ratios are more effective when they utilize tissues that are less vulnerable to metabolic signal alterations, such as fat or skeletal muscle, as reference standards.

Relaxation values

Lesion characterization can also be attempted by calculating lesion T2 relaxation time, though this requires that cumbersome calculations be performed. Reference values for various lesions should be developed at individual imaging sites because of the effect of site-specific hardware and software on expressed T2 differences. There is some overlap in T2 relaxation values between some benign lesions and metastases. A more practical approach in most clinical settings involves the qualitative comparison of lesion signal intensity to reliable internal standards. For example, a lesion that is isointense with

bile or cerebrospinal fluid on a heavily T2-weighted image can usually be considered to represent a cyst or cavernous hemangioma. Malignant hepatic lesions, on the other hand, frequently demonstrate signal intensity characteristics similar to that of splenic tissue. However, like the liver, the spleen is also metabolically active and subject to signal intensity variations that may render this comparison inaccurate.

Contrast agents

Paramagnetic contrast agents such as gadopentetate dimeglumine offer yet another approach to characterization of liver lesions. Cavernous hemangiomas classically demonstrate nodular peripheral enhancement during the bolus phase of contrast material administration, with subsequent progressive centripetal lesion enhancement (Figs. 5-66, *A-C*). This is followed by diffuse retention of contrast material throughout the lesion on delayed images. The nodular appearance of cavernous hemangiomas can suggest the diagnosis of malignancy. Hepatic cysts, on the other hand, are avascular and do not enhance with contrast material.

Metastatic lesions most frequently demonstrate a peripheral enhancing halo on equilibrium phase images (Figs. 5-67, *A* and *B*). However, a ring enhancement pattern is not specific for metastatic lesions; this pattern can also be associated with hepatocellular carcinoma, hepatic abscess, and other lesions.[23,32,54,58,112] Moreover, the enhancement pattern of metastases varies according to their histologic type and tissue of origin, vascularity, necrosis, and other factors. Some metastatic foci demonstrate initial peripheral nodular enhancement and may appear to fill in with contrast material on delayed images, simulating the appearance of cavernous hemangiomas.[135] While such cases are rather unusual, their occurrence mandates that contrast enhancement patterns be closely compared with signal intensity features when lesions are characterized. Marked diffuse nodular enhancement during the bolus phase of contrast material administration can be observed with hepatic adenomas and focal nodular hyperplasia.[123] Intrahepatic cholangiocarcinoma frequently demonstrates initial peripheral contrast enhancement, with subsequent centripetal enhancement similar to cavernous hemangioma (Fig. 5-68).[27] However, unlike hemangiomas, cholangiocarcinomas rarely demonstrate complete opacification on delayed images.

The enhancement patterns of vascular hepatic malignancies such as hepatocellular carcinoma, vascular metastases, and cholangiocarcinoma can also appear similar to that demonstrated by focal nodular hyperplasia.[72] In both situations, prominent enhancement can be observed during the bolus phase. Delayed images following contrast material administration frequently demonstrate a central scar in patients with focal nodular hy-

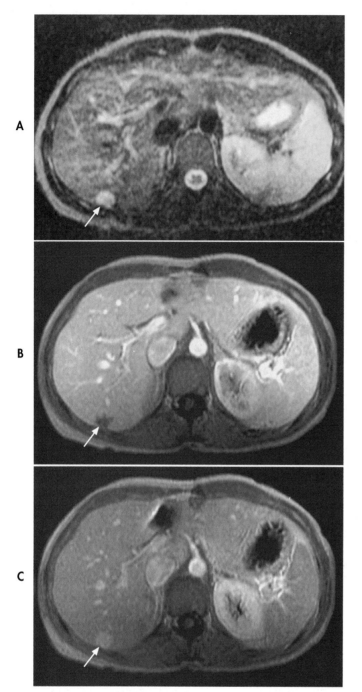

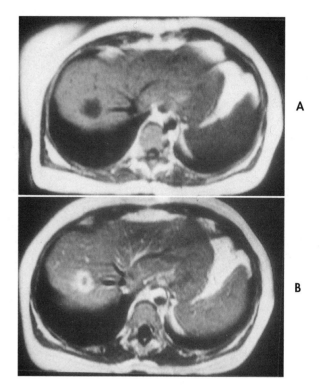

Fig. 5-67. Transaxial T1-weighted rapid acquisition spin echo images obtained before **(A)** and after **(B)** bolus injection of gadolinium chelate contrast material. A 2 cm breast cancer metastasis in the hepatic dome demonstrates prominent ringlike contrast enhancement pattern. (Reprinted from Mirowitz SA, Lee JKT: Radiology 179:612-614, 1991.)

Fig. 5-66. A, Heavily T2-weighted image (TR 3400, TE 120, 2 Nex) demonstrates rounded lesion in posterior segment of right hepatic lobe *(arrow)*. The lesion demonstrates signal intensity equivalent to that of spleen and less than that of fluid within the spinal canal or stomach. The above signal intensity characteristics are most suggestive of malignancy. However, dynamic gadolinium chelate–enhanced rapid gradient echo images (TR 180, TE 4, 90-degree flip angle, 1 Nex) obtained during **(B)** and several minutes following **(C)** bolus contrast material injection depict immediate nodular peripheral enhancement with subsequent centripetal fill-in of the lesion and prolonged contrast material retention. These findings are characteristic for cavernous hemangioma, despite the atypical signal intensity appearance on T2-weighted image.

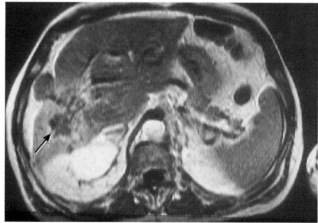

Fig. 5-68. Transaxial T1-weighted rapid acquisition spin echo image obtained 1 minute following bolus injection of gadolinium chelate contrast material. A large mass is present in the posterior segment of the right hepatic lobe *(arrow)*. There is contrast material enhancement along the periphery of the lesion with apparent centripetal fill-in. Although these latter findings are suggestive of cavernous hemangioma, the irregular margination of the lesion and associated hepatic atrophy and umbilication are not. This lesion represents an intrahepatic cholangiocarcinoma. (Reprinted from Mirowitz SA, Lee JKT: Radiology 179:612-614, 1991.)

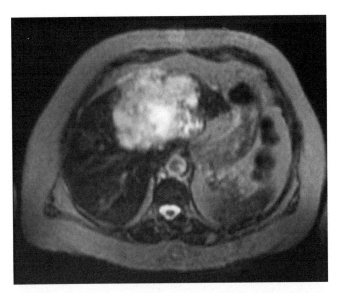

Fig. 5-69. Transaxial T2-weighted image (TR 3400, TE 120, 2 Nex) demonstrates large heterogeneous mass in left hepatic lobe. The majority of the lesion is hypointense relative to CSF, though this was proven to represent a giant cavernous hemangioma on subsequent tagged red blood cell scintigraphy.

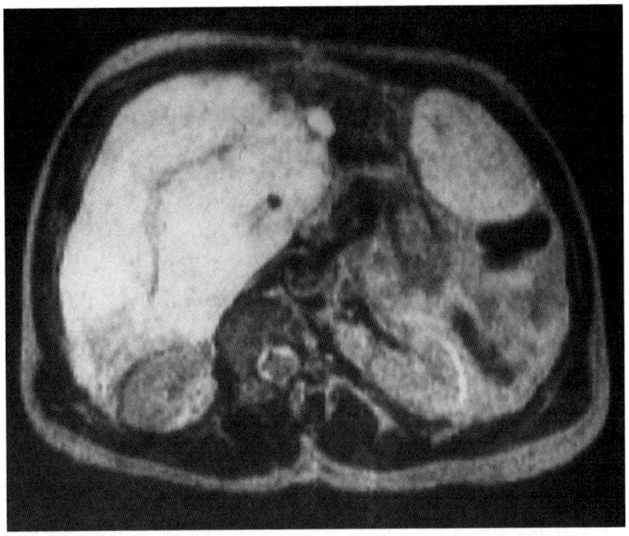

Fig. 5-70. Transaxial T2-weighted image demonstrates giant cavernous hemangioma of the liver. The lesion is markedly hyperintense, although some strandlike soft tissue components are present centrally. A second hemangioma is also evident within the left hepatic lobe.

perplasia. Visualization of such a central scar is rare with malignant lesions, but may occasionally occur.[72]

Lesion morphology

Characterization of liver lesions should also include evaluation of the morphology and internal architecture of the lesion. Benign lesions are usually rounded and have smooth, regular borders. They typically demonstrate uniform signal intensity and lack internal septations or nodules. On the other hand, malignant liver lesions often can have irregular and ill-defined margins, heterogeneous internal signal intensity, and internal soft tissue components. On occasion, cavernous hemangiomas can demonstrate morphologic features that are suggestive of malignancy. They may have a lobular contour, though their margins usually remain smooth and are well defined. Large (i.e., giant) cavernous hemangiomas can have markedly heterogeneous signal characteristics and prominent internal septations that may suggest malignancy[9,17,69,114,115] (Figs. 5-69 and 5-70).

Another morphologic feature that may be useful for characterizing hepatic lesions is observation of retraction of the hepatic capsule overlying the lesion with associated umbilication of the nodular lesion itself. These findings have usually been associated with epithelioid hemangioendothelioma, a rare tumor. However, similar findings have been observed in association with a variety of hepatic metastases that have undergone necrosis and have a desmoplastic reaction.[106] Focal atrophy of liver parenchyma, as occurs in patients with cholangiocarcinoma, can also simulate this finding.[106]

Peritumoral signal intensity alterations

A peripheral ring of peritumoral increased signal intensity can be seen surrounding hepatic metastases on T2-weighted images. These signal intensity alterations often reflect edema, which may be reactive or a result of vascular obstruction, but may contain microscopic tumor invasion.[64,105,115,141] Observation of a peripheral rim of decreased signal intensity may indicate a capsule or pseudocapsule, which is most frequently associated with hepatocellular carcinoma. It has been recognized, however, that both of these features are nonspecific and can be observed with a variety of hepatic lesions.[39,105,115,117,138] For example, a pseudocapsule can occasionally be seen in association with focal nodular hyperplasia.[137]

Similarly, a central stellate region of aberrant signal intensity is classically associated with focal nodular hyperplasia, though malignant lesions can also demonstrate similar findings.[77,115,116,120,132,140] Central scars can be found in association with hepatic adenoma, hepatocellular carcinoma, cholangiocarcinoma, fibrolamellar hepatocellular carcinoma, and giant cavernous hemangioma.[27,37] It has been reported that the central scar associated with fibrolamellar hepatocellular carcinoma often remains hypointense on T2-weighted images, whereas the scar of focal nodular hyperplasia is usually hyperintense.[133] However, this criterion is probably unreliable, since focal nodular hyperplasia may also have an hypointense central scar in some patients.[137]

Focal areas of abnormal hepatic signal intensity can result from vascular obstruction.[50] Areas of abnormal signal intensity can also be observed in patients who have undergone recent partial hepatectomy.[4]

Focal nodular hyperplasia is usually isointense with surrounding liver parenchyma on all pulse sequences. Hepatic adenoma can demonstrate similar signal characteristics.[101] Therefore, these hepatocellular lesions may be difficult to distinguish from one another. Atypical signal intensity features can be associated with focal nodular hyperplasia, including mild hyperintensity on T2-weighted images[37] or hypointensity on T1-weighted images.[26] In fact, atypical features may be observed in at least half of focal nodular hyperplasia lesions. In one series, for example, a central scar was observed in only one of ten patients.[37]

Partial volume effects

Many artifacts can alter the apparent signal intensity of hepatic lesions, resulting in potential misdiagnosis. Partial volume averaging of small cysts or cavernous hemangiomas with adjacent liver parenchyma can cause such benign lesions to simulate malignancy[11,55] (Figs. 5-61, A and B, 5-64, and 5-71, A and B). Therefore characterization of hepatic lesions less than 1 cm in diameter can be less than reliable. Partial volume effects can be countered with the use of reduced section thickness, though signal-to-noise ratio will suffer, and imaging time will be prolonged. Acquisition of images in the coronal or sagittal planes can also be useful for depicting and characterizing some small lesions.

Cross-excitation

Cross-excitation can cause artifactual reduced signal intensity of hepatic lesions, because complete recovery of magnetization between successive radiofrequency excitations does not occur. Respiratory-induced motion of the liver or transmitted cardiac pulsations can cause phase shifts, which lead to artifactual decreases in lesion signal intensity. The latter situation usually affects lesions within the left hepatic lobe.

Opposed magnetization artifact

Short tau inversion recovery (STIR) images are often utilized for detection of hepatic lesions. A thin dark line can be observed along the boundary of tissues of different signal intensity on inversion recovery images.[44]

Regenerative nodules

Regenerative nodules can arise in patients with hepatic cirrhosis. The signal intensity of regenerative nodules is variable, though they are usually hypointense on T2-weighted images. This is due to the iron they contain

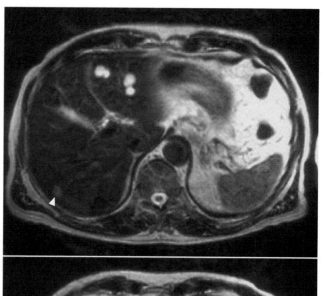

A

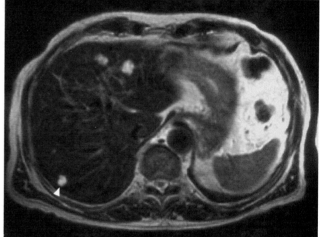

B

Fig. 5-71. A, Transaxial T2-weighted fast spin echo image (TR 4000, effective TE 120, 4 Nex, 16 echo train) depicts cluster of markedly hyperintense cysts in left lobe of liver. There is a moderately intense lesion within the posterior segment of the right lobe, suggestive of metastasis *(arrowhead).* However, this lesion also represented a cyst, with relative decreased signal intensity resulting from partial volume averaging with adjacent liver parenchyma, as depicted on adjacent image **(B).**

as well as to the abnormal increased signal intensity of the cirrhotic liver in which they arise.[93,97,103] The presence of iron can obscure septations within regenerative nodules on T2-weighted and gradient echo images.[93] Although low signal intensity on T2-weighted images is usually seen with siderotic regenerative nodules, hemorrhagic hepatocellular carcinoma or hepatocellular carcinoma arising within a regenerative nodule can present with similar findings.[76,103] A "nodule within a nodule" appearance has been observed in the latter situation.[89] Some regenerative nodules can appear hyperintense on T2-weighted images; however, this finding is suggestive of hepatocellular carcinoma.[93] Regenerative nodules can also have variable signal intensity on T1-weighted images, ranging from hypointense to hyperintense.[60]

Posttherapeutic changes

The signal intensity of hepatic lesions can be altered as a result of medical intervention. For example, decrease in T1 relaxation has been recorded for lesions responding to interferon, whereas this parameter was unaltered in unresponsive lesions.[1,2] Alterations in T2 relaxation were found ineffective for monitoring response in this study. It was proposed that MR signal patterns can be used in conjunction with serial measurements of lesion size to monitor response of hepatic metastases to chemotherapy. Alterations in lesion signal intensity have also been reported following transcatheter chemoembolization of hepatic metastases.[146] T2-weighted images display either an increase or decrease in signal intensity from liquefactive or coagulative tumor necrosis, respectively. A peripheral rim of abnormal signal intensity also frequently surrounds the lesions, representing edema or granulation tissue.

High-intensity lesions on T1-weighted images

Most hepatic lesions are hypointense relative to liver parenchyma on T1-weighted images. Consequently, T1-weighted images are used primarily for detection rather than characterization of liver lesions. However, liver lesions occasionally demonstrate hyperintensity on T1-weighted images (Fig. 5-72, A and B). One cause for increased hepatic signal intensity on T1-weighted images is the presence of fat. While this is most frequently due to focal fatty infiltration, other entities including hepatic adenoma, lipoma, angiomyolipoma, focal nodular hyperplasia, and regenerative nodules can also contain fat.* Surgical defects within the liver may be packed with omental fat.[63] The presence of fat does not indicate that a hepatic lesion is benign, since fatty degeneration may be associated with hepatocellular carcinoma (Figs. 5-73 and 5-74). Hepatocellular carcinoma can also contain paramagnetic copper, which, like fat, results in T1 shortening.[23,58] Fat-suppressed T1-weighted pulse sequences can be used to distinguish these entities. Mitchell et al[87] documented fat as the cause of hyperintensity in only one of five hepatocellular carcinomas that were hyperintense on T1-weighted images.

Blood breakdown products (i.e., methemoglobin) can also result in hyperintensity on T1-weighted images. In the liver, this may be related to posttraumatic or postbiopsy/postsurgical hematomas, hemorrhagic tumors, or thrombosed vessels or aneurysms (Fig. 5-75, A and B). Metastatic melanoma can appear hyperintense on T1-

*References 23, 32, 54, 58, 63, 73, 87, 112.

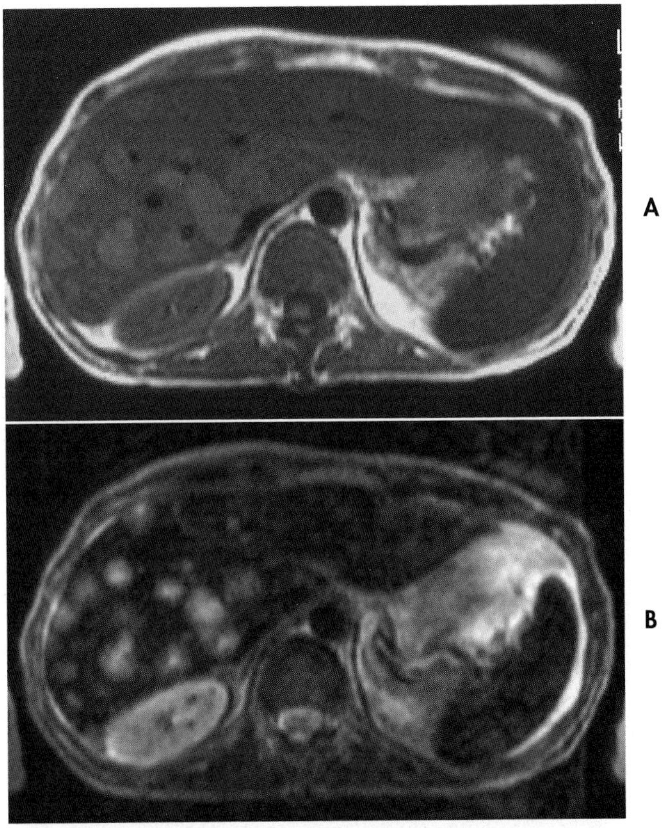

Fig. 5-72. T1-weighted **(A)** (TR 550, TE 12, 4 Nex) and T2-weighted **(B)** (TR 2700, TE 80, 2 Nex) images in patient with breast carcinoma. Multiple metastatic lesions are noted throughout the liver. The lesions appear hyperintense on T1-weighted image relative to the liver, which is of decreased signal intensity because of severe hemosiderosis secondary to previous blood transfusions. The T2-weighted image shows signal intensity loss throughout the liver, spleen, and bone marrow.

weighted images because of the paramagnetic effects of melanin or on the basis of tumoral hemorrhage[23,32,54,58,112] (Fig. 5-76). Cystic liver lesions (e.g., cystic neoplasm, abscess) can be hyperintense on T1-weighted images as a result of proteinaceous contents.

Abnormal decreased signal intensity of the liver on T1-weighted images can occur because of iron overload or hepatic congestion. In this setting, focal liver lesions can appear artifactually hyperintense in the absence of associated hemorrhage or other factors already described.[36]

Diffuse Lesions
Normal appearance

The liver has a T1 relaxation time considerably shorter than that of other abdominal organs (e.g., spleen, kidneys). This is attributed to its high concentration of endoplasmic reticulum and associated proteins.[93] As a re-

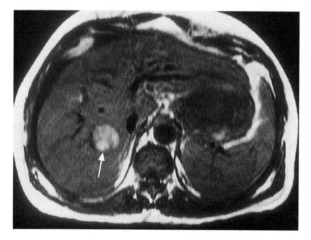

Fig. 5-73. Transaxial T1-weighted image depicts large mass occupying right hepatic lobe. The mass is largely hypointense, though foci of moderate increased signal intensity are noted within its posterior aspect *(arrow)*. The latter findings reflect fatty degeneration within a large hepatocellular carcinoma.

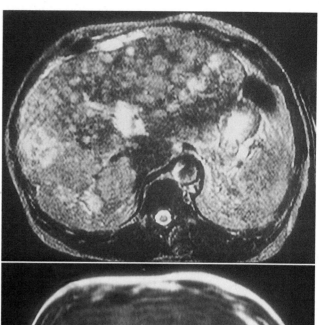

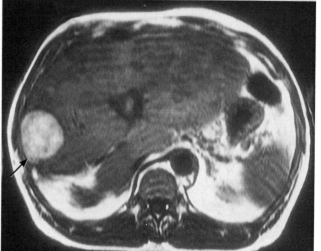

Fig. 5-74. Transaxial T1-weighted image demonstrates hyperintense lesion in right hepatic lobe *(arrow)*, representing fatty degeneration within a hepatocellular carcinoma.

Fig. 5-75. Transaxial T2-weighted **(A)** and T1-weighted **(B)** images at different levels in patient with metastatic carcinoma. There are numerous metastases involving the liver, most of which are better visualized on T2-weighted rather than T1-weighted images. However, a large lesion in posterior segment of right hepatic lobe *(arrow)* demonstrates markedly increased signal intensity on T1-weighted image, as a result of tumoral hemorrhage.

sult, the liver is hyperintense relative to most other abdominal organs on T1-weighted images. Conversely, the liver has a hypointense appearance on T2-weighted images.

Alterations with aging and medication

The T1 relaxation time of hepatic parenchyma decreases with aging.[111] The T1 relaxation of hepatic tissue can be prolonged in women taking oral contraceptives. Irregular foci of variable increased and decreased signal intensity can also be observed in this population, and patchy areas of abnormal contrast material enhancement may occur. These findings can simulate focal liver lesions.

Diffuse heterogeneous signal intensity alterations

The liver can demonstrate diffuse heterogeneous signal intensity alterations in patients with hepatitis, cirrhosis, infiltrative diseases, and vascular conditions such as passive congestion, portal vein thrombosis, and Budd-Chiari syndrome (Fig. 5-77). Radiation therapy and chemotherapy are iatrogenic causes of heterogeneous hepatic signal intensity.[4] Radiation hepatitis can lead to increased signal intensity of the affected portion of the liver on T2-weighted images. These findings have been observed as early as 7 days following initiation of radiation therapy, though there is usually a considerably longer delay.[143] Such signal intensity alterations often re-

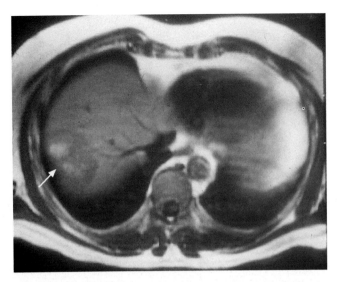

Fig. 5-76. Transaxial T1-weighted image demonstrates melanoma metastasis in hepatic dome *(arrow)*. The lesion is of relative increased signal intensity centrally, because of the paramagnetic effects of melanin and/or intratumoral hemorrhage.

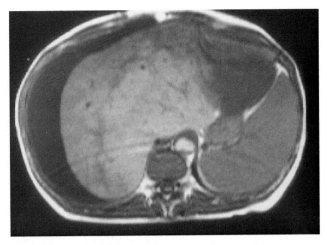

Fig. 5-77. Transaxial T1-weighted image depicts markedly heterogeneous signal intensity throughout the liver parenchyma in patient with Budd-Chiari syndrome. Note that the inferior vena cava and hepatic veins are not visualized. Patient also demonstrates considerable ascites.

solve after approximately 2 months. Areas of diffuse increased signal intensity can result from infiltration of the hepatic parenchyma due to lymphoma or metastatic disease as well as cholestasis, chronic hepatitis, cirrhosis, hepatic congestion, and Budd-Chiari syndrome.[73]

Iron overload

Hepatic iron overload leads to diffuse reduction in signal intensity, particularly on T2-weighted spin echo or gradient echo images. This finding is most frequently observed in patients with hemosiderosis because of previous blood transfusions. Similar findings are also observed in patients with hereditary hemochromatosis. These entities cannot be distinguished through evaluation of the liver alone; other organs must be evaluated for associated signal abnormalities. In patients with hemosiderosis, iron deposition occurs within the reticuloendothelial system. Therefore reduced signal intensity is also observed throughout the spleen[124] (Figs. 5-78, A to 5-79). Hereditary hemochromatosis leads to hepatocellular accumulation of iron as well as possible deposition within other organs such as the pancreas, heart, testes, and pituitary gland. It may be difficult to subjectively determine the presence of hepatic iron overload; therefore, quantitative indexes have been proposed. A liver/fat signal intensity ratio less than 0.29 or 0.21 on T1-weighted or T2-weighted images, respectively, has been used to indicate iron overload.[81] These indexes should be individualized according to the field strength at which imaging is performed, as well as for the particular pulse sequence implemented. Another cause for diffuse decreased signal intensity of the hepatic parenchyma is in-

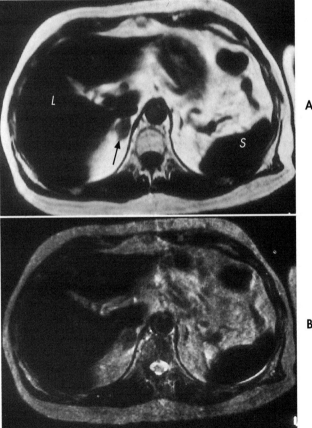

Fig. 5-78. Transaxial T1-weighted **(A)** and T2-weighted **(B)** images show uniform hypointensity throughout liver *(L)* and spleen *(S)* parenchyma as a result of hemosiderosis. A small adenoma of the right adrenal gland is also demonstrated *(arrow)*.

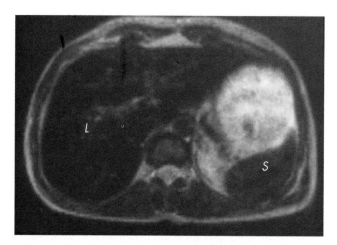

Fig. 5-79. Transaxial T2-weighted image demonstrates uniform hypointensity throughout the liver (*L*) and spleen (*S*) parenchyma in patient with hemosiderosis.

travascular hemolysis, which occurs in patients with paroxysmal nocturnal hemoglobinuria.[124]

The presence of segmental portal venous obstruction can result in focal increased deposition of iron within the parenchyma of the obstructed segment.[57] Vascular obstruction can also cause decreased fat deposition within the affected territory.

Fatty infiltration

Conventional spin echo images are relatively insensitive to depiction of diffuse fatty infiltration of the liver[61,93] (Figs. 5-80, *A-C*). Phase contrast images can be acquired using gradient echo sequences with an appropriate field strength–dependent echo time. Opposed phase images demonstrate decreased signal intensity for voxels containing both water and fat. Consequently, decreased hepatic signal intensity is present in regions affected by fatty infiltration (Fig. 5-84). Decreased signal intensity can also occur on phase contrast gradient echo images as a result of hepatic iron overload. Diffuse fatty infiltration of the hepatic parenchyma can cause the liver to appear hypointense relative to the spleen on a T1-weighted opposed phase image, which is the reverse of the usual situation (Figs. 5-81, *A* and *B*). These entities can be distinguished by noting hepatic signal intensity on T2-weighted spin echo images, with hypointensity indicating iron overload.[93] The use of hepatocellular contrast agents such as manganese-DPDP has not been useful in mapping the distribution of hepatic fatty infiltration.[61] The liver can appear diffusely hyperintense on T1-weighted images acquired by using fat saturation. Diffuse decreased signal intensity throughout the liver and other abdominal organs can occur because of poor penetration of radiofrequency energy, which may be re-

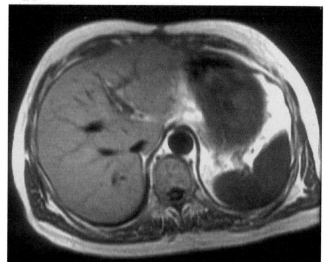

A

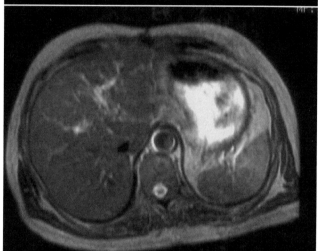

B

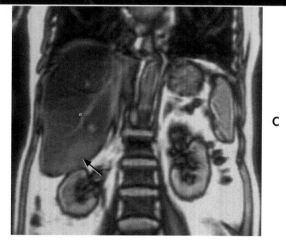

C

Fig. 5-80. Transaxial T1-weighted **(A)** (TR 500, TE 12, 4 Nex) and T2-weighted **(B)** (TR 3400, TE 80, 2 Nex) spin echo images fail to demonstrate signal intensity abnormalities in patient with hepatic fatty infiltration on CT. **C,** Corresponding opposed phase gradient echo image (TR 113, TE 2.6, 90-degree flip angle, 1 Nex) shows marked signal intensity loss throughout liver, reflecting fatty infiltration, with relative sparing peripherally *(arrow)*.

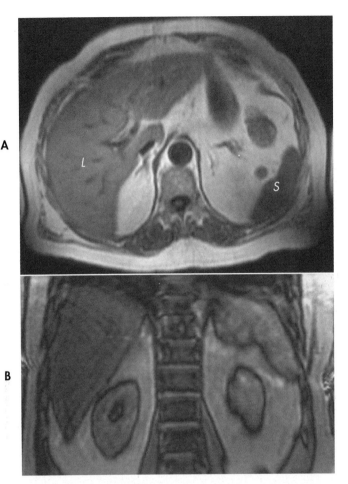

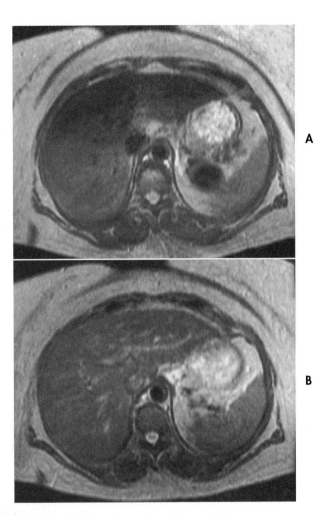

Fig. 5-81. A, Transaxial T1-weighted image (TR 500, TE 12, 4 Nex) demonstrates hyperintensity of the liver (L) relative to the spleen (S), which is normal signal intensity relationship. **B,** Opposed phase coronal T1-weighted gradient echo image (TR 113, TE 2.6, 90-degree flip angle, 1 Nex) shows reversal of liver-spleen signal intensity relationship with relative hypointensity of the liver as compared with the spleen. These findings are due to diffuse hepatic fatty infiltration.

Fig. 5-82. A, Heterogeneous signal intensity is present throughout the liver on transaxial T2-weighted image (TR 3400, TE 80, 2 Nex), with relative decreased signal intensity of left hepatic lobe. This is due to hardware failure resulting in poor radiofrequency penetration. **B,** Repeat of same sequence demonstrates homogeneous hepatic signal profile.

lated to hardware problems, large patient size, or the presence of ascites (Figs. 5-82, A and B). This can also result in apparent heterogeneous signal intensity of the hepatic parenchyma.

Vasculature
Anatomic variations

The right hepatic artery originates from the superior mesenteric artery rather than the celiac artery in approximately 12% of individuals.[6] The positional relationship between the hepatic artery, portal vein, and common hepatic duct can vary.[6] Variations in venous anatomy includes the presence of an accessory inferior right hepatic vein, formation of a common hepatic vein which empties into the right atrium, and variations in the branching

pattern of the hepatic veins[6] (Figs. 5-83, A and B). In one study of 82 children, MR demonstrated an inferior right hepatic vein which was at least as large as the superior right hepatic vein in 23% of the population.[98] The inferior right hepatic vein can provide collateral drainage in patients with obstruction of the high inferior vena cava.

Portal vein thrombosis

MR is useful for evaluating the portal veins for potential thrombosis. Portal venous patency is confirmed when a signal void is present on spin echo images and flow-related enhancement is present on gradient echo images. Slowly flowing blood can lead to relative increased intraluminal signal intensity on spin echo images simu-

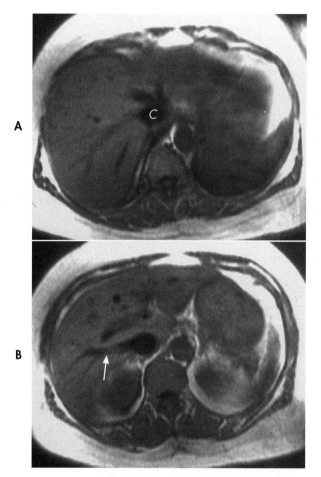

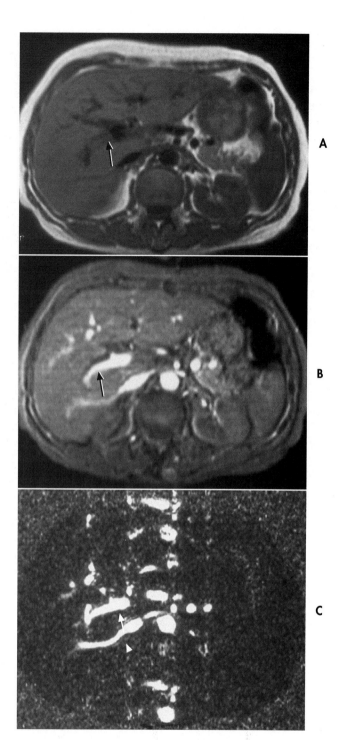

Fig. 5-83. A, Transaxial T1-weighted image (TR 500, TE 12, 4 Nex) demonstrates normal triradiate configuration of hepatic veins as they enter the inferior vena cava (*C*). **B,** Image acquired at lower level demonstrates a large vein draining into the inferior vena cava, representing an accessory inferior right hepatic vein *(arrow).*

lating the appearance of thrombosis[134,147] (Figs. 5-84, *A-C*). Portal venous flow can be particularly slow in patients with portal hypertension. Spatial presaturation radiofrequency pulses assist in reducing intraluminal signal intensity in patients with slow flow. Increased intraluminal signal intensity can be observed on T2-weighted spin echo images because of the even echo rephasing phenomenon or with use of gradient moment nulling for motion artifact suppression. In such situations, the first echo (proton density weighted) and T1-weighted images are helpful in confirming vascular patency. When further confirmation is necessary, the T2-weighted sequence can be repeated using asymmetric echo times and spatial presaturation pulses and without gradient moment rephasing, or gradient echo sequences can be used.

In the presence of very slow blood flow, gradient echo images may fail to demonstrate intraluminal high signal

Fig. 5-84. A, Transaxial T1-weighted image (TR 500, TE 11, 4 Nex) reveals absence of expected flow void in right portal vein, suggestive of thrombosis. Corresponding flow-compensated gradient echo images (TR 40, TE 10, 40-degree flip angle, 1 Nex), with magnitude **(B)** and phase **(C)** reconstructions, confirm that the findings are due to slow flow and that the vessel *(arrow)* is patent. Note accentuation of vascular pulsation artifacts on phase images and improved depiction of right inferior hepatic vein (a normal variant) (arrowhead) as compared with standard magnitude image.

intensity. Flow-related enhancement within the portal veins may also be suboptimally depicted on transaxial gradient echo images, because flow-related enhancement is maximal when imaging is performed perpendicular to the direction of blood flow.[75] For optimal evaluation of the portal venous system, therefore, sagittal or sagittal-oblique images should be considered. An artifactual focus of decreased intraluminal signal intensity simulating thrombus material can be observed within the main portal vein on gradient echo images, probably related to disordered or turbulent blood flow.[126]

Lack of visualization of portal venous structures is an ancillary sign of portal vein thrombosis.[66,134] The portal veins can also appear isointense with surrounding hepatic parenchyma following intravenous contrast material administration in normal individuals. The main portal vein may also demonstrate linear zones of hyperintensity and hypointensity on contrast material–enhanced images, probably because of streaming effects or layering of contrast material.

Phase reconstruction images are another valuable adjunct to magnitude reconstruction spin echo and gradient echo images for evaluating portal venous patency. Phase images are particularly useful for documenting very slow flow, which may not be evident on conventional magnitude images (Fig. 5-88). Flow phenomena and related artifacts are discussed in greater detail elsewhere in this book.

It may be difficult to distinguish portal from hepatic veins on isolated gradient echo images. Careful inspection of adjacent images usually allows these structures to be accurately identified. An alternate means of accomplishing this is to apply radiofrequency presaturation pulses across the portal and mesenteric veins immediately prior to image acquisition.[104] This will cause saturation of flowing spins within the portal vein, whereas the hepatic veins will continue to demonstrate flow-related enhancement.

Direction of portal venous flow

Whereas standard spin echo and gradient echo images may indicate that the portal vein is patent, one cannot determine the direction of portal venous flow on the basis of these images. This is of particular concern in patients with portal hypertension, in whom reversal of portal venous flow is associated with development of varices and other complications. A bolus tracking technique, which involves placement of a spatial radiofrequency presaturation band over the main portal vein immediately prior to performance of a flow sensitive gradient echo sequence, can be useful for evaluating flow direction.[29] On such images, movement of the presaturation band toward the liver indicates hepatopedal flow, whereas hepatofugal flow results in movement of the band away from the liver.

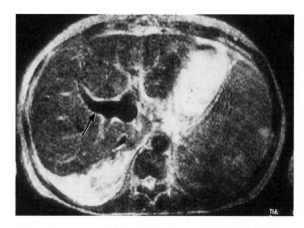

Fig. 5-85. Transaxial T2-weighted image shows relative increased signal intensity along the course of the portal veins *(arrow)* in patient with liver transplant rejection.

Periportal signal changes

Relative increased signal intensity can be observed surrounding the portal vessels in patients with portal vein thrombosis. However, similar findings have also been described in patients with acute viral hepatitis,[53] liver transplant rejection (Fig. 5-85), and other abnormalities.[76] Abnormal enhancement can also be observed on delayed images obtained following contrast material administration in these patients.[43]

GALLBLADDER AND BILIARY TRACT
Gallbladder

Anatomic variations

The gallbladder can be congenitally absent; this condition may be associated with a dilated common bile duct.[6,80] Conversely, duplication of the gallbladder can also be encountered. In some individuals, the gallbladder is suspended on a long mesentery. This predisposes to ectopic location of the gallbladder, such as lateral to the right lobe of the liver[80] or in the left side of the abdomen[6] (Figs. 5-86, *A* and *B*). The gallbladder can also be found in an intrahepatic position.[80] Acquired alterations in gallbladder position can occur in patients who have undergone previous right nephrectomy or partial hepatectomy. When the gallbladder is ectopic, it can simulate lesions such as abscess, lymphocele, or necrotic tumor.

The gallbladder is subject to considerable variation in size, shape, and location.[80] Among the many configurations that the gallbladder may assume is the "boomerang" gallbladder. The normal gallbladder undergoes distention during patient fasting. Septations can traverse the gallbladder lumen, and prominent infolding located near the fundus may form a "phyrigian cap."[80] Prominence

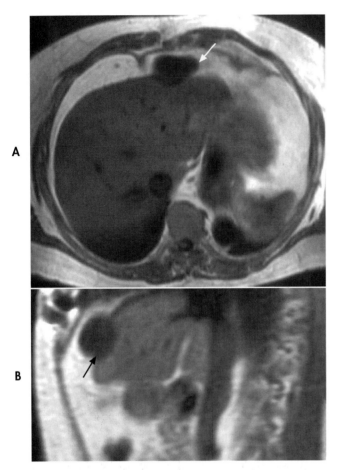

Fig. 5-86. Transaxial T2-weighted image **(A)** (TR 640, TE 12, 4 Nex) and sagittal T1-weighted **(B)** (TR 645, TE 12, 4 Nex) images demonstrate ectopic gallbladder *(arrow)* located ventral to the lateral segment of the left hepatic lobe.

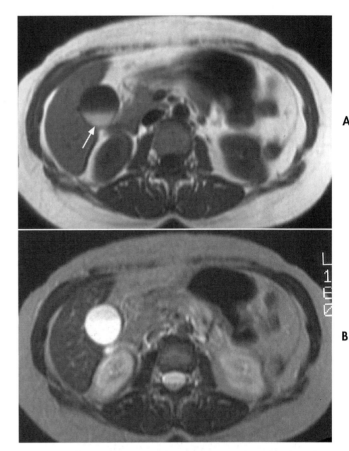

Fig. 5-87. A, Transaxial T1-weighted image (TR 500, TE 12, 4 Nex) demonstrates relative hyperintensity of concentrated bile along the dependent gallbladder lumen *(arrow)*, with corresponding hyperintensity on T2-weighted image **(B)** (TR 3400, TE 80, 2 Nex).

of the valves of Heister is another anatomic variant, though this is usually not evident on MR images.

Lesions

The normal gallbladder often has relatively high signal intensity within its dependent portion on T1-weighted images because of concentrated bile. A fluid-fluid level is usually present, with relatively decreased signal intensity in the nondependent portion of the gallbladder lumen representing less concentrated bile[79] (Figs. 5-87, *A* and *B*). Absence of this fluid-fluid level may indicate that bile cannot be properly concentrated, such as in patients with chronic cholecystitis (Fig. 5-88, *A* and *B*). However, hemorrhagic products and debris within an inflamed gallbladder can produce intraluminal increased signal intensity on T1-weighted images.[139] In this situation, an obstructed and inflamed gallbladder would demonstrate the signal characteristics of a normally functioning gallbladder. Thus bile signal intensity characteristics are not reliable for determination of cholecystitis

on MR images.[139] Instead, observation of morphologic signs including thickening of the gallbladder wall, pericholecystic fluid collections, and gallstones is more reliable.

There may be apparent reversal of the fluid-fluid level in patients with cholelithiasis (Fig. 5-89). In such patients, low signal intensity gallstones usually layer along the dependent aspect of the gallbladder, and increased signal intensity is present superiorly. Gallstones demonstrate variable signal intensity characteristics on MR images.[5,79] One atypical appearance of gallstones consists of high signal intensity foci on T1-weighted images caused by fatty acids.[95] The size of gallstones is artifactually increased on MR images as compared with their size on CT.[139]

Diffuse hypointensity of the gallbladder can indicate mural calcification ("porcelain gallbladder") (Figs. 5-90, *A-C*). Foci of signal void in the gallbladder fossa may be caused by surgical clips in patients who have under-

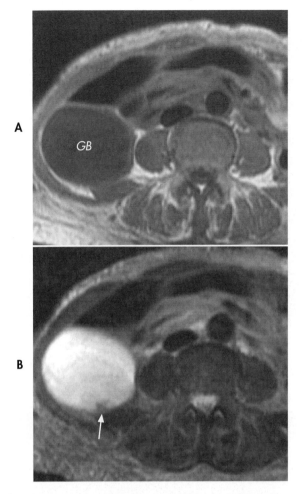

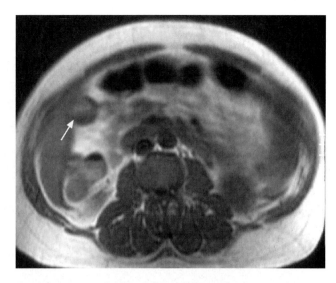

Fig. 5-89. Transaxial T1-weighted image (TR 500, TE 12, 4 Nex) demonstrates relative hypointensity along the dependent portion of the gallbladder lumen *(arrow)* caused by layering gallstones. This is a reversal of the usual signal intensity pattern observed on T1-weighted images.

Fig. 5-88. A, Dilated gallbladder *(GB)* with uniform hypointensity on transaxial T1-weighted image (TR 600, TE 12, 4 Nex) indicates lack of bile concentration consistent with chronic cholecystitis, which was confirmed on DISIDA radionuclide scan. **B,** Corresponding T2-weighted image (TR 3900, TE 80, 2 Nex) shows uniform hyperintensity throughout the gallbladder, except for calculus within dependent portion *(arrow).*

gone cholecystectomy. These artifacts are particularly prominent on gradient echo images, where they can obscure visualization of adjacent tissues.

Biliary Ducts
Ductal dilatation

Nondilated intra- and extrahepatic biliary ducts are routinely visualized on abdominal MR images.[68] Intrahepatic biliary radicles can be difficult to distinguish from vascular structures in some patients.[21] Both are branching, tubular structures that demonstrate low sig-

nal intensity on T1-weighted images and increased signal intensity on gradient compensated T2-weighted images. In problematic cases, T1-weighted gradient echo images can provide such distinction. Such images depict flow enhancement within portal and hepatic veins, as compared with low signal intensity biliary ducts. Alternatively, T2-weighted images performed with spatial presaturation but not gradient moment nulling depict bile ducts as hyperintense as compared with hypointense vessels. These methods can also be useful for distinguishing the common bile duct and main portal vein in selected patients. Dilated biliary ducts can be recognized as an excessive number of intrahepatic tubular branching structures, by their fusiform configuration as compared with hepatic vessels, and by their frequent association with extrahepatic biliary ductal dilatation.

Biliary air

Air can be present within the biliary tree as a result of previous surgery involving implantation of the common bile duct into the gastrointestinal tract or in patients with cholangitis. Biliary air results in susceptibility artifacts, which are manifested as signal void foci with possible peripheral hyperintensity (Fig. 5-91). These findings must be distinguished from biliary tract calculi, which can have a similar appearance. Biliary air should also be distinguished from air within the portal venous system, as can occur in patients with bowel infarction. Biliary air tends to have a more central location within

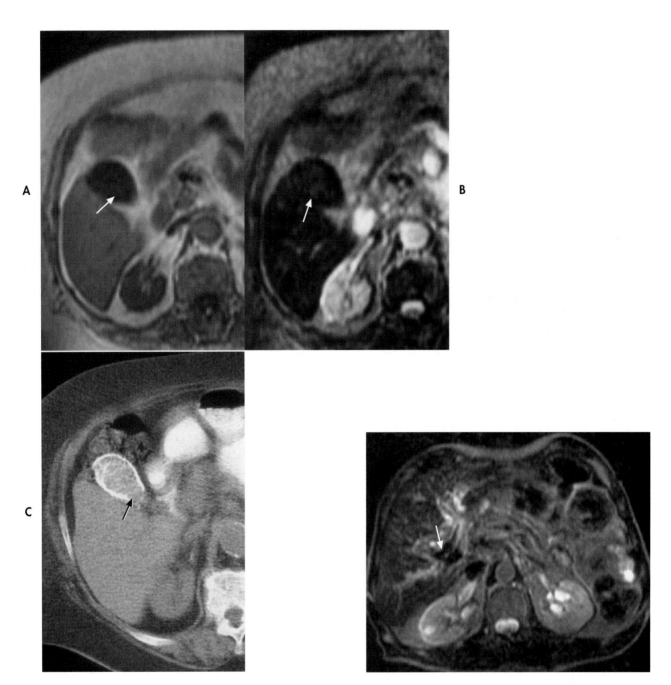

Fig. 5-90. Hypointensity of the gallbladder *(arrow)* is observed on both T1-weighted **(A)** (TR 450, TE 12, 4 Nex) and T2-weighted **(B)** (TR 3300, TE 90, 2 Nex) images. This appearance is due to calcification of the gallbladder wall (i.e., porcelain gallbladder), as confirmed on corresponding CT image **(C)**.

Fig. 5-91. There are multiple foci of markedly decreased signal intensity *(arrow)* within the intrahepatic biliary ducts on transaxial T2-weighted image (TR 3400, TE 120, 2 Nex). While such foci could represent biliary calculi, these findings are due to biliary air in patient who underwent previous Whipple procedure.

the liver than does portal venous air. Drainage catheters and stents located within the biliary tree can also appear as foci of signal void which may simulate pneumobilia.[34]

MR cholangiography

Whereas standard T2-weighted images can usually confirm the presence of dilated biliary ducts, subtle changes in the caliber of these ducts and related lesions may not be evident. This has led to the development of MR cholangiography. This technique involves initial acquisition of a fluid-sensitive sequence, using either a heavily T2-weighted fat-suppressed spin echo or fast spin echo or steady state free precession sequence. The images are subsequently postprocessed using a maximum intensity projection algorithm and reformatted into the coronal or coronal oblique plane to simulate the appearance of a conventional cholangiogram.

Although experience with MR cholangiography is relatively limited at this time, several pitfalls have already been noted. One important limitation is that the length of bile duct strictures has been difficult to determine, and important subtle findings such as asymmetry or mild irregularity at the stricture site may not be evident.[40] Discrepancies between conventional and MR cholangiography may also relate to the lack of distention of the biliary tree with the latter technique. Biliary debris or calculi located proximal to the stricture site can cause the stricture to appear longer than it actually is. Furthermore, any nearby surgical clips, such as in the gallbladder bed, can result in signal void artifacts that can simulate or obscure abnormalities of the bile ducts.[40]

REFERENCES

1. Andersson T, Ericsson A, Eriksson B et al: Relative proton density and relaxation times in liver metastases during interferon treatment, Br J Radiol 62:433-437, 1989.
2. Andersson T, Eriksson B, Hemmingsson A et al: Effect of interferon on T1 relaxation times of liver metastases from endocrine gastrointestinal tumours, Acta Radiol 29:21-25, 1988.
3. Apicella P, Mirowitz SA, Weinreb JC: Extension of vascular structures through hepatic masses on MR and CT images, Radiology 191:135-136, 1994.
4. Arrive L, Hricak H, Goldberg HI et al: MR appearance of the liver after partial hepatectomy, Am J Roentgenol 152:1215-1220, 1989.
5. Baron RL, Shuman WP, Lee SP et al: MR appearance of gallstones in vitro at 1.5 T: correlation with chemical composition, Am J Roentgenol 153:497-502, 1989.
6. Bergman RA, Thompson SA, Afifi AK et al: Compendium of human anatomic variation: text, atlas, and world literature, Baltimore, 1988, Urban & Schwarzenberg.
7. Bernardino ME, Chaloupka JC, Malko JA et al: Are hepatic and muscle T2 values different at 0.5 and 1.5 Tesla? Magn Reson Imaging 7:363-367, 1989.
8. Bernardino ME, Steinberg HV, Pearson TC et al: Shunts for portal hypertension: MR and angiography for determination of patency, Radiology 158:57-61, 1986.
9. Birnbaum BA, Weinreb JC, Megibow AJ et al: Definitive diagnosis of hepatic hemangiomas: MR imaging versus Tc-99m-labeled red blood cell SPECT, Radiology 176:95-101, 1990.
10. Bradley WG, Glenn BJ: The effect of variation in slice thickness and interslice gap on MR lesion detection, Am J Neuroradiol 8:1057-1062, 1987.
11. Brick SH, Hill MC, Lande IM: The mistaken or indeterminate CT diagnosis of hepatic metastases: the value of sonography, Am J Roentgenol 148:723-726, 1987.
12. Brown JJ, Lee JMK, Lee JKT et al: Focal hepatic lesions: differentiation with MR imaging at 0.5 T, Radiology 179:675-679, 1991.
13. Caron KH, Strife JL, Babcock DS et al: Left-lobe hepatic transplants: spectrum of normal imaging findings, Am J Roentgenol 159:497-501, 1992.
14. Catasca JV, Mirowitz SA: T2-weighted MR imaging of the abdomen: fast spin-echo vs conventional spin-echo sequences, Am J Roentgenol 162:61-67, 1994.
15. Chien D, Atkinson DJ, Edelman RR: Strategies to improve contrast in turboFLASH imaging: reordered phase encoding and k-space segmentation, J Magn Reson Imaging 1:63-70, 1991.
16. Chien D, Mulkern RV: Fast spin-echo studies of contrast and small-lesion definition in a liver-metastasis phantom, J Magn Reson Imaging 2:483-487, 1992.
17. Choi BI, Han MC, Park JH et al: Giant cavernous hemangioma of the liver: CT and MR imaging in 10 cases, Am J Roentgenol 152:1221-1226, 1989.
18. Choi BI, Lee GK, Kim ST et al: Mosaic pattern of encapsulated hepatocellular carcinoma: correlation of magnetic resonance imaging and pathology, Gastrointest Radiol 15:238-240, 1990.
19. Dixon WT, Engels H, Castillo M et al: Incidental magnetization transfer contrast in standard multislice imaging, Magn Reson Imaging 8:417-422, 1990.
20. Dodds WJ, Erickson SJ, Taylor AJ et al: Caudate lobe of the liver: anatomy, embryology, and pathology, Am J Roentgenol 154:87-93, 1990.
21. Dooms GC, Fisher MR, Higgins CB et al: MR imaging of the dilated biliary tract, Radiology 158:337-341, 1986.
22. Duerk JL, Pattany PM: Analysis of imaging axes significance in motion artifact suppression technique (MAST): MRI of turbulent flow and motion, Magn Reson Imaging 7:251-263, 1989.
23. Ebara M, Watanabe S, Kita K et al: MR imaging of small hepatocellular carcinoma: effect of intratumoral copper content on signal intensity, Radiology 180:617-621, 1991.
24. Edelman RR, Siegel JB, Singer A et al: Dynamic MR imaging of the liver with Gd-DTPA: initial clinical results, Am J Roentgenol 153:1213-1219, 1989.
25. Ehman RL, McNamara MT, Brasch RC et al: Influence of physiologic motion on the appearance of tissue in MR images, Radiology 159:777-782, 1986.
26. El Rahman M, Li KCP, Ros PR: Hepatic focal nodular hyperplasia: new MR findings, Magn Reson Imaging 7:687-688, 1989.
27. Fan ZM, Yamashita Y, Harada M et al: Intrahepatic cholan-

giocarcinoma: spin-echo and contrast-enhanced dynamic MR imaging, Am J Roentgenol 161:313-317, 1993.

28. Ferrucci JT, Freeny PC, Stark DD et al: Advances in hepatobiliary radiology, Radiology 168:319-338, 1988.

29. Finn JP, Kane RA, Edelman RR et al: Imaging of the portal venous system in patients with cirrhosis: MR angiography vs duplex Doppler sonography, Am J Roentgenol 161:989-994, 1993.

29a. Flickinger FW, Pfeifer EA: Hepatic sarcoidosis: MR findings (letter), Am J Roentgenol 156:1324-1325, 1991.

30. Foley WD, Kneeland JB, Cates JD et al: Contrast optimization for the detection of focal hepatic lesions by MR imaging at 1.5 T, Am J Roentgenol 149:1155-1160, 1987.

31. Fullerton GD, Cameron IL, Ord VA: Frequency dependence of magnetic resonance spin-lattice relaxation of protons in biological materials, Radiology 151:135-138, 1984.

32. Gabata T, Matsui O, Kadoya M et al: MR imaging of hepatic adenoma, Am J Roentgenol 155:1009-1011, 1990.

33. Gendler R, Shapiro RS, Mitty HA et al: CT findings after percutaneous biliary procedures, Radiology 187:373-376, 1993.

34. Girard MJ, Hahn PF, Saini S et al: Wallstent metallic biliary endoprosthesis: MR imaging characteristics, Radiology 184:874-876, 1992.

35. Gore JC, Pope CF, Sostman HD: Errors in the assessment of the efficacy of MRI pulse sequences, Magn Reson Imaging 4:251-255, 1986.

36. Guyader D, Gandon Y: MR of hepatocellular carcinoma in idiopathic hemochromatosis (letter), Am J Roentgenol 151:833, 1988.

37. Haggar AM, Bree RL: Hepatic focal nodular hyperplasia: MR imaging at 1.0 and 1.5 T, J Magn Reson Imaging 2:85-88, 1992.

38. Hahn PF, Stark DD, Ferrucci JT: Accumulation of iron oxide particles around liver metastases during MR imaging, Gastrointest Radiol 17:173-174, 1992.

39. Hahn PF, Stark DD, Saini S et al: The differential diagnosis of ringed hepatic lesions in MR imaging, Am J Roentgenol 154:287-290, 1990.

40. Hall-Craggs MA, Allen CM, Owens CM et al: MR cholangiography: clinical evaluation in 40 cases, Radiology 189:423-427, 1993.

41. Hamed MM, Hamm B, Ibrahim ME et al: Dynamic MR imaging of the abdomen with gadopentetate dimeglumine: normal enhancement patterns of the liver, spleen, stomach, and pancreas, Am J Roentgenol 158:303-307, 1992.

42. Hamm B, Wolf K-J, Felix R: Conventional and rapid MR imaging of the liver with Gd-DTPA, Radiology 164:313-320, 1987.

43. Hammerman AM, Kotner LM Jr, Doyle TB: Periportal contrast enhancement on CT scans of the liver, Am J Roentgenol 156:313-315, 1991.

44. Hearshen DO, Ellis JH, Carson PL et al: Boundary effects from opposed magnetization artifact in IR images, Radiology 160:543-547, 1986.

45. Heiken JP, Weyman PJ, Lee JKT et al: Detection of focal hepatic masses: prospective evaluation with CT, delayed CT, CT during arterial portography, and MR imaging, Radiology 171:47-51, 1989.

46. Hendrick RE, Nelson TR, Hendee WR: Optimizing tissue contrast in magnetic resonance imaging, Magn Reson Imaging 2:193-204, 1984.

47. Henkelman RM, Hardy P, Poon PY et al: Optimal pulse sequence for imaging hepatic metastases, Radiology 161:727-734, 1986.

48. Henkelman RM, Hardy PA, Bishop JE et al: Why fat is bright in RARE and fast spin-echo imaging, J Magn Reson Imaging 2:533-540, 1992.

49. Hopper KD, Kasat RS, Mahraj R: The papillary process of the liver: a pseudotumor on coronal and sagittal MRI, SMRM Book of Abstracts, p 3210, 1992.

50. Itai Y, Ohtomo K, Kokubo T et al: Segmental intensity differences in the liver on MR images: a sign of intrahepatic portal flow stoppage, Radiology 167:17-19, 1988.

51. Ito K, Choji T, Fujita T et al: Imaging of the portocaval space, Am J Roentgenol 161:329-334, 1993.

52. Ito K, Choji T, Fujita T et al: Early-enhancing pseudolesion in medial segment of left hepatic lobe detected with multisection dynamic MR, Radiology 187:695-699, 1993.

53. Itoh H, Sakai T, Takahashi N et al: Periportal high intensity on T2-weighted MR images in acute viral hepatitis, J Comput Assist Tomogr 16:564-567, 1992.

54. Itoh K, Nishimura K, Togashi K et al: Hepatocellular carcinoma: MR imaging, Radiology 164:21-25, 1987.

55. Itoh K, Saini S, Hahn PF et al: Differentiation between small hepatic hemangiomas and metastases on MR images: importance of size-specific quantitative criteria, Am J Roentgenol 155:61-66, 1990.

56. Jones KM, Mulkern RV, Schwartz RB et al: Fast spin-echo MR imaging of the brain and spine: current concepts, Am J Roentgenol 158:1313-1320, 1992.

57. Kawamori Y, Matsui O, Kitagawa K et al: Segmental hepatic iron deposition due to peripheral portal vein tumor thrombus: MR features, J Comput Assist Tomogr 15:1042-1044, 1991.

58. Kitagawa K, Matsui O, Kadoya M et al: Hepatocellular carcinomas with excessive copper accumulation: CT and MR findings, Radiology 180:623-628, 1991.

59. Kneeland JB, Shimakawa A, Wehrli FW: Effect of intersection spacing on MR image contrast and study time, Radiology 158:819-822, 1986.

60. Koslow SA, Davis PL, DeMarino GB et al: Hyperintense cirrhotic nodules on MRI, Gastrointest Radiol 16:339-341, 1991.

61. Kreft B, Tanimoto A, Baba Y et al: Diagnosis of fatty liver with MR imaging, J Magn Reson Imaging 2:463-471, 1992.

62. Kucharczyk W, Crawley AP, Kelly WM et al: Effect of multislice interference on image contrast in T2- and T1-weighted MR images, Am J Neuroradiol 9:443-451, 1988.

63. Lee MJ, Hahn PF, Saini S et al: Differential diagnosis of hyperintense liver lesions on T1-weighted MR images, Am J Roentgenol 159:1017-1020, 1992.

64. Lee MJ, Saini S, Compton CC et al: MR demonstration of edema adjacent to a liver metastasis: pathologic correlation, Am J Roentgenol 157:499-501, 1991.

65. Levenson H, Greensite F, Hoefs J et al: Fatty infiltration of the liver: quantification with phase-contrast MR imaging at 1.5 T vs biopsy, Am J Roentgenol 156:307-312, 1991.

66. Levi HM, Newhouse JH: MR imaging of portal vein thrombosis, Am J Roentgenol 151:283-286, 1988.

67. Li KC, Glazer GM, Quint LE et al: Distinction of hepatic cavernous hemangioma from hepatic metastases with MR imaging, Radiology 169:409-415, 1988.

68. Liddell RM, Baron RL, Ekstrom JE et al: Normal intrahepatic bile ducts: CT depiction, Radiology 176:633-635, 1990.

69. Lombardo DM, Baker ME, Spritzer CE et al: Hepatic hemangiomas vs metastases: MR differentiation at 1.5 T, Am J Roentgenol 155:55-59, 1990.

70. Low RN, Francis IR, Herfkens RJ et al: Fast multiplanar spoiled gradient-recalled imaging of the liver: pulse sequence optimization and comparison with spin-echo MR imaging, Am J Roentgenol 160:501-509, 1993.

71. Low RN, Francis IR, Sigeti JS et al: Abdominal MR imaging: comparison of T2-weighted fast and conventional spin-echo, and contrast-enhanced fast multiplanar spoiled gradient-recalled imaging, Radiology 186:803-811, 1993.

72. Mahfouz A-E, Hamm B, Taupitz M et al: Hypervascular liver lesions: differentiation of focal nodular hyperplasia from malignant tumors with dynamic gadolinium-enhanced MR imaging, Radiology 186:133-138, 1993.

73. Marti-Bonmati L, Menor F, Vizcaino I et al: Lipoma of the liver: US, CT, and MRI appearance, Gastrointest Radiol 14:155-157, 1989.

74. Marti-Bonmati L, Talens A, del Olmo J et al: Chronic hepatitis and cirrhosis: evaluation by means of MR imaging with histologic correlation, Radiology 188:37-43, 1993.

75. Martinoli C, Cittadini G, Pastorino C et al: Gradient echo MRI of portal vein thrombosis, J Comput Assist Tomogr 16:226-234, 1992.

76. Matsui O, Kadoya M, Kameyama T et al: Adenomatous hyperplastic nodules in the cirrhotic liver: differentiation from hepatocellular carcinoma with MR imaging, Radiology 173:123-126, 1989.

77. Mattison GR, Glazer GM, Quint LE et al: MR imaging of hepatic focal nodular hyperplasia: characterization and distinction from primary malignant hepatic tumors, Am J Roentgenol 148:711-715, 1987.

78. Maves CK, Caron KH, Bissett GS III et al: Splenic and hepatic peliosis: MR findings, Am J Roentgenol 158:75-76, 1992.

79. McCarthy S, Hricak H, Cohen M et al: Cholecystitis: detection with MR imaging, Radiology 158:333-336, 1986.

80. Meilstrup JW, Hopper KD, Thieme GA: Imaging of gallbladder variants, Am J Roentgenol 157:1205-1208, 1991.

81. Miller FH, Fisher MR, Soper W et al: MRI of hepatic iron deposition in patients with renal transplant, Gastrointest Radiol 16:229-233, 1991.

82. Mirowitz SA, Heiken JP, Lee JKT: Potential MR pitfall in relying on lesion/liver intensity ratio in presence of hepatic hemochromatosis, J Comput Assist Tomogr 12:323-324, 1988.

82a. Mirowitz SA, Lee JKT: Optimizing MR imaging of the abdomen: one case for rapid-acquisition spin-echo MR imaging, Radiology 179:612-614, 1991.)

83. Mirowitz SA, Lee JKT, Brown JJ et al: Rapid acquisition spin-echo (RASE) MR imaging: a new technique for reduction of artifacts and acquisition time, Radiology 175:131-135, 1990.

84. Mirowitz SA, Lee JKT, Gutierrez E et al: Dynamic gadolinium-enhanced rapid acquisition spin-echo MR imaging of the liver, Radiology 179:371-376, 1991.

85. Mirowitz SA, Gutierrez E, Lee JKT et al: Normal abdominal enhancement patterns with dynamic gadolinium-enhanced MR imaging, Radiology 180:637-640, 1991.

86. Mitchell DG, Burk DL Jr., Vinitski S et al: The biophysical basis of tissue contrast in extracranial MR imaging, Am J Roentgenol 149:831-837, 1987.

87. Mitchell DG, Palazzo J, Hann HW et al: Hepatocellular tumors with high signal on T1-weighted MR images: chemical shift MR imaging and histologic correlation, J Comput Assist Tomogr 15:762-769, 1991.

88. Mitchell DG, Palazzo J, Hann HW et al: Mass-like hepatic hypertrophy: MRI findings with histologic correlation, Magn Reson Imaging 10:541-547, 1992.

89. Mitchell DG, Rubin R, Siegelman ES et al: Hepatocellular carcinoma within siderotic regenerative nodules: appearance as a nodule within a nodule on MR images, Radiology 178:101-103, 1991.

90. Mitchell DG, Ortega H, Mohamed F et al: Aortic ghost artifact in ultrashort-TE multislice gradient echo MR images is not increased by paramagnetic enhancement, Magn Reson Med 29:269-272, 1993.

91. Mitchell DG, Vinitski S, Burk DL Jr et al: Multiple spin-echo MR imaging of the body image contrast and motion-induced artifact, Magn Reson Imaging 6:535-546, 1988.

92. Mitchell DG, Vinitski S, Saponaro S et al: Liver and pancreas: improved spin-echo T1 contrast by shorter echo time and fat suppression at 1.5 T, Radiology 178:67-71, 1991.

93. Mitchell DG: Focal manifestations of diffuse liver disease at MR imaging, Radiology 185:1-11, 1992.

94. Miyake H, Suzuki K, Ueda S et al: Localized fat collection adjacent to the intrahepatic portion of the inferior vena cava: a normal variant on CT, Am J Roentgenol 158:423-425, 1992.

95. Moeser PM, Julian S, Karstaedt N et al: Unusual presentation of cholelithiasis on T1-weighted MR imaging, J Comput Assist Tomogr 12:150-152, 1988.

96. Mulkern RV, Wong ST, Winalski C et al: Contrast manipulation and artifact assessment of 2D and 3D RARE sequences, Magn Reson Imaging 8:557-566, 1990.

97. Murakami T, Nakamura H, Hori S et al: CT and MR of siderotic regenerating nodules in hepatic cirrhosis, J Comput Assist Tomogr 16:578-582, 1992.

98. Ng YY, Finn JP, Hall-Craggs MA: Inferior right hepatic veins: MR assessment of prevalence and potential clinical significance in children, Pediatr Radiol 20:605-607, 1990.

99. Nghiem HV, Herfkens RJ, Francis IR et al: The pelvis: T2-weighted fast spin-echo MR imaging, Radiology 185:213-217, 1992.

100. Ni Y, Marchal G, Yu J et al: Experimental liver cancers: Mn-DPDP-enhanced rims in MR-microangiographic-histologic correlation study, Radiology 188:45-51, 1993.

101. Nokes SR, Baker ME, Spritzer CE et al: Hepatic adenoma: MR appearance mimicking focal nodular hyperplasia, J Comput Assist Tomogr 12:885-887, 1988.

102. Ohtomo K, Itai Y, Matuoka Y et al: Hepatocellular carcinoma: MR appearance mimicking cavernous hemangioma, J Comput Assist Tomogr 14:650-652, 1990.

103. Ohtomo K, Itai Y, Ohtomo Y et al: Regenerating nodules of liver cirrhosis: MR imaging with pathologic correlation, Am J Roentgenol 154:505-507, 1990.

104. Otake S, Matsuo M, Kuroda Y: Distinction of hepatic vein from portal vein by MR imaging, J Comput Assist Tomogr 14:201-204, 1990.

105. Outwater E, Tomaszewski JE, Daly JM et al: Hepatic colorectal metastases: correlation of MR imaging and pathologic appearance, Radiology 180:327-332, 1991.

106. Outwater E: Capsular retraction in hepatic tumors (letter), Am J Roentgenol 160:422, 1993.

107. Paling MR, Abbitt PL, Mugler JP et al: Liver metastases: optimization of MR imaging pulse sequences at 1.0 T, Radiology 167:695-699, 1988.

108. Powers T, Lum A, Patton JA: Abdominal MRI artifacts, Semin Ultrasound, CT, MR 10:2-10, 1989.

109. Rahmouni A, Golli M, Mathieu D et al: Castleman disease mimicking liver tumor: CT and MR features, J Comput Assist Tomogr 16:699-703, 1992.

110. Reinig JW, Dwyer AJ, Miller DL et al: Liver metastases: detection with MR imaging at 0.5 and 1.5 T, Radiology 170:149-153, 1989.

111. Richards MA, Webb JA, Jewell SE et al: In-vivo measurement of spin lattice relaxation time (T1) of liver in healthy volunteers: the effects of age, sex, and oral contraceptive usage, Br J Radiol 61:34-37, 1988.

112. Roberts JL, Fishman EK, Hartman DS et al: Lipomatous tumors of the liver: evaluation with CT and US, Radiology 158:613-617, 1986.

113. Rofsky NM, Weinreb JC, Bernardino ME et al: Hepatocellular tumors: characterization with Mn-DPDP-enhanced MR imaging, Radiology 188:53-59, 1993.

114. Ros PR, Lubbers PR, Olmsted WW et al: Hemangioma of the liver: heterogeneous appearance on T2-weighted images, Am J Roentgenol 149:1167-1170, 1987.

115. Rummeny E, Saini S, Wittenberg J et al: MR imaging of liver neoplasms, Am J Roentgenol 152:493-499, 1989.

116. Rummeny E, Weissleder R, Sironi S et al: Central scars in primary liver tumors: MR features, specificity, and pathologic correlation, Radiology 171:323-326, 1989.

117. Rummeny E, Weissleder R, Stark DD et al: Primary liver tumors: diagnosis by MR imaging, Am J Roentgenol 152:63-72, 1989.

118. Runge VM, Wood ML: Fast imaging and other motion artifact reduction schemes: a pictorial overview, Magn Reson Imaging 6:595-607, 1988.

119. Schertz LD, Lee JKT, Heiken JP et al: Proton spectroscopic imaging (Dixon method) of the liver: clinical utility, Radiology 173:401-405, 1989.

120. Schiebler ML. Hepatocellular carcinoma: MR appearance mimicking focal nodular hyperplasia (letter), Am J Roentgenol 150:472, 1988.

121. Schwaighofer BW, Yu KK, Mattrey RF: Diagnostic significance of interslice gap and imaging volume in body MR imaging, Am J Roentgenol 153:629-632, 1989.

122. Schwartz LH, Seltzer SE, Tempany CMC et al: Prospective comparison of T2-weighted fast spin-echo, with and without fat suppression, and conventional spin-echo pulse sequences in the upper abdomen, Radiology 189:411-416, 1993.

123. Semelka RC, Shoenut JP, Kroeker MA et al: Focal liver disease: comparison of dynamic contrast-enhanced CT and T2-weighted fat-suppressed, FLASH, and dynamic gadolinium-enhanced MR imaging at 1.5 T, Radiology 184:687-694, 1992.

124. Siegelman ES, Mitchell DG, Outwater E et al: Idiopathic hemochromatosis: MR imaging findings in cirrhotic and pre-cirrhotic patients, Radiology 188:637-641, 1993.

125. Silverman PM, Patt RH, Baum PA et al: Ghost artifact on gradient-echo imaging: a potential pitfall in hepatic imaging, Am J Roentgenol 154:633-634, 1990.

126. Silverman PM, Patt RH, Garra BS et al: MR imaging of the portal venous system: value of gradient-echo imaging as an adjunct to spin-echo imaging, Am J Roentgenol 157:297-302, 1991.

127. Slone HW, Bennett WF, Bova JG: MR findings of multiple biliary hamartomas, Am J Roentgenol 161:581-583, 1993.

128. Soyer P, Laissy J-P, Sibert A, Azencot M et al: Hepatic metastases: detection with multisection FLASH MR imaging during gadolinium chelate-enhanced arterial portography, Radiology 189:401-405, 1993.

129. Stark DD, Wittenberg J, Edelman RR et al: Detection of hepatic metastases: analysis of pulse sequence performance in MR imaging, Radiology 159:365-370, 1986.

130. Steinberg HV, Alarcon JJ, Bernardino ME: Focal hepatic lesions: comparative MR imaging at 0.5 and 1.5 T, Radiology 174:153-156, 1990.

131. Te Strake L, Freling NJM, Kamman RL et al: Abdominal applications of fast MR imaging: a comparison of fast field echo (FFE) and spin echo (SE) pulse sequences, Magn Reson Imaging 7:297-303, 1989.

132. Titelbaum DS, Burke DR, Meranze SG et al: Fibrolammelar hepatocellular carcinoma: pitfalls in nonoperative diagnosis, Radiology 167:25-30, 1988.

133. Titelbaum DS, Hatabu H, Schiebler ML et al: Fibrolamellar hepatocellular carcinoma: MR appearance, J Comput Assist Tomogr 12:588-591, 1988.

134. Torres WE, Gaylord GM, Whitmire L et al: The correlation between MR and angiography in portal hypertension, Am J Roentgenol 148:1109-1112, 1987.

135. Van Beers B, Demeure R, Pringot J et al: Dynamic spin-echo imaging with Gd-DTPA: value in the differentiation of hepatic tumors, Am J Roentgenol 154:515-519, 1990.

136. Van Lom KJ, Brown JJ, Perman WH et al: Liver imaging at 1.5 Tesla: pulse sequence optimization based on improved measurement of tissue relaxation times, Magn Reson Imaging 9:165-171, 1991.

137. Vilgrain V, Flegou J-F, Arrive L et al: Focal nodular hyperplasia of the liver: MR imaging and pathologic correlation in 37 patients, Radiology 184:699-703, 1992.

138. von Sinner W, te Strake L, Clark D et al: MR imaging in hydatid disease, Am J Roentgenol 157:741-745, 1991.

139. Weissleder R, Stark DD, Compton CC et al: Cholecystitis diagnosis by MR imaging, Magn Reson Imaging 6:345-348, 1988.

140. Wilbur AC, Gyi B: Hepatocellular carcinoma: MR appearance mimicking focal nodular hyperplasia, Am J Roentgenol 149:721-722, 1987.

141. Wittenberg J, Stark DD, Forman BH et al: Differentiation of hepatic metastases from hepatic hemangiomas and cysts by using MR imaging, Am J Roentgenol 151:79-84, 1988.

142. Wood ML, Runge VM, Henkelman RM: Overcoming motion in abdominal MR imaging, Am J Roentgenol 150:513-522, 1988.

143. Yankelevitz DF, Knapp PH, Henschke CI et al: MR appearance of radiation hepatitis, Clin Imaging 16:89-92, 1992.

144. Yates CK, Streight RA: Focal fatty infiltration of the liver simulating metastatic disease, Radiology 159:83-84, 1986.

145. Yoshikawa J, Matsui O, Takashima T et al: Focal fatty change of the liver adjacent to the falciform ligament: CT and sonographic findings in five surgically confirmed cases, Am J Roentgenol 149:491-494, 1987.

146. Yoshioka H, Nakagawa K, Shindou H et al: MR imaging of the liver before and after transcatheter hepatic chemoembolization for hepatocellular carcinoma, Acta Radiol 31:63-67, 1990.

147. Zirinsky K, Markisz JA, Rubenstein WA et al: MR imaging of portal venous thrombosis: correlation with CT and sonography, Am J Roentgenol 150:283-288, 1988.

6

Spleen, Pancreas, and Gastrointestinal Tract

SPLEEN
Anatomic Variations

While the spleen usually has a smooth contour, it can also have a lobular configuration. The spleen may also exhibit notches or fissures along its surface. These fissures can extend into the substance of the spleen to variable degrees, and in some cases they may appear to divide it. These variations in splenic contour should not be interpreted as evidence of prior splenic insult, such as infarct or trauma.

The spleen can vary in its position and configuration in normal subjects. A "wandering spleen" may be located anterior and inferior to the left kidney. Acquired alterations in splenic position can occur following left nephrectomy. The spleen can extend posteriorly around the left kidney. It can also demonstrate a prominent medial

process, which can simulate a splenic or perisplenic mass lesion (Figs. 6-1 and 6-2).

Congenital absence of the spleen rarely occurs. Accessory spleens—small nodules of functioning splenic tissue—are frequently found adjacent to the spleen proper. Accessory splenic tissue is present in at least 10% of individuals[3] (Figs. 6-3 and 6-4). Its major significance is that it can simulate abnormal lymph nodes or a lesion arising in the left adrenal gland or pancreatic tail. Less typical locations for accessory splenic tissue include the greater omentum or transverse mesocolon, pancreatic

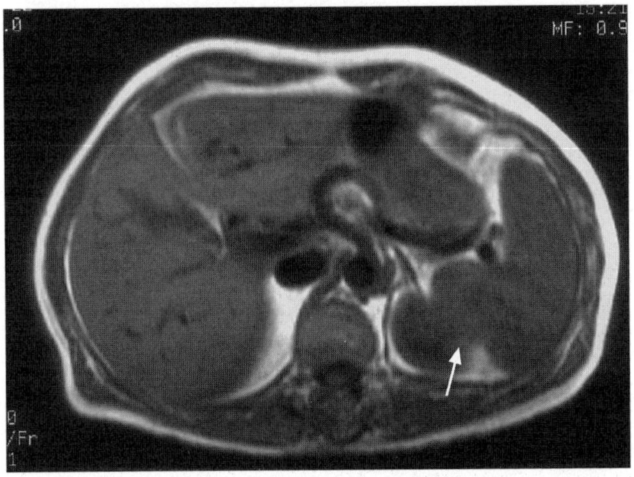

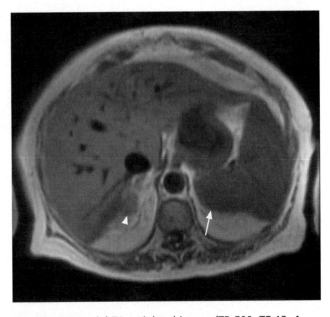

Fig. 6-2. Transaxial T1-weighted image (TR 500, TE 12, 4 Nex) demonstrates a prominent medial process of the spleen *(arrow)*. Also noted is an apparent right adrenal mass, caused by partial volume averaging of the upper pole of the right kidney *(arrowhead)*. (Reprinted from Mirowitz SA: MRI Clin N Am 3:23-37, 1995.)

Fig. 6-1. A prominent medial process of the spleen *(arrow)* is demonstrated on transaxial T1-weighted image (TR 500, TE 12, 4 Nex). The medial process maintains isointensity with remainder of splenic parenchyma, allowing distinction from an exophytic mass lesion.

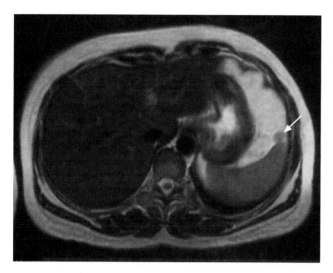

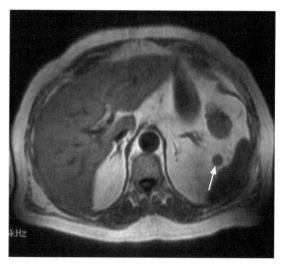

Fig. 6-3. A small accessory spleen is seen anterior to the spleen proper *(arrow)*. Note that the accessory splenic tissue is isointense with the spleen on this fast spin echo T2-weighted image (TR 4000, effective TE 120, 4 Nex, 16 echo train).

Fig. 6-4. Transaxial T1-weighted image (TR 500, TE 12, 4 NEX) demonstrates a small accessory splenic nodule *(arrow)*. (Reprinted from Mirowitz SA: MRI Clin N Am 3:23-37, 1995.)

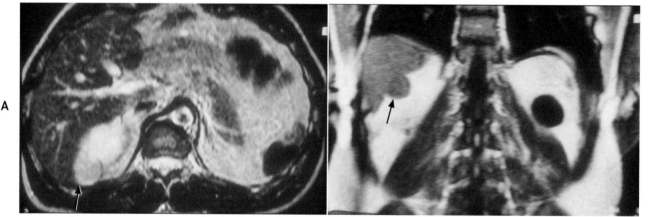

Fig. 6-5. Transaxial T2-weighted **(A)** and coronal contrast material enhanced T1-weighted **(B)** images reveal a nodular structure adjacent to the right hepatic lobe *(arrows)*, which represents splenosis in a patient with splenosis who underwent previous splenectomy.

tail, and a variety of other locations throughout the abdomen.[3]

Following abdominal trauma, dissemination of splenic tissue (splenosis) may occur. In such cases, accessory splenic tissue can be located along the serosal surface of the bowel and within the mesentery and diaphragm, resulting in potential simulation of lymphadenopathy, carcinomatosis, or other lesions[38] (Figs. 6-5, *A* and *B*). Hyperplasia of accessory splenic tissue can be observed in patients who have undergone splenectomy.

Accessory splenic tissue should parallel the spleen proper in its signal intensity on all pulse sequences. Superparamagnetic iron oxide particles, which selectively produce negative enhancement of reticuloendothelial tissues, can provide a more definitive characterization of accessory splenic tissue.[38]

Detection of Splenic Lesions

The splenic artery is frequently tortuous, and its number of branches can vary.[3] Partial volume averaging of the splenic artery or vein with adjacent fat can simulate a nodular lesion in the splenic hilum.

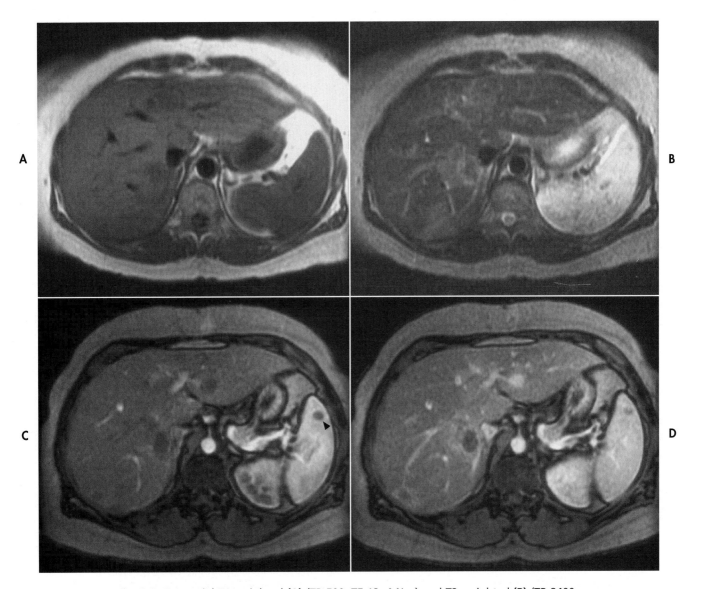

Fig. 6-6. Transaxial T1-weighted **(A)** (TR 500, TE 12, 4 Nex) and T2-weighted **(B)** (TR 3400, TE 80, 2 Nex) spin echo images in a patient with colon cancer metastatic to liver. A small splenic metastasis is poorly visualized on both T1- and T2-weighted images. **C,** The lesion is easily visualized on a dynamic gadolinium chelate enhanced spoiled gradient echo image (TR 150, TE 2.6, 90-degree flip angle, 1 Nex). **D,** Gradient echo image acquired approximately 2 minutes later demonstrates decreased lesion visibility, resulting from equilibration of contrast material between the lesion and surrounding splenic parenchyma (arrowhead).

Splenic lesions are relatively difficult to detect using most cross-sectional imaging studies, including conventional magnetic resonance (MR) sequences, because the relaxation characteristics of splenic lesions are generally similar to those of a normal spleen.[11,19] Hence, there is frequently little or no perceptible differential signal intensity between lesions and the surrounding spleen on either T1- or T2-weighted images (Figs. 6-6, *A-D*). This applies to malignant lesions such as lymphoma[25] and me-

---

ENTITIES THAT MAY SIMULATE SPLENIC LESIONS

- Lobularity, notches, fissures
- Medial process
- Accessory spleen
- Heterogeneous enhancement pattern
- Extension of left hepatic lobe
- Partial volume averaging with stomach, fat

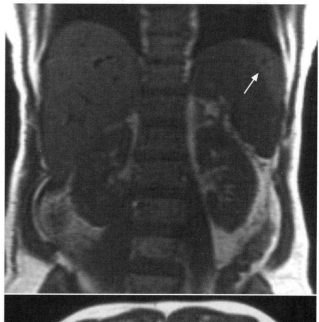

Fig. 6-7. T1-weighted coronal image (TR 500, TE 11, 4 Nex) demonstrates relative increased signal intensity along the superior pole of the spleen *(arrow)*, simulating the appearance of a subcapsular hematoma. This increased signal represents a prominent left hepatic lobe *(L)*, which extends across the midline and overrides the spleen.

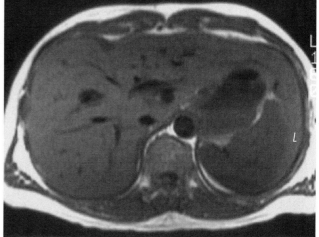

Fig. 6-8. A, Coronal T1-weighted image (TR 267, TE 11, 0.5 Nex) demonstrates differential signal intensity in the region of the spleen *(arrow)*, which may simulate subcapsular splenic hematoma. **B,** Transaxial T1-weighted image (TR 500, TE 12, 4 Nex) reveals a prominent left hepatic lobe that extends lateral and superior to the spleen, resulting in the above appearance. Also note reduced signal-to-noise ratio in **A,** which is caused by limited data acquisition. (Reprinted from Mirowitz SA: MRI Clin N Am 3:23-37, 1995.)

tastases, as well as to benign lesions such as hamartoma.[26]

In addition to its difficulty in depicting focal splenic lesions, MR has also been of limited value for demonstrating diffuse splenic abnormalities and for determining the nature of splenic enlargement (i.e., benign vs. malignant).[40,45] Therefore reactive splenomegaly caused by viral or granulomatous infection frequently cannot be distinguished from that resulting from lymphoma on standard MR images.

The visibility of splenic lesions is maximized on heavily T1- and T2-weighted images. Lesion detection is also enabled when there are signal alterations caused by lesion hemorrhage and/or necrosis. These findings lead to foci of relative increased signal intensity on T1- and/or T2-weighted images. Detection of splenic lesions is also made easier when there is associated deformation of the splenic contour, as can occur with large or peripheral lesions.

The left hepatic lobe can extend lateral to the spleen. When this occurs, the relative increased signal intensity of hepatic compared with splenic tissue on T1-weighted images may cause the hepatic tissue to simulate a subcapsular splenic hematoma or other lesion (Figs. 6-7 to 6-8, *B*).

Hepatic lesions arising in such an aberrant left hepatic lobe may appear to be splenic in origin. Partial volume averaging of fat within the gastrosplenic ligament can simulate an hemorrhagic splenic lesion, particularly on coronal T1-weighted images (Figs. 6-9 and 6-10). Similarly, the spleen can undergo partial volume averaging with the stomach or its liquid contents; the latter can simulate a high signal intensity splenic lesion on T2-weighted images (Fig. 6-11).

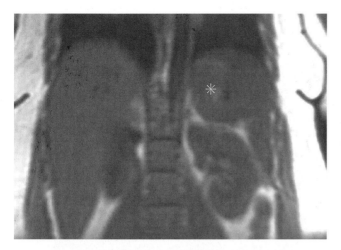

Fig. 6-9. Coronal T1-weighted image (TR 500, TE 12, 4 Nex) demonstrates an apparent high signal intensity lesion involving the spleen *(asterisk)*. This represents partial volume averaging of fat within the gastrosplenic ligament.

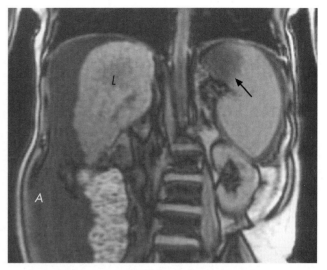

Fig. 6-11. Coronal spoiled gradient echo image (TR 113, TE 2.6, 90-degree flip angle, 1 Nex) demonstrates an apparent mass lesion involving medial aspect of the spleen *(arrow)*. This appearance is due to partial volume averaging with the gastric fundus. Also noted are findings indicating hepatic cirrhosis (*L*) and massive ascites (*A*). (Reprinted from Mirowitz SA: MRI Clin N Am 3:23-37, 1995.)

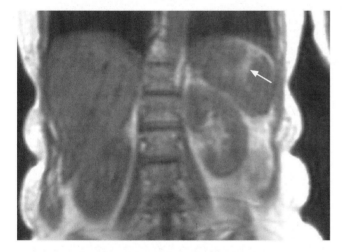

Fig. 6-10. Coronal T1-weighted image (TR 600, TE 12, 4 Nex) demonstrates an apparent ill-defined high signal intensity lesion involving the spleen *(arrow)*. This is due to partial volume averaging of fat within the gastrosplenic ligament.

Contrast Agents

The use of contrast agents has been investigated as a means for improving the detection of focal or diffuse splenic lesions. The bolus administration of paramagnetic agents such as gadopentetate dimeglumine in conjunction with rapid spin echo or gradient echo image acquisition can lead to improved detection of focal splenic lesions (Figs. 6-6, *A-D* and 6-12, *A-F*).[19,33] However, the visibility of such lesions diminishes rapidly within 1 to 2 minutes after contrast material administration, because

of equilibration of the contrast agent between splenic tissue and lesions. Therefore administration of contrast material as a slow infusion or use with relatively long conventional pulse sequences can obscure splenic lesions rather than make them more apparent.

During the bolus phase of contrast material administration, the spleen has a markedly heterogeneous appearance[20,34] (Figs. 6-13, *A* to 6-14, *B*). This is manifested by rounded, linear, or wedge-shaped foci of relative decreased signal intensity as compared with the higher signal intensity of the remainder of the spleen. This pattern reflects a transient lack of equilibration of contrast material between the cords and pulp of splenic parenchyma or between splenic sinusoids and pulp. It has been suggested that irregular splenic enhancement without evidence of a structured pattern may indicate splenic replacement,[34] though further study is necessary to validate this hypothesis. The major significance of this heterogeneous splenic enhancement pattern is that it can simulate focal splenic lesions or obscure their visualization. Conversion to an homogeneous splenic contrast enhancement pattern generally occurs approximately 1 minute after contrast is injected (Figs. 6-15, *A-C*). True splenic lesions are usually identified as foci of abnormal enhancement that persist on images acquired 1 minute after contrast administration. This 1 minute image is critically important, since splenic lesions may become obscured as contrast material undergoes further equilibration, as described previously.

Superparamagnetic iron oxide particles are expected

A   C   E

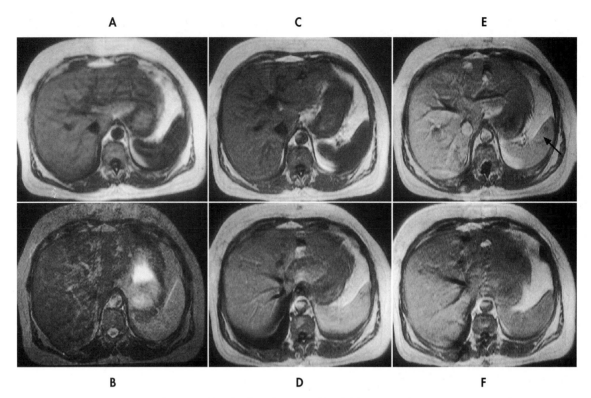

B   D   F

Fig. 6-12. Transaxial T1-weighted **(A)** and T2-weighted **(B)** images demonstrate normal appearance of spleen. However, corresponding rapid acquisition spin echo images obtained before **(C)**, during **(D)**, and 1 minute **(E)** and 5 minutes **(F)** after bolus injection of gadolinium chelate contrast material demonstrate 1 cm metastasis within the anterior spleen (*arrow*). Note that the lesion is maximally conspicuous during or immediately after contrast material injection and becomes obscured on a delayed contrast enhanced image.

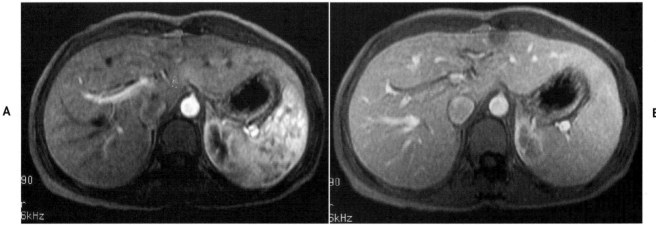

Fig. 6-13. A, Transaxial spoiled gradient echo image (TR 180, TE 4, 90-degree flip angle, 1 Nex) obtained during bolus injection of gadolinium chelate contrast material. There is markedly heterogeneous contrast material enhancement throughout the splenic parenchyma. This converted to an homogeneous pattern on a delayed image **(B)**.

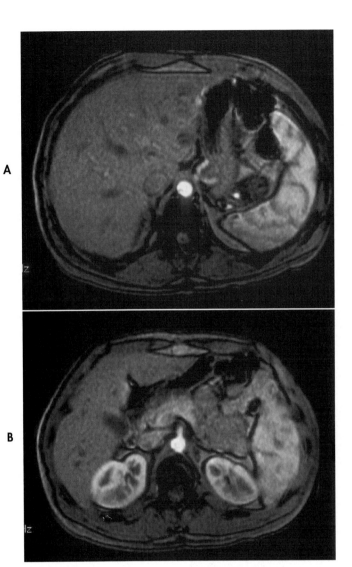

A

B

Fig. 6-14. Rapid spoiled gradient echo images (TR 117, TE 2.8, 60-degree flip angle, 1 Nex) acquired during bolus injection of gadolinium chelate contrast material at two different levels. These images demonstrate a heterogeneous splenic enhancement pattern, which is variable at different levels within the spleen. Image acquired near the upper-mid spleen **(A)** shows curvilinear regions of relative decreased enhancement, whereas a more caudal image **(B)** shows relatively decreased enhancing foci to be more nodular. The spleen appeared homogeneous on images acquired 20 seconds later. (Reprinted from Mirowitz SA: MRI Clin N Am 3:23-37, 1995.)

to improve detection of focal splenic lesions as well as diffuse splenic replacement. This contrast agent selectively accumulates in reticuloendothelial cells, such as those of normal splenic parenchyma, decreasing their signal intensity. This renders splenic lesions more conspicuous by increasing their relative signal intensity as compared with normal splenic tissue. This agent also

provides the best opportunity for detection of diffuse splenic replacement and distinction of benign from malignant causes of splenomegaly.

Characterization of Splenic Lesions

When splenic lesions are observed on MR images, their appearance is often nonspecific. Therefore, distinction between malignant and benign lesions is usually not possible. For example, benign entities such as splenic hamartomas and splenic peliosis can resemble malignant tumors (Figs. 6-16, *A* and *B*). Splenic infarcts, which frequently have a hemorrhagic component, can simulate hemorrhagic metastases or paramagnetic melanoma lesions (Fig. 6-17). Patients with Gaucher disease can manifest focal splenic nodules, which may be confused for metastatic lesions, in addition to splenic infarcts.[13] Splenic cysts and cavernous hemangiomas have prolonged T2 relaxation, similar to their hepatic counterparts, and can be mistaken for necrotic neoplasms.

Most splenic lesions are hyperintense relative to surrounding splenic parenchyma on T2-weighted images. However, splenic lesions have variable signal intensity patterns, and some lesions, such as lymphoma, can be hypointense[11] (Figs. 6-18, *A* and *B*). In patients with cirrhosis, multiple nodular low signal intensity foci often indicate siderotic Gamna-Gandy bodies rather than neoplasm.[18,31] Susceptibility related signal loss caused by these lesions is increased on gradient echo images.

A number of benign lesions may be incidentally encountered in the spleen. Among these are splenic cysts and hemangiomas, which display imaging features similar to their counterparts in the liver (Figs. 6-19 to 6-20, *B*), and splenic hamartomas (see Figs. 6-16, *A* and *B*).

The spleen is typically hyperintense on T2-weighted images relative to the liver, exhibiting signal intensity similar to that of the kidneys. However, diffuse reduction of splenic signal intensity is frequently observed[11] (Figs. 6-21 and 6-22). This signal alteration appears to be a nonspecific phenomenon, which may relate to accumulation of iron secondary to erythrocyte breakdown. Splenic signal intensity may also be reduced in response to some administered medications, such as chemotherapeutic agents (Figs. 6-23, *A* and *B*). Diffuse homogeneous reduction of splenic signal intensity on T2-weighted images should not be interpreted as indicating splenic infiltration or replacement by tumor. In fact, the presence of such signal alterations can potentially improve the conspicuousness of focal splenic lesions, serving as an inherent contrast agent similar in mechanism to the superparamagnetic iron oxide agents already discussed (Figs. 6-24, *A* and *B* to 6-25).

Following splenectomy, fluid collections are frequently observed within the splenic bed.[19] These fluid collections can simulate a postoperative abscess (Figs. 6-26, *A* and *B*).

Text continued on p. 166

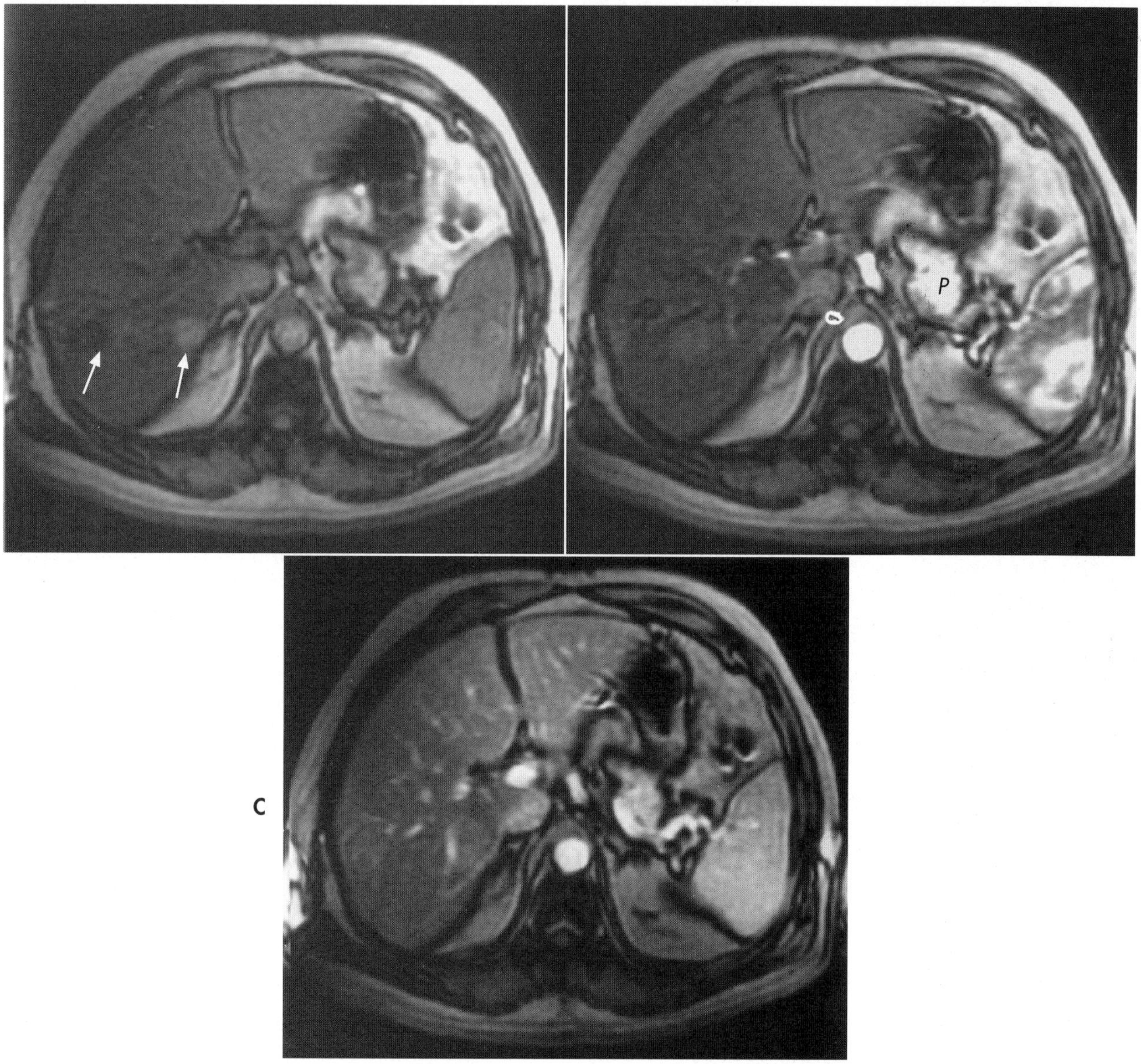

Fig. 6-15. Rapid spoiled gradient echo images (TR 113, TE 2.6, 90-degree flip angle, 1 Nex) before **(A)**, during **(B)**, and 1 **(C)** and minute following bolus injection of gadolinium chelate contrast material. Markedly heterogeneous splenic enhancement is noted during the bolus phase, with rapid conversion to a homogeneous pattern. Prominent enhancement of the pancreas *(P)* is also demonstrated. Also note paradoxic relative decreased prominence of aortic pulsation artifacts *(arrows)* projecting over the right lobe of the liver following contrast material administration, as compared with precontrast image. (Reprinted from Mirowitz SA: MRI Clin N Am 3:23-37, 1995.)

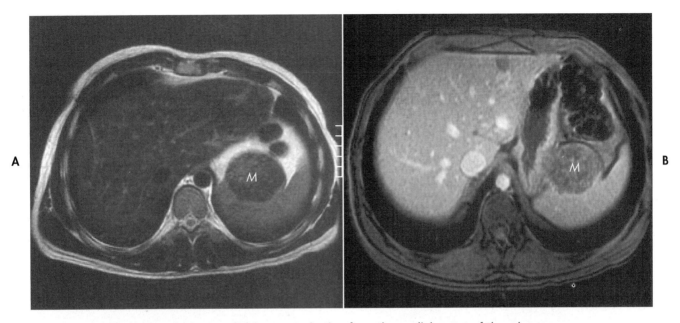

Fig. 6-16. A large mass (*M*) is seen projecting from the medial aspect of the spleen on the transaxial fast spin echo T2-weighted (TR 4000, effective TE 120, 4 Nex, 16 echo train) (**A**) and contrast enhanced gradient echo (**B**) images. This solid lesion represents a presumed splenic hamartoma.

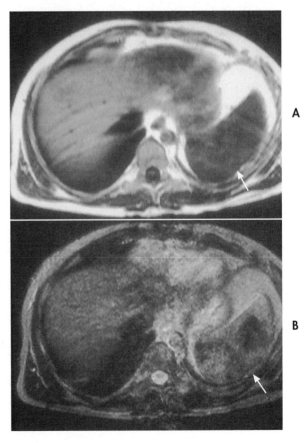

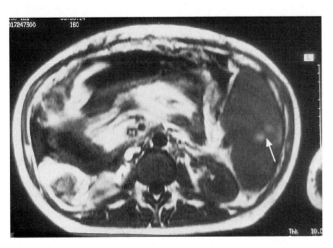

Fig. 6-17. Transaxial T1-weighted image demonstrates an enlarged spleen with a focus of relative increased signal intensity peripherally *(arrow)*, representing a hemorrhagic splenic infarct.

Fig. 6-18. T1-weighted (**A**) and T2-weighted (**B**) transaxial images demonstrate heterogeneous foci of relative decreased signal intensity within the splenic parenchyma (arrows), representing lymphomatous involvement.

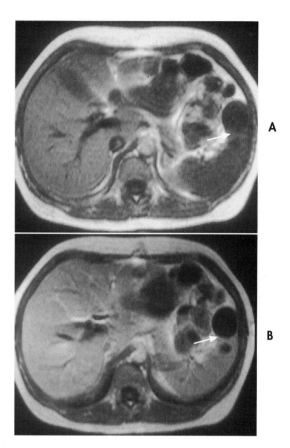

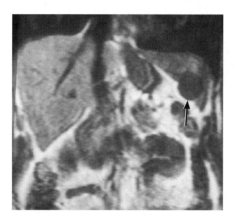

Fig. 6-19. Coronal contrast enhanced T1-weighted image demonstrates a cyst projecting from the caudal aspect of the spleen *(arrow)*.

Fig. 6-20. Transaxial T1-weighted rapid acquisition spin echo images obtained before **(A)** and after **(B)** intravenous gadolinium chelate contrast material administration. Two cysts are seen involving the anterior aspect of the spleen *(arrows)*.

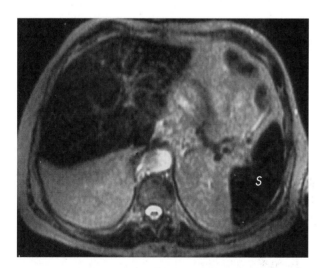

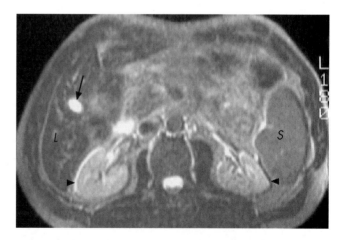

Fig. 6-21. Transaxial T2-weighted image (TR 3600, TE 120, 2 Nex) demonstrates uniform reduced signal intensity throughout the spleen *(S)* in a patient who had undergone previous liver transplantation.

Fig. 6-22. The spleen *(S)* is only slightly hyperintense relative to the liver *(L)* on this transaxial T2-weighted image (TR 3400, TE 120, 2 Nex). Note that splenic parenchyma is considerably reduced in signal intensity as compared with that of the kidneys. An apparent high signal intensity hepatic lesion *(arrow)* represents partial volume averaging with the gallbladder. Note chemical shift misregistration artifact paralleling the renal capsules *(arrowheads)*.

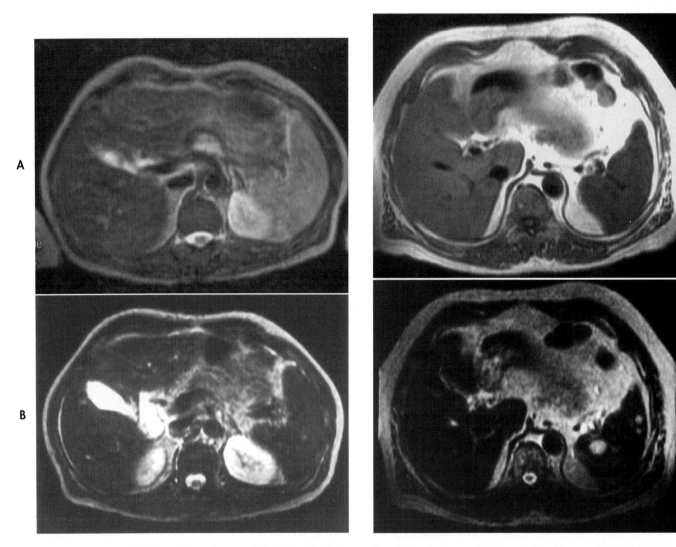

Fig. 6-23. Transaxial T2-weighted images (TR 3400, TE 80, 2 Nex) obtained before **(A)** and 3 months following **(B)** initiation of chemotherapy for lymphoma. The initial image demonstrates normal hyperintensity of the spleen relative to the liver. However, after chemotherapy administration, the liver and spleen are isointense. Note that renal parenchyma is unchanged in signal intensity. The patient was doing well at the time of the second examination and had experienced a regression of the lymphoma.

Fig. 6-24. A, Transaxial T1-weighted image (TR 550, TE 12, 4 Nex) in patient with lymphoma demonstrates a normal appearing spleen. **B,** Corresponding T2-weighted image (TR 3400, TE 80, 2 Nex) reveals multiple nodular foci of lymphomatous splenic involvement. These foci are isointense with the expected signal intensity of the spleen and are only visualized in this patient because of markedly reduced intensity of background splenic parenchyma resulting from iron overload.

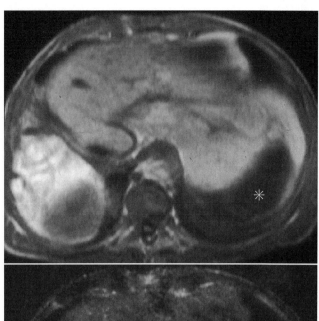

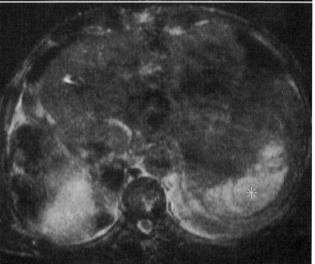

Fig. 6-25. Transaxial T1-weighted image demonstrates uniform hypointensity throughout the liver (*L*) and spleen (*S*) parenchyma in patient with hemosiderosis.

Fig. 6-26. Transaxial T1-weighted **(A)** and T2-weighted **(B)** images demonstrate an apparent normal appearing spleen *(asterisks)*. However, this represents a splenic bed hematoma in a patient who underwent recent splenectomy. The hematoma assumes the expected configuration and signal intensity of the spleen on both images.

PANCREAS
Anatomic Variations

The pancreas can be diffusely prominent in some patients in the absence of pathology. In such cases, the normal lobular architecture and signal intensity of the pancreas are retained, the pancreatic duct is not dilated, and there are no alterations in the peripancreatic fat. These findings distinguish a prominent normal pancreas from one affected by pancreatitis. This is particularly important because the signal intensity of the pancreas may not be noticeably altered in many patients with acute pancreatitis.[33]

Focal prominence of a portion of the pancreas can also be observed as a normal variant. For example, mass-like enlargement of the pancreatic head or tail can occur (Figs. 6-27, *A* to 6-28, *B*). The pancreatic tail can simulate a mass or adenopathy when it is prominent or redundant. The segment of focal pancreatic prominence should again conform to the signal intensity characteristics of the remainder of the pancreas on all pulse sequences, demonstrate a normal architecture and ductal pattern, and show no peripancreatic abnormalities.

Accessory pancreatic tissue can be located within the mesentery, stomach or duodenum, gallbladder, or spleen.[3] An accessory pancreas can be formed by an uncinate process that has failed to unite with the rest of the gland.[3] Annular pancreas is a congenital anomaly in which tissue related to the pancreatic head surrounds and narrows the descending portion of the duodenum.[3]

The pancreatic tail can vary in its cephalocaudal position and may be bifid.[3] The pancreatic tail can extend around the lateral margin of the left kidney in some patients (Fig. 6-29). The distal pancreas can also undergo alteration in position in patients who have undergone previous left nephrectomy. Variations in the branching pattern of the pancreatic ducts and variable presence of accessory ducts occur, but these are usually not discernible on MR images.

Pancreatic Contour

The contour of the pancreas is frequently not smooth but rather characterized by a lobular and sometimes nodular appearance[42] (Figs. 6-30 to 6-31, *B*). This lobular appearance becomes more prominent with increasing patient age.[10] Contour irregularity of a portion of the pancreas, such as the pancreatic head, can also occur as

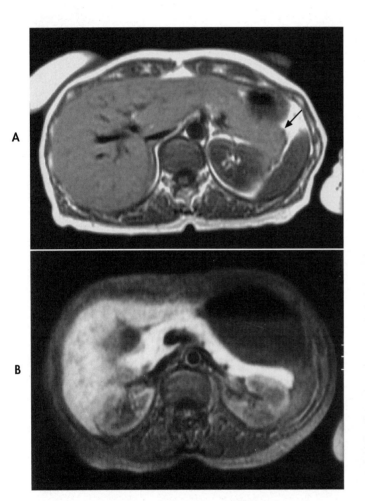

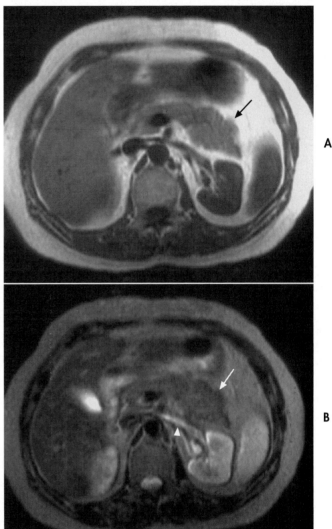

Fig. 6-27. A, Initial T1-weighted image (TR 470, TE 12, 4 Nex) demonstrates apparent fullness of the pancreatic tail *(arrow)*. **B,** Repeat imaging with use of fat saturation and following water distention of the stomach indicates no evidence of mass in this location. Note relative hyperintensity of the pancreatic parenchyma on fat suppressed as compared to conventional T1-weighted image. In addition, improved renal corticomedullary differentiation is demonstrated on the fat-suppressed image.

Fig. 6-28. Focal prominence of the pancreatic tail *(arrows)* is demonstrated on transaxial T1-weighted **(A)** (TR 500, TE 11, 4 Nex) and T2-weighted **(B)** (TR 3400, TE 80, 2 Nex) images as a normal variant. Note that the pancreatic tail follows the signal intensity of the remainder of pancreatic tissue on both pulse sequences. Also noted is relative increased signal intensity within the left renal vein proximal to the superior mesenteric artery on the flow-compensated T2-weighted image *(arrowhead)*. This is related to relative slow blood flow and/or use of gradient moment nulling. (Reprinted from Mirowitz SA: MRI Clin N Am 3:23-37, 1995.)

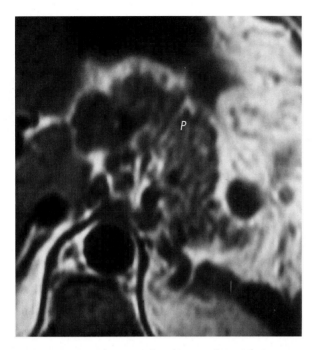

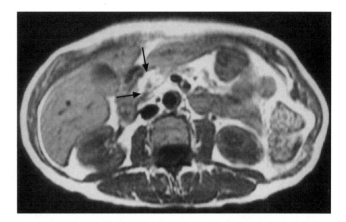

Fig. 6-29. Transaxial T1-weighted image (TR 500, TE 12, 4 Nex) demonstrates lobular contour of normal pancreas (*P*). Heterogeneous increased signal intensity caused by fatty replacement is also noted.

Fig. 6-30. Transaxial T1-weighted image (TR 500, TE 11, 4 Nex) demonstrates focal increased signal intensity of the pancreatic head *(arrows)* compared with remainder of the pancreas. These findings indicate focal fatty replacement of the pancreatic head. (Reprinted from Mirowitz SA: MRI Clin N Am 3:23-37, 1995.)

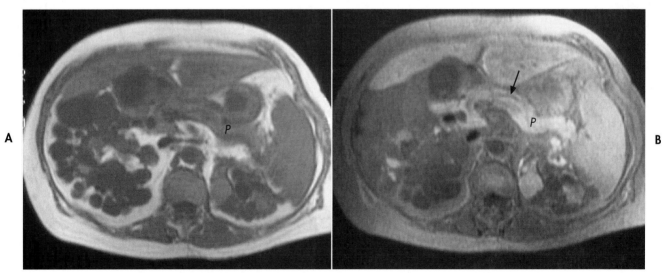

Fig. 6-31. Transaxial T1-weighted images (TR 500, TE 11, 4 Nex) obtained without **(A)** and with **(B)** fat saturation. Note relative increased signal intensity of pancreatic tissue (*P*) on the fat-suppressed image. A normal pancreatic duct can be visualized *(arrow)*. There are innumerable renal cysts bilaterally in this patient with adult polycystic kidney disease. (Reprinted from Mirowitz SA: MRI Clin N Am 3:23-37, 1995.)

a normal variant.[23] The margins of the pancreas may demonstrate apparent irregularity because of the effects of respiratory and gastrointestinal peristaltic motion.[29]

Pancreatic Duct

While the normal pancreatic duct was usually not visible on early MR images, the introduction of more effective motion suppression techniques and newer pulse sequences allows this small structure to be frequently visualized even when nondilated (Figs. 6-32, *A* and *B*). The pancreatic duct is particularly likely to be visible on high-resolution fast spin echo images, dynamic contrast-enhanced images, and fat-suppressed T1-weighted images. It should measure no more than 2 mm in diameter in normal individuals.

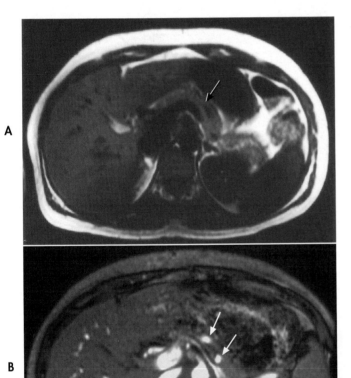

A

B

Fig. 6-32. A, Transaxial T1-weighted image (TR 500, TE 12, 4 Nex) demonstrates apparent focal dilatation of the pancreatic duct *(arrow)*. This is due to partial volume averaging of the pancreas with adjacent splenic vessels *(arrows)*, confirmed on corresponding spoiled gradient echo image **(B)** (TR 50, TE 12, 60-degree flip angle, 2 Nex). (Reprinted from Mirowitz SA: MRI Clin N Am 3:23-37, 1995.)

The fat plane separating the posterior margin of the pancreas from the splenic vein can appear to represent a dilated pancreatic duct, particularly on T2-weighted images. However, flow within the splenic vein should be easily recognizable, particularly when gradient echo sequences are utilized. The splenic artery or vein can also simulate a dilated pancreatic duct, particularly when these vessels are tortuous and undergo volume averaging with the pancreas (Figs. 6-33, *A-D*).

Physiologic Changes

The pancreas undergoes volume loss and progressive replacement of parenchymal tissue by fat as a normal part of the aging process. Therefore the pancreas may appear small and relatively hyperintense on T1-weighted images in elderly patients. Physiologic pancreatic atrophy should be distinguished from that which occurs distal to an obstructing pancreatic lesion. In the latter situation, dilatation of the pancreatic duct is frequently evident within the atrophic segment, which also demonstrates abnormal signal intensity characteristics. Pancreatic size can also be reduced in patients with diabetes mellitus.[10] While fatty replacement of pancreatic tissue is most frequently a diffuse process, focal fatty changes within the pancreas can also be encountered in some individuals (Figs. 6-34, *A* and *B*).

Signal Intensity Characteristics

The normal pancreas is hyperintense relative to the liver on all pulse sequences and is hyperintense relative to the spleen on T1 but not T2-weighted images.[29] The pancreas can be difficult to identify in some patients on T2-weighted images because of isointensity with surrounding fat.[29,33] Even when focal lesions cannot be identified, a pancreas that is hypointense relative to the liver on a T1-weighted image should be considered suspicious.[23] Relative hyperintensity of the pancreas on T2-weighted images can cause pancreatic lesions to be difficult to identify on the basis of isointensity with surrounding normal pancreatic tissue.[8,33] Islet cell tumors, however, are often hyperintense relative to surrounding normal pancreatic tissue.[33]

ENTITIES THAT MAY SIMULATE PANCREATIC LESIONS

- Focal/diffuse prominence
- Lobular contour
- Fatty involution
- Respiratory/gastrointestinal motion artifacts
- Adjacent bowel loops
- Volume averaging with splenic vessels

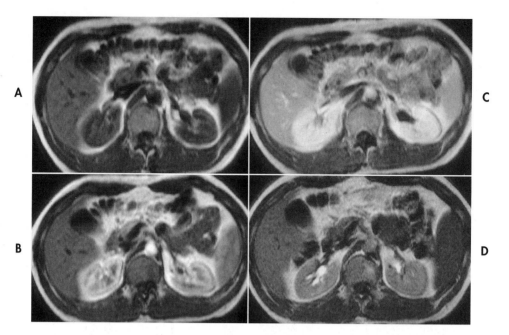

Fig. 6-33. Transaxial T1-weighted rapid acquisition spin echo images obtained before **(A)**, during **(B)**, and 1 minute **(C)** and 5 minutes **(D)** following the bolus injection of intravenous gadolinium chelate contrast material. During the bolus phase of contrast material administration, there is prominent renal cortical enhancement. Note that enhancement within the liver and pancreas is relatively uniform. Hepatic vessels are hypointense relative to the liver during this phase. Mildly delayed image reveals hyperintensity of the hepatic vessels as well as uniform enhancement throughout the renal parenchyma. Relative decreased intensity of the liver, spleen, pancreas and renal parenchyma is demonstrated on the more delayed image, where contrast material is seen filling the renal collecting system.

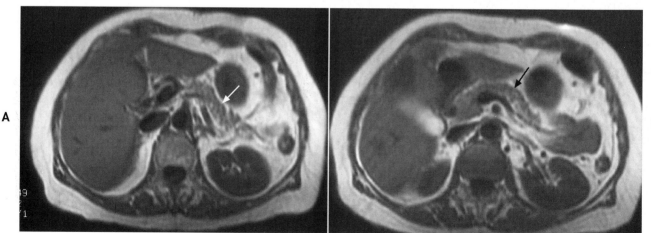

Fig. 6-34. Transaxial T1-weighted images (TR 550, TE 12, 4 Nex) at two consecutive levels demonstrate a lobular contour of the pancreas *(arrow)* in 80-year-old female. Also note interspersed foci of relative increased signal intensity representing fatty replacement.

The pancreas routinely appears relatively hyperintense on T1-weighted images acquired using fat suppression[24,36] (see Fig. 6-32, A and B). This appearance is observed even in patients with fatty replacement of the pancreas.[23] These signal intensity characteristics are related to suppression of signal intensity from surrounding abdominal fat, with secondary expansion of the dynamic range for tissue contrast display. The hyperintense appearance of the normal pancreas on fat-suppressed T1-weighted images provides favorable conditions for identification of focal pancreatic lesions. Such lesions will appear conspicuously hypointense relative to surrounding normal pancreatic parenchyma.

Contrast Enhancement Behavior

Further increase in pancreatic signal intensity is observed when intravenous paramagnetic contrast agents such as gadopentetate dimeglumine are administered.[20] The pancreas normally undergoes homogeneous and diffuse contrast enhancement (Figs. 6-15 and 6-35). Pancreatic carcinoma demonstrates variable contrast enhancement following contrast material administration. In most patients, such tumors enhance less intensely than normal pancreatic tissue, though marked enhancement can occur.[23] Heterogeneous pancreatic enhancement following bolus administration of paramagnetic contrast material can also occur in patients with chronic pancreatitis.[33] Enhancement of the pancreas can also occur after administration of manganese-DPDP, an agent that primarily accumulates within hepatocellular tissue.[8,9]

Simulation of Pancreatic Masses

An apparent mass in the region of the pancreatic head can be created by fluid, air, and/or debris within the descending duodenum or within a duodenal diverticulum. Prominence of the duodenal papilla represents another potential cause for a pseudolesion of the pancreatic head. Proximal jejunal loops located adjacent to the pancreas can simulate a mass arising from the pancreatic body or tail (Figs. 6-36, A and B).

Gastrointestinal tract structures can simulate pancreatic lesions because of their proximity and frequent isointensity with the pancreas. The latter situation is due to the lack of a widely utilized contrast agent for marking the gastrointestinal tract on MR images. A number of practical materials can be used to distinguish pancreatic masses and gastrointestinal tract structures. For example, water, effervescent granules, barium, kaolin clay preparations, and nutritional support formulae are simple, widely available, and effective methods for accomplishing these objectives (Figs. 6-37 to 6-38, B).

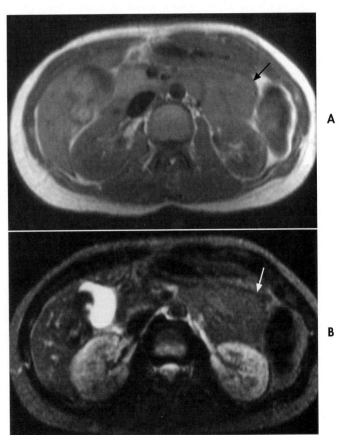

A

B

Fig. 6-36. An apparent lobular mass arising *(arrows)* from the distal pancreatic body and tail is depicted on transaxial T1-weighted **(A)** (TR 500, TE 11, 4 Nex) and T2-weighted **(B)** (TR 3400, TE 120, 2 Nex) images. However, this finding is due to a cluster of small bowel loops located adjacent to the pancreas. Slight differential signal intensity between these bowel loops and the pancreatic head is noted on both images.

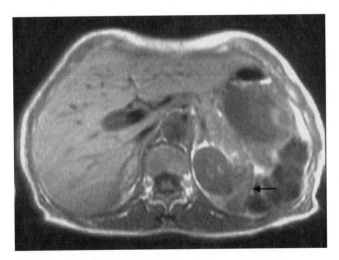

Fig. 6-35. The pancreatic tail extends around the lateral aspect of the left kidney *(arrow)* on this T1-weighted transaxial image (TR 500, TE 12, 4 Nex). (Reprinted from Mirowitz SA: MRI Clin N Am 3:23-37, 1995.)

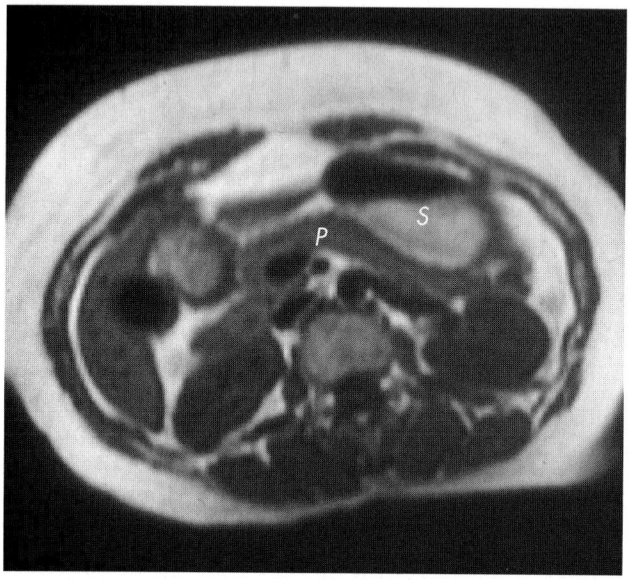

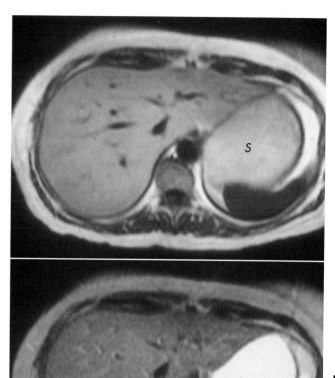

Fig. 6-37. Transaxial T1-weighted image (TR 600, TE 12, 2 Nex) obtained following administration of nutritional support formula. There is excellent distinction between the stomach (*S*) and adjacent pancreas (*P*), allowing for markedly improved delineation of these structures compared with unenhanced images. (Reprinted from Mirowitz SA: J Comput Assist Tomogr 16:908-915, 1992.)

Characterization of Pancreatic Lesions

Diagnostic difficulties can be encountered in attempting to characterize pancreatic lesions. One frequent source of difficulty is the distinction between focal pancreatitis and pancreatic carcinoma. Both entities can result in masslike focal enlargement and abnormal signal intensity of the pancreas.[44] Diffuse decreased signal intensity throughout the pancreas on fat-suppressed T1-weighted images, diffuse decreased intensity on dynamic contrast-enhanced imaging, small cystic areas, and absence of a discrete focus of masslike enlargement or abnormal signal intensity are signs suggestive of pancreatitis.[33]

Pancreatic calcifications are frequently present in patients with chronic pancreatitis; however, such calcifications can be obscure on conventional MR images.[33,41] Breath-hold gradient echo techniques can be useful for improving depiction of pancreatic calcifications. Vascular encasement has been considered an indication of pancreatic malignancy. However, vascular encasement can also be seen in patients with benign pancreatic lesions.[1]

Small carcinomas that result in distal pancreatitis can be particularly difficult to recognize on MR images because of their small size and because they may be obscured by associated inflammatory changes.[33] Periampullary carcinomas are often small at the time of presentation because they lead to ductal obstruction; these too can be difficult to visualize on MR.[33] Ductal

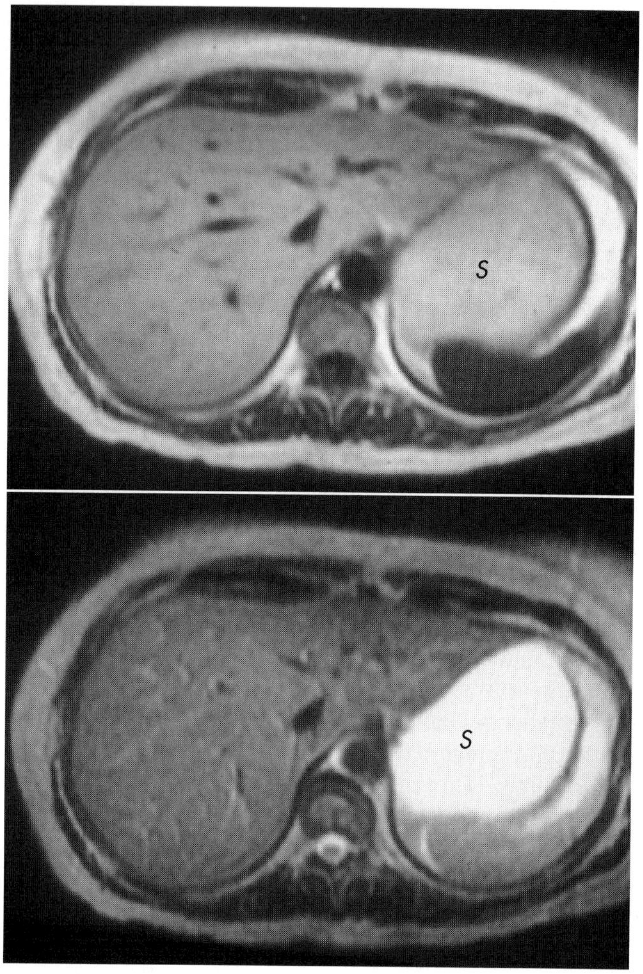

Fig. 6-38. Transaxial T1-weighted **(A)** (TR 500, TE 12, 4 Nex) and T2-weighted **(B)** (TR 2500, TE 90, 2 Nex) images following administration of nutritional support formula. This agent results in a marked increased signal intensity and in excellent distention of the gastric lumen (*S*), allowing for accurate evaluation of gastric wall thickness and differentiation from adjacent structures. (Reprinted from Mirowitz SA: J Comput Assist Tomogr 16:908-915, 1992.)

ENTITIES THAT MAY SIMULATE GASTROINTESTINAL TRACT LESIONS

- Esophagogastric junction/pylorus
- Hiatal hernias
- Retained food products
- Indwelling tubes/postoperative changes
- Diverticula
- Underdistention
- Motion artifacts
- Gelatin sponge

adenocarcinoma can have a similar appearance to cholangiocarcinoma when the latter involves the intrapancreatic portion of the distal common bile duct.[33]

The presence of pancreatic or peripancreatic fluid collections is usually due to pseudocyst formation in a patient with pancreatitis. However, pancreatic cystadenomas and necrotic tumors such as sarcomas display fluid-like internal signal characteristics, potentially simulating pseudocysts. A rare low-grade pancreatic malignant tumor—the solid and papillary epithelial neoplasm—can also appear as a well-defined cystic lesion, which can also be suggestive of a pseudocyst.[27] Therefore, when a cystic pancreatic lesion is identified, correlation with clinical history and laboratory results should be performed to assess for pancreatitis. In addition, secondary findings of inflammation, edematous changes in the peripancreatic fat, or extension of fluid into the left pararenal space should be sought. Cases that remain problematic may require follow-up MR evaluation, endoscopic retrograde cholangiopancreatography, or biopsy.

Pancreatic transplants frequently demonstrate apparent enlargement and heterogeneous signal characteristics.[43,48,49] These findings can result in a false diagnosis of graft rejection. Conversely, when such rejection occurs, it can be difficult to visualize on MR images.[6]

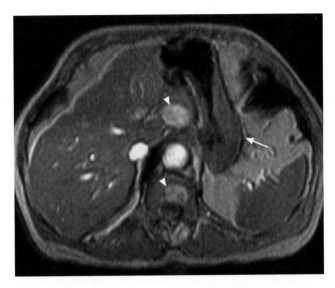

Fig. 6-39. There is apparent thickening of the inferior gastric wall *(arrow)* on this transaxial gradient echo image (TR 33, TE 5, 30-degree flip angle, 2 Nex). This finding is related to underdistention of the stomach. Also noted is a series of hyperintense rounded increased signal intensities *(arrowheads)*, some of which overlie the liver and simulate lesions. These latter findings are due to aortic pulsation artifacts. (Reprinted from Mirowitz SA: MRI Clin N Am 3:23-37,1995.)

GASTROINTESTINAL TRACT
Simulation of Lesions

Many entities can simulate masses related to the gastrointestinal tract. The muscular components of the esophagastric junction can appear thickened and masslike in normal individuals. The pyloric muscle may be relatively prominent, simulating a mass involving the distal stomach.

Hiatal hernias are common and can simulate a gastric or distal esophageal mass. This is most likely to occur when the hernia sac is not fully distended with air or when it contains food debris. Soft tissue thickening, suggestive of a mass, can be observed in the region of the esophagogastric junction in patients who have undergone previous surgical repair of a hiatal hernia.

Retained food products within the gastric lumen can appear to represent a mass. This is usually encountered in patients who have recently eaten; who have gastroparesis related to diabetes, vagotomy, or other causes; or who have mechanical gastric outlet obstruction. Food products can have highly variable signal intensity, depending on their composition. In many cases, food within the stomach has high signal intensity on T1-weighted images, because of fat and/or proteinaceous contents. When a gastric mass is suspected, some patients will require reexamination after fasting or nasogastric suction.

Indwelling nasogastric tubes, nasoenteric or percutaneous feeding tubes, or long decompression tubes can create foci of decreased signal intensity within the stomach and/or small bowel, potentially simulating lesions.

Gastric diverticula arising from the gastric fundus can simulate an exophytic gastric mass or a mass arising from the pancreas or left adrenal gland. Duodenal diverticula are very common; these can simulate lesions arising from the duodenum, stomach, or pancreatic head. Prominence of the duodenal papilla can occasionally simulate a small mass in the descending duodenum. The stomach as well as the spleen and left hepatic lobe can be partially retroperitoneal in location.[3]

Apparent thickening of the gastric mucosal folds and/or gastric wall can be due to nondistention of the stomach (Fig. 6-39). These findings can simulate gastritis or infiltrative tumors of the gastric wall such as adenocarcinoma or lymphoma. In some patients, focal masslike gastric wall thickening is observed, suggestive of gastric carcinoma. Apparent thickening of the gastric wall resulting from nondistention frequently terminates abruptly near the location of a gastric air-fluid level[12] (Fig. 6-40). This sign can be useful in distinguishing true thickening from pseudothickening caused by underdistention. However, definitive exclusion of underlying gastric pathology may require repeat image acquisition following distention of the stomach with water, air, or

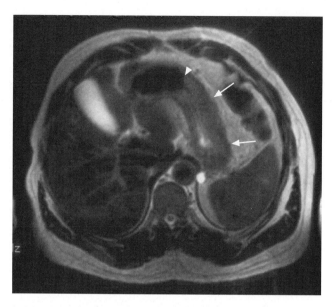

Fig. 6-40. Transaxial fast spin echo T2-weighted image (TR 3500, effective TE 120, 4 Nex, 16 echo train) demonstrates apparent thickening of the gastric wall *(arrows)* that terminates abruptly at the level of an air fluid level *(arrowhead).* Note that above this level the gastric wall assumes a normal thickness.

contrast material. Absence of signal intensity alterations within the apparently thickened segment of the gastric wall is supportive of pseudothickening, though mural signal alterations may not be evident in some patients with gastritis or some infiltrative neoplasms.

Anatomic Variations

The gastrointestinal tract can undergo nonrotation or partial or complete malrotation. Malalignment of the superior mesenteric artery and vein, when observed on transaxial images, may indicate such malrotation. However, the pancreas can displace the mesenteric vessels, resulting in their apparent malalignment.[37] The small bowel loops can also undergo acquired alterations in location. For example, jejunal loops may fill the left renal fossa in patients who have undergone previous left nephrectomy. The colon may be interposed between the anterior surface of the liver and the anterior abdominal wall (Chilaiditi syndrome). The hepatic flexure can be located lateral to the right hepatic lobe, and the ascending colon can present in the hepatorenal fossa or in a retrorenal position.[16] The presence of bowel within any of these atypical locations may simulate a subphrenic or mesenteric abscess or neoplasm. The presence of air and fecal material within the colon results in a heterogeneous mottled appearance similar to that of an abscess.

A Meckel diverticulum, arising from the distal ileum, occurs in approximately 1% to 2% of the population and

can contain ectopic gastric mucosa and pancreatic glands.[3] Colonic diverticulosis is frequently present, particularly in older individuals.

The ileocecal valve may be prominent and appear as a filling defect. Increased signal intensity on T1-weighted images can be observed within the ileocecal valve as a result of lipomatous tissue. Lipomas can also be encountered elsewhere throughout the colon.[46] The appendix may be absent or duplicated or found in a variety of unusual locations throughout the abdomen.[3]

Motion Artifacts

Artifacts related to peristaltic bowel motion are frequent and are usually manifested as blurring of anatomic detail.[4,7,42] When regular or periodic bowel contractions occur, more structured ghost artifacts can occur along the phase-encoding direction of the image. The prominence of these motion artifacts is proportional to the signal intensity of intraluminal bowel contents. Therefore, in the presence of intraluminal fluid, peristaltic artifacts are accentuated on T2-weighted images. These artifacts can be particularly severe on images acquired using the STIR technique, because they depict fluid as hyperintense and because of their low signal-to-noise ratio.[7,30]

The presence of gastrointestinal motion artifacts can be reduced when a hypotonic agent such as glucagon is administered.[4,7,42] The effectiveness of glucagon is of limited duration, however, and examination times must be relatively short or the drug may have to be administered repeatedly for optimal results. Intravenous administration of glucagon is not recommended because of the reduced duration of effectiveness; instead, the agent should be given as a subcutaneous or preferably intramuscular injection.

Signal Intensity Patterns

The gastrointestinal tract can demonstrate a variety of intraluminal signal intensity patterns on MR images, ranging from markedly hypointense (e.g., from air, fecal material) to markedly hyperintense (e.g., from lipids and proteinaceous contents on T1-weighted images and fluid secretions on T2-weighted images). Small bowel loops frequently demonstrate signal intensity characteristics similar to those of soft tissue. This may cause such loops to simulate enlarged lymph nodes or other abdominal masses. High intensity may be observed along the mucosal surface of the gastrointestinal tract, presumably because of proteinaceous mucous secretions (Fig. 6-41).

While a number of oral MR contrast agents have been investigated, none has yet achieved widespread acceptance for routine usage. Such agents are useful, however, as problem solving tools in selected patients. Gastrointestinal contrast agents may provide either positive or negative intraluminal enhancement effects. Positive con-

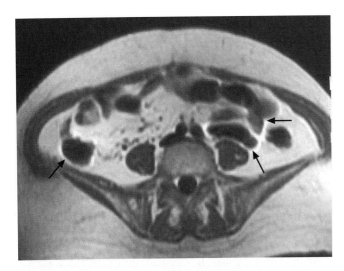

Fig. 6-41. Hyperintensity is observed along the mucosal surface of the small and large bowel *(arrows)* on transaxial T1-weighted image (TR 500, TE 12, 4 Nex). This is presumed due to mucus-like contents along the bowel mucosa.

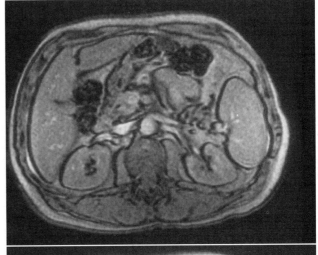

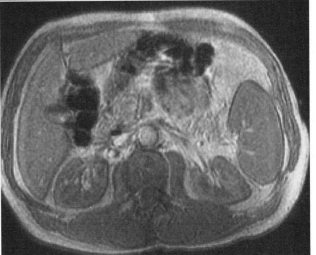

Fig. 6-42. Foci of relative decreased signal intensity are seen surrounding the viscera (liver, spleen, kidney), bowel, vessels, and fascial planes. These findings represent chemical shift phase cancellation artifact on an opposed phase spoiled gradient echo image **(A)** (TR 118, TE 2.8, 60-degree flip angle, 1 Nex). These findings are largely eliminated with use of an in-phase echo time **(B)** (TR 135, TE 4.2, 90-degree flip angle, 1 Nex).

trast agents result in increased intraluminal signal intensity and include orally administered gadopentetate dimeglumine solutions, solutions containing ferric ammonium citrate and other paramagnetic trace metals, nutritional support formula, and suspensions of oils (Figs. 6-40 and 6-41). The latter agents are not miscible with gastrointestinal tract secretions, which can contribute to nonuniform intraluminal enhancement. All positive enhancement agents share the limitation of increasing motion artifacts related to bowel peristalsis. These artifacts can simulate or obscure a gastrointestinal tract or other abdominal pathology. The active component of some agents may undergo absorption and/or dilution as they traverse the small bowel, leading to reduced effectiveness.[21]

Negative oral contrast agents such as air, clays, barium, iron oxides, and perfluorochemicals result in reduced intraluminal signal intensity. These agents may also be either miscible or immiscible with bowel contents. Negative enhancing agents have the advantage of reducing rather than accentuating peristaltic motion artifacts. However, the presence of bowel wall thickening may be less conspicuous because of similar low signal intensity of intraluminal contents and the adjacent bowel wall. Iron oxide preparations can lead to susceptibility artifacts, particularly on gradient echo images, which can obscure the bowel wall and surrounding structures. The concentration of iron must be optimized to avoid these susceptibility effects and yet maintain effective contrast enhancement.[15]

Markedly decreased signal intensity is observed along the serosal surface of the gastrointestinal tract on gradient echo images acquired using an echo time at which fat and water protons are of opposed phase. These are referred to as chemical shift phase cancellation artifacts, and they can potentially obscure subtle serosal tumor invasion (Figs. 6-42, *A* and *B*). Susceptibility artifacts may also result from air within the unenhanced gastrointestinal tract and can similarly obscure the gastrointestinal tract or other abdominal organs[39] (Figs. 6-43, *A* and *B* and 6-44). These artifacts can be minimized with the use of short echo times, use of T1-weighted rather than T2-weighted pulse sequences, and substitution of spin echo for gradient echo pulse techniques.[5] In addition, use of a higher resolution imaging matrix and reduced slice thick-

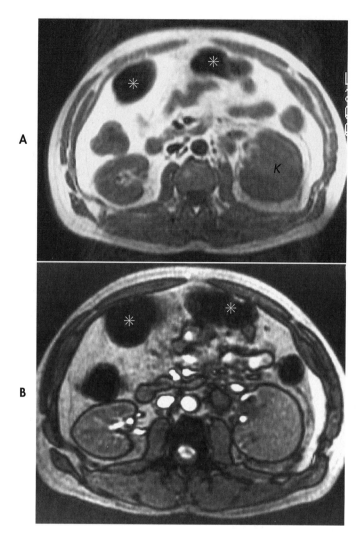

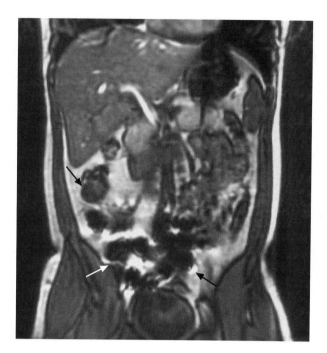

Fig. 6-44. Coronal spoiled gradient echo image (TR 120, TE 3, 90-degree flip angle, 1 Nex) demonstrates areas of artifactual signal void caused by susceptibility artifact related to bowel gas *(arrows)*. (Reprinted from Mirowitz SA: MRI Clin N Am 3:23-37, 1995.)

Fig. 6-43. Transaxial T1-weighted spin echo **(A)** (TR 580, TE 11, 4 Nex) and gradient echo **(B)** (TR 50, TE 12, 60-degree flip angle, 2 Nex) images. Areas of decreased signal intensity represent susceptibility artifacts arising from air within the bowel lumen *(asterisks)*. Note the blooming effect of these artifacts on the gradient echo image. Susceptibility artifacts also result in poor visualization of the fat plane between the hepatic flexure and abdominal wall. Also noted is a left renal cell carcinoma (*K*).

ness can help to decrease the prominence of susceptibility artifacts.[47] Air-containing structures such as bowel that are out of the plane of gradient echo image acquisition can also result in foci of artifactual signal loss.[32]

The signal intensity of barium sulfate varies according to its concentration. High-density barium sulfate suspension produces low signal intensity on all pulse sequences.[17] However, at lower concentrations hyperintensity can occur.[2] The optimal concentration of barium sulfate is between 170% and 220% weight/volume.

While oral administration of barium can help delineate abnormalities of the upper gastrointestinal tract, this material can also be administered rectally to improve evaluation of the rectum and colon.[28]

Kaolin clay preparations manifest different signal behavior on T1- and T2-weighted sequences. This material results in positive intraluminal contrast on short TE T1-weighted images, whereas negative contrast is present on T2-weighted images.[23] These features are favorable for depiction of gastrointestinal tract abnormalities on both sequences.

Enhancement of the gastrointestinal tract can also occur following intravenous contrast material administration. Following gadopentetate dimeglumine injection, relatively modest and inconspicuous mural enhancement occurs on conventional T1-weighted images[35] (Figs. 6-45, *A* and *B*). However, when contrast-enhanced fat-suppressed T1-weighted images are acquired, mural enhancement can appear prominent and can simulate abnormal enhancement associated with inflammatory or neoplastic conditions[22] (Figs. 6-46 to 6-48, *B*). Such enhancement is usually most prominent within the small bowel loops and least prominent in the stomach. Because of simultaneous enhancement of adjacent abdominal viscera, it can be difficult to distinguish enhancing bowel loops from other organs or adjacent lesions.

Gelatin sponge material may be placed within the

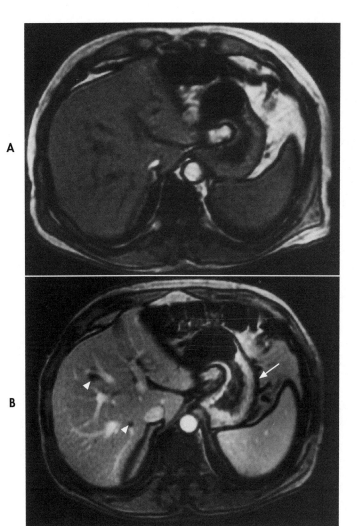

Fig. 6-45. Transaxial spoiled gradient echo images (TR 114, TE 2.6, 90-degree flip angle, 1 Nex) obtained before **(A)** and after **(B)** intravenous gadolinium chelate administration. There is prominent enhancement of the gastric wall (arrow) following bolus injection of 0.1 mmol/kg gadolinium chelate contrast material. These images were photographed using identical window and level settings. Two small hepatic cysts (arrowheads) are also noted. (Reprinted from Mirowitz SA: MRI Clin N Am 3:23-37, 1995.)

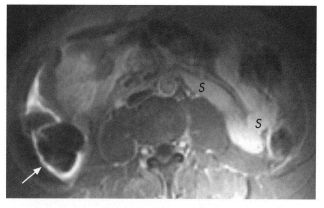

Fig. 6-46. There is marked diffuse enhancement throughout the small bowel loops (*S*) as well as enhancement of the colonic wall (arrow) on this transaxial contrast-enhanced fat-suppressed T1-weighted image (TR 600, TE 12, 4 Nex) in a patient without bowel disease. (Reprinted from Mirowitz SA: MRI Clin N Am 3:23-37, 1995.)

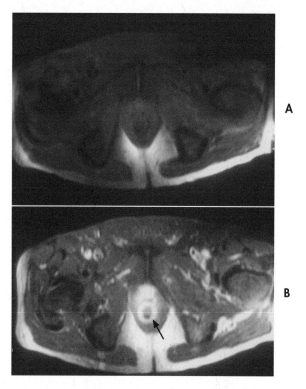

Fig. 6-47. Fat-suppressed T1-weighted images obtained before **(A)** and after **(B)** intravenous gadolinium chelate contrast material administration. There is prominent enhancement of the rectal wall (arrow) in this patient without gastrointestinal tract abnormality. (Reprinted from Mirowitz SA: Abdom Imaging 18:215-219, 1993.)

peritoneal cavity to promote hemostasis during abdominal surgery. Its presence can simulate an abdominal mass or abscess in recent postoperative patients.[14] This material has heterogeneous decreased signal intensity on T1-weighted images and increased intensity on T2-weighted images. Multiple small signal void foci can be observed, representing air within the sponge. This appearance can simulate an abdominal abscess or necrotic neoplasm. The sponge material demonstrates more homogeneous signal characteristics over the several weeks following surgery,

while it loses its marginal definition because of progressive resorption.

Decreased signal intensity throughout the central abdomen can be observed in patients with extensive ascites

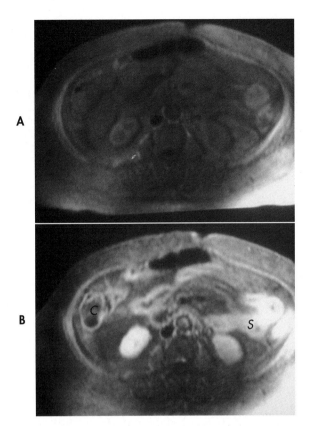

Fig. 6-48. Transaxial fat-suppressed T1-weighted images obtained before **(A)** and after **(B)** intravenous gadolinium chelate contrast material administration. There is prominent mural enhancement throughout all small bowel loops (*S*) as well as the colon (*C*) in this patient without gastrointestinal tract abnormality. (Reprinted from Mirowitz SA: Abdom Imaging 18:215-219, 1993.

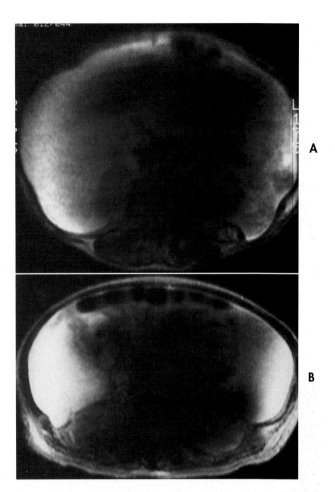

Fig. 6-49. Transaxial T2-weighted images (TR 3000, TE 90, 2 Nex) in two different patients with extensive ascites. Artifactual reduced signal intensity is noted throughout the central abdomen on both images, caused by poor radiofrequency penetration.

(Figs. 6-49, *A* and *B*). This is due to the inability to achieve adequate radiofrequency penetration and is particularly noticeable on T2-weighted images. The presence of ascitic fluid can also generate considerable phase errors (i.e., ghosting artifacts), which obscure abdominal structures and lesions.

REFERENCES

1. Baker ME, Cohan RH, Nadel SN et al: Obliteration of the fat surrounding the celiac axis and superior mesenteric artery is not a specific CT finding of carcinoma of the pancreas, Am J Roentgenol 155:991-994, 1990.
2. Ballinger JR, Ros PR: High density barium sulfate suspension for MRI optimization of concentration for bowel opacification, Magn Reson Imaging 10:637-640, 1992.
3. Bergman RA, Thompson SA, Afifi AK et al: Compendium of human anatomic variation: text, atlas, and world literature, Baltimore, 1988, Urban & Schwarzenberg.
4. Brown JJ, Duncan JR, Heiken JP et al: Perflouroctylbromide as a gastrointestinal contrast agent for MR imaging: use with and without glucagon, Radiology 181:455-460, 1991.
5. Czervionke LF, Daniels DL, Wehrli FW et al: Magnetic susceptibility artifacts in gradient-recalled echo MR imaging, Am J Neuroradiol 9:1149-1155, 1988.
6. del Pilar Fernandez M, Bernardino ME, Neylan JF et al: Diagnosis of pancreatic transplant dysfunction: value of gadopentetate dimeglumine-enhanced MR imaging, Am J Roentgenol 156:1171-1176, 1991.
7. Ehman RL, McNamara MT, Brasch RC et al: Influence of physiologic motion on the appearance of tissue in MR images, Radiology 159:777-782, 1986.
8. Gehl H-B, Urhahn R, Bohndorf K et al: Mn-DPDP in MR imaging of pancreatic adenocarcinoma: initial clinical experience, Radiology 186:795-798, 1993.
9. Gehl H-B, Vorwerk D, Klose K-C et al: Pancreatic enhancement after low-dose infusion of Mn-DPDP, Radiology 180:337-339, 1991.
10. Gilbeau J-P, Poncelet V, Libon E et al: The density, contour, and thickness of the pancreas in diabetics: CT findings in 57 patients, Am J Roentgenol 159:527-531, 1992.
11. Hahn PF, Weissleder R, Stark DD et al: MR imaging of focal splenic tumors, Am J Roentgenol 150:823-827, 1988.

12. Hammerman AM, Mirowitz SA, Susman N: The gastric air-fluid sign: aid in CT assessment of gastric wall thickening, Gastrointest Radiol 14:109-112, 1989.

13. Hill SC, Damaska BM, Ling A et al: Gaucher disease: abdominal MR imaging findings in 46 patients, Radiology 184:561-566, 1992.

14. Hoeffner EG, Crowley MG, Soulen RL: MR imaging appearance of intraperitoneal gelatin sponge in mice, J Magn Reson Imaging 2:63-67, 1992.

15. Holtas S, Wallengren NO, Ericsson A et al: Signal alterations, artifacts and image distortion induced by a superparamagnetic contrast medium. A phantom study in a 0.3 tesla MR system, Acta Radiol 31:213-216, 1990.

16. Hopper KD, Sherman JL, Luethke JM et al: The retrorenal colon in the supine and prone patient, Radiology 162:443-446, 1987.

17. Marti-Bonmati L, Vilar J, Paniagua JC et al: High density barium sulphate as an MRI oral contrast, Magn Reson Imaging 9:259-261, 1991.

18. Minami M, Itai Y, Ohtomo K et al: Siderotic nodules in the spleen: MR imaging of portal hypertension, Radiology 172:681-684, 1989.

19. Mirowitz SA, Brown JJ, Lee JKT et al: Dynamic gadolinium-enhanced MR imaging of the spleen: normal enhancement patterns and evaluation of splenic lesions, Radiology 179:681-686, 1991.

20. Mirowitz SA, Gutierrez E, Lee JKT et al: Normal abdominal enhancement patterns with dynamic gadolinium-enhanced MR imaging, Radiology 180:637-640, 1991.

21. Mirowitz SA, Susman N: Use of nutritional support formula as a gastrointestinal contrast agent for MRI, J Comput Assist Tomogr 16:908-915, 1992.

22. Mirowitz SA: Contrast enhancement of the gastrointestinal tract on MR images using intravenous gadolinium-DTPA, Abdom Imaging 18:215-219, 1993.

22a. Mirowitz SA: MR pitfalls and variants in the extrahepatic abdomen, MRI Clin N Am 3:23-37, 1995.

23. Mitchell DG, Shapiro M, Schuricht A et al: Pancreatic disease: findings on state-of-the-art MR images, Am J Roentgenol 159:533-538, 1992.

24. Mitchell DG, Vinitski S, Saponaro S et al: Liver and pancreas: improved spin-echo T1 contrast by shorter echo time and fat suppression at 1.5 T, Radiology 178:67-71, 1991.

25. Nyman R, Rhen S, Ericsson A et al: An attempt to characterize malignant lymphoma in spleen, liver, and lymph nodes with magnetic resonance imaging, Acta Radiol 28:527-533, 1987.

26. Ohtomo K, Fukuda H, Mori K et al: CT and MR appearances of splenic hamartoma, J Comput Assist Tomogr 16:425-428, 1992.

27. Ohtomo K, Furui S, Onoue M et al: Solid and papillary epithelial neoplasm of the pancreas: MR imaging and pathologic correlation, Radiology 184:567-570, 1992.

28. Panaccione JL, Ros PR, Torres GM et al: Rectal barium in pelvic MR imaging initial results, J Magn Reson Imaging 1:605-607, 1992.

29. Piccirillo M, Bourque A, McCarthy S et al: High field imaging of the normal pancreas, Mag Reson Imaging 7:457-461, 1989.

30. Porter BA: High-field-strength STIR imaging: limitations (letter), Am J Roentgenol 153:1104, 1989.

31. Sagoh T, Itoh K, Togashi K et al: Gamma-Gandy bodies of the spleen: evaluation with MR imaging, Radiology 172:685-687, 1989.

32. Schick RM, Wismer GL, Davis KR: Magnetic susceptibility effects secondary to out-of-plane air in fast MR scanning, Am J Neuroradiol 9:439-442, 1988.

33. Semelka RC, Ascher SM: MR imaging of the pancreas, Radiology 188:593-602, 1993.

34. Semelka RC, Shoenut JP, Lawrence PH et al: Spleen: dynamic enhancement patterns on gradient-echo MR images enhanced with gadopentetate dimeglumine, Radiology 185:479-482, 1992.

35. Semelka RC, Shoenut JP, Silverman R et al: Bowel disease: prospective comparison of CT and 1.5- T pre- and postcontrast MR imaging with T1-weighted fat-suppressed and breath-hold FLASH sequences, J Magn Reson Imaging 1:625-632, 1991.

36. Semelka RC, Simm FC, Recht MP et al: MR imaging of the pancreas at high field strength: comparison of six sequences, J Comput Assist Tomogr 15:966-971, 1991.

37. Shatzkes D, Gordon DH, Haller JO et al: Malrotation of the bowel: malalignment of the superior mesenteric artery-vein complex shown by CT and MR, J Comput Assist Tomogr 14:93-95, 1990.

38. Storm BL, Abbitt PL, Allen DA et al: Splenosis: superparamagnetic iron oxide-enhanced MR imaging, Am J Roentgenol 159:333-335, 1992.

39. Te Strake L, Freling NJM, Kamman RL et al: Abdominal applications of fast MR imaging: a comparison of fast field echo (FFE) and spin echo (SE) pulse sequences, Magn Reson Imaging 7:297-303, 1989.

40. Thomsen C, Josephsen P, Karle H et al: Determination of T1- and T2-relaxation times in the spleen of patients with splenomegaly, Magn Reson Imaging 8:39-42, 1990.

41. Tjon A, Tham RTO, Heyerman HGM et al: Cystic fibrosis: MR imaging of the pancreas. Radiology 179:183-186, 1991.

42. Tscholakoff D, Hricak H, Thoeni R et al: MR imaging in the diagnosis of pancreatic disease, Am J Roentgenol 148:703-709, 1987.

43. Vahey TN, Glazer BM, Francis IR et al: MR diagnosis of pancreatic transplant rejection, Am J Roentgenol 150:557-560, 1988.

44. Vellet AD, Romano W, Bach DB et al: Adenocarcinoma of the pancreatic duct: comparative evaluation with CT and MR imaging at 1.5 T, Radiology 183:87-95, 1992.

45. Weissleder R, Elizondo G, Stark DD et al: The diagnosis of splenic lymphoma by MR imaging: value of superparamagnetic iron oxide, Am J Roentgenol 152:175-180, 1989.

46. Younathan CM, Ros PR, Burton SS: MR imaging of colonic lipoma, J Comput Assist Tomogr 15:492-494, 1991.

47. Young IR, Cox IJ, Bryant DJ et al: The benefits of increasing spatial resolution as a means of reducing artifacts due to field inhomogeneities, Magn Reson Imaging 6:585-590, 1988.

48. Yuh WTC, Hunsicker LG, Nghiem DD et al: Pancreatic transplants: evaluation with MR imaging, Radiology 170:171-177, 1989.

49. Yuh WTC, Wiese JA, Abu-Yousef MM et al: Pancreatic transplant imaging, Radiology 167:679-683, 1988.

7

Adrenals, Kidneys, Retroperitoneum

ADRENAL GLANDS
Anatomic Variations

The adrenal glands typically demonstrate a slender Y-shaped configuration. However, these structures can be quite variable in their size and shape. Reported variations include pyramidal, quadrilateral, foliate, and spherical configurations.[7] The configuration of the right and left adrenal glands is frequently different in the same individual. Normal adrenal glands may appear nodular or elongated as normal variations.

Congenital absence of the adrenal gland rarely occurs. Another rare occurrence is the presence of accessory adrenal tissue in ectopic locations such as the renal capsule, kidney, liver, or pelvis.[7] The blood supply to the adrenal glands is highly variable in terms of the number and site of origin of adrenal arteries and veins.[7] While retroperitoneal cysts are most frequently associated with the kidney, adrenal cysts can also be incidentally discovered in asymptomatic individuals.[54]

Simulation of Adrenal Masses

Several anatomic structures can simulate the appearance of an adrenal mass. Adrenal pseudotumors are more frequently encountered on the left rather than the right side. The splenic vein, a tortuous splenic artery, or a splenic artery aneurysm may each project into the left suprarenal region and simulate a nodular left adrenal mass[17] (Fig. 7-1). The splenic vasculature can be recognized by intraluminal flow void appearance on spin echo images; however, this may not be apparent because of slow flow or when there is partial volume averaging of the vessel with adjacent fat. Gradient echo images can be used to confirm the vascular nature of such pseudomasses by demonstrating intraluminal flow-related enhancement.

The pancreatic tail can extend into the left suprarenal region, where it can also simulate an adrenal mass (Figs.

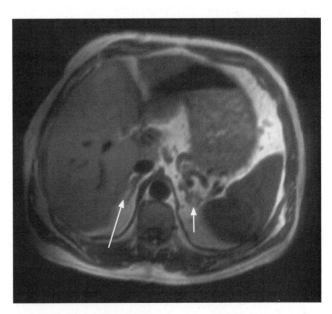

Fig. 7-1. Fat interposed between the adrenal crura simulates a high signal intensity adrenal lesion (*arrow*) on this transaxial T1-weighted image (TR 500, TE 12, 4 Nex). Partial volume averaging with tortuous splenic artery simulates a nodule involving the left adrenal gland in same patient (*small arrow*).

ENTITIES THAT MAY SIMULATE ADRENAL LESIONS

- Morphologic variations
- Splenic artery/vein/aneurysm
- Pancreatic tail
- Gastric diverticulum
- Posterior gastric wall
- Exophytic hepatic mass
- Colon in hepatorenal fossa
- Upper pole kidney, renal lesions, hypertrophied renal tissue
- Diaphragmatic crus

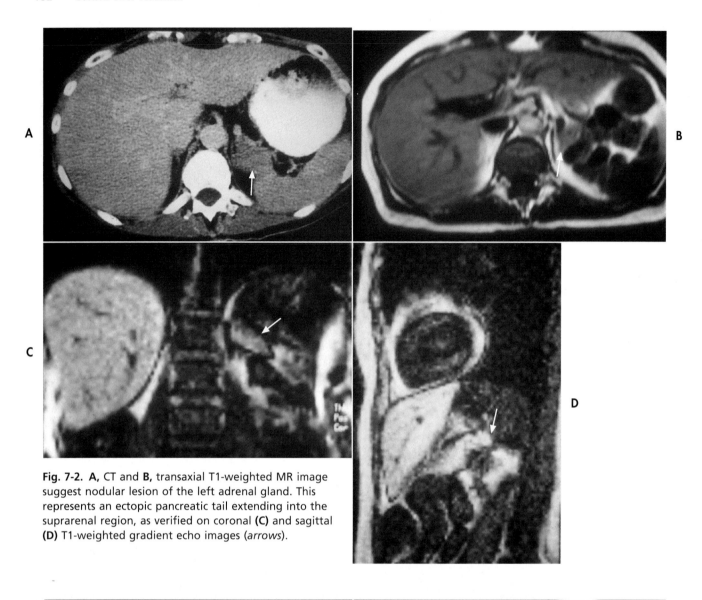

Fig. 7-2. **A,** CT and **B,** transaxial T1-weighted MR image suggest nodular lesion of the left adrenal gland. This represents an ectopic pancreatic tail extending into the suprarenal region, as verified on coronal **(C)** and sagittal **(D)** T1-weighted gradient echo images (*arrows*).

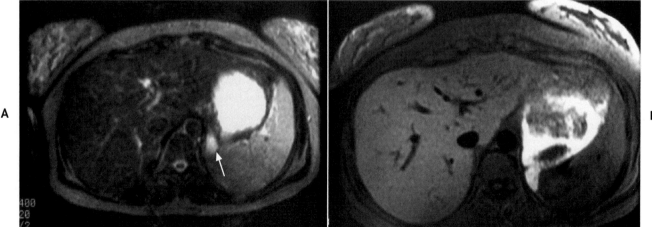

Fig. 7-3. **A,** Transaxial T2-weighted image (TR 3400, TE 120, 2 Nex) in patient with suspected pheochromocytoma. There is an apparent 2 cm high signal intensity left adrenal mass (*arrow*). **B,** T1-weighted fat-suppressed image (TR 500, TE 11, 4 Nex) acquired after oral administration of contrast material (nutritional support formula) demonstrates that the apparent lesion represents a posterior gastric diverticulum.

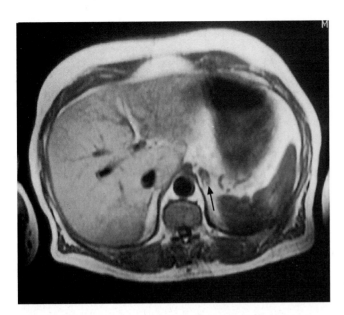

Fig. 7-4. Transaxial T1-weighted image (TR 500, TE 12, 4 Nex) demonstrates an apparent left adrenal mass (*arrow*), caused by volume averaging with the gastric antrum. The left adrenal gland was visualized to be normal on additional images.

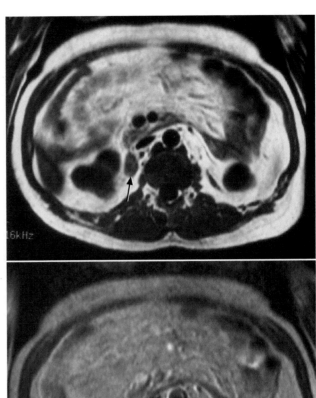

A

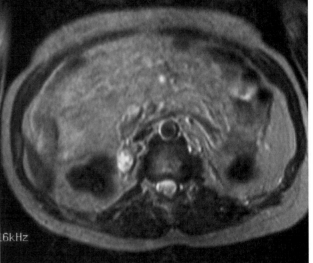

B

7-2, *A-D*). Pancreatic tissue can be identified on fat-suppressed T1-weighted images, where it is hyperintense relative to most other abdominal tissues. Accessory splenic tissue can appear to represent a nodular left adrenal mass; it can usually be recognized because of its isointensity with the spleen proper on all pulse sequences. Yet another cause for left adrenal pseudolesion is a gastric diverticulum, which can have variable signal characteristics depending on whether it contains primarily air or fluid (Figs. 7-3, *A* and *B*). Partial volume averaging of the left adrenal gland with the posterior gastric wall can also simulate an adrenal mass (Fig. 7-4).

Causes of apparent lesions related to the right adrenal gland include an exophytic hepatic mass, colon within the hepatorenal fossa[17] (Figs. 7-5, *A* and *B* and 7-6) or extension of the duodenum into the suprarenal region in patients who have undergone nephrectomy. Exophytic masses projecting from the upper pole of the kidneys or focal renal hypertrophy resulting from previous scarring may simulate an adrenal mass on either side (Figs. 7-7, *A* and *B* and 7-8, *A* and *B*). In one reported case, a leiomyosarcoma originating in the renal hilus simulated an adrenal tumor.[24] Partial volume averaging of the upper pole of a normal kidney with either the left or the right adrenal gland can also simulate an adrenal mass (Fig. 7-9).

Coronal images are often helpful in determining whether a retroperitoneal mass is renal or adrenal in origin. Dynamic contrast-enhanced imaging is also useful

Fig. 7-5. Apparent 2 cm nodular mass involving the right adrenal gland (*arrow*) on transaxial T1-weighted **(A)** (TR 500, TE 11, 4 Nex) and T2-weighted **(B)** (TR 3400, TE 80, 2 Nex) images. The apparent mass demonstrates increased signal intensity on a T2-weighted image, which is suspicious for neoplasm. However, this represents a portion of the duodenum that has extended into the superrenal region, as verified by continuity with the gastrointestinal tract on adjacent images.

for distinguishing focal renal hypertrophy from adrenal masses. Hypertrophied renal tissue demonstrates peripheral cortical enhancement during the bolus phase of contrast material administration, similar to the remainder of the kidney. Another source for adrenal pseudolesions on either side is the diaphragmatic crus, which can have a nodular configuration and project into the suprarenal region. A rare cause of apparent adrenal malignancy is inclusion of ectopic renal tissue within the adrenal gland.[5]

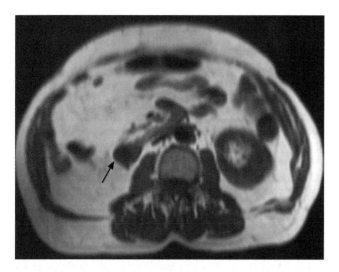

Fig. 7-6. A portion of the duodenum extends into the right superrenal region, simulating an adrenal mass (*arrow*), on this transaxial T1-weighted image (TR 400, TE 15, 4 Nex) in patient who has undergone previous right nephrectomy.

Characterization of Adrenal Masses
T2-weighted images

Magnetic resonance (MR) is frequently used to characterize adrenal masses. A benign adrenal adenoma is typically of decreased signal intensity on T2-weighted images. While quantitative indexes have been proposed for characterization of adrenal lesions, this determination is usually based on visual inspection in most clinical settings. It is useful to have an internal standard against which the signal intensity of adrenal masses can be compared. The liver frequently serves as such an internal standard. Adrenal lesions that are isointense or hypointense relative to hepatic parenchyma are suggestive of

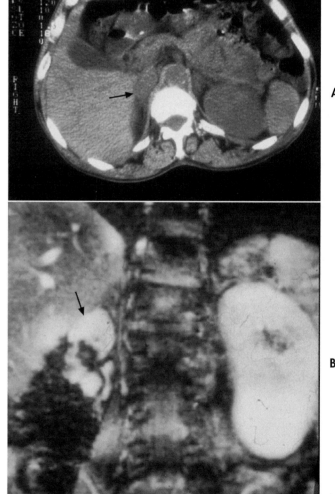

Fig. 7-8. CT **(A)** and corresponding transaxial MR images (not shown) demonstrate apparent right adrenal mass (*arrow*). However, this represents focal compensatory hypertrophy of the upper pole of the right kidney in patient with renal atrophy, as verified on corresponding coronal contrast enhanced gradient echo image (*arrow*) **(B).**

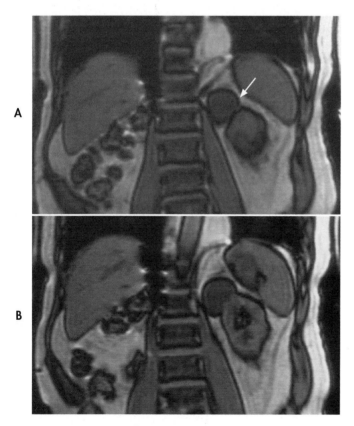

Fig. 7-7. A, Coronal spoiled gradient echo image (TR 113, TE 2.6, 90-degree flip angle, 1 Nex) demonstrates cystic lesion that appears to arise from the left adrenal gland (*arrow*). **B,** Adjacent image demonstrates interface of lesion with upper pole of left kidney documenting that it represents a renal cyst.

adrenal adenoma, whereas hyperintensity relative to liver indicates the possibility of adrenal malignancy. However, such determinations should be made cautiously, since the liver is a metabolically active organ that can undergo signal intensity alterations from a variety of conditions. For example, a benign adrenal lesion could appear hyperintense relative to liver parenchyma that is affected by iron overload. In this situation, the lesion would be incorrectly assumed to represent malignancy. Conversely, if the hepatic parenchyma is of unusually increased signal intensity because of fatty infiltration, hepatitis, or other conditions, a malignant adrenal lesion could be diagnosed as benign. The use of a tissue that is less subject to signal intensity alterations, such as paravertebral muscle, provides more consistent results and can serve as a double check system in conjunction with evaluation of the liver. The paravertebral muscles display somewhat lower signal intensity on T2-weighted images than liver, so diagnosis of benignancy will be based on more stringent criteria when this standard is used.

Characterization of adrenal masses is also affected by the pulse sequence parameters used for image acquisition.[3,21,28,42] The criteria already discussed were primarily based on experience with moderately T2-weighted images, using echo times on the order of 60 to 80 msec. These criteria have not been validated for use with more heavily T2-weighted images (e.g., 120 to 160 msec echo times) or other implementations of T2-weighted imaging such as those using fast spin echo or other recently introduced techniques. While it is expected that adenomas will remain relatively hypointense as compared with malignant adrenal lesions, these techniques should be used cautiously until the results of controlled studies become available.

Most adrenal adenomas that are incidentally discovered do not produce symptoms related to active hormonal secretion (i.e., nonhyperfunctioning adenomas). Hyperfunctioning adrenal adenomas may secrete excessive quantities of corticosteroids or mineralocorticoids. While these lesions are benign, they can demonstrate signal intensity characteristics suggestive of malignancy on T2-weighted MR images.[11] Therefore correlation with clinical examination for Cushing syndrome, hypertension, or other manifestations of adrenal hypersecretion, as well as laboratory findings, is important in avoiding a false diagnosis of a malignant adrenal mass.

Some nonhyperfunctioning adrenal adenomas may also occasionally demonstrate aberrant signal characteristics that can simulate malignancy [3,4,21,41,42] (Figs. 7-10 and 7-11). While biopsy may be necessary in such situations, the observation of small size (<3 cm diameter), homogeneous signal intensity, and stability over the course of serial examinations are features suggestive of benign lesions. Both adrenal glands may be enlarged, with increased signal intensity on T2-weighted images, as a result of adrenal hyperplasia. These findings can simulate bilateral metastatic lesions.[39] Simulation of metastatic disease is likely particularly in the presence of nodular adrenal hyperplasia. Heterogeneous signal alterations within adrenal adenomas can be caused by hemorrhagic breakdown products, resulting in confusion with a malignant lesion.[3]

T1-weighted images

While T2-weighted images are most frequently used to characterize adrenal masses, malignant and benign adrenal lesions also differ in their T1 relaxation properties.[11] However, such differences are usually less perceptible than T2 relaxation differences, hence T1-weighted images are used primarily for detection rather than characterization of adrenal masses.

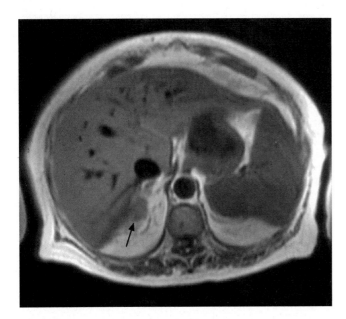

Fig. 7-9. Transaxial T1-weighted image (TR 500, TE 12, 4 Nex) demonstrates apparent right adrenal mass (*arrow*), caused by partial volume averaging with upper pole of right kidney.

PITFALLS IN CHARACTERIZATION OF ADRENAL LESIONS

- Alterations in hepatic signal intensity (e.g., iron overload, hepatitis, cirrhosis, fatty infiltration)
- Nonstandard pulse sequence parameters
- Hyperfunctioning adenomas
- Nodular adrenal hyperplasia
- Hemorrhagic adenoma
- Lipid-containing malignancies
- Absence of fat in some benign lesions
- Chemical shift phase cancellation artifact

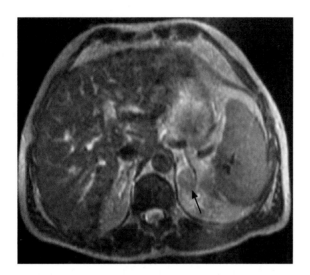

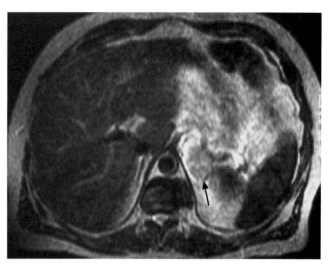

Fig. 7-10. Transaxial T2-weighted image (TR 3400, TE 80, 2 Nex) demonstrates left adrenal mass with signal intensity somewhat greater than that of liver and muscle and equivalent to that of spleen (*arrow*). However, the mass was unchanged on multiple examinations and represents a presumed adenoma, despite somewhat atypical signal intensity characteristics.

Fig. 7-11. A 4 cm left adrenal mass (*arrow*) is demonstrated on this transaxial T2-weighted image (TR 2500, TE 80, 2 Nex). The mass is hyperintense relative to the liver and paravertebral muscle, although it was proven to represent a benign adenoma pathologically.

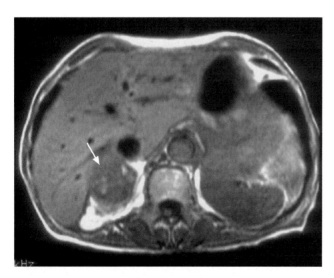

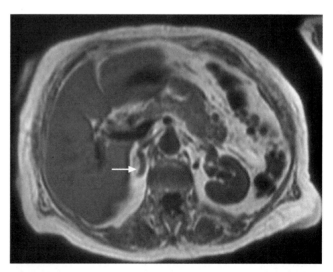

Fig. 7-12. A 4 cm right adrenal mass is demonstrated on transaxial T1-weighted image (TR 460, TE 12, 4 Nex)(*arrow*). There are multiple foci of relative increased signal intensity within the lesion, which could represent areas of fat within a benign adrenal myelolipoma. However, these represent foci of subacute hemorrhage in a lung cancer metastasis.

Fig. 7-13. An apparent high signal intensity lesion (*arrow*) is demonstrated in the right adrenal gland on this transaxial T1-weighted image (TR 500, TE 11, 2 Nex). However, this represents fat interposed between the adrenal crura and may be mistaken for myelolipoma or hemorrhagic lesion.

The appearance of an adrenal mass on T1-weighted images may, however, yield important clues as to its nature. For example, the atypical observation of hyperintensity within an adrenal mass on T1-weighted images suggests the presence of fatty material, such as occurs in association with adrenal myelolipoma. In some cases, the entire myelolipoma exhibits signal intensity characteristics concordant with those of fat. However, soft tissue components may comprise a variable portion of the lesion, and in some cases no fat is evident.[34]

Hyperintensity on T1-weighted images can also indicate the presence of methemoglobin, which may be seen in association with benign or malignant hemorrhagic adrenal lesions [35,42] (Fig. 7-12). Foci of lipid within an adrenal mass will demonstrate isointensity with mesenteric and subcutaneous fat, whereas hemorrhagic products will often vary from fat signal intensity. Fat suppression techniques such as fat saturation and phase contrast imaging can provide definitive identification of lipid products. In patients with simple adrenal hemorrhage, follow-up MR examination will document the progressive reduction in size of the affected gland(s) as well as signal alterations compatible with the evolution of blood breakdown products.[27] The presence of normal retroperitoneal fat interposed between the crura of a normal adrenal gland can simulate the appearance of a small adrenal myelolipoma (Figs. 7-1 and 7-13). The absence of mass effect on the adrenal gland can be used to distinguish these entities.

Fat suppression methods

As noted previously, conventional T2-weighted images may demonstrate considerable overlap between benign and malignant adrenal masses.[33] The use of fat suppression techniques can assist in the characterization of adrenal masses, since benign adrenal lesions including adenomas often contain microscopic foci of lipid material. While fat saturation sequences may be used, phase contrast methods have shown greater promise. For example, gradient echo images acquired using an echo time at which fat and water protons are out-of-phase with one another can be acquired rapidly during suspended respiration. Determination of the appropriate echo time must be based on the field strength at which imaging is performed. On these "opposed phase" images, voxels containing both fat and water display reduced signal intensity as compared with their signal on a corresponding "in-phase" image.

It has been found that adrenal adenomas, nodular hyperplasia, and myelolipomas exhibit significantly lower signal intensity than metastases or pheochromocytomas on opposed phase images.[33,52] Tsushima et al[52] proposed

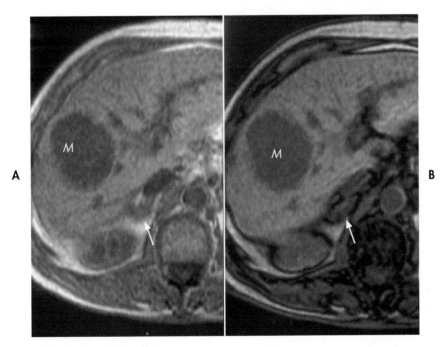

Fig. 7-14. Transaxial spoiled gradient echo image obtained using in-phase **(A)** (TR 178, TE 4.2, 1 Nex) and opposed-phase **(B)** (TR 153, TE 2.6, 1 Nex) parameters in patient with hepatic metastatic disease (*M*). A right adrenal metastasis (*arrow*) demonstrates decreased signal intensity on opposed-phase image, suggestive of adrenal adenoma. This artifactual loss of signal intensity is related to partial volume averaging of fat and tumor on images acquired using relatively large slice thickness (10 mm) and a rectangular (128 × 256) imaging matrix.

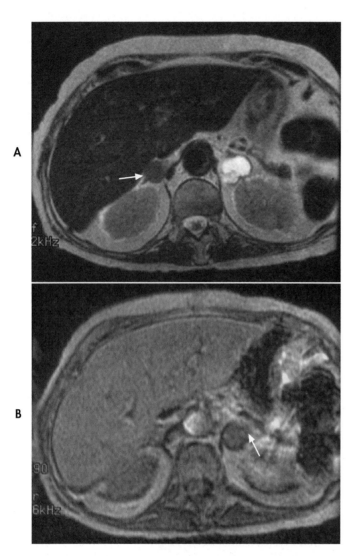

Fig. 7-15. A, Transaxial fast spin echo T2-weighted image (TR 3500, effective TE 120, 4 Nex, 16 echo train) demonstrates 2 cm right adrenal mass (*arrow*), which is approximately isointense with hepatic parenchyma. A left-sided 3.5 cm adrenal mass is markedly hyperintense relative to liver. **B,** The corresponding opposed-phase gradient echo image (TR 124, TE 3.4, 90-degree flip angle, 1 Nex) depicts the left-sided lesion (*arrow*) to be hypointense relative to liver, suggestive of lipid components within a benign adrenal adenoma. However, such hypointensity is due to fluid-like components in an area of necrosis within this adrenal metastasis on a relatively T1-weighted gradient echo image. Although the right-sided lesion is relatively isointense with the liver on T2-weighted image, absence of perceptible signal loss on the opposed-phase gradient echo image indicates adrenal metastasis.

use of a lesion/diaphragmatic crus ratio as a means of objectively discriminating these two groups, with a ratio of less than 1.16 and greater than 1.23 indicative of adenoma/hyperplasia and metastasis/pheochromocytoma, respectively. The use of opposed phase gradient echo images has yielded more accurate results in the characterization of adrenal masses than T2 relaxation values.[53]

The basis for distinction of adrenal adenomas from malignant adrenal lesions using phase contrast techniques relies on the presence of lipid within the former lesions and the absence of lipids in the latter. However, lipid material has been found in some metastatic lesions, such as those arising from primary renal carcinoma.[43,53] Lipids have also been found in some cases of primary adrenal carcinoma and pheochromocytoma. Liposarcoma and hepatocellular carcinoma are additional abdominal malignancies that contain lipid material.[53] In such cases, misdiagnosis of a malignant lesion as a benign one could occur. On the other hand, the lack of identifiable fat can occur with many adrenal lesions, including inflammatory processes, adrenal hemorrhage, cyst, as well as most metastases and pheochromocytomas.[53] In one series, neither opposed phase gradient echo images nor T2 calculations could reliably differentiate between hyperfunctioning and nonhyperfunctioning adrenal adenomas, though the former had somewhat less lipid material.[53]

Another limitation of phase contrast imaging for adrenal mass characterization is the presence of artifactual signal loss at fat-water interfaces. These chemical shift phase cancellation artifacts can potentially cause small malignancies to appear to represent benign lesions[33] (Figs. 7-14, *A* and *B*). Lesions must generally be greater than 8 mm in diameter in order to generate reliable results.[53] The presence of necrosis within an adrenal malignancy can result in marked decreased signal intensity on relatively T1-weighted opposed phase gradient echo images; it is important that this low signal intensity not be mistaken for that caused by lipid contents (Figs. 7-15, *A* and *B*).

Contrast-enhanced imaging

Dynamic contrast material–enhanced gradient echo imaging has also been implemented in an effort to improve characterization of adrenal masses. In their series of 52 masses, Krestin et al. found that the addition of dynamic contrast-enhanced imaging to conventional images improved accuracy of adrenal mass characterization from 71% to 88%.[31] Using this technique, benign adenomas typically demonstrate only moderate contrast enhancement, with return of signal intensity to baseline levels after 10 minutes. This compares with more rapid and prolonged enhancement for malignant adrenal lesions.

Following bolus administration of paramagnetic contrast material, the normal adrenal glands demonstrate

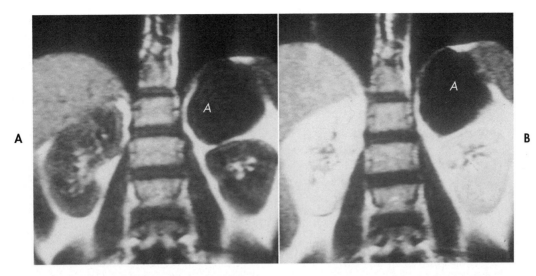

Fig. 7-16. Coronal T1-weighted rapid acquisition spin echo images obtained before **(A)** and following **(B)** intravenous gadolinium chelate contrast material administration. There is a large cyst (*A*) of the left adrenal gland without associated abnormal contrast material enhancement.

prominent enhancement (see Figs. 6-15, *A-C*). Increase in adrenal signal intensity of 300% over baseline values has been noted on dynamic enhanced gradient echo imaging.[48] Modest enhancement on the order of 50% over baseline values is usually present on delayed T1-weighted spin echo images.

Adrenal cysts may be encountered as an incidental finding; they display imaging features similar to their renal counterparts (Figs. 7-16, *A* and *B*).

KIDNEYS
Anatomic Variations

Lack of visualization of a kidney may be caused by congenital absence. However, in such circumstances search for an ectopic kidney should be prompted, particularly if compensatory hypertrophy of the contralateral kidney is not evident. When a kidney is absent, the renal fossa can be occupied by bowel loops as well as pancreas, liver, spleen, or other abdominal organs. These structures can simulate the appearance of various renal abnormalities. An ectopic kidney may be discovered in the contralateral renal fossa (crossed fused ectopia), in the lower abdomen, or in the true pelvis. While inferior descent of an ectopic kidney is more frequent, ectopia may also occur in a cephalad direction, resulting in a "thoracic" kidney.

The kidneys frequently demonstrate rotational abnormalities along their anatomic axis. When the kidneys assume a horizontal position, transaxial images may suggest focal or diffuse renal enlargement (Figs. 7-17, *A* and *B*). However, the basis for such apparent abnormalities

can usually be appreciated if coronal images are acquired. Medial deviation of the lower poles of both kidneys suggests the presence of a "horseshoe kidney" (Figs. 7-18, *A* and *B*). The isthmus of renal parenchyma that unites the two kidneys can be visualized traversing the midline of the abdomen, where it can simulate adenopathy or other masses. A poorly defined mass of renal tissue may be apparent in patients with a "cake kidney."

Following nephrectomy, bowel may extend into the renal fossa. If one is unaware that a nephrectomy has been performed, this bowel extension can potentially simulate various renal abnormalities (Figs. 7-19 and 7-20).

ENTITIES THAT MAY SIMULATE RENAL LESIONS

- Rotational abnormalities
- Crossed fused ectopia
- "Cake kidney"
- Postoperative changes
- Renal lobulations
- "Dromedary hump"
- Splenic impression
- "Column of Bertin"
- Prominent hilar lip
- Compensatory renal hypertrophy
- Spleen/accessory spleen
- Cortical defects
- Chemical shift misregistration artifact
- Concentrated contrast material in collecting system
- Motion artifacts

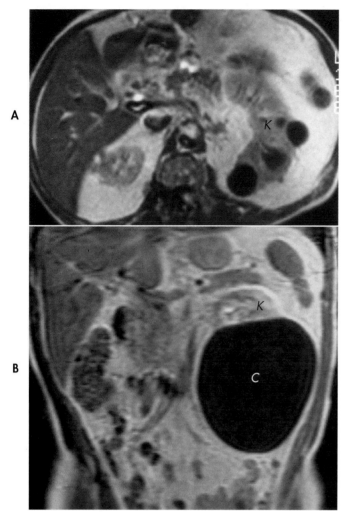

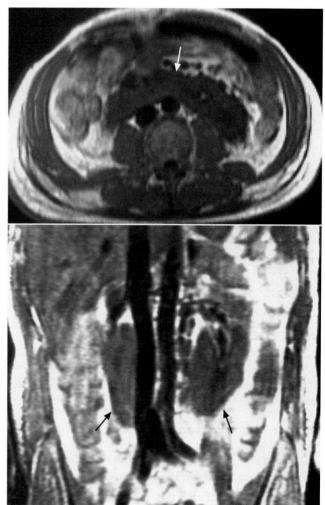

Fig. 7-17. A, There is apparent enlargement of the left kidney (*K*) on transaxial gadolinium chelate enhanced T1-weighted image (TR 267, TE 11, 0.5 Nex). In addition, multiple renal cysts are demonstrated. **B,** Coronal image using same parameters demonstrates the left kidney (*K*) to be smaller than the right kidney. Apparent enlargement on previous image was due to altered rotation of the kidney secondary to a 13 cm lower pole cyst (*C*).

Fig. 7-18. A, Soft tissue extends across the midabdomen anterior to the aorta and inferior vena cava on transaxial T1-weighted image (TR 400, TE 12, 2 Nex) (*arrow*). This represents the isthmus of a "horseshoe kidney," with the medially placed lower poles of both kidneys visualized on a coronal T1-weighted image **(B)** (TR 600, TE 17, 2 Nex) (*arrows*).

Renal Pseudotumors

The renal contour, while most frequently smooth and regular, may be affected by several anatomic variations. The presence of an undulating renal surface is frequently due to retained fetal lobulations. Focal prominence of renal tissue along the lateral aspect of the left kidney may be attributable to a splenic impression or "dromedary hump." Focal asymmetric prominence of renal cortex along the lateral aspect of the kidney may also occur as a normal variant. The junctional zone separating renal cortex from medulla may be relatively prominent in some patients, and focal invagination of cortical tissue can result in the "column of Bertin." Along the medial aspect of the kidney, a prominent renal hilar lip may be observed.

Each of these entities can simulate a focal renal mass. Nonstandard MR techniques may prove useful in distinguishing these pseudotumors from actual renal lesions. For example, fat suppressed T1-weighted images result in heightened renal corticomedullary differentiation as compared with conventional T1-weighted images[46] (Figs. 7-21, *A* and *B*). As a result, focal prominence of renal cortex can frequently be recognized and distinguished from other abnormalities. Another useful method

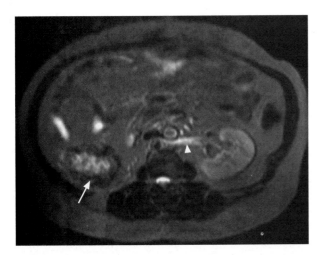

Fig. 7-19. A heterogeneous signal intensity "mass" in the right renal fossa (*arrow*) on transaxial T2-weighted image (TR 3560, TE 120, 22 Nex) represents colon in patient who has undergone previous right nephrectomy. Also noted is retroaortic left renal vein with relative increased intraluminal signal intensity within its proximal segment (*arrowhead*). The latter finding is related to relatively slow blood flow due to second echo rephasing, and to use of flow compensating gradients.

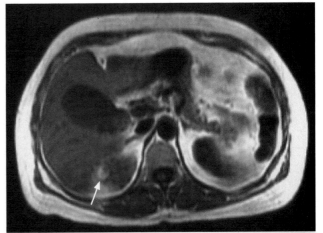

A

B

Fig. 7-21. T1-weighted transaxial images (TR 400, TE 15, 2 Nex) obtained without (**A**) and with (**B**) fat saturation. There is improved renal corticomedullary differentiation apparent on the fat-suppressed image. In addition, relative hyperintensity of the liver and pancreas is noted on the fat-suppressed as compared with the conventional image. A hyperintense lesion involving the upper pole of the right kidney is demonstrated in **A** (*arrow*). Differential diagnosis includes hemorrhagic/proteinaceous cyst, other hemorrhagic lesions, or a fat-containing lesion. Decrease in signal intensity of the lesion on a fat-suppressed image documents that it represents an angiomyolipoma (*arrow*).

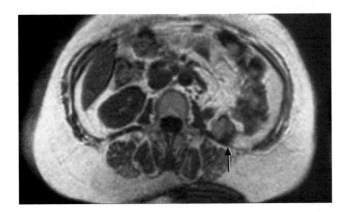

Fig. 7-20. Transaxial T1-weighted image (TR 266, TE 11, 0.5 Nex) shows the descending colon to be located within the left renal fossa (*arrow*) in a patient who has undergone previous left nephrectomy.

for characterizing renal pseudotumors is dynamic contrast-enhanced rapid imaging, using rapid spin echo or gradient echo techniques. Intense enhancement of the renal cortex is observed during the bolus phase of contrast material administration[32] (Figs. 7-22 and 7-23). This allows for distinction of focally prominent or ectopic renal cortical tissue from renal neoplasms. Equilibration of

contrast material throughout the renal parenchyma occurs 1 to 2 minutes after contrast material is injected. Because conventional T1-weighted spin echo acquisition times exceed this time window, they are not useful for recognizing renal pseudotumors on the basis of contrast enhancement patterns.

Scarring caused by chronic pyelonephritis, infarct, or other renal insults can result in volume loss in a portion of a kidney, with compensatory hypertrophy of remaining viable renal tissue (see Fig. 7-8). Such locally hypertrophied renal tissue can simulate a renal mass. This

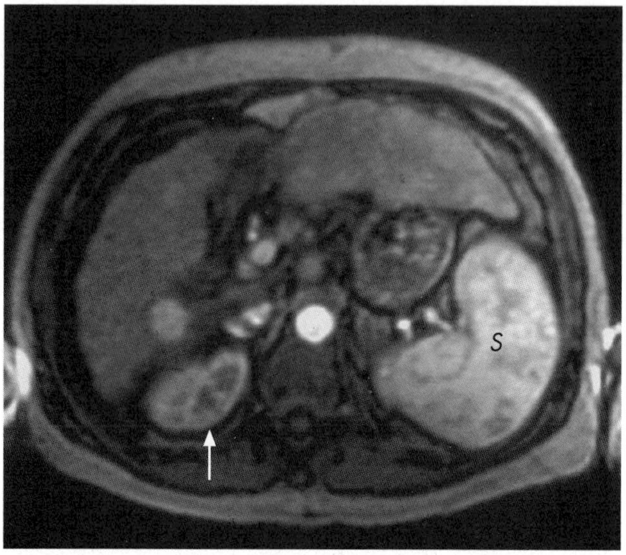

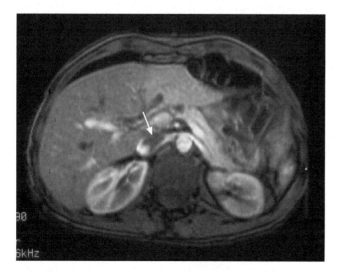

Fig. 7-22. Transaxial spoiled gradient echo image (TR 120, TE 3, 90-degree flip angle, 1 Nex) acquired during bolus injection of gadolinium chelate contrast material demonstrates marked enhancement of the renal cortex (*arrow*). Also noted is heterogeneous enhancement of the spleen (*S*), which converted to a homogeneous pattern 1 minute later.

entity can also be resolved through the use of dynamic contrast-enhanced imaging techniques. In such cases, the hypertrophic tissue demonstrates contrast enhancement features identical to those of the remaining renal parenchyma in terms of timing, intensity, and pattern of enhancement. This is in distinction to renal neoplasms, which usually undergo decreased intensity of enhancement relative to normal renal tissue during the bolus phase of contrast material administration and also frequently demonstrate a heterogeneous enhancement pattern.[18]

The caudal extent of the spleen or accessory splenic tissue can simulate an exophytic renal mass. Partial volume averaging of the spleen with renal parenchyma can also result in apparent renal lesions. Congenital or acquired defects in the renal cortex may be filled with fat;

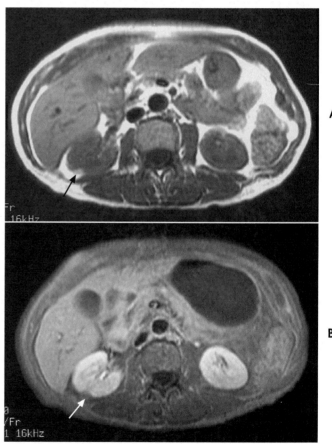

Fig. 7-23. Spoiled gradient echo image (TR 153, TE 2.6, 90-degree flip angle, 1 Nex) obtained during bolus injection of paramagnetic contrast material. There is intense cortical enhancement of the kidneys. Also noted is enhancement of most vascular structures, with an apparent defect suggestive of thrombus within the inferior vena cava (*arrow*). This latter finding is artifactual, resulting from turbulence at the confluence of the renal veins.

Fig. 7-24. A, A focus of increased signal intensity is observed along the posterolateral right kidney (*arrow*) on transaxial T1-weighted image (TR 500, TE 11, 4 Nex). This represents fat filling a focal renal cortical defect. This finding simulates a hyperintense renal lesion such as angiomyolipoma (*arrow*) on this conventional and gadolinium chelate–enhanced fat-suppressed T1-weighted image (TR 500, TE 11, 4 Nex)(**B**).

this can simulate an angiomyolipoma, complex cyst, or a hemorrhagic renal neoplasm (Figs. 7-24, *A* and *B*).

Corticomedullary Differentiation

T1-weighted images usually depict the renal cortex as hyperintense relative to the medulla. Absence of differentiation between renal cortex and medulla on such images is associated with a variety of medical renal diseases including glomerulonephritis, interstitial nephritis, and many others. This finding has also been used to indicate the presence of rejection in a transplanted kidney. However, absence of corticomedullary differentiation is highly nonspecific and has also been observed in association with acute tubular necrosis and cyclosporine toxicity.[23,57] The conspicuousness of corticomedullary distinction also varies with hydrational status.

Collecting System

The renal collecting system may demonstrate anatomic variation. The number of calyces can vary between 6 and 14.[7] Direct extension of the infundibula into the ureter can occur without formation of a true renal pelvis.[7] The renal pelvis may be somewhat dilated and project into the peripelvic fat, creating a so-called extrarenal pelvis. This entity may lead to a false diagnosis of hydronephrosis. However, the renal calyces are nondilated with a simple extrarenal pelvis, as opposed to most patients with hydronephrosis. The extrarenal pelvis may also be mistaken for a peripelvic renal cyst, though in the latter entity there is no continuity between the cyst and the ureter. Renal duplication can result in an obstructed upper pole moiety, which can simulate a mass as it displaces the lower pole moiety inferiorly (Figs. 7-25, *A* and *B*).

Abundant lipomatous tissue may be present within the renal sinus (renal sinus lipomatosis), which can attenuate the renal collecting system. The renal pelvis, calyces, and infundibula can each be duplicated. Calyceal diverticula may simulate cystic renal lesions.

Vasculature

The left renal vein may pass behind rather than in front of the aorta. Retroaortic renal vein is present in 1.5% to 8.7% of the normal population.[20] In some patients, preaortic and retroaortic branches of the left renal vein unite prior to entering the inferior vena cava, resulting in a circumaortic renal vein (Figs. 7-26, *A* and *B*). An anatomically normal left renal vein may appear relatively distended proximal to its passage between the aorta and superior mesenteric artery as a result of extrinsic pressure effects exerted by the superior mesenteric artery. The proximal left renal vein also frequently demonstrates relative increased signal intensity in this location on flow-compensated T2-weighted images, presum-

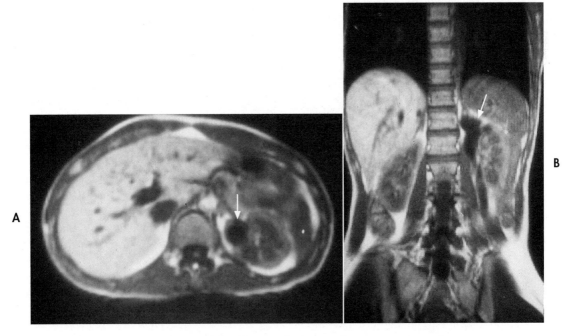

Fig. 7-25. A, Transaxial T1-weighted image demonstrates an apparent cystic mass involving the anteromedial aspect of the left kidney (*arrow*). This represents a duplicated kidney with obstruction of the upper pole moiety, as verified on coronal T1-weighted image (*arrow*)(**B**).

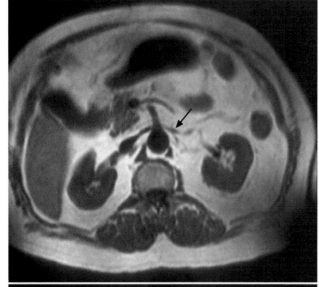

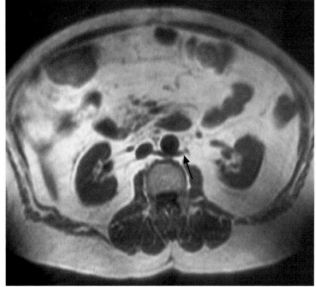

Fig. 7-26. A, Transaxial T1-weighted images (TR 500, TE 12, 4 Nex) at two different levels demonstrate preaortic (*arrow*) and **B,** retroaortic (*arrow*) components of a circumaortic left renal vein.

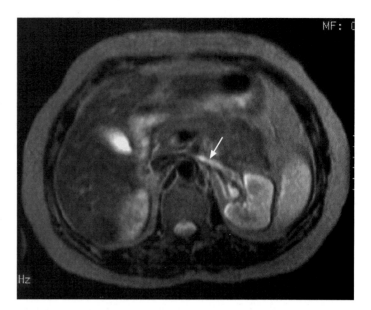

Fig. 7-27. Flow-compensated T2-weighted transaxial image (TR 3400, TE 80, 2 Nex) demonstrates increased signal intensity within the left renal vein proximal to the superior mesenteric artery (*arrow*). This represents physiologic slowing of blood flow and/or the effect of gradient moment nulling. Whereas these findings may simulate thrombus, additional spin echo and gradient echo images demonstrated this vessel to be patent.

ably because of slow and in-plane flow (Fig. 7-27). Multiple renal veins can be present and are more frequent on the right.

The renal arteries can arise from variable positions along the abdominal aorta or from the proximal iliac arteries.[7] Accessory renal arteries are present in approximately 25% of individuals and can originate from the aorta or suprarenal or inferior phrenic arteries.[7] The right renal artery may extend anterior rather than posterior to the inferior vena cava.[7]

The renal arteries are highly tortuous in some patients. Such vessels can undergo volume averaging with adja-

cent fat, simulating perirenal adenopathy or exophytic renal lesions. The lateral arcuate ligaments of the diaphragm may extend into the posterior pararenal space, where they can simulate a nodular mass.[47]

Chemical Shift Misregistration Artifact

Chemical shift misregistration artifact frequently leads to signal alterations surrounding the kidneys. Artifactual displacement of signal intensity occurs along the frequency-encoding direction at fat-water interfaces because of inherent differences in the precessional frequencies of fat and water protons. Chemical shift artifact results in a curvilinear zone of hyperintensity along the lateral margin of one kidney, with a corresponding hypointense zone along the lateral aspect of the contralateral kidney. These artifacts may simulate a small perirenal fluid collection or hematoma. Such artifacts may also obscure peripheral renal parenchyma and any small cortical lesions in this location.

Chemical shift misregistration artifacts are more prominent on images acquired on high field rather than low field systems. Their prominence is also increased when a narrow receiver bandwidth is used to improve the signal-to-noise ratio. Narrow bandwidth techniques should therefore not be used for renal imaging, except in conjunction with fat suppression methods. The promi-

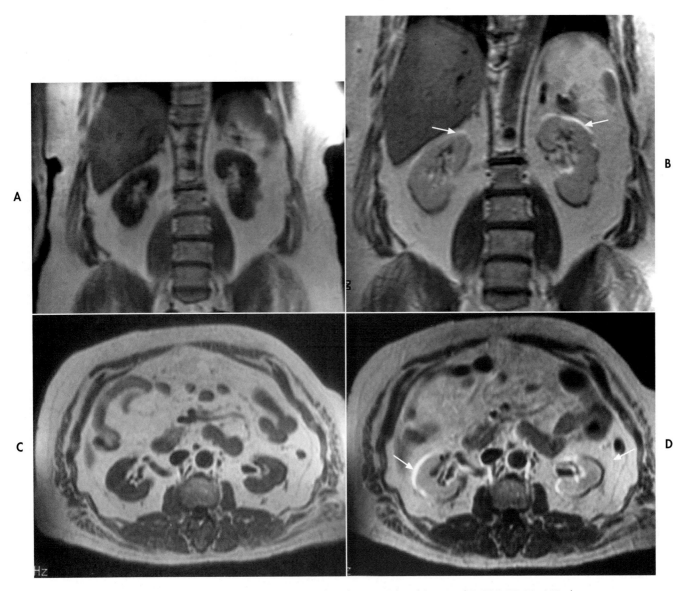

Fig. 7-28. Coronal **(A, B)** and transaxial **(C, D)** T1-weighted images (TR 500, TE 11, 4 Nex) obtained before **(A, C)** and after **(B, D)** intravenous gadolinium chelate administration. There is accentuation of chemical shift misregistration artifact along the frequency-encoding axis (superior-inferior in coronal images and right-left in transaxial images) on the contrast-enhanced images (*arrows*).

nence of chemical shift misregistration artifacts is also proportionate to the signal intensity of renal parenchyma. Therefore, such artifacts are accentuated on T2- as compared with T1-weighted images, and they are also more prominent on T1-weighted images obtained following paramagnetic contrast material administration[1] (Figs. 7-28, *A-D*, 7-29, *A* and *B*, and 7-30, *A* and *B*).

When chemical shift misregistration cannot be confidently established as the source of aberrant perirenal signal intensity, the pulse sequence may be repeated following reassignment of the phase and frequency encoded gradients. Because chemical shift misregistration

occurs along the frequency-encoding axis, reorientation of this axis (e.g., from right-left to anterior-posterior) will cause such artifacts to undergo corresponding displacement. This will allow the previously obscured regions to be more accurately evaluated.

Chemical shift misregistration has been noted to occur along the slice select as well as frequency encode direction.[55] This is expressed as aberrant signal intensity along the upper poles of the kidneys on transaxial T2-weighted images (Figs. 7-31, *A* and *B*). These artifacts can simulate a mass arising from the upper pole of the kidney or adrenal gland.[55]

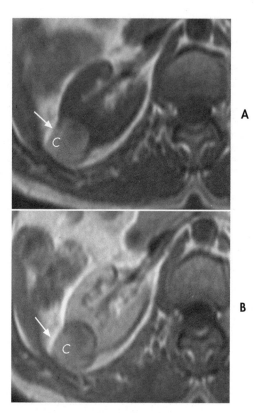

Fig. 7-29. Transaxial T1-weighted images (TR 550, TE 11, 4 Nex) obtained before **(A)** and after **(B)** intravenous gadolinium chelate administration in patient with 3 cm hemorrhagic cyst (*C*) projecting from right kidney. Accentuation of chemical shift misregistration artifact is noted on the contrast-enhanced image surrounding renal parenchyma as well as the mass (*arrows*). Visualization of such chemical shift misregistration indicates that the mass contains fluid contents rather than fat, which would not result in these findings.

Chemical Shift Phase Cancellation Artifact

Another type of chemical shift artifact may occur in the perirenal region and elsewhere throughout the abdomen on gradient echo images. This phenomenon, known as chemical shift phase cancellation artifact, is a reflection of the TE-dependent cyclic variation in relative phase of fat and water protons. Gradient echo images acquired using a field-strength specific "opposed phase" TE demonstrate artifactual decreased signal intensity at all fat-water interfaces. Unlike the chemical shift misregistration artifact, chemical shift phase cancellation occurs in both the phase and the frequency encoding directions, and it is manifested as a dark etching outlining abdominal organs, bowel loops, and fascial planes (Figs. 7-32, *A* and *B*). Sampling of the echo when fat and water protons have coherent phase will eliminate this artifact. Chemical shift phase cancellation artifacts are not observed on conventional spin echo images, because of the rephasing effects of the 180-degree radiofrequency pulse.

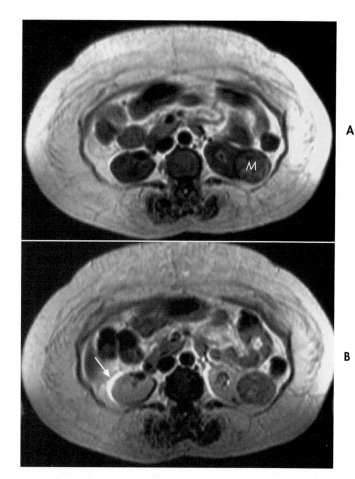

Fig. 7-30. Transaxial T1-weighted images (TR 600, TE 11, 4 Nex) obtained before **(A)** and after **(B)** gadolinium chelate administration. A solid mass (*M*) is seen projecting from the left kidney, with foci of hyperintensity suggestive of hemorrhagic renal neoplasm. Fat-suppressed image (not shown) indicated that these foci represented fat within an angiomyolipoma. Contrast enhancement is noted throughout the lesion, and accentuation of chemical shift misregistration artifact surrounding the kidneys is also visualized on a contrast-enhanced image (*arrow*).

Detection of Renal Masses

Perhaps the most important limitation of conventional MR imaging for evaluation of the kidneys is its frequently poor depiction of solid renal masses.[19,22,26,40] This is due to similar T1 and T2 relaxation values between many renal neoplasms and normal renal parenchyma. As a result, renal masses may go undetected on T1- and T2-weighted images unless they can be visualized on the basis of signal changes resulting from intratumoral hemorrhage or necrosis or if they perceptibly deform the renal contour or result in a mass effect. Therefore conventional spin echo sequences cannot be relied on for the exclusion of renal neoplasms; alternative methods must be used.

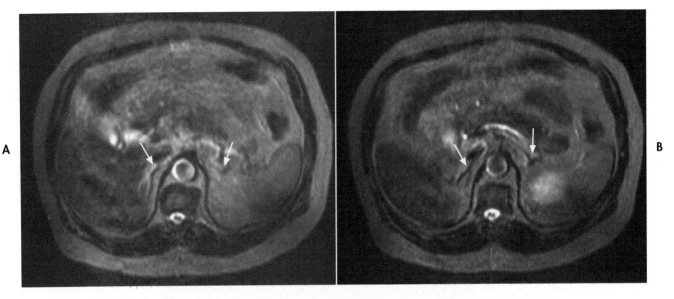

Fig. 7-31. Transaxial T2-weighted images (TR 3650, TE 120, 2 Nex) at two consecutive levels. **A** demonstrates the adrenal glands (*arrows*) to be uniformly hyperintense, whereas on the contiguous image **(B)** they are markedly hypointense (*arrows*). These findings are due to chemical shift misregistration effects occurring along the slice selection direction.

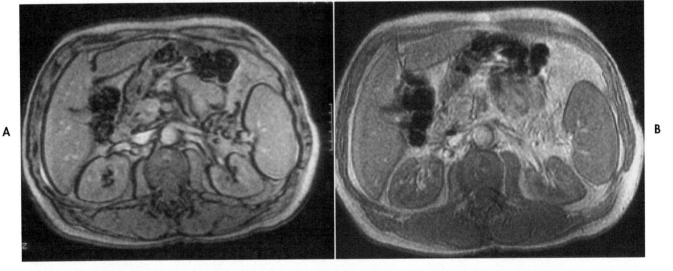

Fig. 7-32. Spoiled gradient echo images obtained using opposed-phase **(A)** (TR 118, TE 2.8, 60-degree flip angle, 1 Nex) and in-phase **(B)** (TR 135, TE 4.2, 90-degree flip angle, 1 Nex) imaging parameters. Dark lines outline the abdominal viscera, bowel, vessels, and fascial planes on an opposed-phase image, representing chemical shift phase cancellation artifact. These findings are not evident using an in-phase echo time.

Contrast Material

Paramagnetic contrast material has proven to be quite useful for the detection of renal masses (Figs. 7-33, *A-C*, 7-34, *A* and *B*, 7-35, *A* and *B*, and 7-36, *A-C*). Prominent enhancement of renal parenchyma occurs following contrast material administration, with relatively less intense enhancement of solid renal masses. This differential enhancement allows such masses to be more conspicuously depicted on enhanced as compared with unenhanced images. T1-weighted images acquired using either spin echo or gradient echo methods may be used.

Dynamic contrast-enhanced rapid imaging is useful for characterization of renal pseudotumors, as discussed previously. However, there does not appear to be a substantive advantage in terms of solid renal lesion detection for using rapid as compared with conventional contrast-enhanced techniques. Rapid imaging techniques

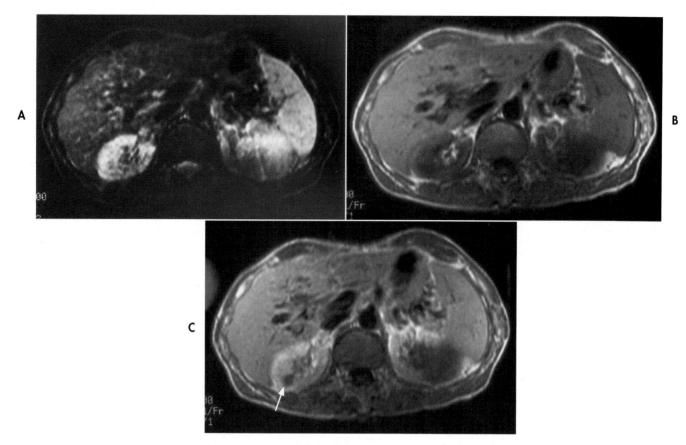

Fig. 7-33. Transaxial T2-weighted **(A)** (TR 3400, TE 80, 2 Nex) and T1-weighted (TR 500, TE 11, 2 Nex) images obtained before **(B)** and after **(C)** gadolinium chelate administration. The right kidney demonstrates a normal appearance on unenhanced T1-weighted and T2-weighted images. A 2 cm right renal cyst (*arrow*) is visualized only on the contrast-enhanced T1-weighted image.

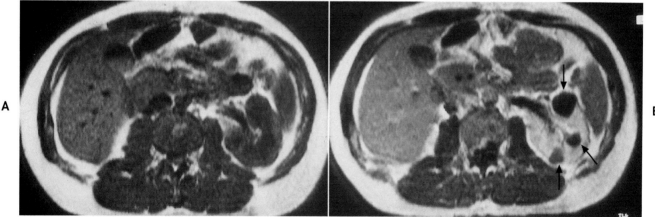

Fig. 7-34. Transaxial T1-weighted rapid acquisition spin echo images obtained before **(A)** and following **(B)** intravenous contrast material administration. Multiple cysts (*arrows*) involving the left kidney are poorly visualized on unenhanced image, although they are easily seen following contrast material administration.

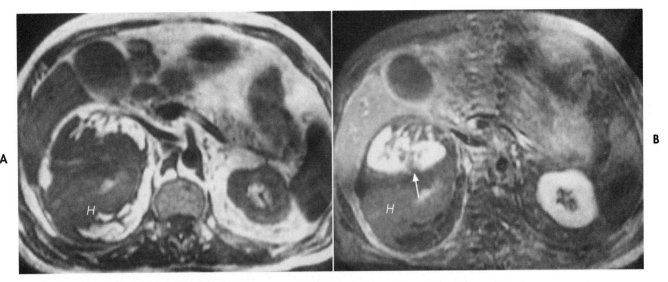

Fig. 7-35. A, Transaxial T1-weighted image demonstrates extensive right perirenal hematoma (*H*) that deviates the kidney anteriorly. There are no focal renal lesions identified on this or on a corresponding T2-weighted image. **B,** Fat-suppressed T1-weighted image obtained following intravenous gadolinium chelate contrast material administration demonstrates small focus of decreased signal intensity within posterior renal cortex (*arrow*), representing a renal cell carcinoma that has undergone hemorrhage.

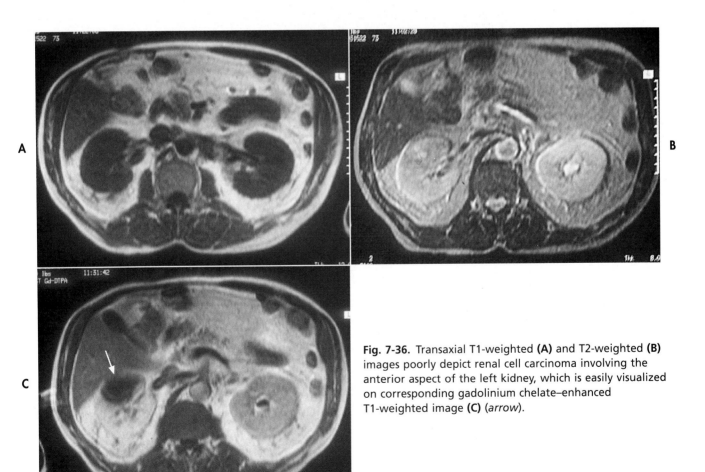

Fig. 7-36. Transaxial T1-weighted **(A)** and T2-weighted **(B)** images poorly depict renal cell carcinoma involving the anterior aspect of the left kidney, which is easily visualized on corresponding gadolinium chelate–enhanced T1-weighted image **(C)** (*arrow*).

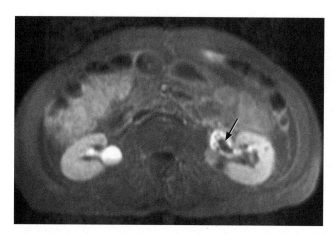

Fig. 7-37. Transaxial fat-suppressed T1-weighted image (TR 350, TE 12, 2 Nex) obtained following gadolinium chelate administration. A dilated left extrarenal pelvis is visualized, containing a focus of markedly decreased signal intensity (*arrow*). This represents a renal calculus, as documented by additional images and CT, and is similar in appearance to concentrated gadolinium contrast material.

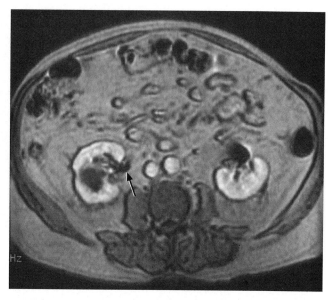

Fig. 7-38. Transaxial spoiled gradient echo image (TR 120, TE 3, 90-degree flip angle, 1 Nex) following gadolinium chelate contrast material administration. There is marked hypointensity within the right renal pelvis caused by concentrated contrast material (*arrow*). This appearance may simulate urinary tract calculi. Bilateral renal cysts are also demonstrated.

are advantageous for reducing or eliminating respiratory motion artifacts, since images can be acquired during suspended respiration. During the bolus phase of dynamic contrast-enhanced imaging, prominent enhancement is noted within the renal cortex, which is followed by diffuse enhancement throughout the renal parenchyma (see Fig. 7-23).

Foci of transiently decreased signal intensity are observed within the renal medulla on dynamic contrast-enhanced gradient echo images. These foci represent T2 shortening effects of gadopentetate dimeglumine that occurs when the contrast agent becomes highly concentrated within the renal tubules and collecting system.[9,12,18,29,45] These findings should not be interpreted as evidence of hemorrhage, iron deposition, or calcification, all of which can result in similar signal loss on gradient echo images (Figs. 7-37 and 7-38). Alterations in these renal enhancement patterns can occur in the presence of urinary tract obstruction or vascular compromise.

The T1 shortening effects of gadopentetate dimeglumine are more conspicuous when fat suppression techniques are used, because the dynamic range for tissue contrast display is expanded when the normally high signal intensity of fat is eliminated. The use of contrast-enhanced fat suppression imaging has shown improved depiction of renal lesions as compared with conventional T1-weighted sequences. Image quality is also improved with fat suppression because of reduced prominence of respiratory motion artifacts.

Renal Calculi

Renal calculi are difficult to visualize on conventional spin echo pulse sequences. Depiction of such calculi is improved on gradient echo sequences, which more sensitively depict areas of signal loss caused by alterations in magnetic susceptibility relating to the presence of calcium.

Renal Cysts

Renal cysts are routinely encountered and may be broadly considered in the context of normal variation. It has been estimated that renal cysts are present in approximately half of the adult population. Simple renal cysts appear as rounded structures with homogeneous low signal intensity on T1-weighted images and marked hyperintensity on T2-weighted images. The signal intensity of a cyst should be similar to that of other fluid, such as bile or cerebrospinal fluid. The cyst wall is so thin as to be imperceptible and demonstrates no evidence of nodularity or septations. Finally, cysts demonstrate no enhancement following intravenous contrast material administration.

When all of the above criteria are met, the diagnosis of renal cysts is straightforward, and no further investigation is required. However, a number of conditions may render the characterization of renal cysts more difficult. For example, some renal cysts demonstrate relative increased signal intensity on T1-weighted images and/or relative decreased signal intensity on T2-weighted images as compared with fluid. This is usually due to hemorrhagic or proteinaceous contents within the cyst, which

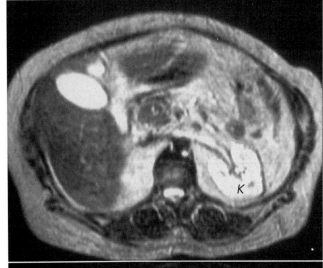

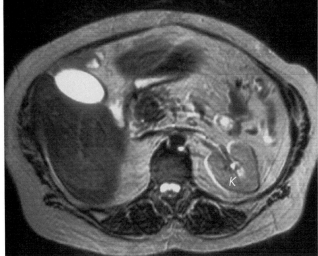

Fig. 7-39. Transaxial conventional **(A)** (TR 3400, TE 80, 2 Nex) and fast spin echo **(B)** (TR 4000, effective TE 120, 4 Nex, 16 echo train) T2-weighted images. There is markedly reduced renal signal intensity (*K*) on the fast spin echo image as compared to its conventional spin echo counterpart.

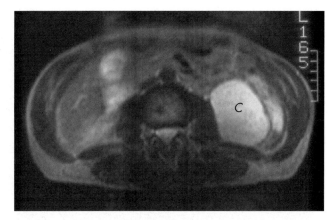

Fig. 7-40. A large cyst (*C*) is seen projecting from the left kidney on transaxial T2-weighted image (TR 3400, TE 80, 2 Nex). Artifactual reduced signal intensity is noted within the cyst on the basis of motion-related phase shifts.

may be related to previous episodes of trauma or infection. Clot within the cyst can simulate a soft tissue component, further heightening suspicion for malignancy. Wall thickening, septations, or nodularity may be observed in some atypical cysts. In spite of their aberrant signal intensity and morphologic characteristics, atypical cysts should continue to demonstrate a well-defined contour and lack of contrast material enhancement. Complex renal cysts, which appear intense on T1-weighted images as a result of proteinaceous or hemorrhagic contents, can appear similar to angiomyolipoma (see Fig. 7-21). Differentiation can be made with the use of fat suppressed T1-weighted images.

The use of inadequately T1-weighted or T2-weighted pulse sequences can cause renal cysts and solid renal neoplasms to have similar signal intensity characteristics. Therefore the minimum TE that can be achieved should be chosen for performance of T1-weighted sequences, and a TE of 90 to 120 msec should be used to acquire T2-weighted images. These parameters allow for improved distinction between cysts and solid lesions on the basis of signal characteristics. Improved distinction between renal cysts and solid neoplasms can also be achieved with use of heavily T2-weighted fast spin echo (i.e., RARE) sequences.[10] The renal parenchyma appears markedly hyperintense on conventional T2-weighted spin echo images. However, it appears of relatively decreased signal intensity on T2-weighted fast spin echo images (Figs. 7-39, *A* and *B*). Artifactual loss of signal intensity within a renal cyst on T2-weighted images can result from motion, thereby simulating a solid lesion (Fig. 7-40).

Renal cell carcinomas can appear well defined and in some cases may be cystic, simulating a benign cyst. As mentioned before, under no circumstances should a renal cyst undergo contrast material enhancement. However, hypovascular renal carcinomas, such as those of the papillary type can undergo relatively subtle enhancement (Figs. 7-41, *A-C*). Such enhancement may not be visually apparent and can only be recognized with the use of quantitative measurements. The use of quantitative measurements of lesion signal intensity before and after contrast administration may provide misleading results. Because the receiver radiofrequency transmitter and gain settings are usually adjusted prior to the performance of each individual pulse sequence, and because of the relative scaling of signal intensities on MR images, quantitative measurements of signal intensity may have little significance. If measurements are to be meaningful, ratios that compare a particular tissue with another refer-

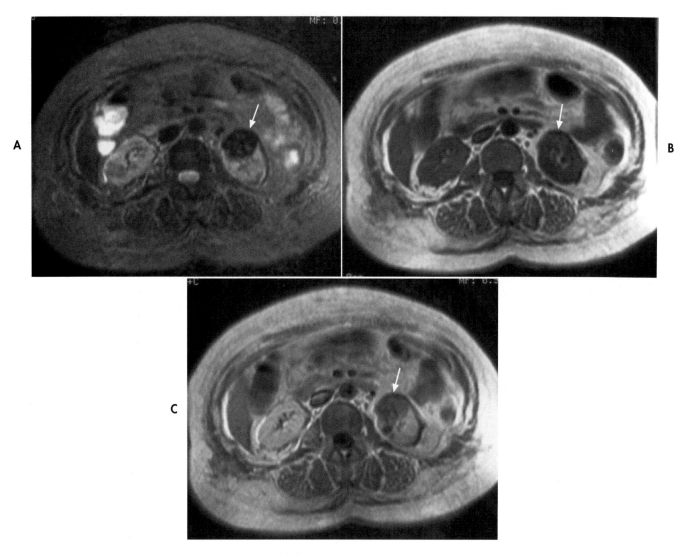

Fig. 7-41. Transaxial T2-weighted **(A)** (TR 2500, TE 80, 1 Nex) and T1-weighted (TR 550, TE 11, 2 Nex) images obtained before **(B)** and after **(C)** gadolinium chelate administration. Renal cell carcinoma arising from left kidney (*arrow*) is markedly hypointense on T2-weighted image. Mild hyperintensity is noted on T1-weighted image obtained before contrast material administration, with minimal apparent lesion enhancement.

ence tissue or phantom should be used. While pre- and post-contrast-enhanced images may be performed without adjusting the receiver gain, this is not recommended because the increased signal that occurs following contrast material administration may overwhelm the capacity of the receiver. This results in "overshoot artifacts" in which the gray scale appearance of the image becomes distorted.

Accurate interpretation of contrast-enhanced images mandates that unenhanced images using identical imaging parameters be acquired. When such images are unavailable, benign nonenhancing lesions having intrinsic increased signal intensity on T1-weighted images (e.g., from fat or hemorrhage) may be interpreted as enhancing malignant lesions.[44]

Motion Artifacts and Partial Volume Effects

Motion artifacts, particularly those relating to respiratory motion, disperse aberrant signal intensity along the phase encoding direction of the image. These phase errors are more prominent on contrast-enhanced images. When the high signal intensity components of such artifacts overlie the kidneys, abnormal enhancement could be simulated. Partial volume averaging of renal cysts with adjacent enhanced parenchyma or with perirenal fat can also simulate abnormal contrast enhancement.

Characterization of Renal Lesions

Even after a renal mass has been determined to be solid rather than cystic, its precise nature may still not be apparent. Benign renal adenomas and oncocytomas usually display features identical to those of renal cell carcinoma.[36]

Most renal carcinomas are isointense to hyperintense relative to renal parenchyma on T2-weighted images. However, atypical renal carcinomas can appear hypointense on T2-weighted images. Such lesions could be mistaken for other benign low-intensity lesions, such as renal fibroma.[13,51]

Fibrous tissue and/or compressed renal parenchyma can create the appearance of a pseudocapsule surrounding renal cell carcinomas on T1- or T2-weighted images.[50] While visualization of such a pseudocapsule indicates that tumor invasion into the adjacent perirenal fat is unlikely, microscopic tumor invasion can still be present.

High signal intensity on T1-weighted images can be associated with benign as well as malignant renal lesions. Hemorrhagic/proteinaceous renal cysts demonstrate T1 shortening, as described above. Renal cell carcinoma is typically highly vascular and may also undergo spontaneous hemorrhage. Hemorrhagic products can be observed in association with benign or malignant lesions that have undergone previous biopsy, as well as in patients who have undergone recent lithotripsy.[6] Metastases from melanoma can demonstrate T1 shortening because of the paramagnetic effects of melanin.

Another cause for increased signal intensity on T1-weighted images is the presence of fat. Documentation of fat within a renal lesion is virtually diagnostic of angiomyolipoma, a benign entity that may occur spontaneously or in association with tuberous sclerosis. Other renal lesions containing fat, such as dermoid, teratoma, or liposarcoma, are exceedingly rare. Renal cell carcinoma may engulf surrounding perirenal fat, thereby simulating the appearance of angiomyolipoma.[14,15] Postoperative defects in the renal cortex may also be filled with fat.[37] Fat suppression techniques can be used to distinguish fat from other causes of T1 shortening. Angiomyolipoma may simulate hemorrhagic renal cell carcinoma and can also appear to represent a solid renal lesion when it contains little observable fat.

Renal cell carcinomas can rarely contain small amounts of fat.[15,25,49] This may relate to foci of osseous metaplasia[25] and can be associated with calcification.[49] In such cases, confusion for angiomyolipoma may occur. Other renal lesions that can also contain fat include Wilms tumor,[15] teratomas, lipoma, liposarcoma, oncocytoma, and xanthogranulomatous pyelonephritis.[49]

> **ENTITIES THAT MAY SIMULATE LYMPH NODES**
>
> - Diaphragmatic crus
> - Anterior vertebral osteophytes
> - Retroaortic/circumaortic renal vein
> - Left-sided/duplicated inferior vena cava
> - Tortuous aorta/aortic aneurysm
> - Psoas muscle
> - Retroperitoneal fibrosis

RETROPERITONEUM

Lymph Nodes

Normal lymph nodes

Lymph nodes can be visualized within the intraperitoneal and retroperitoneal compartments of the abdomen in normal individuals. However, such lymph nodes should be small—less than 1 cm—and relatively few in number. Lymph nodes within the retrocrural space represent an exception to the 1 cm rule; malignancy should be suspected when these nodes exceed 6 mm in diameter.

Simulation of enlarged lymph nodes

Many structures can simulate enlarged lymph nodes. The diaphragmatic crura and psoas muscles may have a nodular and/or asymmetric appearance that suggests retroperitoneal lymphadenopathy (Figs. 7-42, A-C and 7-43). Prominent anterior vertebral osteophytes can project into the retroperitoneum and simulate lymph nodes. Recognition of both of these entities is facilitated on coronal or sagittal images.

Among the vascular causes of pseudoadenopathy are collateral retroperitoneal veins, retroaortic or circumaortic renal veins, and a left-sided or duplicated inferior vena cava (Figs. 7-44 and 7-45). Intermediate signal intensity within these vascular structures may be due to relative slow blood flow or entry phenomenon on T1-weighted images, or it may be found when gradient moment nulling is used for artifact reduction on T2-weighted images. The absence of a flow void within these vessels further contributes to confusion for soft tissue structures. A tortuous and ectatic aorta that undergoes volume averaging with adjacent retroperitoneal fat or a saccular aortic aneurysm containing thrombus can also simulate enlarged retroperitoneal lymph nodes (Figs. 7-46, A and B and 7-47, A and B). The use of gradient echo images or phase reconstructions allows the vascular nature of these entities to be appreciated.

Oil-based contrast agents can accumulate within retroperitoneal lymph nodes following conventional x-ray

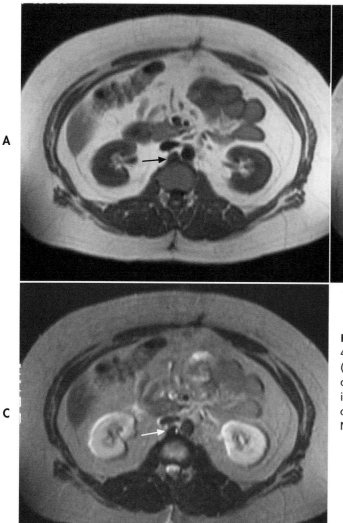

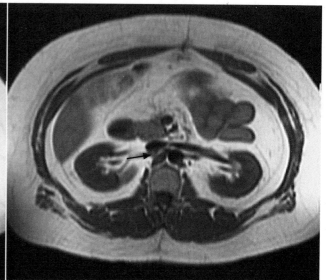

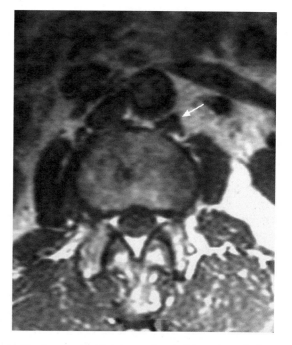

Fig. 7-42. Transaxial T1-weighted image **(A)** (TR 500, TE 12, 4 Nex) demonstrates apparent periaortic lymph node (*arrow*), which is shown to represent the diaphragmatic crus (*arrow*) on adjacent image **(B).** The apparent nodule is isointense with the paravertebral muscle (*arrow*) on corresponding T2-weighted image **(C)** (TR 3400, TE 80, 2 Nex).

lymphangiography. This can result in diminished conspicuity of such nodes on T1-weighted images, as a result of their isointensity with surrounding fat.[8]

Characterization of enlarged lymph nodes

The underlying basis for lymph node enlargement is not reliably determined on MR images. Nodal enlargement caused by reactive changes or granulomatous involvement demonstrates similar morphologic and signal intensity features as nodes replaced by a tumor.[16] Quantitative measurements of T1 and T2 relaxation times do not allow for distinction of benign versus malignant lymphadenopathy. This important limitation will be addressed with the clinical implementation of reticuloendothelial contrast agents such as ultrasmall superparamagnetic iron oxide crystals. This agent accumulates in normal nodal tissue, where it induces signal loss. The

Fig. 7-43. An apparent retroperitoneal lymph node located posterolateral to the aorta (*arrow*) on transaxial T1-weighted image (TR 500, TE 13, 4 Nex) represents the diaphragmatic crus.

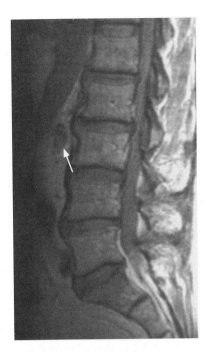

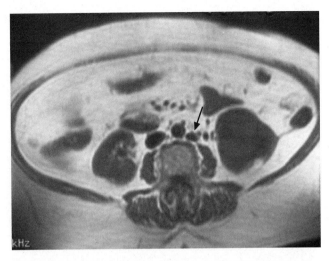

Fig. 7-44. An intermediate signal intensity structure (*arrow*) suggestive of a retroperitoneal lymph node is demonstrated on sagittal proton density–weighted image (TR 2000, TE 30, 1 Nex). This represents a retroaortic left renal vein, with relative increased intraluminal signal intensity on the basis of slow flow.

Fig. 7-45. Transaxial T1-weighted image (TR 500, TE 12, 4 Nex) demonstrates nodular structure in the left periaortic region (*arrow*), suggestive of an enlarged lymph node. This represents the proximal portion of a left retroaortic renal vein, as verified on contiguous images and other sequences.

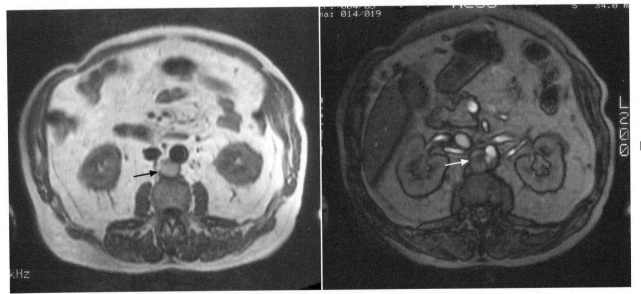

Fig. 7-46. A, Transaxial T1-weighted image (TR 500, TE 12, 4 Nex) in patient undergoing staging for prostate cancer demonstrates an apparent enlarged aorticocaval lymph node (*arrow*). However, this represents thrombus material within a saccular abdominal aortic aneurysm (*arrow*), as indicated by a corresponding spoiled gradient echo image **(B)** (TR 50, TE 12, 60-degree flip angle, 2 Nex) and verified surgically.

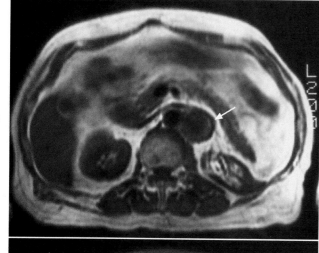

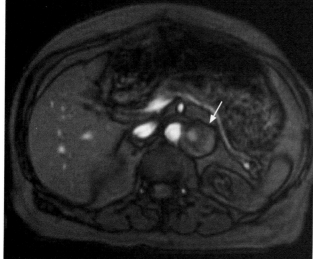

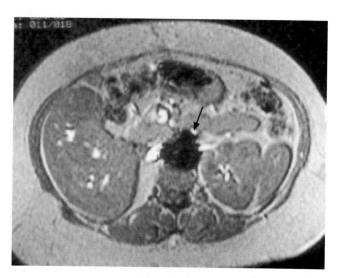

Fig. 7-48. Transaxial gradient echo image (TR 50, TE 5, 40-degree flip angle, 2 Nex) demonstrates a large area of signal void in the periaortic region (*arrow*) caused by vascular clips that limit visualization of periaortic adenopathy and obscure visualization of the aorta and renal vessels.

Fig. 7-47. A, A 3 cm rounded mass (*arrow*) is demonstrated in the left periaortic region on transaxial T1-weighted image (TR 500, TE 20, 4 Nex). The mass demonstrates intermediate signal intensity peripherally and decreased signal intensity centrally. This could potentially represent a large necrotic periaortic lymph node. **B,** Corresponding gradient echo image (TR 50, TE 12, 30-degree flip angle, 2 Nex) reveals flow related enhancement within the center of this lesion, verifying that it represents a saccular abdominal aortic aneurysm (*arrow*).

inability of the agent to accumulate in regions of nodal replacement results in foci of relative increased signal intensity.[56]

Vascular Structures

The aorta usually bifurcates at approximately the L-4 level, though the bifurcation can occur at a lower or higher position. The abdominal aorta may be highly tortuous. A large number of accessory vessels can originate from the abdominal aorta.

The inferior vena cava can be located to the left of the abdominal aorta, rather than to its right. In patients with such transposition of the inferior vena cava, the cava usually crosses to the right at approximately the level of the left renal vein.[20] The inferior vena cava may be duplicated, with the two cavas being symmetric or more often asymmetric in size. The left cava usually unites with the right-sided cava at the level of the renal veins.[20] Distinction of a left-sided inferior vena cava from a dilated left gonadal vein is made by observing extension of the gonadal vein through the inguinal canal.[20] The inferior vena cava may be congenitally absent, with return of blood flow from the lower extremities via a dilated azygos/hemiazygos venous system. In patients with retrocaval ureter—actually an anomaly of the inferior vena cava—the proximal right ureter loops partially (retrocaval) or completely (circumcaval) around the inferior vena cava.

Artifactual signal void may be observed within the retroperitoneum as a result of the presence of surgical clips or a caval filter, though the Vena Tech filter appears to generate relatively little artifact[30] (Fig. 7-48).

In the presence of a large abdominal mass, it may be difficult to determine whether the mass is intraperitoneal or retroperitoneal in origin (Figs. 7-49, *A-C*).

Diaphragm

The diaphragmatic crus can appear nodular or irregular in normal subjects, simulating adenopathy (Fig. 7-50). Small nodular foci can be observed in the pararenal space, particularly in elderly patients[38] (Fig. 7-51). These

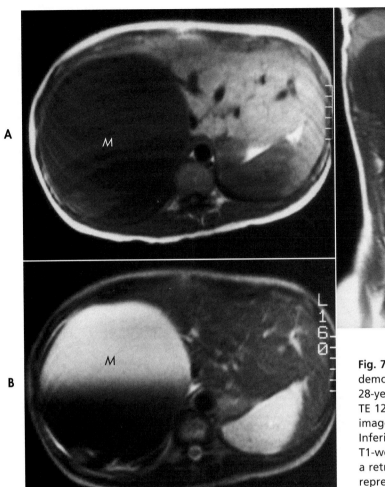

A

B

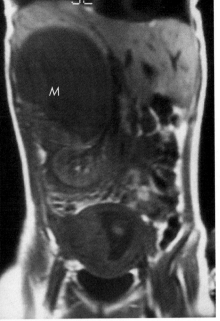

C

Fig. 7-49. A large hemorrhagic cystic mass (*M*) is demonstrated within the right upper quadrant in 28-year-old pregnant female on T1-weighted **(A)** (TR 550, TE 12, 4 Nex) and T2-weighted **(B)** (TR 3700, TE 80, 2 Nex) images. It is difficult to determine the origin of this mass. Inferior displacement of the right kidney on coronal T1-weighted image **(C)** indicates that this likely represents a retroperitoneal lesion. The lesion was proved to represent a hemorrhagic adrenal cyst pathologically. A gravid uterus is also noted.

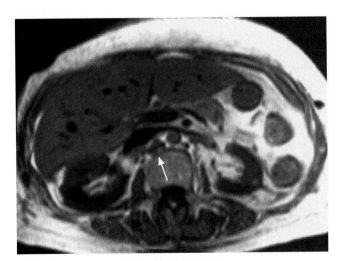

Fig. 7-50. Transaxial T1-weighted image (TR 500, TE 12, 4 Nex) depicts apparent nodular lesion in right periaortic region (*arrow*). This represents a nodular projection from the diaphragmatic crus.

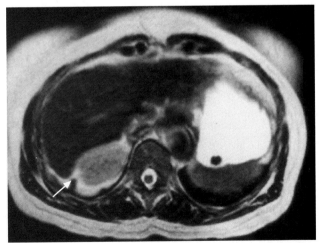

Fig. 7-51. A low signal intensity nodule is seen posterolateral to the right kidney (*arrow*). This represents a nodular infolding of the diaphragm. The apparent lesion demonstrates signal intensity equivalent to that of muscle.

nodules represent a portion of the diaphragmatic muscle that is infolded during deep inspiration or hypertrophied, and they can simulate neoplasm.

Psoas Muscles

The psoas muscles may be prominent and can also simulate enlarged retroperitoneal nodes, particularly when they are asymmetric in size. Similarly, a psoas hematoma or abscess can simulate bulky lymphadenopathy.

Retroperitoneal Fibrosis

Retroperitoneal fibrosis can have variable signal intensity characteristics. Distinction between benign and malignant causes of retroperitoneal fibrosis can be difficult.[2]

REFERENCES

1. Apicella PL, Mirowitz SA, Borrello J: Chemical shift misregistration artifacts: increased conspicuity following intravenous administration of gadopentetate dimeglumine, Magn Reson Imaging, 12:675-678, 1994.
2. Arrive' L, Hricak H, Tavares NJ et al: Malignant versus nonmalignant retroperitoneal fibrosis: differentiation with MR imaging, Radiology 172:139-143, 1989.
3. Baker ME, Blinder R, Spritzer C et al: MR evaluation of adrenal masses at 1.5 T, Am J Roentgenol 153:307-312, 1989.
4. Baker ME, Spritzer C, Blinder R et al: Benign adrenal lesions mimicking malignancy on MR imaging: report of two cases, Radiology 163:669-671, 1987.
5. Barr RG, Lorig RJ: Renal tissue within the adrenal gland simulating an adrenal mass (letter), Am J Roentgenol 155:656, 1990.
6. Baumgartner BR, Dickey KW, Ambrose SS et al: Kidney changes after extracorporeal shock wave lithotripsy: appearance on MR images, Radiology 163:531-534, 1987.
7. Bergman RA, Thompson SA, Afifi AK et al: Compendium of human anatomic variation: text, atlas, and world literature, Baltimore, 1988, Urban & Schwarzenberg.
8. Buckwalter KA, Ellis JH, Baker DE et al: Pitfall in MR imaging of lymphadenopathy after lymphangiography, Radiology 161:831-832, 1986.
9. Carvlin MJ, Arger PH, Kundel HL et al: Use of Gd-DTPA and fast gradient-echo and spin-echo MR imaging to demonstrate renal function in the rabbit, Radiology 170:705-711, 1989.
10. Catasca J, Mirowitz SA: T2-weighted MR imaging of the abdomen: fast spin-echo vs conventional spin-echo sequences, Am J Roentgenol 162:61-67, 1994.
11. Chezmar JL, Robbins SM, Nelson RC et al: Adrenal masses: characterization with T1-weighted MR imaging, Radiology 166:357-359, 1988.
12. Choyke PL, Frank JA, Girton ME et al: Dynamic Gd-DTPA-enhanced MR imaging of the kidney: experimental results, Radiology 170:713-720, 1989.
13. Cormier P, Patel SK, Turner DA et al: MR imaging findings in renal medullary fibroma, Am J Roentgenol 153:83-84, 1989.
14. Curry NS, Schabel SI, Garvin AJ et al: Intratumoral fat in a renal oncocytoma mimicking angiomyolipoma, Am J Roentgenol 154:307-308, 1990.
15. Davidson AJ, Davis CJ Jr: Fat in renal adenocarcinoma: never say never, Radiology 188:316, 1993.
16. de Lange EE, Fechner RE, Edge SB et al: Preoperative staging of rectal carcinoma with MR imaging: surgical and histopathologic correlation, Radiology 176:623-628, 1990.
17. Dunnick NR: Adrenal imaging: current status, Am J Roentgenol 154:927-936, 1990.
18. Eilenberg SS, Lee JKT, Brown JJ et al: Renal masses: evaluation with gradient-echo Gd-DTPA-enhanced dynamic MR imaging, Radiology 176:333-338, 1990.
19. Fein AB, Lee JKT, Balfe DM et al: Diagnosis and staging of renal cell carcinoma: a comparison of MR imaging and CT, Am J Roentgenol 148:749-753, 1987.
20. Friedland GW, de Vries PA Nino-Murcia M, et al: Congenital anomalies of the inferior vena cava: embryogenesis and MR features, Urol Radiol 13:237-248, 1992.
21. Glazer GM, Woolsey EJ, Borrello J et al: Adrenal tissue characterization using MR imaging, Radiology 158:73-79, 1986.
22. Glazer GM: MR imaging of the liver, kidneys, and adrenal glands, Radiology 166:303-312, 1988.
23. Hanna S, Helenon O, Legendre C et al: MR imaging of renal transplant rejection, Acta Radiol 32:42-46, 1991.
24. Harris RD, Heany JA, Sueoka BL et al: Retroperitoneal leiomyosarcoma: a rare cause of adrenal pseudotumor on CT and MRI, Urol Radiol 10:186-188, 1988.
25. Helenon O, Chretien Y, Paraf F et al: Renal cell carcinoma containing fat: demonstration with CT, Radiology 188:429-430, 1993.
26. Hricak H, Thoeni RF, Carroll PR et al: Detection and staging of renal neoplasms: a reassessment of MR imaging, Radiology 166:643-649, 1988.
27. Itoh K, Yamashita K, Satoh Y et al: MR imaging of bilateral adrenal hemorrhage, J Comput Assist Tomogr 12:1054-1056, 1988.
28. Kier R, McCarthy S: MR characterization of adrenal masses: field strength and pulse sequence considerations, Radiology 171:671-674, 1989.
29. Kikinis R, von Schultess GK, Jager P et al: Normal and hydronephrotic kidney: evaluation of renal function with contrast-enhanced MR imaging, Radiology 165:837-842, 1987.
30. Kiproff PM, Deeb ZL, Contractor FM et al: Magnetic resonance characteristics of the LGM vena cava filter: technical note, Cardiovasc Intervent Radiol 14:254-255, 1991.
31. Krestin GP, Freidmann G, Fishbach R et al: Evaluation of adrenal masses in oncologic patients: dynamic contrast-enhanced MR vs CT, J Comput Assist Tomogr 15:104-110, 1991.
32. Mirowitz SA, Gutierrez E, Lee JKT et al: Normal abdominal enhancement patterns with dynamic gadolinium-enhanced MR imaging, Radiology 180:637-640, 1991.
33. Mitchell DG, Crovello M, Matteucci T et al: Benign adrenocortical masses: diagnosis with chemical shift MR imaging, Radiology 185:345-351, 1992.
34. Musante F, Derchi LE, Bazzocchi M et al: MR imaging of adrenal myelolipomas, J Comput Assist Tomogr 15:111-114, 1991.

35. Musante F, Derchi LE, Zappasodi F et al: Myelolipoma of the adrenal gland: sonographic and CT features, Am J Roentgenol 151:961-964, 1988.

36. Palmer WE, Chew FS: Renal oncocytoma, Am J Roentgenol 156:1144, 1991.

37. Papanicolaou N, Harbury OL, Pfister RC: Fat-filled postoperative renal cortical defects: sonographic and CT appearance, Am J Roentgenol 151:503-505, 1988.

38. Parienty RA, Marichez M, Pradel J et al: Pararenal pseudotumors of the diaphragm: computed tomographic features, Gastrointest Radiology 12:131-133, 1987.

39. Premkumar A, Chow CK, Choyke PL et al: Stress-induced adrenal hyperplasia simulating metastatic disease: CT and MR findings (letter), Am J Roentgenol 159:675-676, 1992.

40. Quint LE, Glazer GM, Chenevert TL et al: In vivo and in vitro MR imaging of renal tumors: histopathologic correlation and pulse sequence optimization, Radiology 169:359-362, 1988.

41. Reinig JW, Doppman JL, Dwyer AJ et al: MRI of indeterminate adrenal masses, Am J Roentgenol 147:493-496, 1986.

42. Reinig JW, Doppman JL, Dwyer AJ et al: Adrenal masses differentiated by MR, Radiology 158:81-84, 1986.

43. Reinig JW: MR imaging differentiation of adrenal masses: has the time finally come? Radiology 185:339-340, 1992.

44. Semelka RC, Hricak H, Stevens SK et al: Combined gadolinium-enhanced and fat-saturation MR imaging of renal masses, Radiology 178:803-809, 1991.

45. Semelka RC, Hricak H, Tomei E et al: Obstructive nephropathy: evaluation with dynamic Gd-DTPA-enhanced MR imaging, Radiology 175:797-803, 1990.

46. Semelka RC, Chew W, Hricak H et al: Fat-saturation MR imaging of the upper abdomen, Am J Roentgenol 155:1111-1116, 1990.

47. Silverman PM, Cooper C, Zeman RK: Lateral arcuate ligaments of the diaphragm: anatomic variations at abdominal CT, Radiology 185:105-108, 1992.

48. Small WC, Bernardino ME: Gd-DTPA adrenal gland enhancement at 1.5 T, Magn Reson Imaging 9:309-312, 1991.

49. Strotzer M, Lehner KB, Becker K: Detection of fat in a renal cell carcinoma mimicking angiomyolipoma, Radiology 188:427-428, 1993.

50. Sui-Qiao H, Shi-Shun Z, Qi-Lun H: MR appearance of the pseudocapsule of renal cell carcinoma and its pathologic basis, Urol Radiol 13:158-161, 1992.

51. Sussman SK, Glickstein MF, Krzymowski GA: Hypointense renal cell carcinoma: MR imaging with pathologic correlation, Radiology 177:495-497, 1990.

52. Tsushima Y, Ishizaka H, Kato T et al: Differential diagnosis of adrenal masses using out-of-phase FLASH imaging: a preliminary report, Acta Radiol 33:262-265, 1992.

53. Tsushima Y, Ishizaka H, Matsumoto M: Adrenal masses: differentiation with chemical shift, fast low-angle shot MR imaging, Radiology 186:705-709, 1993.

54. Tung GA, Pfister RC, Papanicolaou N et al: Adrenal cysts: imaging and percutaneous aspiration, Radiology 173:107-110, 1989.

55. Wachsberg RH, Mitchell DG, Rifkin MD et al: Chemical shift artifact along the section-select axis, J Magn Reson Imaging 2:589-591, 1992.

56. Weissleder R, Eliozondo G, Josephson L et al: Experimental lymph node metastases: enhanced detection with MR lymphography, Radiology 171:835-839, 1989.

57. Winsett MZ, Amparo EG, Fawcett HD et al: Renal transplant dysfunction: MR evaluation, Am J Roentgenol 150:319-323, 1988.

Section Three

PELVIS

8

General Pelvis, Bladder, Rectum

GENERAL PELVIS
Anatomic Variations

Among the most frequent anatomic variations involving the bony pelvis are nonunion of the pubic and ischial rami, absence of the acetabular notch, and presence of an accessory ischial spine.[4] The configuration of the bony pelvis differs in males and females.

The pelvic muscles also vary among individuals. The levator ani muscles are particularly subject to variation in size and composition.[4] Some muscles of the pelvic floor, such as the transversus perinei superficialis and profundus, may be hypoplastic or absent.[4] The coccygeal muscle may be fused with the levator ani muscles.[4] Fat may separate the rectus abdominus muscles (Fig. 8-1).

The gonadal arteries can be duplicated or absent; the origin and course of these vessels are also variable. The gonadal artery can arise from the renal, suprarenal, or lumbar arteries or from various positions along the course of the abdominal aorta.[4] The right gonadal artery can be found posterior rather than anterior to the inferior vena cava.[4] The internal and external iliac arteries can arise directly from the aorta, without formation of the common iliac arteries.[7] There is marked variation in the number, origin, and course of the internal iliac artery branches. Pelvic veins can also be duplicated or absent or have an anomalous origin or course.

Pelvic Lipomatosis

In patients with pelvic lipomatosis, abundant pelvic fat can deviate the seminal vesicles medially, and prominent fat deposits can become interposed between the prostate and anterior rectal wall. The bladder base can be elevated, and ureteral obstruction may occur.[14] Fat demonstrates characteristic signal intensity on standard pulse sequences, allowing for its recognition and distinction from most neoplasms. In equivocal cases, fat suppression techniques can be used for confirmation.

Extensive pelvic fat may be present in obese patients and in patients receiving corticosteroids (Fig. 8-2).

Lymph Nodes

Small pelvic lymph nodes, measuring less than 1 cm in diameter, can be observed in normal individuals. Pelvic lymph nodes are most frequently present in the inguinal region, where they usually represent reactive nodes related to minor inflammatory processes involving the lower extremities. However, lymph node pathology can only be suspected on the basis of nodal size on magnetic resonance (MR) images, since signal charac-

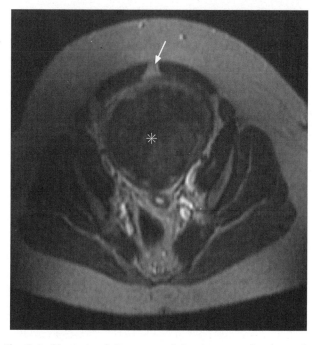

Fig. 8-1. Diastasis of the rectus abdominus muscles *(arrow)* is demonstrated on transaxial T2-weighted image (TR 3300, TE 90, 2 Nex) in patient with large myomatous uterus *(asterisk).*

213

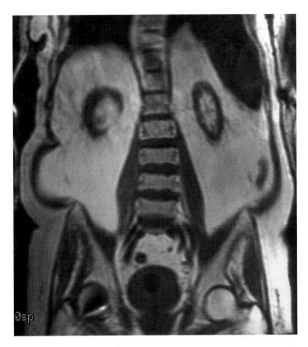

Fig. 8-2. Extensive intraabdominal fat deposition is evident on coronal T1-weighted image (TR 300, TE 12, 4 Nex) in patient receiving high-dose steroid therapy.

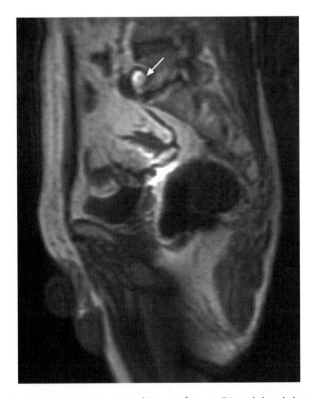

Fig. 8-3. The initial sagittal image from a T1-weighted data set (TR 400, TE 20, 1 Nex) demonstrates increased signal intensity within the iliac vein *(arrow)* as a result of entry phenomenon. It simulates the presence of adenopathy in this patient being evaluated for staging prostate cancer.

teristics do not distinguish benign from malignant nodes. Superparamagnetic iron oxide contrast agents have shown some promise for refining diagnosis of lymph node replacement, though these agents are not yet available for clinical use. An unusual cause for pelvic lymphadenopathy is Castleman disease, for which MR imaging findings have been reported.[24]

Several entities can simulate enlarged pelvic lymph nodes. The iliac veins can demonstrate intermediate signal intensity, similar to that of soft tissue, because of relatively slow blood flow, entry phenomenon, or even echo rephasing (Figs. 8-3 to 8-5). These flow phenomena are discussed in detail in Chapter 2. Vessels can be recognized by their tubular nature, which allows them to be visualized over several successive images. Flow sensitive gradient echo images can be used in problematic cases. The venous plexuses surrounding pelvic organs can also simulate lymphadenopathy (Figs. 8-6, *A* and *B*).

Some pelvic musculotendinous structures can also simulate enlarged lymph nodes. For example, a fat plane separating the iliacus and psoas muscles can cause the former structure to appear as a rounded soft tissue mass in the vicinity of the iliac lymph node chain (Fig. 8-4). A similar phenomenon may occur in some patients related to the psoas major and psoas minor muscles. An inguinal or femoral hernia can also simulate enlarged lymph nodes, particularly when the hernia contains bowel (Figs. 8-7, *A* and *B*).

Loops of bowel are another entity that may potentially simulate enlarged pelvic lymph nodes. The signal intensity of gastrointestinal tract structures on MR images is highly variable and may be similar to that of soft tissue.

ENTITIES THAT MAY SIMULATE PELVIC MASSES/LYMPH NODES

- Vascular structures
  Slow flow
  Even echo rephasing
  Gradient moment nulling
  Entry phenomenon
- Musculotendinous structures
  Iliacus muscle
  Psoas minor muscle
- Hernias
  Inguinal
  Femoral
- Postoperative changes
  Gelatin sponge
  Urinary conduits
  Altered position seminal vesicles, cervix
- Pelvic kidney

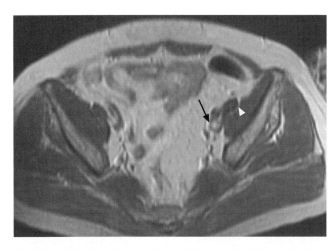

Fig. 8-4. Gadopentetate-enhanced transaxial T1-weighted image (TR 500, TE 12, 2 Nex) demonstrates intermediate signal intensity structure in left external iliac region *(arrow)* in a patient undergoing staging for prostate cancer. While this could represent adenopathy, it is due to slow flow within the external iliac vein. Also note fat plane separating left psoas from iliacus muscles *(arrowhead)*, which could also contribute to simulation of a lymph node.

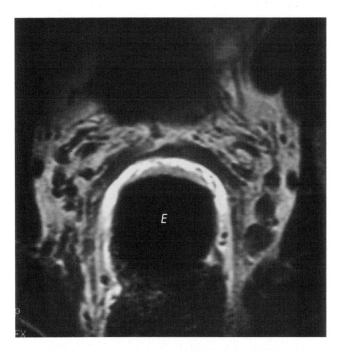

Fig. 8-5. Transaxial T1-weighted (TR 600, TE 20, 2 Nex) endorectal coil image demonstrates multiple nodular structures of intermediate signal intensity in both obturator regions. While these structures appear to represent lymph nodes, they are actually prominent vessels with relatively slow flow. Note high signal intensity artifact present at surface of endorectal coil (*E*).

The use of gastrointestinal contrast agents is helpful for marking the bowel and in distinguishing it from other structures (Figs. 8-8, *A* and *B* and 8-9, *A* and *B*).

The presence of renal tissue within the pelvis (i.e., pelvic kidney) can also simulate a pelvic mass (Figs. 8-10 and 8-11). However, this entity is usually easily recognized on the basis of reniform configuration, visualization of corticomedullary differentiation, and absence of tissue within the renal fossa.

Postoperative Changes

Gelatin sponge is often used to promote hemostasis in patients who have undergone surgery; this material can simulate a mass on MR images.[20,21] Because it absorbs fluids and often contains air bubbles, gelatin sponge is most likely to simulate a pelvic abscess. The sponge ma-

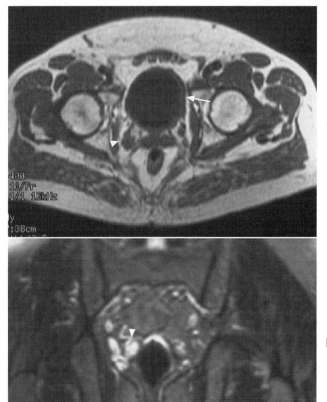

Fig. 8-6. A, Transaxial T1-weighted image (TR 400, TE 11, 4 Nex) demonstrates apparent enlarged lymph node adjacent to right seminal vesicle *(arrowhead)*. This represents an asymmetrically prominent venous plexus, as documented on coronal fat-suppressed fast spin echo T2-weighted image **(B)** (TR 4000, effective TE 96, 4 Nex, 16 echo train length). Note chemical shift misregistration artifact resulting in apparent thickening of the bladder wall on the patient's left side *(arrow,* **A**).

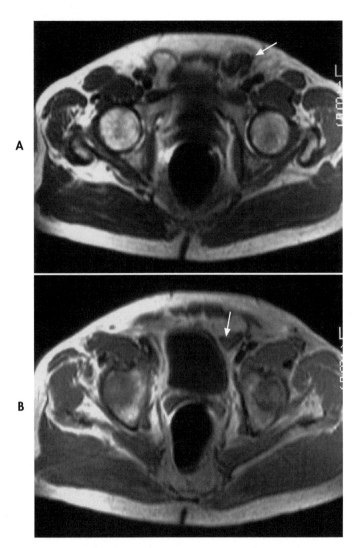

Fig. 8-7. Transaxial T1-weighted images (TR 550, TE 12, 2 Nex) in patient evaluated for prostate cancer staging. There is an apparent soft tissue mass suggestive of adenopathy in the left inguinal **(A)** and iliac **(B)** regions *(arrows)*. These represent a bowel loop contained within an inguinal hernia.

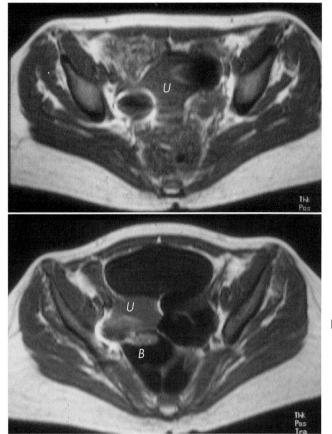

Fig. 8-8. Transaxial T1-weighted images of the pelvis acquired before **(A)** and after **(B)** oral administration of perfluorooctylbromide contrast agent. The unenhanced image demonstrates isointensity between the uterus *(U)* and surrounding bowel loops. However, following contrast material administration, negative enhancement of bowel loops *(B)* results in improved discrimination between these structures.

terial is visible on MR images for 2 to 4 weeks after its placement.[20]

In the postoperative patient, lymphoceles can appear hyperintense on T1-weighted images because of their proteinaceous content.[22] This appearance can simulate hematoma. In patients who have undergone cystectomy, urinary conduits can appear as lobular high signal intensity structures on T2-weighted images subjacent to the anterior abdominal wall or in the right iliac fossa,[22] where they can simulate an abscess. Small soft tissue nodules are frequently observed in the gluteal region, representing injection granulomas.

Signal Intensity Characteristics

Initial studies using T2-weighted fast spin echo imaging indicate that it provides better depiction of pelvic anatomy and pathology than conventional T2-weighted images.[30,35] Skeletal muscle and the smooth muscle comprising uterine myomas are less intense on fast spin echo images than on conventional images.[35] Fast spin echo sequences provide good tissue contrast, spatial resolution, and edge definition.[8,28] Fat demonstrates considerably higher signal intensity on T2-weighted images acquired using a fast spin echo image rather than conventional spin echo technique. This is probably due to a number of interrelated mechanisms including magnetization transfer effects, decoupling of J-modulation, stimulated echoes, and others.[9] Fast spin echo images demonstrate greater blurring than conventional spin echo

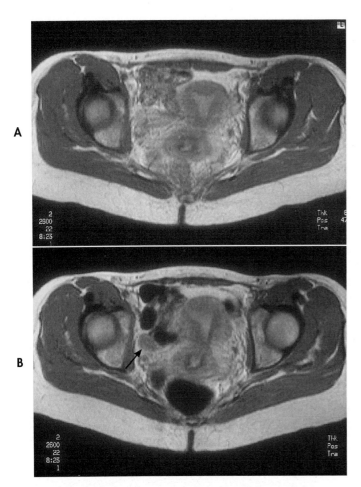

Fig. 8-9. Transaxial proton density–weighted (TR 2600, TE 22) images obtained before **(A)** and after **(B)** oral administration of perfluorooctylbromide. Distinction between bowel loops and adnexal structures is difficult on the precontrast image, because of isointensity between these structures. However, with negative enhancement of the bowel lumen, the right ovary *(arrow)* is easily identified.

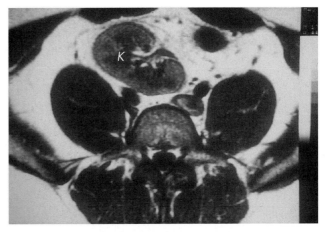

Fig. 8-10. Transaxial T1-weighted image of the pelvis demonstrates a pelvic kidney *(K)*.

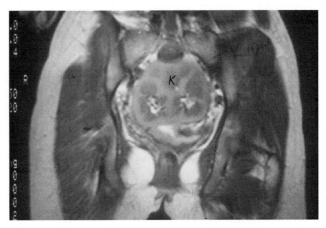

Fig. 8-11. A pelvic "cake" kidney *(K)* is demonstrated on this coronal T1-weighted image.

images, particularly when a long echo train or short echo time are used.[8,28,35]

Fat suppression sequences are also used to evaluate many pelvic abnormalities. These sequences provide improved tissue contrast as a result of expansion of the dynamic range for image display. Other major advantages include a decrease in chemical shift misregistration artifacts and decreased prominence of respiratory motion artifacts. Limitations of these sequences include reduced number of imaging slices per unit time, decreased signal-to-noise ratio leading to grainy image appearance, and increased prominence of susceptibility artifacts related to metal or air. Fat saturation can result in uneven suppression of fat signal throughout the field-of-view, particularly when there are inhomogeneities in the magnetic

field such as those that may introduced by bowel gas, surgical clips, and other sources.

Surface Coils

Specialized local coils are another recent advance for pelvic MR imaging. Endocavitary coils placed within the rectum or vagina provide high signal-to-noise ratio for evaluation of the prostate, seminal vesicles, cervix, and rectum using small fields-of-view. When a local coil is used, signal intensity diminishes rapidly with increasing distance from the coil. Nonuniform signal profiles can degrade image quality and cause structures or lesions situated beyond the sensitive range of the coil to be obscured (Figs. 8-12 and 8-13, *A* and *B*). When a body coil image is obtained with an endocavitary coil in place, susceptibility artifacts are observed (see Fig. 8-5). Multicoil arrays, positioned externally around the pelvis, also

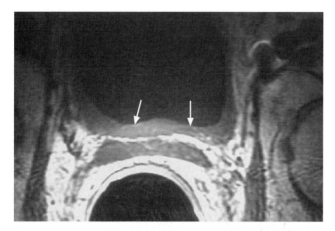

Fig. 8-12. Transaxial T1-weighted image (TR 600, TE 20, 2 Nex) acquired using an endorectal coil demonstrates thickening of the posterior bladder wall caused by bladder carcinoma *(arrows)*. However, the anterior extent of the lesion cannot be determined because of rapid loss of signal intensity with increasing distance from the local coil.

generate high signal-to-noise ratio for pelvic imaging and provide a more uniform signal profile throughout the pelvis.

URINARY BLADDER
Anatomic Variations

The bladder demonstrates relatively little anatomic variation. In some individuals the bladder can have an hourglass configuration.[4] Duplication or absence of the bladder or urethra rarely occurs.[4] In patients with ureteral duplication, the ureter can open ectopically into the vagina, seminal vesicle, or prostatic urethra.[4] The ureter can vary in its position; it may be located posterior to the inferior vena cava (retrocaval ureter) or between the inferior vena cava and abdominal aorta.[4] The kidney and its associated ureter may be located entirely within the pelvis in some individuals.

Postoperative Changes

The bladder may shift in position as a result of pelvic surgery. For example, it can shift posteriorly in patients who have undergone abdominoperineal resection (Figs. 8-14 and 8-15, *A* and *B*). In patients with extensive ascites, fluid layering within the pelvis can appear to represent the urinary bladder (Figs. 8-16, *A* and *B*).

Lesion Detection and Characterization

Thickening of the urinary bladder wall can indicate neoplastic involvement. However, other entities lead to similar findings, including inflammatory disease (i.e., cystitis), pelvic radiation therapy,[36] and chronic bladder

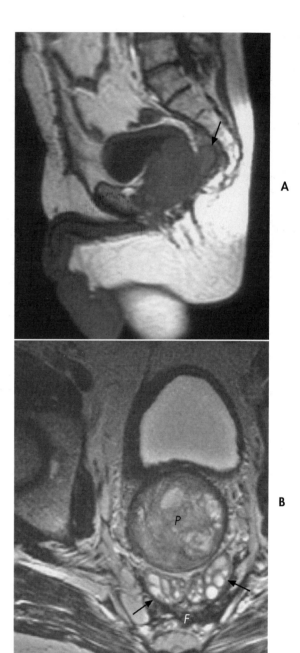

Fig. 8-13. A, A presacral soft tissue mass *(arrow)* is suggested on sagittal T1-weighted image (TR 400, TE 20, 1 Nex). This represents the seminal vesicles, which are posteriorly displaced in patient who has undergone previous abdominoperineal resection, as demonstrated by fast spin echo T2-weighted image *(arrows)* **(B)** (TR 7000, effective TE 108, 4 Nex). Presacral fibrosis *(F)* related to previous surgery is also noted on transaxial T2-weighted image. There is marked prostatic enlargement and heterogeneous signal intensity *(P)* caused by benign prostatic hyperplasia, as well as associated bladder wall thickening resulting from chronic outlet obstruction. These images were acquired using a local coil positioned beneath the patient. Note deformity of the soft tissues and attenuation of signal intensity with increasing distance from the surface coil in **A.**

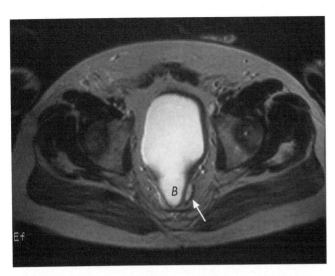

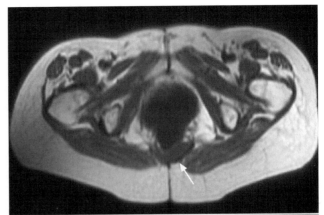

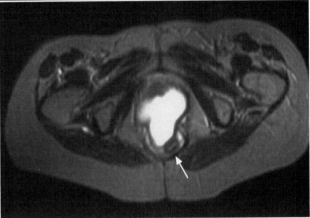

Fig. 8-14. Transaxial T2-weighted fast spin echo image (TR 4000, effective TE 119, 4 Nex, 16 echo train) of pelvis in patient who underwent previous abdominoperineal resection. The bladder (B) extends posteriorly into the presacral space with the seminal vesicles partially visualized lateral to the bladder (arrow).

Fig. 8-15. A, An apparent presacral soft tissue mass (arrow) is noted on transaxial T1-weighted image (TR 550, TE 12, 4 Nex) in a woman who underwent previous abdominoperineal resection of rectal cancer. **B,** Corresponding T2-weighted image (TR 2800, TE 120, 2 Nex) demonstrates the "mass" to be the uterine cervix (arrow), which has extended posteriorly as a result of previous surgery, along with the posterior wall of the urinary bladder.

outlet obstruction, usually caused by prostatic enlargement (Figs. 8-17 and 8-18). Chronic bladder outlet obstruction is also associated with bladder wall irregularity and diverticulae.

Following radiotherapy, increased signal intensity is often observed throughout the pelvis, including in muscles and fascial planes, on T2-weighted images. High signal intensity can also be observed in the bladder mucosa.[22] In patients with bladder carcinoma, these findings can simulate extramural tumor extension into the perivesical fat.[36] Radiation therapy may also result in thickening of the bladder wall, which must be distinguished from neoplastic involvement (Fig. 8-19).

The bladder wall can also appear to be thickened in normal individuals when the bladder lumen is not well distended.[23] Whereas a full bladder leads to patient discomfort and motion artifacts, the bladder should be imaged when it is partially distended. One method that has been recommended is to have the patient void 2 hours before the examination and not again until imaging has been completed.[3] Overdistention of the bladder lumen can obscure some mural lesions.[3,29] The intramural portions of the ureters can simulate a mural lesion of the bladder, though their symmetry and characteristic location near the bladder trigone should allow for distinction.

Focal wall thickening and increased signal intensity on T2-weighted images reflect mural edema, which occurs following recent biopsy or tumor resection. This can simulate the appearance of residual or recurrent tumor involvement.[3] In addition, inflammatory

---

NONNEOPLASTIC BLADDER WALL THICKENING/SIGNAL ALTERATIONS

- Cystitis
- Radiation therapy
- Bladder outlet obstruction
- Underdistention
- Recent biopsy/resection
- Chemical shift misregistration artifact

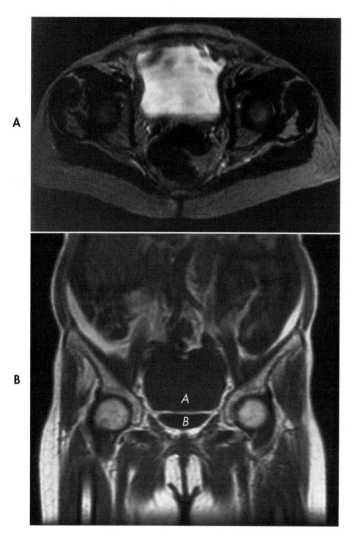

A

B

Fig. 8-16. A, Transaxial T2-weighted fast spin echo image (TR 3500, effective TE 119, 4 Nex, 16 echo train) demonstrates an apparent fluid-fluid level within the urinary bladder. This fluid collection actually represents ascites *(A)* that has layered above the urinary bladder *(B)*, as shown on corresponding coronal T1-weighted image, **B.**

APPARENT FILLING DEFECTS IN BLADDER THAT MAY SIMULATE A TUMOR

- Intramural ureters
- Partial volume averaging with bladder wall, prostate, bowel
- Paramagnetic contrast material
- Blood clot
- Calculi
- Catheters
- Ureteral jet phenomenon

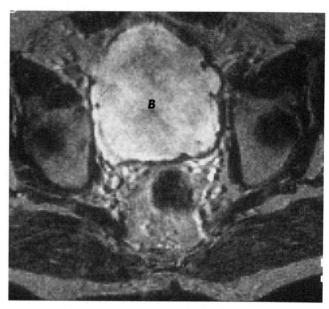

Fig. 8-17. Transaxial T2-weighted image in patient with benign prostatic hyperplasia demonstrates marked trabeculation of the urinary bladder *(B)* wall resulting from chronic bladder outlet obstruction.

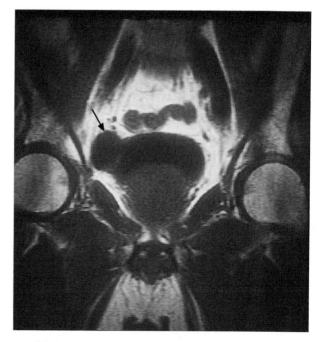

Fig. 8-18. Coronal T1-weighted image in patient with benign prostatic hyperplasia demonstrates diverticulum *(arrow)* projecting from the right superolateral aspect of the urinary bladder.

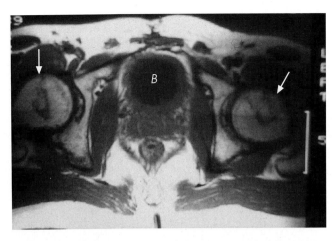

Fig. 8-19. Marked concentric thickening of the urinary bladder *(B)* wall is demonstrated on this transaxial T1-weighted image in a patient who has undergone previous radiation therapy for prostatic rhabdomyosarcoma. Also note avascular necrosis involving both femoral heads *(arrows)*.

changes surrounding tumors can result in their overstaging on MR images.[29] Another cause for overstaging is partial volume averaging of a tumor with the bladder wall or surrounding soft tissues.[29]

Chemical Shift Misregistration Artifact

Chemical shift misregistration artifact is another cause for apparent bladder wall thickening[1,27] (Figs. 8-6 and 8-20, *A* and *B*). The different precessional frequency of fat and water protons leads to misregistration of signal intensity along the frequency-encoding direction of the image at fat-water interfaces, such as at the junction of bladder wall and perivesical fat. The result is apparent thinning of the bladder wall on one side, with corresponding apparent wall thickening on the contralateral side. While this artifact is usually easily recognized, it is desirable to minimize chemical shift misregistration because of its potential to obscure as well as to simulate bladder wall pathology. Chemical shift misregistration artifact can be reduced when imaging is performed using low field strength systems, wide receiver bandwidths, and small voxel sizes.[1,27] Chemical shift misregistration is generally more prominent on T2- versus T1-weighted images.

When chemical shift artifacts persist despite the above measures, the phase- and frequency-encoding gradients can be reoriented, which will redirect these artifacts along the anterior and posterior bladder walls. Images acquired using conventional and reversed gradient orientations will allow the entire bladder wall to be accurately evaluated. Images can also be acquired in an alternate plane, such as the coronal or sagittal plane. This can be useful for evaluating lesions located along the bladder

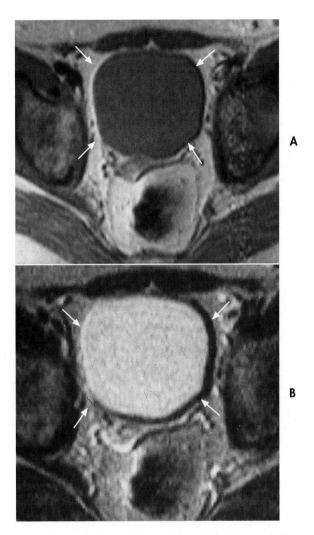

Fig. 8-20. Transaxial T1-weighted **(A)** and T2-weighted **(B)** images of the pelvis. Chemical shift misregistration artifacts *(arrows)* at the bladder-fat interface are demonstrated on both images. Note that the thickness of the chemical shift band is accentuated on the T2-weighted as compared with the T1-weighted image.

dome and base, though lateral wall lesions will be poorly visualized.

As mentioned before, chemical shift misregistration artifacts can obscure extravesical tumor extension and lead to understaging. Another cause for understaging is the presence of microscopic tumor invasion into or through the bladder wall, which cannot be visualized on MR images.[29]

Contrast Enhancement Patterns

Paramagnetic contrast agents, such as gadopentetate dimeglumine, provide enhancement of mural tumor, which may not be evident on unenhanced T1- and T2-

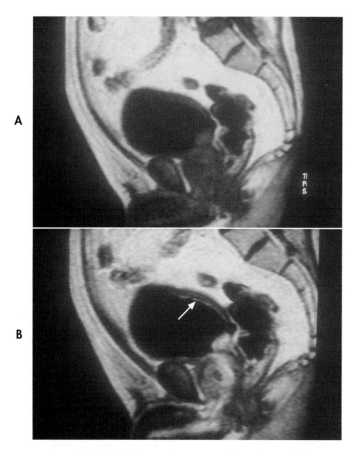

Fig. 8-21. Sagittal T1-weighted images obtained before **(A)** and after **(B)** intravenous gadopentetate dimeglumine administration in a patient with superficial bladder carcinoma. The tumor is relatively inapparent on the precontrast image, because of similar signal intensity as urine. However, following contrast material administration, enhancement of the lesion results in improvement in its conspicuousness *(arrow).*

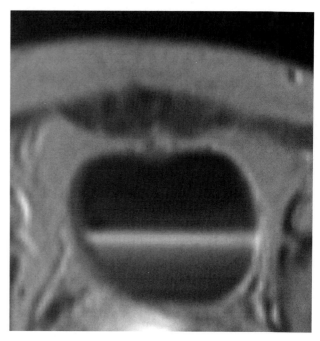

Fig. 8-22. Transaxial T1-weighted image (TR 500, TE 12, 2 Nex) obtained following gadopentetate dimeglumine administration. There are three signal intensity zones depicted within the lumen of the urinary bladder. The dependent zone represents concentrated contrast material, the intermediate hyperintense zone represents dilute contrast material, and the supernatant represents urine.

weighted images because of isointensity with surrounding urine or bladder wall. Contrast administration is particularly helpful for superficial tumors. The bladder wall undergoes mild contrast enhancement in normal individuals. Dynamic bolus contrast-enhanced imaging may be helpful in further improving distinction of tumor and surrounding uninvolved bladder wall and in determining the depth of bladder wall invasion[37] (Figs. 8-21, *A* and *B*). The plane of image acquisition should be optimized according to the known or suspected site of tumor involvement based on preliminary images or results of other procedures.[29] Images are optimally acquired perpendicular to the tumor site in order to best assess the depth of mural invasion. Abnormal enhancement of the bladder wall can be observed following radiation therapy.[22]

A trilaminar appearance is observed within the blad-

der lumen following contrast material administration[16] (Figs. 8-22 and 8-23, *A* and *B*). The dependent layer appears markedly hypointense because of highly concentrated contrast material. The T2 shortening effects of concentrated gadopentetate dimeglumine overwhelm its corresponding shortening of T1 relaxation. The middle layer appears hyperintense because of the T1 shortening effects of a dilute contrast material solution. Moderate reduced signal intensity is observed in the nondependent layer, representing unenhanced urine. While three layers are typically observed on T1-weighted images, the middle and upper layers are usually indistinguishable on T2-weighted images.

Dilute contrast material within the bladder can appear to represent an hemorrhagic intraluminal lesion on T1-weighted images, particularly when the typical laminar appearance described above is not evident. Relative increased signal intensity on unenhanced T1-weighted images and decreased intensity on T2-weighted images can be seen along the dependent aspect of the bladder in patients with proteinuria or pyuria (Fig. 8-24). An intravesical blood clot, which may be due to trauma, instrumentation, urinary tract calculi, or bleeding from bladder carcinoma or upper urinary tract lesions, can appear to

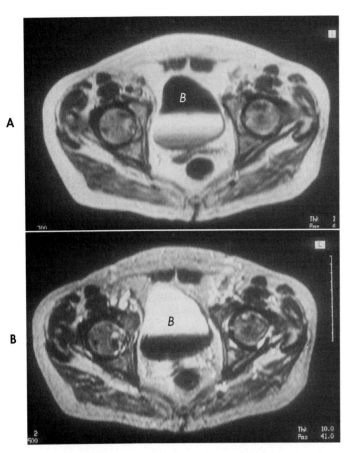

A

B

Fig. 8-23. Transaxial T1-weighted **(A)** (TR 700, TE 15) and T2-weighted **(B)** (TR 2500, TE 90) images of the pelvis obtained following intravenous gadopentetate dimeglumine administration. A trilaminar appearance is noted within the lumen of the urinary bladder *(B)* on the T1-weighted image, whereas a bilaminar appearance is demonstrated on the corresponding T2-weighted image. The dependent layers represent concentrated and dilute contrast material, whereas the supernatant represents urine.

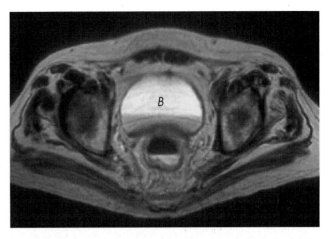

Fig. 8-24. Transaxial fast spin echo T2-weighted image (TR 4000, effective TE 117, 4 Nex, 16 echo train) demonstrates fluid-fluid level in urinary bladder *(B)*. This is due to sedimentation of proteinaceous cellular contents in patient with severe bacteriuria.

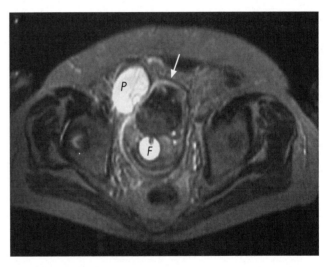

Fig. 8-25. A large low signal intensity structure *(arrow)* is noted within the urinary bladder on transaxial T2-weighted image (TR 3800, TE 120, 2 Nex). This represents a blood clot. A Foley balloon catheter *(F)* is also present. High signal intensity structure located anterolateral to the urinary bladder represents a reservoir for an inflatable penile prosthesis *(P)*.

represent a nodular mass lesion (Fig. 8-25). A transurethral (Foley) catheter or suprapubic catheter within the bladder lumen can also simulate a nodular mass on isolated images (Fig. 8-25). Partial volume averaging of the bladder with an enlarged prostate gland, the uterus, or adjacent small bowel loops can create the appearance of an intravesical mass (Figs. 8-26 and 8-27). A region of altered intravesicular signal intensity is occasionally observed because of inflow of urine into the bladder from the ureteral orifices (i.e., ureteral jet)[6,10] (Fig. 8-28). Bladder diverticulum can simulate a mass adjacent to the urinary bladder (Figs. 8-29, *A* and *B*). Benign lesions involving the wall of the urinary bladder, such as leiomyoma, can also simulate bladder carcinoma.[40]

RECTUM
Lesion Detection and Characterization

The major indication for MR imaging of the rectum is to stage the extent of rectal cancer and to evaluate response to therapy. Some apparent thickening of the rectal wall can be related to underdistention of the rectal lumen; this can lead to overestimation of the size of rec-

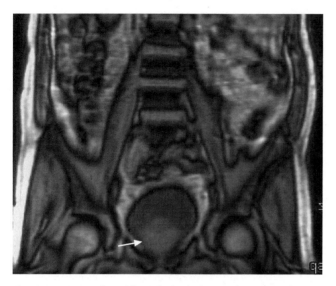

Fig. 8-26. Coronal rapid spoiled gradient echo image (TR 113, TE 2.6, 90-degree flip angle, 1 Nex) demonstrates apparent rounded mass within the inferior aspect of the urinary bladder *(arrow)*. These findings are due to partial volume averaging of the bladder with an enlarged prostate gland.

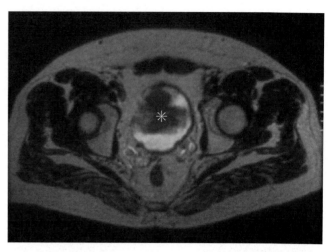

Fig. 8-27. T2-weighted fast spin echo transaxial image (TR 4000, effective TE 120, 4 Nex, 16 echo train) demonstrates an apparent mass *(asterisk)* within the urinary bladder. This is due to partial volume averaging of the bladder with overlying small bowel loops.

tal tumors. Fecal material within the rectum can also simulate a polypoid or sessile mass. These situations can be avoided through the use of cleansing enemas prior to MR imaging and inflation of the rectum with air or a balloon device. Endocavitary surface coils have been used to evaluate patients with rectal cancer. These coils provide distention of the rectal lumen as well as improved signal-to-noise ratio. Balloons or endocavitary coils can flatten large rectal masses, causing their size to be underestimated.

Lesion Staging

Some pitfalls can also be encountered in staging rectal tumors. For example, strandlike signal alterations can occur in the perirectal fat and can simulate local extramural tumor involvement.[7] When nodular or asymmetric irregular soft tissue thickening greater than several millimeters is observed, tumor invasion should be suspected. Perirectal soft tissue thickening also occurs in patients who have received preoperative radiation therapy, also resulting in potential overstaging by MR.[11,12,36]

Limitations related to detection of tumor involvement within nonenlarged lymph nodes was discussed previously and also applies to the staging of rectal carcinoma.[7]

Accurate detection and staging of rectal tumors can be affected by gastrointestinal tract motion artifacts. These artifacts are diminished in patients who are fasting and following administration of glucagon.[5,39] Deep pelvic structures undergo relatively little respiratory-related motion, though the use of respiratory ordered

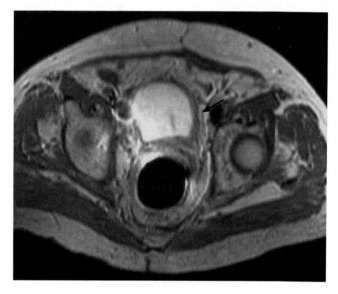

Fig. 8-28. Transaxial gadopentetate-enhanced T1-weighted image (TR 550, TE 12, 2 Nex) demonstrates asymmetric thickening of the posterior left lateral bladder wall caused by carcinoma *(arrow)*. A linear region of decreased signal intensity within the bladder lumen is noted near the trigone. This latter finding is due to turbulence caused by the ureteral jet phenomenon.

phase encoding, spatial presaturation, and gradient moment nulling can contribute to improved overall image quality.

Postoperative and Postradiation Changes

MR has been used to characterize presacral soft tissue masses in patients who have undergone previous sur-

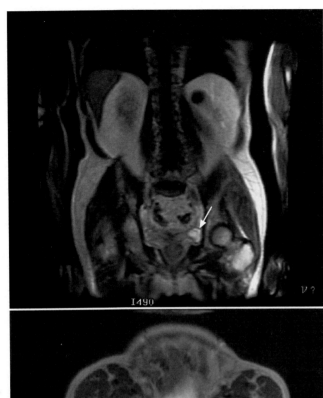

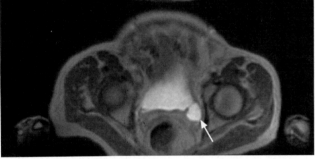

Fig. 8-29. A, A 2 cm enhancing mass *(arrow)* is noted within the left obturator region on a coronal gadopentetate enhanced T1-weighted image (TR 270, TE 11, 0.5 Nex). **B,** The corresponding transaxial gadopentetate enhanced image (TR 270, TE 11, 0.5 Nex) demonstrates continuity of the "mass" with the urinary bladder, indicating that it represents a bladder diverticulum *(arrow).*

gery for rectal carcinoma. The two major considerations when such masses are encountered are posttherapeutic fibrosis or residual/recurrent tumor. Thickening of the perirectal fascia and presacral soft tissues as well as edematous changes throughout the deep pelvic musculature and marrow space of the sacrum are seen in patients who have received pelvic irradiation.[36] Distinction between presacral fibrosis and residual/recurrent tumor is generally made on T2-weighted images. A mass that has uniform low signal intensity (e.g., isointense with normal paravertebral muscles) indicates fibrosis, whereas a tumor generally displays relative increased signal intensity. However, desmoplastic forms of rectal adenocarcinoma do occur and can potentially simulate benign fibrosis. Conversely, benign postoperative changes can simulate a tumor when MR is performed before complete transformation of granulation tissue into mature fibro-

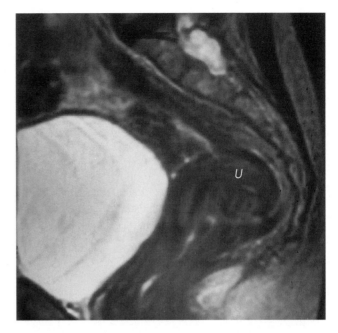

Fig. 8-30. A markedly retroverted and retroflexed uterus *(U)* extends into the presacral space on sagittal T2-weighted fast spin echo image (TR 4000, effective TE 120, 4 Nex, 8 echo train).

sis.[13,15,18,38] Tissue that has been recently treated with radiation demonstrates increased signal intensity on T2-weighted spin echo or STIR images and enhancement following paramagnetic contrast material administration. These findings can be seen as early as 6 weeks following commencement of therapy and can persist for over 1 year.[17] These soft tissue alterations generally have well-defined margins, corresponding to the therapy port. While MR may not allow for definitive distinction between fibrosis and a tumor in all patients, foci of relative increased signal intensity on T2-weighted images can serve to guide needle placement for biopsy in equivocal cases.[32]

Following abdominoperineal resection, the seminal vesicles may extend posteriorly into the presacral space, where they can simulate a mass[19,33] (see Fig. 8-13). The seminal vesicles are recognized by their characteristic high signal intensity and honeycomb architecture on T2-weighted images. The uterine cervix can assume a comparable position in female patients and is recognized by low signal intensity fibrous stroma surrounding central high signal endocervical glands and secretions (see Fig. 8-15). Marked retroflexion of the uterus can cause uterine tissue to simulate a presacral soft tissue lesion (Fig. 8-30).

Contrast Enhancement Patterns

Inflammatory or neoplastic lesions lead to thickening of the bowel wall, as well as increased mural enhancement when intravenous contrast material is given.[34] Abnormal enhancement of the bowel wall is most sensitively depicted on fat suppressed T1-weighted spin echo images. Prominent enhancement of the rectal wall can also be observed on contrast-enhanced fat suppressed images in normal individuals.[26]

Contrast agents have been administered per rectum to improve staging of rectal cancer. Rectally administered barium sulfate suspension can provide distention as well as negative contrast enhancement of the rectal lumen.[31] A progressive decrease in intraluminal signal intensity occurs on spin echo and gradient echo sequences as the concentration of barium sulfate is increased. The optimal concentration of barium sulfate suspension has been determined to be between 170% to 220% weight/volume.[2] In this concentration, decreased intraluminal signal intensity occurs on T1- and T2-weighted spin echo and STIR images.[25]

REFERENCES

1. Babcock EE, Brateman L, Weinreb JC et al: Edge artifacts in MR images: chemical shift effect, J Comput Assist Tomogr 9:252-257, 1985.
2. Ballinger JR, Ros PR: High density barium sulfate suspension for MRI: optimization of concentration for bowel opacification, Magn Reson Imaging 10:637-640, 1992.
3. Barentsz JO, Ruijs SHJ, Strijk SP: The role of MR imaging in carcinoma of the urinary bladder, Am J Roentgenol 160:937-947, 1993.
4. Bergman RA, Thompson SA, Afifi AK et al: Compendium of human anatomic variation: text, atlas, and world literature, Baltimore, 1988, Urban & Schwarzenberg.
5. Brown JJ, Duncan JR, Heiken JP et al: Perflourooctylbromide as a gastrointestinal contrast agent for MR imaging: use with and without glucagon, Radiology 181:455-460, 1991.
6. Burge HJ, Middleton WD, McClennan BL et al: Ureteral jets in healthy subjects and in patients with unilateral ureteral calculi: comparison with color Doppler US, Radiology 180:437-442, 1991.
7. Chan TW, Kressel HY, Milestone B et al: Rectal carcinoma: staging at MR imaging with endorectal surface coil: work in progress, Radiology 181:461-467, 1991.
8. Chien D, Mulkern RV: Fast spin-echo studies of contrast and small-lesion definition in a liver-metastasis phantom, J Magn Resonan Imaging 2:483-487, 1992.
9. Constable RT, Anderson AW, Zhong J et al: Factors influencing contrast in fast spin-echo MR imaging, Magn Reson Imaging 10:497-511, 1992.
10. Cox IH, Erickson SJ, Foley WD et al: Ureteric jets: evaluation of normal flow dynamics with color Doppler sonography, Am J Roentgenol 158:1051-1005, 1992.
11. de Lange EE, Fechner RE, Edge SB et al: Preoperative staging of rectal carcinoma with MR imaging: surgical and histopathologic correlation, Radiology 176:623-628, 1990.
12. de Lange EE, Fechner RE, Spaulding CA et al: Rectal carcinoma treated by preoperative irradiation: MR imaging and his-

13. de Lange EE, Fechner RE, Wanebo HJ: Suspected recurrent rectosigmoid carcinoma after abdominoperineal resection: MR imaging and histopathologic findings, Radiology 170:323-328, 1989.
14. Demas BE, Avallone A, Hricak H: Pelvic lipomatosis: diagnosis and characterization by magnetic resonance imaging, Urol Radiol 10:198-202, 1988.
15. Ebner F, Kressel HY, Mintz MC et al: Tumor recurrence versus fibrosis in the female pelvis: differentiation with MR imaging at 1.5 T, Radiology 166:333-340, 1988.
16. Elster AD, Sobol WT, Hinson WH: Pseudolayering of Gd-DTPA in the urinary bladder, Radiology 174:379-381, 1990.
17. Fletcher BD, Hanna SL, Kun LE: Changes in MR signal intensity and contrast enhancement of therapeutically irradiated soft tissue, Magn Reson Imaging 8:771-777, 1990.
18. Gomberg JS, Friedman AC, Radecki PD et al: MRI differentiation of recurrent colorectal carcinoma from postoperative fibrosis, Gastrointest Radiol 11:361-363, 1986.
19. Haggar AM, Alpern MB, Froelich JW: MR identification of seminal vesicles simulating a presacral mass after abdominal perineal resection, Am J Roentgenol 151:519-520, 1988.
20. Hoeffner EG, Crowley MG, Soulen RL: MR imaging appearance of intraperitoneal gelatin sponge in mice, J Magn Reson Imaging 2:63-67, 1992.
21. Hoeffner EG, Soulen RL, Christensen CW: Gelatin sponge mimicking a pelvic neoplasm on MR imaging, Am J Roentgenol 157:1227-1228, 1991.
22. Hricak H: Postoperative and postradiation changes in the pelvis, Magn Reson Q 6:276-297, 1990.
23. Husband JES, Olliff JFC, Williams MP et al: Bladder cancer: staging with CT and MR imaging, Radiology 173:435-440, 1989.
24. Luburich P, Nicolau C, Ayuso MC et al: Pelvic Castleman disease: CT and MR appearance, J Comput Assist Tomogr 16:657-659, 1992.
25. Marti-Bonmati L, Vilar J, Paniagua JC et al: High density barium sulphate as an MRI oral contrast, Magn Reson Imaging 9:259-261, 1991.
26. Mirowitz SA: Contrast enhancement of the gastrointestinal tract on MR images using intravenous gadolinium-DTPA, Abdom Imaging 18:215-219, 1993.
27. Mitchell DG, Vinitski S, Rifkin MD et al: Sampling bandwidth and fat suppression: effects on long TR/TE MR imaging of the abdomen and pelvis at 1.5 T, Am J Roentgenol 153:419-425, 1989.
28. Mulkern RV, Wong STS, Winalski C et al: Contrast manipulation and artifact assessment of 2D and 3D RARE sequences, Magn Reson Imaging 8:557-566, 1990.
29. Narumi Y, Kadota T, Inoue E et al: Bladder tumors: staging with gadolinium-enhanced oblique MR imaging, Radiology 187:145-150, 1993.
30. Nghiem HV, Herfkens RJ, Francis IR et al: The pelvis: T2-weighted fast spin-echo MR imaging, Radiology 185:213-217, 1992.
31. Panaccione JL, Ros PR, Torres GM et al: Rectal barium in pelvic MR imaging: initial results, J Magn Reson Imaging 1:605-607, 1991.

32. Rafto SE, Amendola MA, Gefter WB: MR imaging of recurrent colorectal carcinoma versus fibrosis, J Comput Assist Tomogr 12:521-523, 1988.

33. Secaf E, Nuruddin RN, Hricak H et al: MR imaging of the seminal vesicles, Am J Roentgenol 156:989-994, 1991.

34. Semelka RC, Shoenut JP, Silverman R et al: Bowel disease: prospective comparison of CT and 1.5- T pre- and postcontrast MR imaging with T1-weighted fat-suppressed and breath-hold FLASH sequences, J Magn Reson Imaging 1:625-632, 1991.

35. Smith RC, Reinhold C, Lange RC et al: Fast spin-echo MR imaging of the female pelvis. Part I. Use of a whole-volume coil, Radiology 184:665-669, 1992.

36. Sugimura K, Carrington BM, Quivey JM et al: Postirradiation changes in the pelvis: assessment with MR imaging, Radiology 175:805-813, 1990.

37. Tanimoto A, Yuasa Y, Imai Y et al: Bladder tumor staging: comparison of conventional and gadolinium-enhanced dynamic MR imaging and CT, Radiology 185:741-747, 1992.

38. Wetzel LH, Levine E: MR imaging of sacral and presacral lesions, Am J Roentgenol 154:771-775, 1990.

39. Winkler ML, Hricak H: Pelvis imaging with MR: technique for improvement, Radiology 158:848-849, 1986.

40. Yoon IJ, Kim KH, Lee BH: Leiomyoma of the urinary bladder: MR findings (letter), Am J Roentgenol 161:449-450, 1993.

9

Male Pelvis

PROSTATE GLAND
Anatomic Variations

The prostate can display a number of variations in its lobar anatomy. These include absence of the "median lobe" and persistent independence of the "lateral lobes."[2] The ejaculatory ducts have variable branching patterns, and the prostatic utricle can be either absent or enlarged.[2]

A network of fine linear structures can be seen in the peripheral zone of the prostate, particularly on endorectal coil images (Fig. 9-1). These represent ejaculatory ducts, rather than scarring or other abnormalities. The periprostatic venous plexus, which surrounds the prostatic capsule, routinely demonstrates increased signal intensity on T2-weighted images, rather than the flow void observed in most vessels.[19] This is due to very slow flow, which leads to second echo rephasing.[20]

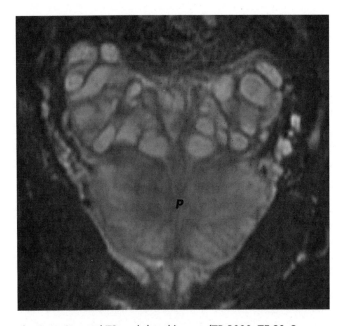

Fig. 9-1. Coronal T2-weighted image (TR 3000, TE 80, 2 Nex) acquired using endorectal coil demonstrates a network of fine linear hypointense structures radiating throughout the otherwise hyperintense peripheral zone of the prostate (*P*), representing ejaculatory ducts. The characteristic architecture of the seminal vesicles is also shown.

Prostatic Cysts

Prostatic cysts may be encountered as incidental findings in asymptomatic individuals. Mullerian duct or utricle cysts are midline lesions that have high signal intensity on T2-weighted and also frequently on T1-weighted images[30,32,34,39] (Fig. 9-2). These cysts are distinguished from Wolffian duct cysts, which have a more irregular contour and are not located along the midline of the gland.[30] These benign cystic lesions can simulate mucinous forms of prostate carcinoma or prostate abscess.

Zonal Anatomy

The anatomically distinct central and transitional zones of the prostate cannot be distinguished from one another on MR images. These zones are represented as a relatively large region of intermediate to low signal intensity (on T2-weighted images) and are collectively referred to as the central gland. The transitional zone is the predominant site for development of benign prostatic

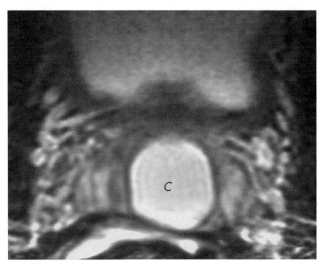

Fig. 9-2. Transaxial T2-weighted endorectal coil image (TR 3000, TE 80, 2 Nex) demonstrates a large cyst (*C*) arising from the midline of the prostate gland.

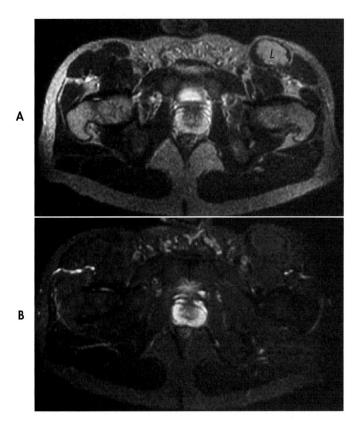

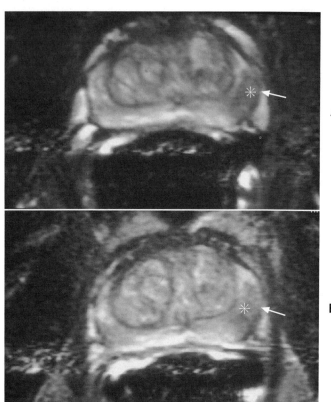

Fig. 9-3. Transaxial T2-weighted images (TR 2500, TE 80, 2 Nex) acquired without **(A)** and with **(B)** fat suppression. The fat suppressed image demonstrates improved depiction of prostatic zonal anatomy and prostatic margins. Note relative increased signal intensity of vascular structures on fat suppressed image. There is a lipoma (L) within the right rectus femoris muscle, which is not apparent with fat suppression.

Fig. 9-4. Corresponding transaxial T2-weighted endorectal coil images obtained with **(A)** and without **(B)** fat saturation. Note that the focus of hypointensity within the left peripheral zone (asterisk), caused by prostate cancer, is more conspicuous, and motion artifacts are somewhat less conspicuous on the fat saturated image. Although the prostate capsule (arrow) appears to be intact on both of these images, there was pathologic evidence of microscopic transcapsular tumor penetration.

hyperplasia. Surrounding the central gland is the comparatively hyperintense peripheral zone, from which most prostate cancers arise. Distinction between the central gland and peripheral zone on the basis of signal intensity differences is evident on T2-weighted images, but not on T1-weighted images. Fat suppression techniques may allow for further improvement in depiction of prostatic zonal anatomy on T2-weighted images[15,36] (Figs. 9-3, A and B). This is due to improvement in the dynamic range for tissue contrast display, as well as to reduction of motion and chemical shift misregistration artifacts (Figs. 9-4, A and B).

Physiologic Changes

The prostate gland undergoes many alterations as a result of normal aging. Enlargement of the gland routinely occurs with aging, due to benign prostatic hyperplasia. Signal intensity differences between the central gland and peripheral zone on T2-weighted images generally increase in prominence with aging, and the ante-

rior fibromuscular stroma and periprostatic venous plexus become less prominent.[1] Prostatic glandular secretions can calcify, creating low signal intensity foci, particularly near the junction of the central gland and peripheral zone.

Contrast Enhancement Patterns

The central gland often appears markedly heterogeneous after intravenous contrast material administration[14] (Figs. 9-5, A and B). This appearance is attributable to benign prostatic hyperplasia. Adenomatous foci enhance more intensely than the remainder of the central gland, whereas cystic foci may undergo little or no enhancement. This pattern differs from that of the peripheral zone, which undergoes more homogeneous and less intense enhancement.[14] These regional differences in contrast enhancement improve the depiction of prostatic zonal anatomy on contrast enhanced T1-weighted im-

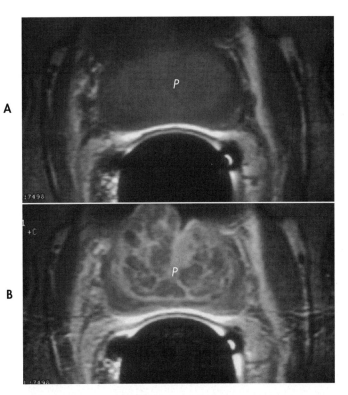

A

B

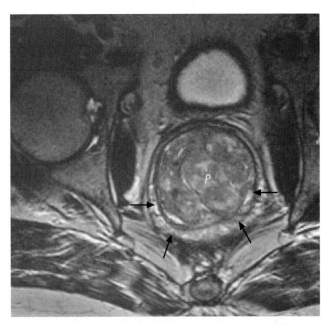

Fig. 9-6. Massive hypertrophy of the central gland of the prostate *(P)* is present with markedly heterogeneous signal intensity caused by benign hyperplasia on transaxial fast spin echo T2-weighted image (TR 7000, effective TE 108, 4 Nex, 16 echo train). The compressed peripheral zone *(arrows)* is similar in appearance to the periprostatic venous plexus. However, the plexus does not extend directly posterior to the prostate gland, allowing for distinction of these structures.

Fig. 9-5. Corresponding T1-weighted endorectal coil images obtained before **(A)** and after **(B)** intravenous gadopentetate dimeglumine administration. There is marked heterogeneous enhancement throughout the central prostate gland *(P)* in this patient with benign prostatic hyperplasia. Note improved differentiation between the central gland and peripheral zone of the prostate on the enhanced as compared with unenhanced image.

ages, compared with similar unenhanced images (Fig. 9-5). However, prostatic zonal anatomy generally is best defined on T2-weighted images. The periprostatic venous plexus enhances prominently, again reflective of very slow flow rates.[14,20]

Prostate Capsule

The prostate capsule is very thin and not reliably visualized on body coil images.[19] This is primarily due to limited spatial resolution, which occurs when relatively large fields-of-view, slice thickness, and interslice gaps are used. Chemical shift misregistration artifact occurs along the frequency encoded direction of the image (usually right-left for transaxial pelvic images), creating artifactually increased signal intensity along one lateral margin of the prostate and corresponding decreased signal intensity on the contralateral side. This can further obscure visualization of the prostate capsule.

The prostate capsule is much better discerned when images are acquired using endorectal surface coils. These

coils provide improved signal-to-noise ratio, which allows images to be acquired using significantly smaller voxel sizes. Small voxel sizes improve spatial resolution and also reduce the prominence of chemical shift misregistration effects.

The prostate capsule is also better depicted on T1-weighted images following contrast material administration.[14] This is because the nonenhancing capsule is interposed between prostatic tissue and the periprostatic venous plexus, both of which undergo prominent enhancement.[14] However, the capsule is usually best visualized on T2-weighted images. We have not found fat suppression to be advantageous for visualizing the prostate capsule or other anatomic features of the prostate.[16]

Benign Prostatic Hyperplasia

Benign prostatic hyperplasia affects most elderly males. While this condition is highly prevalent, its prominence and clinical impact vary substantially among individuals. Benign prostatic hyperplasia results in changes in morphology and signal intensity throughout the central prostate gland. In addition to enlargement and nodularity of the central gland, foci of relative increased and decreased signal intensity on T2-weighted images are observed[4,26] (Figs. 9-6 and 9-7, *A* and *B*). These findings

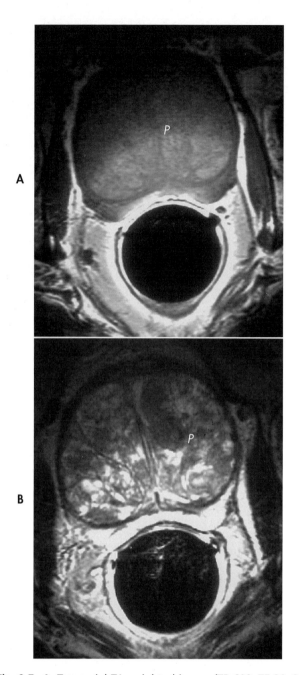

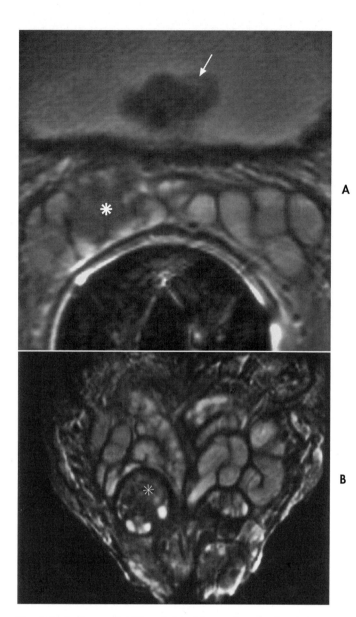

Fig. 9-7. A, Transaxial T1-weighted image (TR 600, TE 20, 2 Nex) acquired using endorectal coil demonstrates massive prostatic enlargement *(P).* There is reduced signal intensity throughout the anterior half of the prostate because of its distance from the coil. **B,** Improved signal-to-noise ratio on T2-weighted fast spin echo image (TR 4500, effective TE 114, 4 Nex, 16 echo train) results in somewhat better visualization of this region and demonstrates marked heterogeneous signal intensity throughout the central gland because of benign prostatic hyperplasia.

Fig. 9-8. A, Transaxial T2-weighted fast spin echo image (TR 4500, effective TE 114, 4 Nex, 16 echo train) through the seminal vesicles demonstrates apparent tumor replacement within the right seminal vesicle *(asterisk).* This finding is due to partial volume averaging of the seminal vesicle with a large prostatic BPH nodule, as depicted on the corresponding coronal T2-weighted image **(B).** Note hypointense periphery surrounding BPH nodules in addition to diffuse heterogeneous signal intensity throughout the central gland. Fig. 9-8**A** also demonstrates volume averaging with a prominent "median lobe" of prostate, simulating bladder invasion *(arrow).* Trabeculation and thickening of the bladder wall are due to chronic bladder outlet obstruction.

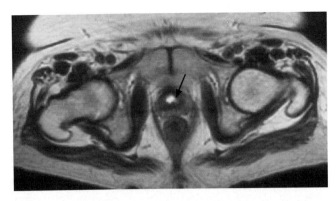

Fig. 9-9. Transaxial T2-weighted fast spin echo image (TR 4000, effective TE 117, 4 Nex, 16 echo train) demonstrates focus of increased signal intensity within the prostate *(arrow),* representing pooled urine in a transurethral resection defect. This should not be confused for a midline prostate cyst.

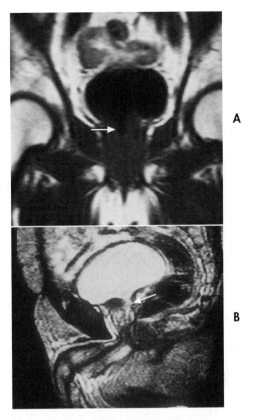

Fig. 9-10. Coronal T1-weighted **(A)** and sagittal T2-weighted **(B)** images demonstrate pooling of urine within the prostatic urethra *(arrow)* in a patient who has undergone previous transurethral prostatic resection.

represent cystic adenomatous and stromal forms of hyperplasia, respectively. Foci of relative increased intensity on T1-weighted images can be observed, caused by proteinaceous and/or hemorrhagic cystic contents. Although multiple small nodules are most frequent, large dominant nodules can also be observed. The appearance of paired lateral lobes flanking the prostatic urethra is frequent. Benign prostatic hyperplasia nodules are frequently surrounded by a low signal intensity pseudocapsule, which can assist in their recognition (Figs. 9-8, *A* and *B*). This contrasts with internal septations, which do not form complete rings and can be seen with prostate cancer.[25] Following transurethral resection of benign prostatic hyperplasia, a focus of increased intensity representing pooled urine is observed in the region of the prostatic urethra (Figs. 9-9 and 9-10, *A* and *B*). Hypertrophy of the peripheral zone of the prostate can occasionally occur following transurethral resection of prostatic tissue (Fig. 9-11).

Detection and Characterization of Prostatic Lesions
Central gland cancers

Benign prostatic hyperplasia and prostatic carcinoma cannot be distinguished on the basis of their signal intensity characteristics.[8,13] Rather, the location of nodular signal abnormalities within the prostate gland is critical for their characterization. Although prostate cancer usually arises in the peripheral zone, it has its origin in the central gland in approximately 15% of patients. Detection of prostate cancer within the central gland is difficult for two reasons. First, the signal intensity of prostate cancer and that of the central gland are similar, hindering lesion visualization.[13] Second, morphologic and signal alterations within the central gland resulting from benign prostatic hyperplasia can obscure visualiza-

---

PITFALLS IN DETECTION OF PROSTATE CANCER

- Recent needle biopsy (hemorrhage)
- Prostatitis/prostate abscess
- Benign prostatic hyperplasia
- Prostatic cyst
- Mucinous carcinoma, cystic ectasia
- Prostatic calculi
- Altered prostate signal intensity due to aging, radiation, hormone therapy
- Central gland tumors
- Apical tumors
- Diffuse tumor infiltration
- Granulomatous disease

---

tion of coincident carcinoma. For both of these reasons, central gland cancers are rarely detected on magnetic resonance (MR) images. However, if a homogeneous region of relative decreased signal intensity is observed centrally, prostate cancer should be considered.[35]

When the central gland is enlarged as a result of severe hyperplasia, the peripheral zone can become com-

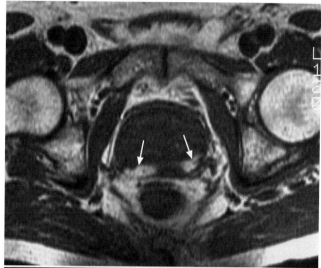

Fig. 9-11. Transaxial T2-weighted image (TR 3000, TE 80, 2 Nex) acquired using endorectal coil in patient who underwent previous transurethral prostate resection. There is complete absence of the central prostate gland because of previous surgery, and significant hypertrophy of the peripheral zone has occurred. A large focus of relative decreased signal intensity within the peripheral zone *(asterisk)* represents a site of prostate cancer.

pressed.[29] This can inhibit visualization of prostatic zonal anatomy and of prostate cancer.

Prostate apex

The prostatic apex is another location where detection of prostate cancers can be difficult.[5,25] This is often due to failure to adequately inspect this region of the gland. However, the apex can suffer from reduced signal-to-noise ratio when an endorectal coil system is used, as a result of rapid attenuation of the signal with increasing distance from the coil[25] (Fig. 9-11). The combined use of an endorectal and anterior surface coil or an external multicoil array improves signal intensity uniformity throughout the image.[11] There are also software algorithms that normalize the signal intensity profile across the field-of-view for surface coil images.[17]

Post-biopsy hemorrhage

MR examinations of the prostate are usually performed after a diagnosis of prostate cancer has been established by needle biopsy. Blood breakdown products resulting from the previous biopsy are frequently observed on MR images. Subacute hemorrhagic products (i.e., methemoglobin) appear as foci of increased signal intensity on T1-weighted images, with decreased or increased signal intensity on T2-weighted images (Figs. 9-12, A and B). Biopsy related hemorrhage can obscure visualization of underlying prostate carcinoma.[3,28,29] Therefore, postbiopsy MR images are not reliable for detection of carcinoma but are performed for purposes of

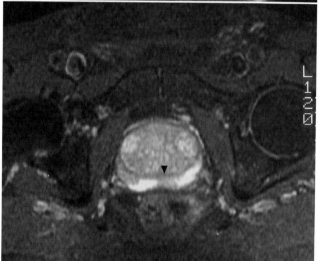

Fig. 9-12. Transaxial T1-weighted **(A)** and T2-weighted **(B)** images in patient with prostate cancer who underwent recent prostatic needle biopsy. The T1-weighted image demonstrates foci of relative increased signal intensity *(arrows)* within the peripheral zone, caused by subacute blood products related to the recent biopsy. The corresponding T2-weighted image demonstrates these areas to be hyperintense, with a focus of relative hypointensity to the left of midline *(arrowhead)* representing the patient's prostate cancer. Note that on the T1-weighted image blood products are not identified within the tumor site.

staging. It has been observed that postbiopsy hemorrhage tends to localize in prostatic tissue that does not contain tumor, rather than within the tumor itself[25] (Figs. 9-12, A and B). When inversion recovery (i.e., STIR) imaging is used, the signal intensity of blood products as well as fat may be nulled. This can create a discrete focus of marked decreased signal intensity within the prostate gland, which simulates the appearance of cancer.[25]

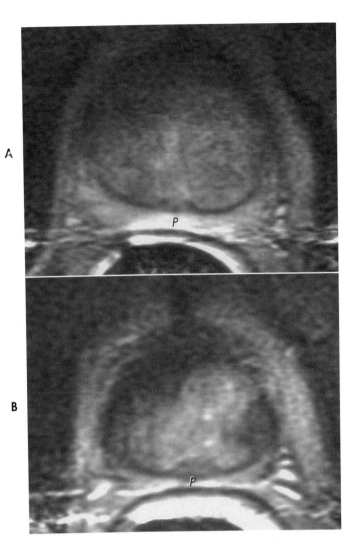

Fig. 9-13. Transaxial T2-weighted endorectal coil images (TR 3000, TE 80, 2 Nex) of the prostate obtained before **(A)** and after **(B)** administration of hormonal therapy for prostate cancer. Following therapy the prostate is of reduced size and signal intensity compared with the baseline image. The peripheral zone (*P*) demonstrates marked volume loss. Note artifacts related to motion of the local coil within the rectum.

Diffuse tumor infiltration

When prostate cancer diffusely infiltrates the gland, it is difficult to detect.[4] Whereas diffuse reduction in signal intensity throughout the peripheral zone on T2-weighted images may raise suspicion of tumor involvement, such findings can also be caused by hormonal or radiation therapy, fibrosis, or unknown reasons.[19] When the peripheral zone is diffusely hypointense, it can blend together with the central gland. In this situation, the high signal intensity periprostatic venous plexus can appear to represent the peripheral zone (see Fig. 9-6). However,

the periprostatic plexus does not extend around the posterior aspect of the gland, unlike the peripheral zone.

Radiation changes

In patients treated with radiation therapy, the peripheral zone can appear isointense with surrounding fat on T2-weighted images.[6] In some patients, the peripheral zone can become hypointense relative to the central gland, creating a reversal of the normal zonal signal intensity pattern.[6] These findings are due to atrophy of glandular tissue with conversion to fibrosis and are potentiated by concomitant administration of hormonal therapy or by orchiectomy[6] (Figs. 9-13, *A* and *B*).

Signal intensity characteristics

Although prostate cancer typically appears as a low signal intensity lesion, mucinous forms can appear markedly hyperintense on T2-weighted images.[4,10,18,29] These findings can cause prostate cancer to simulate a cyst, abscess, or cystic benign prostatic hyperplasia.[18] The hyperintensity of mucinous carcinoma may be indistinguishable from surrounding peripheral zone tissue or periprostatic venous plexus, causing the cancer to be overlooked.[18] Another cause for focal increased signal intensity within the central gland or peripheral zone on T2-weighted images is cystic atrophy, which can be associated with foci of prostatic cancer.[13] Cystic ectasia can result in increased signal intensity within the peripheral zone on T2-weighted images. This can cause the normal peripheral zone tissue to appear abnormally hypointense, simulating cancer.[35]

Tumor volume

Previous episodes of prostatitis can result in fibrosis within the peripheral zone. The resultant decreased signal intensity can be indistinguishable from prostate cancer.[13,22] This situation can also result from atrophy within the peripheral zone, which results in decreased glandular tissue and therefore decreased signal intensity.[35]

Although benign prostatic hyperplasia usually arises in the central gland, on occasion it can arise in the peripheral zone, where it simulates carcinoma. This may occur in the form of fibrous, muscular, or fibromuscular hyperplasia and atypical adenomatous hyperplasia.[25] Granulomatous disease is another rare cause for focal decreased signal intensity within the peripheral zone that can simulate cancer.[25] Biopsy related hemorrhage can obscure visualization of prostate cancer, as discussed previously. In addition, blood breakdown products that appear hypointense on T2-weighted images (i.e., deoxyhemoglobin, intracellular methemoglobin, hemosiderin) can simulate tumor.

The volume of a prostatic tumor is frequently difficult to determine on MR images, particularly those ac-

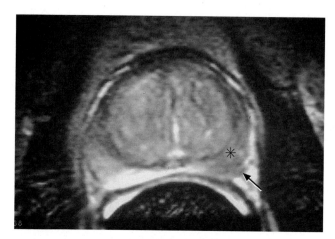

Fig. 9-14. Transaxial T2-weighted endorectal coil image demonstrates a focus of confluent hypointensity within the peripheral zone of the prostate on the left *(asterisk),* representing a site of prostatic carcinoma. Note that there is some apparent irregularity of the prostate capsule in the region of the neurovascular bundle adjacent to the tumor *(arrow),* suggestive of transcapsular tumor penetration. However, at prostatectomy, the prostate capsule was found to be intact.

quired using the body coil.[4,23] A tumor can infiltrate between prostatic glands, rather than replacing them, causing tumor volume to be underestimated.[10] Biopsy related hemorrhage can also contribute to inaccuracy in estimating tumor volume and result in either overestimation or underestimation of actual volume.[3,28,29,35]

Staging of Prostate Cancer

The determination of prostate cancer extent guides therapy options. When a tumor is confined to the prostate gland (stages A, B), radical prostatectomy is believed to offer the best opportunity for cure. However, patients with a tumor spread beyond the prostate capsule (stage C) or with distant metastases (stage D) are usually not considered surgical candidates and are offered hormonal and/or radiation therapy instead. Entities that restrict visualization of the prostate capsule were discussed previously; these also limit visualization of extracapsular tumor spread. Identification of subtle capsular tumor penetration is limited on body coil images. Microscopic tumor invasion of the prostate capsule is not reliably detected even on high-resolution endorectal coil images[27,29,38] (see Fig. 9-4). Initial evaluation of the use of gadopentetate dimeglumine for local prostate cancer staging indicates that this agent does not contribute significantly to the data available on unenhanced T2-weighted endorectal coil images.[15]

Bulging or distortion of the prostate capsule can indicate capsular tumor invasion or penetration, even when

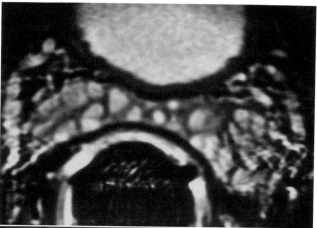

A

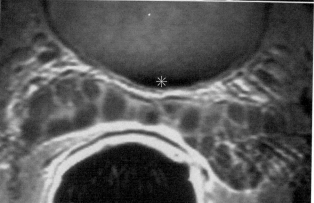

B

Fig. 9-15. A, Transaxial T2-weighted image (TR 3000, TE 80, 2 Nex) demonstrates normal appearance of seminal vesicles. There is marked hyperintensity of internal contents, with a honeycomb-like architecture. **B,** Gadopentetate enhanced T1-weighted image (TR 600, TE 20, 2 Nex) demonstrates similar architectural features, though the relative signal intensity of tubular walls versus intraluminal contents is reversed as compared with the T2-weighted image. Note signal intensity loss related to concentrated gadopentetate in the dependent aspect of the urinary bladder *(asterisk).*

LIMITATIONS IN LOCAL STAGING OF PROSTATE CANCER

- Microscopic disease
- Recent needle biopsy
- Motion artifacts
- Partial volume averaging
- Benign prostatic hyperplasia
- Limited signal-to-noise ratio
- Limited spatial resolution

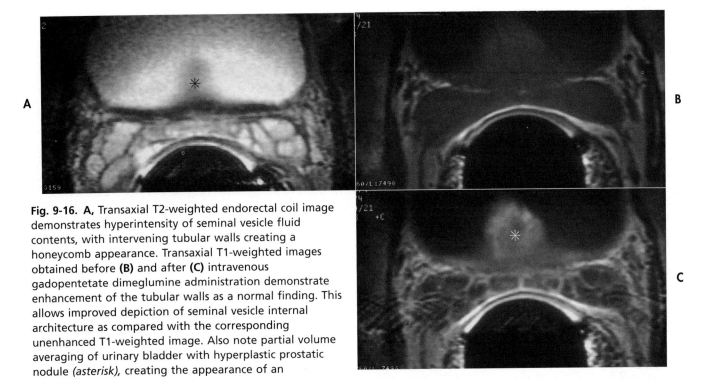

Fig. 9-16. A, Transaxial T2-weighted endorectal coil image demonstrates hyperintensity of seminal vesicle fluid contents, with intervening tubular walls creating a honeycomb appearance. Transaxial T1-weighted images obtained before **(B)** and after **(C)** intravenous gadopentetate dimeglumine administration demonstrate enhancement of the tubular walls as a normal finding. This allows improved depiction of seminal vesicle internal architecture as compared with the corresponding unenhanced T1-weighted image. Also note partial volume averaging of urinary bladder with hyperplastic prostatic nodule *(asterisk),* creating the appearance of an intraluminal bladder lesion.

abnormal pericapsular soft tissue is not visualized.[31] Irregular bulging of the capsule is highly indicative of stage C disease, although smooth bulging does not necessarily indicate tumor invasion. Focal alteration in prostatic contour can also occur in patients with benign prostatic hyperplasia.

Recent prostatic needle biopsy can lead to alterations in the periprostatic fat, which simulate transcapsular tumor penetration[29] (Fig. 9-14). Apparent abnormality in the periprostatic soft tissues can also result from artifacts caused by vascular pulsation, bowel peristalsis, or gross patient motion.[38] Rectal motion artifacts are more severe when an endorectal coil is used (Fig. 9-13). These artifacts are reduced with appropriate inflation of the endorectal balloon and with use of intramuscular glucagon. Pulsation artifacts related to the obturator vessels are also accentuated on endorectal coil images. The impact of motion artifacts can be reduced with the use of gradient reorientation, so that the phase encoded direction is aligned along the right/left axis of the body. In addition, fat suppression techniques can reduce the signal intensity of some motion artifacts.[25]

Overstaging can also occur when an enlarged "median prostate lobe" protrudes into the bladder base, simulating tumor invasion (see Fig. 9-8). Partial volume effects can result in reduced signal intensity of the periprostatic venous plexus, which simulates tumor invasion.

SEMINAL VESICLES
Signal Intensity Characteristics

The normal seminal vesicles appear markedly intense on T2-weighted images because of their fluid contents. Hyperintensity of the seminal vesicles is further accentuated on fat suppressed T2-weighted images. On T1-weighted images the seminal vesicles usually appear slightly hyperintense relative to other fluids, such as urine. This is due to their relatively proteinaceous contents, which leads to shortening of T1 relaxation. The seminal vesicles have a distinct honeycomb internal architecture, with a series of fluid-containing tubules with surrounding convoluted walls (Figs. 9-15, *A* and *B* and 9-16, *A-C*).

Seminal Vesicle Size

While the seminal vesicles are usually symmetric in size, asymmetry can occur as a normal variant (Figs. 9-17, *A* and *B* and 9-18), and agenesis of a seminal vesicle may rarely occur.[2] When the seminal vesicle is absent, the surrounding high signal intensity venous plexus can simulate the seminal vesicle.[33] The seminal vesicles usually have a "bow-tie" configuration, though their morphology varies somewhat.

The seminal vesicles can be markedly prominent in some asymptomatic individuals. Observation of normal internal architecture and signal features allows prominent

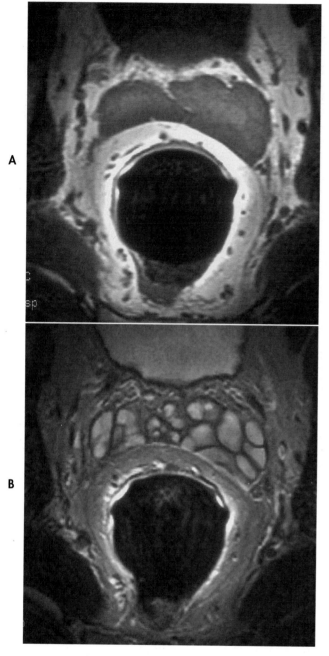

A

B

Fig. 9-17. A, Transaxial T1-weighted endorectal coil image (TR 600, TE 20, 2 Nex) in patient with prostate cancer. There is asymmetric enlargement of the left seminal vesicle. While this finding raises suspicion of possible tumor involvement, the corresponding fast spin echo T2-weighted image **(B)** (TR 4500, effective TE 114, 4 Nex, 16 echo time) confirms that no tumor is present.

or asymmetric seminal vesicles to be distinguished from those that are pathologic. Enlargement of the seminal vesicles can also be caused by cystic dilatation of the seminal vesicle tubules.[12] Discrete cysts can arise within the seminal vesicles on a congenital basis.[7] Seminal

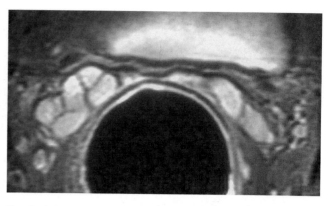

Fig. 9-18. Transaxial T2-weighted image (TR 3000, TE 80, 2 Nex) acquired using endorectal coil demonstrates asymmetry of the seminal vesicles, with the right seminal vesicle considerably larger than the left.

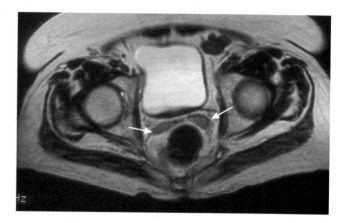

Fig. 9-19. Transaxial T2-weighted fast spin echo image (TR 4000, effective TE 117, 4 Nex, 16 echo train) demonstrates uniform reduced signal intensity throughout both seminal vesicles *(arrows)* in an elderly male.

vesicle dilatation can also result from intrinsic or extrinsic obstruction of the ejaculatory duct.[33]

Seminal Vesicle Position

The position of the seminal vesicles may be altered following pelvic surgery. In patients who have undergone abdominoperineal resection, the seminal vesicles may extend into the presacral space, where they can simulate a mass.[9,33] (See Fig. 8-13.) The distinct architecture and signal characteristics of the seminal vesicles should, however, allow for their recognition on T2-weighted MR images.

Signal Intensity Alterations

The appearance of the seminal vesicles changes as a function of patient age.[33] In prepubertal and elderly males, the seminal vesicles are smaller and of reduced

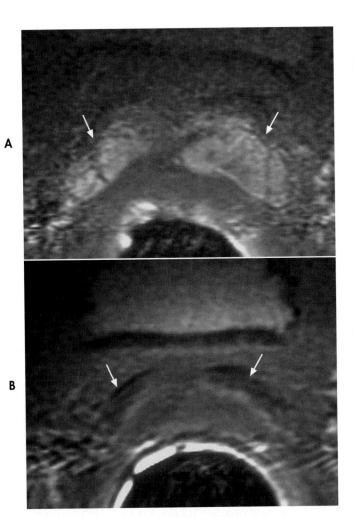

A

B

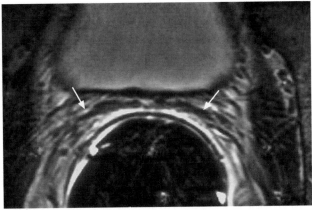

Fig. 9-21. Transaxial fast spin echo T2-weighted endorectal coil image (TR 4500, effective TE 114, 4 Nex, 16 echo train) demonstrates atrophy of the seminal vesicles *(arrows)* with related marked decreased signal intensity in patient being treated with hormonal therapy for prostate carcinoma.

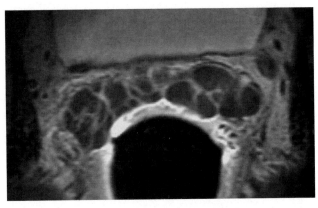

Fig. 9-20. Transaxial T2-weighted images (TR 3000, TE 80, 2 Nex) of the seminal vesicles *(arrows)* obtained before **(A)** and after **(B)** administration of hormonal therapy for prostate cancer. The seminal vesicles are of normal size and signal intensity on the baseline image. However, following hormonal therapy initiation, they demonstrate marked decrease in size and are uniformly hypointense.

Fig. 9-22. Gadopentetate enhanced T1-weighted endorectal coil image (TR 600, TE 20, 2 Nex). Prominent enhancement of the walls of the seminal vesicle tubules is displayed, resulting in a honeycomb pattern similar to that observed on T2-weighted images.

signal intensity on T2-weighted images as compared with those of reproductive age men[19,33] (Fig. 9-19). Similar alterations are also observed in patients who have received pelvic irradiation, castration, or estrogen as treatment for prostate cancer[6,33] (Figs. 9-20, *A* and *B* and 9-21). These findings reflect atrophy of seminal vesicle tubules, with replacement by fibrosis.

In these situations, the reduced signal intensity of the seminal vesicles can simulate tumor invasion, particularly in patients with known prostate cancer. However, the presence of bilaterally symmetric signal alterations, concomitant decrease in seminal vesicle size, and correlation with patient age and medical history should allow false-positive diagnoses to be avoided.

Detection and Characterization of Lesions

The most frequent indication for evaluating the seminal vesicles with MR is to evaluate for possible tumor invasion in patients with prostate carcinoma. Seminal vesicle tumor invasion indicates stage C disease, which is associated with poorer prognosis and can restrict a patient from consideration as a candidate for surgical treatment. Seminal vesicle tumor invasion is usually depicted as foci of relative reduced signal intensity within the vesicle(s) on T2-weighted images. These findings indicate replacement of high signal intensity fluid by solid tumor tissue, which has shorter T2 relaxation.

Seminal vesicle tumor invasion is generally not apparent on T1-weighted images because of isointensity between vesicular fluid and tumor. Use of intravenous ga-

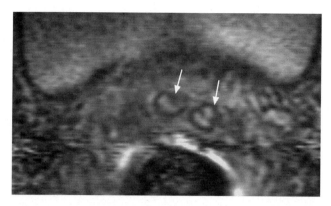

Fig. 9-23. Transaxial T2-weighted endorectal coil image (TR 3000, TE 80, 2 Nex) of the seminal vesicles. The ampullae of the vas deferens *(arrows)* are depicted as foci of hyperintensity with peripheral hypointense borders representing their muscular walls. Phase encoding artifact caused by motion of the coil within the rectum is also apparent.

dopentetate dimeglumine can improve visualization of seminal vesicle architecture and pathology on T1-weighted images.[15] This agent results in prominent enhancement of the tubular walls, whereas the intervening fluid contents do not enhance (Figs. 9-15, *A* and *B*, 9-16, *A-C*, and 9-22). When tumor invasion is present, contrast enhancement is observed within the tubule lumina. While early studies indicate that gadopentetate dimeglumine does not significantly improve detection of seminal vesicle tumor invasion compared with T2-weighted images, it can be useful as a problem-solving tool in problematic cases.[15] Microscopic tumor invasion of the seminal vesicles cannot be visualized using any available techniques, and it is a significant cause for understaging on MR examinations.[25]

Several entities can simulate invasion of the seminal vesicles by prostate carcinoma. Benign prostatic hyperplasia can result in marked enlargement and cephalad ex-

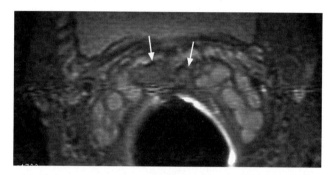

Fig. 9-24. Transaxial T2-weighted endorectal coil image (TR 3000, TE 80, 2 Nex) demonstrates symmetric foci of relative decreased signal intensity *(arrows)* involving proximal seminal vesicles, suggestive of tumor invasion. There was no seminal vesicle invasion at the time of prostatectomy. These findings represent the muscular walls of the ampullae of the vas deferens.

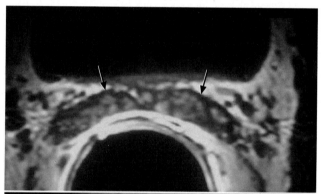

A

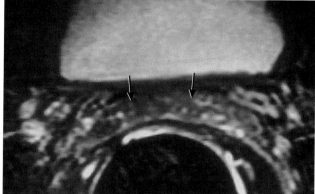

B

Fig. 9-26. Corresponding transaxial T1-weighted **(A)** and T2-weighted **(B)** endorectal coil images of the seminal vesicles in patient who underwent recent prostatic needle biopsy. There is relative increased signal intensity noted throughout the seminal vesicles on the T1-weighted image with corresponding areas of hypointensity on the T2-weighted image *(arrows)*. While the latter findings could result from tumor invasion, findings in this patient were attributable to blood products related to the recent biopsy.

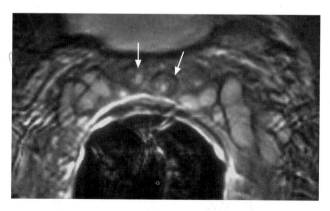

Fig. 9-25. Transaxial endorectal fast spin echo T2-weighted image (TR 4500, effective TE 114, 4 Nex, 16 echo train) demonstrates symmetric foci of decreased signal intensity *(arrows)* within the proximal seminal vesicles. These represent the muscular walls of the ampullae of the vas deferens.

tension of the central prostate gland. The central gland can then undergo partial volume averaging with the proximal seminal vesicles on transaxial images, resulting in apparent foci of decreased signal intensity suggesting tumor involvement[27] (Fig. 9-8). Coronal and/or sagittal images can help clarify the nature of these apparent abnormalities. Partial volume averaging of the seminal vesicles with adjacent bowel loops can also occur, with similar results.

The ampullae of the vas deferens, located within the proximal seminal vesicles, can appear hypointense on T2-weighted images because of their surrounding muscular fibers. This can simulate bilateral tumor invasion of the seminal vesicles (Figs. 9-23 to 9-25). The ampullae of the vas deferens can be recognized on the basis of their characteristic location, bilateral symmetry, and central increased signal intensity within the ampullary lumina, resulting in a target appearance.

The presence of epithelial hyperplasia within the seminal vesicles can result in hypointensity simulating tumor invasion. Calculi can form within the seminal

vesicles, which result in foci of decreased signal intensity potentially simulating tumor invasion.[25] Motion artifacts caused by bowel peristalsis, patient movement, or vascular pulsation can result in blurring and structured high and low signal intensity artifacts that can cause seminal vesicle tumor invasion to be simulated or obscured. Thickening of the walls of the seminal vesicle tubules can indicate early tumor invasion, even when tubular fluid contents are not replaced.[29]

Following prostate needle biopsy, secondary hemorrhage can simulate seminal vesicle tumor invasion[15,19,33] (Figs. 9-26, *A* and *B* and 9-27, *A* and *B*). Hemorrhagic products can occur within the seminal vesicles through two mechanisms. First, the seminal vesicles may be inadvertently encountered by the needle during biopsy, resulting in hemorrhage. Second, retrograde transport of hemorrhagic products from the site of prostatic biopsy to the seminal vesicles may occur via the ejaculatory ducts.[15] Hemorrhagic breakdown products can appear hyperintense on T1-weighted images (methemoglobin) and hypointense on T2-weighted images (deoxyhemoglobin, intracellular methemoglobin, or hemosiderin), with the latter findings simulating tumor invasion.

Distinction between seminal vesicle hemorrhage and tumor invasion rests on several observations. First, the distribution of hemorrhagic products frequently does not correspond to the expected location for prostatic tumor invasion. Prostate cancer tends to invade the seminal vesicles in a proximal to distal progression, except in patients with extensive direct transcapsular invasion. On the other hand, hemorrhagic products display random localization within the seminal vesicles and are frequently more prominent distally. Second, hemorrhagic breakdown products can appear hyperintense on T1-weighted images, which is unusual for tumor invasion. Furthermore, hemorrhagic products are usually more hypoin-

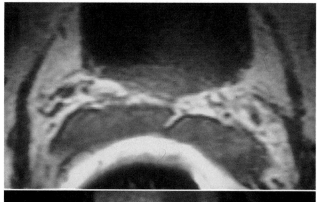

A

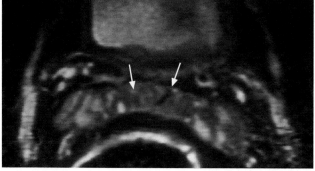

B

Fig. 9-27. Corresponding T1-weighted **(A)** and T2-weighted **(B)** endorectal coil images of the seminal vesicles in patient who underwent recent needle biopsy of the prostate. Foci of marked hypointensity *(arrows)* are noted within the seminal vesicles on the T2-weighted image, without correlate on the T1-weighted image. While these findings are suspicious for tumor involvement, they represent blood products within the seminal vesicles resulting from needle biopsy.

PITFALLS IN DETECTION OF SEMINAL VESICLE TUMOR INVASION

- Prominent/asymmetric seminal vesicles
- Seminal vesicle cyst
- Signal alterations related to age, irradiation, hormone therapy
- Microscopic tumor invasion
- Partial volume averaging
- Ampullae of vas deferens
- Epithelial hyperplasia
- Seminal vesicle calculi
- Motion artifacts
- Post-biopsy hemorrhage
- Other causes of seminal vesicle hemorrhage
- Amyloid deposits

tense on T2-weighted images than tumor tissue. Prostatic tumor invasion can occasionally precipitate seminal vesicle hemorrhage. Therefore, the presence of T1 and T2 shortening is not completely reliable in excluding tumor involvement. Other conditions that can result in seminal vesicle hemorrhage include seminal vesiculitis, genitourinary tract tumors, trauma, vascular malformations, anticoagulation, and hypertension. Third, in patients with biopsy-related seminal vesicle hemorrhage, hemorrhagic breakdown products are apparent within the prostate at the biopsy site(s). Fourth, the use of gadopentetate dimeglumine should result in intratubular enhancement in patients with seminal vesicle tumor invasion, though hemorrhagic products do not enhance. When these criteria do not allow for confident distinction of tumor invasion versus biopsy-related hemorrhage in a potential surgical candidate, the seminal vesicles can be biopsied under sonographic guidance or follow-up MR imaging can be performed.

Amyloid deposits can also occur within the seminal vesicles and simulate tumor invasion on MR images. Amyloid deposition can lead to diffuse decreased signal intensity throughout the seminal vesicles and usually occurs in a bilaterally symmetric fashion.[24] This is related to the aging process and does not indicate systemic amyloidosis.

SCROTUM/TESTES/PENIS

The penis is rarely bifid or duplicated.[2] One or both testes may be congenitally absent or can be present in the form of a small tissue remnant.[2] Polyorchidism is rarely observed and is characterized by supernumerary testes.[2] The testes are more frequently variable in their location rather than number. During their descent into the scrotal sac, they may become arrested in the abdominal cavity, inguinal canal, or perineum.[2] The penile corpora undergo prominent enhancement following intravenous contrast material administration.

Cysts of the tunica albuginea can demonstrate a complex architecture and can appear to represent an exophytic lesion arising from the testis.[21] Acquisition of images in multiple planes usually allows an extratesticular origin to be verified.

Ectasia of the seminiferous tubules of the testis can result in a masslike appearance in the region of the mediastinum testis.[37] This appears isointense with the testis on both T1- and T2-weighted images.

REFERENCES

1. Allen KS, Kressel HY, Arger PH et al: Age-related changes of the prostate: evaluation by MR imaging, Am J Roentgenol 152:77-81, 1989.
2. Bergman RA, Thompson SA, Afifi AK et al: Compendium of human anatomic variation: text, atlas, and world literature, Baltimore, 1988, Urban & Schwarzenberg.
3. Bezzi M, Kressel HY, Allen KS et al: Prostatic carcinoma: staging with MR imaging at 1.5 T, Radiology 169:339-346, 1988.
4. Carrol CL, Sommer FG, McNeal JE et al: The abnormal prostate: MR imaging at 1.5 T with histopathologic correlation, Radiology 163:521-525, 1987.
5. Carter HB, Brem RF, Tempany CM et al: Nonpalpable prostate cancer: detection with MR imaging, Radiology 178:523-525, 1991.
6. Chan TW, Kressel HY: Prostate and seminal vesicles after irradiation: MR appearance, J Magn Reson Imaging 1:503-511, 1991.
7. Gevenois PA, Van Sinoy ML, Sintzoff SA Jr et al: Cysts of the prostate and seminal vesicles: MR imaging findings in 11 cases, Am J Roentgenol 155:1021-1024, 1990.
8. Griebel J, Hess CF, Schmiedl U et al: MR characteristics of prostatic carcinoma and benign prostatic hyperplasia at 1.5 T, J Comput Assist Tomogr 12:988-994, 1988.
9. Haggar AM, Alpern MB, Froelich JW: MR identification of seminal vesicles simulating a presacral mass after abdominal perineal resection, Am J Roentgenol 151:519-520, 1988.
10. Kahn T, Burrig K, Schmitz-Drager B et al: Prostatic carcinoma and benign prostatic hyperplasia: MR imaging with histopathologic correlation, Radiology 173:847-851, 1989.
11. Kier R, Wain S, Troiano R: Fast spin-echo MR images of the pelvis obtained with a phased-array coil: value in localizing and staging prostatic carcinoma, Am J Roentgenol 161:601-606, 1993.
12. Littrup PJ, Lee F, McLeary RD et al: Transrectal US of the seminal vesicles and ejaculatory ducts: clinical correlation, Radiology 168:625-628, 1988.
13. Lovett K, Rifkin MD, McCue PA et al: MR imaging characteristics of noncancerous lesions of the prostate, J Magn Resonan Imaging 2:35-39, 1992.
14. Mirowitz SA, Brown JJ, Heiken JP: Evaluation of the prostate and prostatic carcinoma with gadolinium-enhanced endorectal coil MR imaging, Radiology 186:153-157, 1993.
15. Mirowitz SA: Seminal vesicles: biopsy-related hemorrhage simulating tumor invasion at endorectal MR imaging, Radiology 185:373-376, 1992.
16. Mirowitz SA, Heiken JP, Brown JJ: Endorectal MR imaging of the prostate: evaluation of fat saturation technique, Magn Resonan Imaging 12:743-747, 1994.
17. Narayana PA, Brey WW, Kulkarni MV et al: Compensation for surface coil sensitivity variation in magnetic resonance imaging, Magn Reson Imaging 6:271-274, 1988.
18. Outwater E, Schiebler ML, Tomaszewski JE et al: Mucinous carcinomas involving the prostate: atypical findings at MR imaging, J Magn Reson Imaging 2:597-600, 1992.
19. Phillips ME, Kressel HY, Spritzer CE et al: Normal prostate and adjacent structures: MR imaging at 1.5 T, Radiology 164:381-385, 1987.
20. Poon PY, Bronskill MJ, Poon CS et al: Identification of the periprostatic venous plexus by MR imaging, J Comput Assist Tomogr 15:265-268, 1991.
21. Poster RB, Spirt BA, Tamsen A et al: Complex tunica albuginea cyst simulating an intratesticular lesion, Urol Radiol 13:129-132, 1991.

22. Quint LE, Van Erp JS, Bland PH et al: Prostate cancer: correlation of MR images with tissue optical density at pathologic examination, Radiology 179:837-842, 1991.
23. Quint LE, Van Erp JS, Bland PH et al: Carcinoma of the prostate: MR images obtained with body coils do not accurately reflect tumor volume, Am J Roentgenol 156:511-516, 1991.
24. Ramchandani P, Schnall MD, LiVolsi VA et al: Senile amyloidosis of the seminal vesicles mimicking metastatic spread of prostatic carcinoma on MR images, Am J Roentgenol 161:99-100, 1993.
25. Schiebler ML, Schnall MD, Pollack HM et al: Current role of MR imaging in the staging of adenocarcinoma of the prostate, Radiology 189:339-352, 1993.
26. Schiebler ML, Tomaszewski JE, Bezzi M et al: Prostatic carcinoma and benign prostatic hyperplasia: correlation of high-resolution MR and histopathologic findings, Radiology 172:131-137, 1989.
27. Schiebler ML, Yankaskas BC, Tempany CE et al: MR imaging in adenocarcinoma of the prostate: interobserver variation and efficacy for determining stage C disease, Am J Roentgenol 158:559-562, 1992.
28. Schmidt JD: MR imaging in adenocarcinoma of the prostate in stage C disease (commentary), Am J Roentgenol 158:563, 1992.
29. Schnall MD, Imai Y, Tomaszewski J et al: Prostate cancer: local staging with endorectal surface coil MR imaging, Radiology 178:797-802, 1991.
30. Schnall MD, Pollack HM, Van Arsdalen K et al: The seminal tract in patients with ejaculatory dysfunction: MR imaging with an endorectal surface coil, Am J Roentgenol 159:337-341, 1992.
31. Schnall MD, Tomaszweski J, Pollack HM et al: The bulging prostate gland—a sign of capsular involvement, SMRM Book of Abstracts, 1991, p 279.
32. Schwartz JM, Bosniak MA, Hulnick DH et al: Computed tomography of midline cysts of the prostate, J Comput Assist Tomogr 12:215-218, 1988.
33. Secaf E, Nuruddin RN, Hricak H et al: MR imaging of the seminal vesicles, Am J Roentgenol 156:989-994, 1991.
34. Sener RN, Farmaka H, Ozaksoy D: Midline cyst of the prostate (letter), Am J Roentgenol 155:656-657, 1990.
35. Sommer FG, Nghiem HV, Herfkens R et al: Determining the volume of prostatic carcinoma: value of MR imaging with an external-array coil, Am J Roentgenol 161:81-86, 1993.
36. Tamler B, Sommer FG, Glover GH et al: Prostatic MR imaging performed with the three-point Dixon technique: work in progress, Radiology 179:43-47, 1991.
37. Tartar VM, Trambert MA, Balsara ZN et al: Tubular ectasia of the testicle: sonographic and MR imaging appearance, Am J Roentgenol 160:539-542, 1993.
38. Tempany CMC, Rahmouni AD, Epstein JI et al: Invasion of the neurovascular bundle by prostate cancer: evaluation with MR imaging, Radiology 181:107-112, 1991.
39. Thurnher S, Hricak H, Tanagho EA: Mullerian duct cyst: diagnosis with MR imaging, Radiology 168:25-28, 1988.

10

Female Pelvis

UTERUS
Anatomic Variations

The uterus varies considerably in its position and orientation. Variable degrees of anteversion or retroversion are commonly present and may be associated with anteflexion or retroflexion (Fig. 10-1). A tilted and/or flexed uterus can appear to be of increased prominence on transaxial images (Figs. 10-2, *A* and *B*). Oblique images may be acquired along the true long and short axes of the uterus to facilitate evaluation of such a uterus. Alternatively, routine orthogonal images may be retrospectively reformatted along the true axis of the uterus using a software interpolation algorithm (Figs. 10-3, *A* and *B*).[1] The orientation and position of the uterus can also be affected by adjacent structures. For example, the uterus may be displaced by a distended urinary bladder.

The normal uterus demonstrates narrowing at the site of the internal uterine os. Diverticula of the uterus rarely occurs.[9] Many anomalies that affect the uterus are related to alterations in mullerian duct development and/or fusion and are associated with infertility.[9] Magnetic resonance (MR) provides excellent depiction of such uterine

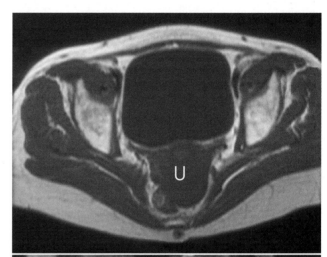

A

B

Fig. 10-2. A, Transaxial T1-weighted image (TR 400, TE 11, 4 Nex) demonstrates apparent prominence of the uterus (U) in 61-year-old female. This appearance is due to marked retroflexion of the uterine corpus, as verified on midsagittal fast spin echo T2-weighted image **(B)** (TR 4000, effective TE 120, 4 Nex, 8 echo train). Uterine zonal anatomy is poorly depicted in this postmenopausal female as compared with Fig. 10-1.

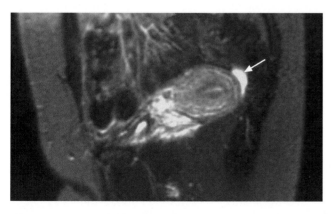

Fig. 10-1. Sagittal fast spin echo T2-weighted image (TR 5500, effective TE 100, 4 Nex, 16 echo train) demonstrates retroflexion of the uterus. A physiologic volume of fluid is present within the pelvic cul-de-sac *(arrow).*

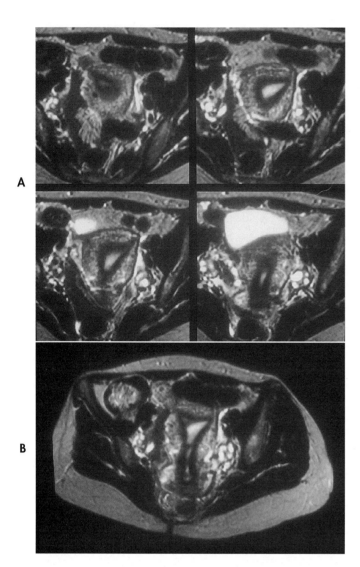

Fig. 10-3. A, An anteverted uterus is segmentally visualized over several adjacent fast spin echo T2-weighted images (TR 4500, effective TE 120, 16 echo train), making evaluation of the entire structure difficult. **B,** The reformatted image from the same data set demonstrates the entire uterus and cervix on a single image, allowing for improved evaluation.

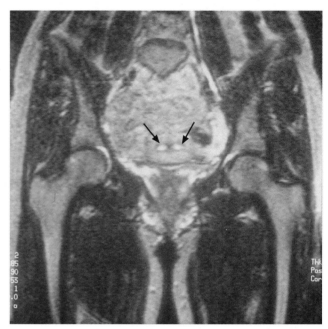

Fig. 10-4. Coronal T2-weighted image in patient with uterine didelphys demonstrates two adjacent uterine horns *(arrows)* separated by myometrium.

anomalies and often contributes information that is complementary to or exceeds what can be obtained with hysterosalpingography.[14,21,35,102] Mullerian duct anomalies include uterine agenesis or hypoplasia, caused by incomplete development of the mullerian ducts; unicornuate uterus, resulting from incomplete development of one mullerian duct; septate uterus, caused by failure of resorption of the septum separating the mullerian ducts; bicornuate uterus, a result of partial failure of mullerian duct fusion that may or may not extend to involve the cervix (bicollis and unicollis, respectively); and uterus didelphys, caused by nonfusion of the mullerian ducts,

with separated uterine horns, separate cervices, and septated proximal vagina (Fig. 10-4). Detailed descriptions of these anomalies are available in many references and therefore are not included here.

MR is particularly useful for providing information regarding the internal structure as well as external morphology of the uterus, as in patients with suspected uterine septae.[69] The ability of MR to distinguish fibrous from myometrial uterine septae is important for treatment planning. The septum of a septate uterus has relative low signal intensity, whereas intermediate signal intensity—equivalent to that of myometrium—is observed between the horns of a bicornuate uterus.[65] MR also allows for direct visualization of the uterine surface, which is continuous in patients with septate uterus, as compared with the focal fundal depression seen in patients with bicornuate uterus.[97] Slight indentation of the uterine fundus may be observed in patients with arcuate uterus.[64,69]

In patients with the Mayer-Rokitansky-Kuster-Hauser syndrome, the uterus is absent, though mullerian remnants may be visualized in its expected position.[22] The ovaries are present, though a rudimentary vagina and renal agenesis may be observed.

Although MR is very useful in documenting many anatomic causes for female infertility, it has some important limitations. For example, MR images provide very limited ability to determine patency of the fallopian tubes and inflammatory or other conditions that may affect these structures. Furthermore, MR is relatively insensitive for depiction of small implants of endometriosis, which may contribute to infertility.[21]

Considerable deformity of the uterus may be observed in patients who received in utero exposure to diethylstilbesterol. MR images may reveal a hypoplastic uterine cavity, possibly with a distinct T-shaped appearance, and focal constrictions can result from thickening of the junctional zone.[93] Furthermore, the fallopian tubes may be dilated or demonstrate a variety of abnormalities, and foci of high signal intensity within the vagina may indicate adenosis.

Zonal Anatomy

The zonal anatomy of the uterus is exquisitely depicted on MR images. T2-weighted images depict a high signal intensity central zone, representing the endometrium and any fluid that may be present within the endometrial cavity. Surrounding this is a curvilinear region of decreased signal intensity known as the junctional zone, which is then surrounded by intermediate signal intensity myometrium. A very thin hypointense zone may also be observed along the periphery of the uterus. Because of its shorter T1 relaxation behavior, slight relative hyperintensity of the junctional zone may be observed on T1-weighted images.[61] However, the zonal anatomy of the uterus is generally poorly depicted on T1- or proton density–weighted images because of isointensity of the various uterine zones on such images.

The nature of the junctional zone and the cause for its unique signal intensity on MR images have been debated in the literature. Whereas it was initially speculated that this represented either the basal layer of the endometrium or a unique layer separating the endometrium and myometrium, subsequent investigation has shown that the junctional zone actually represents the innermost layer of myometrium.[74] The basic distinction between the junctional zone and the "myometrium proper" relates to relative decreased water content within the junctional zone, accounting for its shorter T2 relaxation time.[61] Histologic studies indicate that the smooth muscle cells that compose the junctional zone are highly compact and that the junctional zone contains relatively sparse extracellular matrix as compared with the remainder of the myometrium.[11] The size and number of smooth muscle nuclei are also increased as compared with the remainder of the myometrium.[74] It is likely that all of these factors contribute to the unique appearance of the junctional zone on MR images.

Contrast enhanced MR images also depict regional differences related to uterine zonal anatomy. The zonal anatomy of the uterus is not visualized in many patients on T1-weighted spin echo images obtained following contrast material administration.[34] However, rapid gradient echo images acquired during or shortly after bolus injection of gadolinium chelate contrast material (i.e., dynamic contrast enhanced imaging) are able to capture transient differences in uterine enhancement. Initial images demonstrate mild enhancement in the region of the junctional zone, which is subsequently followed by enhancement of the remainder of the myometrium.[100] The myometrium usually enhances more rapidly than the endometrium; however, in some patients, equivalent early enhancement of endometrium and myometrium is seen, and occasionally endometrial enhancement is greater than that of the myometrium.[34]

Measurement of uterine zones on MR images may not correlate with measurements obtained using ultrasound. Decreased thickness of the endometrium and increased thickness of the junctional zone is often indicated based on MR versus ultrasound measurements, as a result of differences in the depiction of zonal boundaries on the two modalities.[66]

Physiologic Changes
Menstrual cycle

Changes in hormonal status have a profound effect on the appearance of the uterus on MR images. The uterus is relatively prominent in neonates, because of maternal estrogen stimulation, and it undergoes significant decrease in size during the first month of life.[60] Increase in size of the uterus occurs at puberty, when it attains a craniocaudal length up to 7 cm.

In females of reproductive age, the uterine corpus is approximately twice the size of the cervix. However, in premenarchal and postmenopausal females these structures are of similar size.[60] In reproductive age women taking oral contraceptives or gonadotropin-releasing hormone analogs, the corpus/cervix relationship is similar to that observed in postmenopausal women. Conversely, in postmenopausal women receiving estrogen, these structures assume a premenopausal relationship.

As with uterine size, uterine zonal anatomy as depicted on MR images is also a function of hormonal status. Distinction between uterine zones is poorly developed in premenarchal or postmenopausal females, as compared with those of reproductive age (Fig. 10-2).[17,62] Specifically, the junctional zone is often not apparent in pre- or postmenopausal subjects. Once again, hormonal therapy may alter depiction of zonal anatomy. The uterus of postmenopausal patients receiving estrogen replacement therapy demonstrates an appearance similar to that of reproductive age females.[5,32]

In reproductive age females, uterine zonal anatomy varies during the course of the menstrual cycle. During the follicular phase, the endometrial stripe is approximately 6 mm wide, enlarging to 10 mm during the secretory phase.[60] The myometrium also increases in thickness throughout the follicular phase, concordant with the increase in endometrial thickness. In patients receiving oral contraceptives, the endometrium is only approximately 2 mm thick. In postmenopausal women the endometrial stripe is no more than 3 mm thick, and the interface between it and adjacent myometrium may be indistinct.[60] Alteration in the thickness of the junctional zone was observed by Janus et al,[43] and it generally paralleled the growth of the endometrium during the proliferative and secretory phases. However, other authors indicate that the junctional zone does not vary significantly in width during the menstrual cycle, averaging 5 mm wide.[60] Myometrial edema causes relative increased myometrial signal intensity during the midsecretory phase of the menstrual cycle in women receiving oral contraceptives.[60] Small blood clots may be observed within the endometrial cavity during menstruation.[13]

The contrast enhancement pattern of the uterus also varies with hormonal status. During the proliferative phase, maximal endometrial enhancement is observed on images acquired immediately after gadolinium chelate administration. However, during the secretory phase endometrial enhancement is more prominent on relatively delayed images. No significant alterations in the pattern of myometrial enhancement are observed throughout the menstrual cycle. Yamashita et al observed three patterns of enhancement on dynamic contrast enhanced imaging of the uterus: (1) slight initial subendometrial enhancement (in region of junctional zone but not correlating exactly with it) with subsequent myometrial enhancement; (2) marked initial enhancement in region of junctional zone; and (3) predominant enhancement of outer myometrium.[98] They referred to these as type I, II, and III enhancement patterns, respectively. The type I pattern was most commonly observed during the proliferative stage of the menstrual cycle and in postmenopausal women, whereas types II and III were most common during the secretory or menstrual phases, respectively. There

was little immediate enhancement of the endometrium, though marked enhancement was seen on delayed images.

Observation of excessive fluid within the endometrial cavity can be associated with various abnormalities, including endometrial carcinoma and endometritis. However, a small amount of fluid is frequently observed within the endometrial cavity in normal subjects. In some patients, pooling of fluid within the endometrial cavity may be due to stenosis of the cervical os resulting from childbirth or previous instrumentation. Whereas large fluid collections within the rectouterine space (pelvic cul-de-sac) can also indicate neoplastic or inflammatory processes, a small amount of fluid within the pelvic cul-de-sac can also be observed in normal individuals (Fig. 10-1).

Pregnancy

During pregnancy, the uterus enlarges and undergoes an increase in signal intensity. Engorgement of vessels in and around the uterus is also observed (Fig. 10-5).

MR has been used to evaluate complex fetal anomalies that cannot be resolved by ultrasound. However, fetal motion is a significant limiting factor (Fig. 10-6).[35,93] In some situations, sedatives have been administered intravenously to the mother or directly into the amniotic cavity in an effort to reduce fetal motion. Another approach is to use very rapid imaging techniques, such as echo planar imaging, to improve in utero depiction of fetal anatomy and pathology.[82]

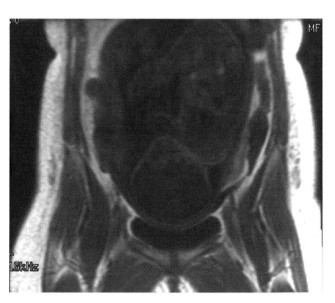

Fig. 10-6. Coronal T1-weighted image (TR 410, TE 12, 2 Nex) in patient imaged during third trimester of pregnancy. While the fetus can be visualized in the vertex position, details relating to fetal anatomy are obscured because of fetal motion.

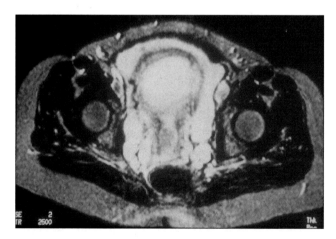

Fig. 10-5. Transaxial T2-weighted image (TR 2500, TE 90, 2 Nex) demonstrates marked engorgement of pelvic vessels in patient imaged during third trimester of pregnancy.

Elevated serum levels of human chorionic gonadotropin and uterine enlargement may indicate ectopic pregnancy, incomplete abortion, or gestational trophoblastic disease. Distinction between these entities is of considerable importance, because of their markedly different treatments. Observations on MR images can be similar in patients with these entities. However, endometrial distention is often greater in patients with incomplete abortion than in those with persistent gestational trophoblastic disease or ectopic pregnancy.[6] Disruption of the junctional zone of the uterus is observed less frequently in patients with ectopic pregnancy than in those with the other conditions. With the above exceptions, however, MR findings among these patients may be nonspecific.

Posttherapy and Postpartum Changes
Postpartum period

Immediately following delivery, the uterus remains enlarged and contains a significant volume of fluid and blood products (Figs. 10-7 and 10-8).[17,39] Intrauterine air is manifested as foci of signal void that are most sensitively depicted on gradient echo images. Although uterine air can indicate endometritis, a small amount of air can be seen immediately following uncomplicated vaginal delivery. The significant alterations observed in the recent postpartum pelvis have the potential to simulate an inflammatory process, particularly when imaging is performed for evaluation of postpartum fever and pain. However, neither parametrial edema nor pelvic mass effect should be observed on MR images following uncomplicated vaginal delivery or cesarean section.[96] When such findings are observed, an inflammatory process should be strongly suggested. Edema surrounding the ovarian vein can indicate ovarian vein thrombosis, another potential postpartum complication. Such perivascular edema should not be observed on images acquired immediately following uncomplicated vaginal delivery or cesarean section.[96]

Cesarean section

The uterine incision site is depicted with signal intensity characteristics of subacute blood breakdown products (i.e., methemoglobin) on MR images acquired soon after cesarean section.[96] Subacute hemorrhage is also frequently observed within the endometrial cavity, and hematoma of the bladder flap is usually seen in patients with a low transverse incision.

Characteristic uterine deformity can be observed in women who have undergone previous cesarean section.[46] The cervix appears elongated and fixed to the anterior abdominal wall. The uterine isthmus is angulated, and the long axis of the uterus may assume a vertical orientation. These findings result from incision of the lower uterine segment during pregnancy. It is possible that these deformities may contribute to infertility in some patients who have undergone cesarean section.

Dilatation and curettage

MR images acquired soon after uterine dilatation and curettage reveal curvilinear areas of decreased signal in-

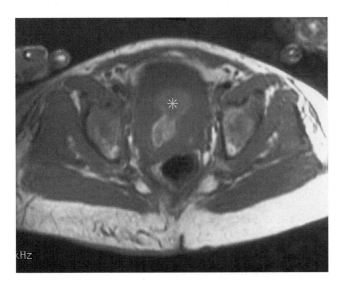

Fig. 10-7. Transaxial T1-weighted image (TR 500, TE 11, 4 Nex) demonstrates increased signal intensity caused by subacute hemorrhagic products *(asterisk)* within the endometrial cavity in patient who underwent recent transvaginal delivery.

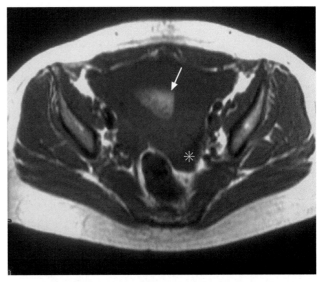

Fig. 10-8. Transaxial T1-weighted image (TR 500, TE 11, 4 Nex) in patient who underwent recent cesarean section demonstrates extensive subacute blood products within the endometrial cavity *(arrow)*. In addition, filling defects within the endometrial cavity are demonstrated consistent with hemorrhagic debris and/or air. A small amount of fluid is also noted in the pelvic cul-de-sac *(asterisk)*.

tensity within the endometrial cavity.[5] These findings probably represent blood clots, and they generally resolve or significantly decrease in size 1 week following the procedure. In the absence of procedural complications, there are no changes in endometrial thickness or in the appearance of the junctional zone.

Radiation therapy

Decreased uterine size and decreased signal intensity are observed in patients who have received pelvic radiation therapy.[2,33] Decreased myometrial signal intensity on T2-weighted images can be observed 1 month following therapy, followed by loss of zonal distinction and decreased uterine size after 3 months. Approximately 6 months following therapy, the endometrium appears decreased in thickness and signal intensity. Many of these changes are similar to those observed in normal postmenopausal women. In postmenopausal women undergoing radiation therapy, the appearance of the uterus is not significantly altered.

Medications

The use of oral contraceptives affects the appearance of the uterus on MR images, as noted previously. Other hormonal medications such as provera, danazol, and diethylstilbestrol can alter uterine signal intensity. Leuprolide, a gonadotropin-releasing hormone agonist, is sometimes used to reduce the size of uterine leiomyomas; this agent also results in a generalized decrease in uterine size.[55] Treatment with clomiphene citrate alters the thickness of the junctional zone in the periovulatory period as compared with untreated controls.[41]

Leiomyomas
Typical appearance

Leiomyomas are extremely common uterine masses, estimated to occur in approximately 20% to 30% of women.[65] Although myomas can be responsible for excessive bleeding, pain, infertility, and other clinical problems, they are frequently encountered as incidental findings in asymptomatic women. In such situations, it is important that they be distinguished from other entities, particularly malignancies.

Because of their tightly bundled smooth muscle fibers, myomas typically appear as well-defined spherical masses and are characterized by uniform decreased signal intensity on T2-weighted images.[14,64] T1-weighted images do not reliably depict all myomas, since on such images myomas may be of similar signal intensity as surrounding myometrium.[103] Contrast agents are being used with increasing frequency for MR evaluation of pelvic abnormalities. When gadolinium chelate contrast agents are administered, the intensity and pattern of enhancement of uterine myomas are highly variable.[57] Myomas may enhance more or less intensely than surrounding un-involved myometrium,[34] and the enhancement pattern of leiomyomas and that of malignancies may appear similar.

Simulation of myomas

A number of entities can simulate uterine myomas on MR images. Bowel loops located adjacent to the uterus appear rounded and show decreased signal intensity because of contained air; these findings can be mistaken for a subserosal or pedunculated uterine leiomyoma (Fig. 10-9). The low signal intensity of the cervical fibrous stroma can simulate a myoma, particularly in patients with distorted pelvic anatomy or when partial volume averaging of the cervix with the uterine corpus occurs (Fig. 10-9). Adnexal lesions having low signal intensity on T2-weighted images, such as ovarian fibroma or Brenner tumor, can also simulate a pedunculated myoma (Fig. 10-10).[65]

Dilated vessels within or adjacent to the uterus can simulate intramural or subserosal uterine myomas because of their flow void appearance on spin echo images. Dilated veins are often observed in association with larger uterine myomas.[5,32,103] Vascular malformations involving the uterus also exhibit flow void within multiple dilated vascular channels of the uterus (Figs. 10-11, A and B). Flow-sensitive gradient echo images can be used to distinguish between vessels or vascular lesions and myomas.

Whereas low signal intensity foci within the endometrial cavity are frequently due to myomas, this appearance is not specific and can be seen with a variety of abnormalities. Among the entities that can exhibit low signal intensity are endometrial carcinoma, endometrial blood clot, endometrial hamartoma, intrauterine pregnancy, and retained products of conception.[13] Because of their signal intensity characteristics, each of these entities can potentially simulate submucosal leiomyomas.

ENTITIES THAT CAN SIMULATE MYOMAS

- Adjacent bowel loops
- Partial volume averaging with cervical stroma
- Low signal intensity adnexal lesions (ovarian fibroma, Brenner tumor)
- Dilated uterine/periuterine vessels
- Endometrial carcinoma
- Endometrial blood clot
- Endometrial hamartoma
- Intrauterine pregnancy
- Focal adenomyosis
- Retained products of conception
- Intrauterine device
- Myometrial contractions

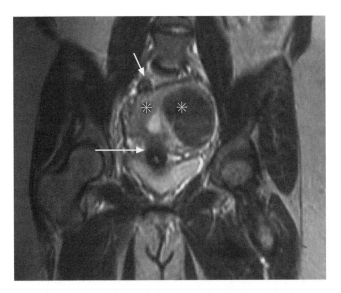

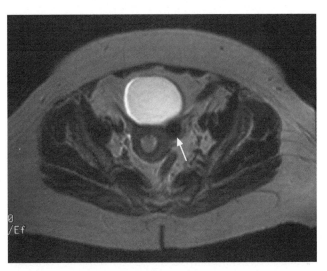

Fig. 10-9. Coronal T2-weighted image (TR 2200, TE 80, 2 Nex) in patient with two intramural leiomyomas *(asterisks)*. There is a bowel loop situated cephalad to the uterus *(small arrow)*, with signal characteristics that could suggest an additional subserosal leiomyoma. Furthermore, the uterine cervix, displayed immediately inferior to the uterine corpus *(arrow)*, may also simulate an exophytic leiomyoma.

Fig. 10-10. Transaxial fast spin echo T2-weighted image (TR 4000, effective TE 120, 4 Nex, 16 echo train) demonstrates uniformly hypointense left adnexal mass *(arrow)*, representing a presumed ovarian fibroma. This appearance can simulate a pedunculated leiomyoma. Note increased fluid within the endometrial cavity.

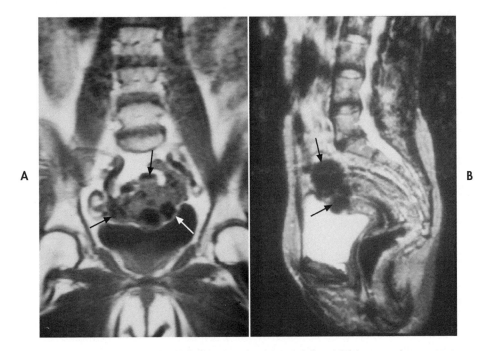

Fig. 10-11. Coronal T1-weighted **(A)** and sagittal T2-weighted **(B)** images demonstrate multiple hypointense foci involving the uterine corpus *(arrows)*. These represent prominent blood vessels in a patient with uterine arteriovenous malformation. The flow void depicted by these vessels can simulate uterine myomas.

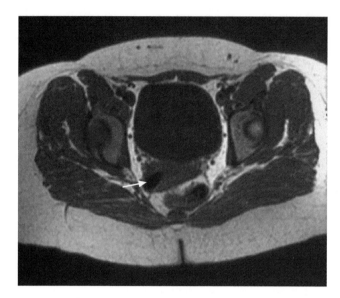

Fig. 10-12. Transaxial T1-weighted image (TR 460, TE 12, 2 Nex) demonstrates rounded low signal intensity structure projecting in the region of the uterine cervix *(arrow)*. While this could appear to represent a myoma, this is due to a tampon located within the posterior vaginal fornix.

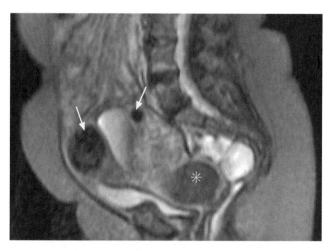

Fig. 10-13. Sagittal T2-weighted image (TR 2700, TE 90, 2 Nex) demonstrates multiple uterine myomas in 51-year-old patient. While most of the myomas demonstrate marked hypointensity *(arrows)*, a large myoma with relative increased signal intensity is also noted posteriorly *(asterisk)*. Such signal variations reflect the presence of myomatous degeneration.

However, evaluation of lesion morphology is very useful in making these distinctions. Leiomyomas are well circumscribed and have a broad base of attachment along the endometrial-myometrial junction.[13] Other entities (listed above) usually appear heterogeneous and unconnected to the myometrium. Of course, clinical correlation is also very helpful in identifying the correct diagnosis when these or other nonspecific findings are observed. Administration of paramagnetic contrast material may be useful in some situations, since some entities such as blood clots do not undergo enhancement. Other causes for low signal intensity foci that may simulate myomas include intrauterine contraceptive devices[56,64,69] and tampons projecting within the vaginal fornix (Fig. 10-12).

Contraction of the myometrium occurs in normal nongravid women and can result in apparent distortion of the endometrium on MR images.[86,87] The contracting portion of the myometrium appears to bulge and demonstrates focal decreased signal intensity on T2-weighted or contrast enhanced T1-weighted images. This combination of findings can simulate leiomyoma or adenomyosis. Because of the transient nature of myometrial contractions, repeat imaging at a later time usually demonstrates a normal appearance.

Atypical myomas

Uterine myomas—particularly large ones—can undergo hyaline degeneration, resulting in atypical signal intensity features. Myomatous degeneration leads to irregular central regions of relative increased signal inten-

sity on T2-weighted images; hyperintense foci on T1-weighted images may also be observed (Fig. 10-13). These findings are due to necrosis and/or hemorrhage within the lesion and can simulate the appearance of an aggressive lesion such as leiomyosarcoma.[17,39,84] However, degenerated myomas maintain a round or oval morphology and well-defined margins, which can help to distinguish them from some malignancies.[65] Degenerative subserosal myomas can simulate hemorrhagic ovarian cysts or ovarian carcinoma.[17,39,64,69]

Relatively increased signal intensity can also be observed within some nondegenerative cellular leiomyomas. These entities should be distinguished since hormonal therapy can be used to reduce the size of cellular, but not degenerated, leiomyomas. Dynamic contrast enhanced imaging can be used to demonstrate more intense early enhancement of cellular as compared with degenerated leiomyomas.[101] Areas of mild hyperintensity within nondegenerated myomas may also be due to prominent vascularity.

A peripheral rim of relative increased signal intensity may surround uterine myomas in the absence of myomatous degeneration (Fig. 10-14).[40] This is due to surrounding edema, usually observed in association with larger myomas. Peripheral increased signal intensity can also represent dilated vascular or lymphatic channels.[65]

Following medical treatment with gonadotrophic releasing hormone, myomas undergo a decrease in size and signal intensity as a result of interruption of their vascular supply.[17,39] These alterations are accompanied by myometrial and endometrial atrophy.

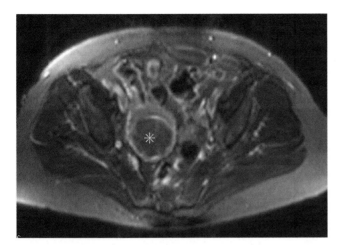

Fig. 10-14. Transaxial fast spin echo T2-weighted image (TR 2600, effective TE 100, 4 Nex, 16 echo train) demonstrates 4 cm uterine myoma *(asterisk)* with surrounding rim of hyperintensity.

> ### ENTITIES THAT CAN SIMULATE ENDOMETRIAL CARCINOMA
>
> - Adenomatous hyperplasia
> - Uterine adenofibromas
> - Endometrial polyps
> - Mesenchymal uterine tumors
> - Metastases
> - Blood clot
> - Necrotic debris
> - Leiomyoma

Adenomyosis

Adenomyosis refers to the presence of endometrial glandular tissue within the myometrium. This condition is associated with abnormal bleeding, pain, or infertility. Foci of adenomyosis are often microscopic, though the inflammatory reaction they incite is often quite extensive.[65] Adenomyosis is usually manifested on MR images as diffuse widening and lack of definition of the junctional zone.[89] Because of its predominance of compact smooth muscle cells, the signal intensity of adenomyosis is similar to that of the junctional zone.[100]

Distinction between relatively mild forms of diffuse adenomyosis and the normal junctional zone may be difficult.[4,100] The normal junctional zone is usually less than 3 mm wide; widening of the junctional zone beyond 5 mm indicates adenomyosis. However, the diagnosis of adenomyosis may be difficult when the junctional zone measures between 3 and 5 mm. Repeat imaging during a different phase of the menstrual cycle may be considered, under the presumption that the normal junctional zone will vary in its thickness. However, the normal junctional zone usually does not undergo significant change in thickness during the menstrual cycle. Observation of punctate hyperintensities within a mildly expanded junctional zone can be seen with adenomyosis, resulting from areas of hemorrhage or endometrial tissue.[100]

Discrete areas of decreased uterine signal intensity can be observed on T2-weighted images in patients with focal adenomyosis. Focal adenomyosis can therefore potentially simulate leiomyoma, which can also have a similar clinical presentation.[35] Because treatment of these entities is quite different, their distinction is impor-

tant. However, these entities can usually be distinguished from one another, since leiomyomas usually appear more discrete with uniformly low signal intensity, whereas adenomyosis is often more diffuse and ill-defined and can demonstrate small hyperintense foci.[91]

Endometrial Carcinoma
Detection

Endometrial carcinoma is usually identified as an expanded and heterogeneous signal intensity endometrial cavity on T2-weighted images.[18,28,40,44] The diagnosis of endometrial carcinoma is usually established by dilatation and curettage performed before MR imaging. This procedure can produce clots within the endometrial cavity, simulating the appearance of tumor tissue.[14,64] Even in the absence of recent intervention, it can be very difficult to distinguish between a viable tumor, necrotic debris, and blood clots within the endometrial cavity.[3,40,85]

Although the signal intensity of endometrial cancer is usually greater than that of the myometrium, its signal characteristics are highly variable.[68] In some patients, endometrial carcinoma appears isointense with normal endometrial tissue and fluid secretions, obscuring visualization of tumor[73]; contrast material may be useful in this distinction. MR images fail to demonstrate an abnormality in nearly 20% of patients with endometrial carcinoma[68]; most of these inapparent lesions are superficial.

The earliest observation in patients with endometrial carcinoma is often thickening of the endometrial stripe. This structure is normally less than 1 cm wide in premenopausal women and less than 3 mm in postmenopausal women.[73] In patients with early endometrial cancer, the endometrial stripe may be of uniform high signal intensity, or it can appear heterogeneous.

Other uterine masses can also appear identical to endometrial carcinoma on MR images. These lesions include adenomatous hyperplasia, uterine adenofibromas, endometrial polyps, mesenchymal uterine tumors, and metastases.[3,35,68,73,93]

Hyperintensity within the endometrial cavity can be observed on T1-weighted images as a result of subacute hemorrhage from endometrial carcinoma or other causes. T1 shortening can also be seen in patients with lipomatous uterine tumors. Fat suppressed T1-weighted images are helpful in distinguishing these tissues. Benign uterine stromal nodules and their sarcomatous counterparts may have a similar appearance.[68]

Staging

The major role of MR imaging in patients with endometrial carcinoma is not detection but rather staging. Specifically, information regarding the depth of myometrial tumor invasion is important prognostically and for treatment planning. The basis for determination of deep myometrial tumor invasion is observation of focal disruption of the junctional zone on T2-weighted images. However, this has not proved to be a highly accurate criterion, with false positive results particularly frequent.[73]

For example, in postmenopausal women in whom the junctional zone is poorly visualized, a false diagnosis of deep myometrial invasion may be made.[40,91] This is of major significance, since endometrial carcinoma is predominantly encountered in the postmenopausal age group. Similarly, when the junctional zone is visible but appears indistinct, the depth of tumor invasion can again be overestimated. Other factors that can contribute to overstaging of endometrial carcinoma invasion include the presence of a blood clot adjacent to the tumor and myometrial atrophy.[89] In some patients, endometrial tumors are relatively isointense with underlying myometrium, creating difficulty in determining the precise depth of tumor invasion.[68] The level of myometrial invasion is also difficult to determine when there is marked endometrial distention and myometrial thinning.[73] Although endocervical canal widening may be seen in patients with cervical invasion of endometrial cancer, this is a nonspecific finding.[73]

Contrast material

The use of paramagnetic contrast material can improve staging accuracy in patients with endometrial carcinoma.[37,77,85] On contrast-enhanced T1-weighted images, tumor generally appears hypointense relative to enhanced normal myometrial tissue. Distinction between tumor and myometrium is usually optimal on images acquired immediately following contrast material injection, though in some patients delayed images are superior. Discontinuity of subendometrial enhancement is observed in patients with myometrial invasion of endometrial cancer.[98] This sign is particularly useful in patients with poorly visualized junctional zones on T2-weighted images. However, when imaging is performed during the secretory or menstrual phases, this sign cannot be assessed, and difficulty may be experienced in evaluating

this sign in women with myomas or endometrial distention.

In addition to improved staging accuracy, detection of small endometrial cancers is also assisted by the use of dynamic gadolinium chelate enhanced imaging.[31] Contrast enhanced images also allow for improved distinction between viable tumor and necrotic debris, which can be problematic on unenhanced images.[37,98]

CERVIX
Anatomic Variations

The cervix may be affected by various mullerian duct anomalies, as described previously. These anomalies can result in either absence or duplication of the cervix. In patients who have undergone abdominoperineal resection for rectal carcinoma, the cervix may extend posteriorly into the presacral space, analogous to the seminal vesicles in postoperative male patients (Fig. 10-15).

Zonal Anatomy

The zonal anatomy of the cervix is poorly depicted on T1-weighted images but easily seen on T2-weighted images. Central high signal intensity is due to endocervical glands as well as mucus within the endocervical canal.[60] High-resolution images may demonstrate a zone of slightly decreased signal intensity just deep to the endocervical canal, representing the plicae palmatae (Fig. 10-16). The cervical fibrous stroma is continuous with the junctional zone of the uterus and shows marked decreased signal intensity on all pulse sequences. The stroma is surrounded by tissue of relatively increased in-

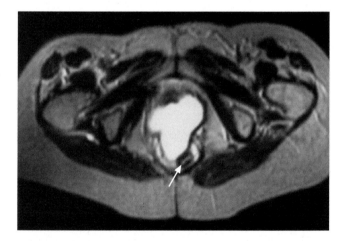

Fig. 10-15. The cervix—distinguished by its characteristic zonal anatomy (arrow)—is identified within the presacral space in this 70-year-old female who underwent previous abdominoperineal resection of rectal carcinoma. There is also associated deformity of the posterior urinary bladder.

tensity on T2-weighted images. An outer cervical zone is variably identified and appears continuous with myometrium. It represents a portion of the cervical fibrous stroma that has relatively reduced cellular density.

Supporting ligaments of the cervix, including the broad ligament, cardinal ligament, round ligaments, vesicouterine ligaments, and uterosacral ligaments, are usually poorly visualized on standard MR images.[60]

Physiologic Changes

The width and length of the cervix average approximately 2.7 cm and do not vary significantly during the menstrual cycle.[60] The internal cervical os appears somewhat widened during the proliferative phase of the menstrual cycle and somewhat smaller during the secretory phase.[35] The signal intensity pattern of the cervix may be altered by changes in hormonal status. Distinction of cervical zonal anatomy is often obscured in postmenopausal females.[88] Shortening and increased signal intensity of the cervix are observed during the third trimester of pregnancy.

Cervical Carcinoma

The major indication for evaluation of the cervix with MR imaging is cervical carcinoma. Detection of cervical cancer is usually made by clinical examination and cytologic smears; MR is used primarily to stage previously diagnosed tumors. Cervical carcinoma is usually

manifested as a focus of relatively increased cervical signal intensity, frequently accompanied by masslike cervical enlargement. Whereas most larger cervical cancers are detectable on MR images, small lesions and particularly carcinoma in situ usually are not.[70] Microinvasive (stage IA) lesions usually are not distinguishable from the high signal intensity of the endocervical canal,[68,73] and therefore MR has shown limited ability to demonstrate subtle tumor infiltration of the cervix (e.g., <5 mm depth).[54] For this reason, lesions visualized on MR, particularly using body coil images, almost invariably have an invasive component.[73] Cervical carcinoma is often exophytic in younger patients, though in older women it may be endocervical.[73]

Tumor size

Determination of tumor size is important for treatment planning and correlates with prognosis. MR provides the most accurate noninvasive means for determining the size of cervical tumors. However, MR images may underestimate the actual extent of superficial cervical cancer.[70] Conversely, the size of some larger tumors is overestimated using MR.[42]

Lesion characterization

Foci of increased signal intensity, as well as morphologic alteration, can be observed in patients who have undergone recent cervical biopsy (Fig. 10-17). Similar changes can also be caused by inflammatory processes involving the cervix. In both situations, findings may simulate cervical carcinoma.

Nabothian cysts are cystically dilated endocervical glands; they are commonly present in asymptomatic women and usually have no clinical significance (Figs.

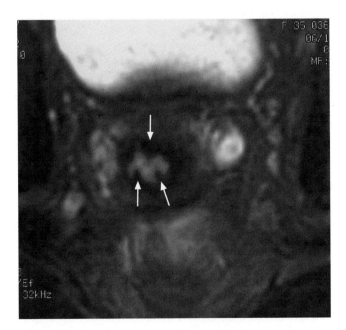

Fig. 10-16. High-resolution transaxial fast spin echo T2-weighted image (TR 4000, effective TE 100, 4 Nex, 16 echo train) demonstrates multiple polypoid extensions projecting from the cervical wall *(arrows)* into the endocervical canal, representing normal plicae palmatae.

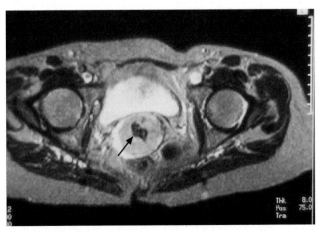

Fig. 10-17. Transaxial T2-weighted image demonstrates cervical mass with focus of marked decreased signal intensity centrally (arrow). The latter findings are due to clot formation following recent cervical biopsy.

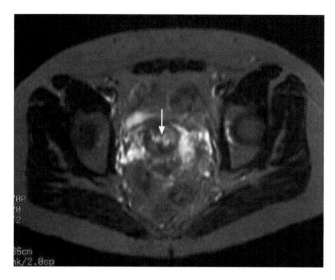

Fig. 10-18. Transaxial T2-weighted image (TR 3700, TE 120, 2 Nex) in 46-year-old female demonstrates multiple small hyperintensities within the uterine cervix *(arrow)*, representing incidental nabothian cysts.

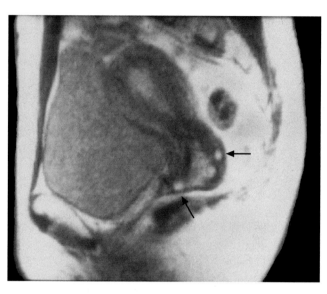

Fig. 10-19. Midsagittal T2-weighted image depicts small hyperintense foci within the cervix *(arrows)*, representing nabothian cysts.

10-18 and 10-19). They are most frequently observed in multiparous women. Nabothian cysts appear as foci of cervical hyperintensity on T2-weighted images.[33,47] Although they are usually small and their fluid composition is evident, larger nabothian cysts can potentially simulate cervical carcinoma, particularly when they undergo partial volume averaging with adjacent cervical stroma.

Although squamous cervical carcinoma is certainly the most frequently encountered cervical mass, it is important to keep in mind that other mass lesions are also encountered in this location. For example, reports describe the appearance of cavernous hemangioma[30] and primary lymphoma of the cervix on MR images.[16]

Adenoma malignum is a well-differentiated form of cervical adenocarcinoma that is organized into cystic nodules.[99] This tumor can be highly aggressive and has a poor prognosis. Adenoma malignum can appear as multiple foci of markedly increased signal intensity within the uterine cervix on T2-weighted images and may be indistinguishable from nabothian cysts. In patients with histologic or cytologic evidence of cervical malignancy, observation of apparent nabothian cysts on MR images should be considered potential sources of malignancy, particularly if typical cervical carcinoma is not evident.

Imaging techniques

In preparation for imaging, the urinary bladder should be emptied to decrease artifacts from motion.[60] Though a vaginal tampon has been occasionally used to facilitate identification of the vagina and cervix on CT imaging, it is unnecessary for MR and may result in

distortion of local anatomy.[60] In patients without contraindications to its use, intramuscular glucagon should be administered to assist in the reduction of peristaltic bowel motion artifacts.[68]

Evaluation of the cervix and surrounding structures has usually been performed using the body coil. However, several new coils are now available that provide superior signal-to-noise ratio and allow for acquisition of higher resolution images of the female pelvis. Despite their advantages, there are also some important limitations presented by each of these coil designs. Multicoil phased arrays provide an excellent signal-to-noise ratio for pelvic imaging. Their limitations include a reduced craniocaudal field-of-view, which can restrict evaluation for pelvic lymph nodes, and marked accentuation of signal intensity of tissues located close to the coil (i.e., subcutaneous fat), resulting in a heterogeneous signal profile across the image. The latter situation can be alleviated with the use of software algorithms or fat suppression.[34] Other disadvantages include an increase in respiratory ghosting artifacts, caused by movement of the coil or accentuated signal intensity of body wall fat, and relative decreased signal-to-noise ratio within the central pelvis in large patients.[68]

Endocavitary surface coils can be positioned within the rectum or vagina to allow for acquisition of even higher resolution (i.e., smaller field-of-view) images with high signal-to-noise ratio (Fig. 10-20). These coils improve evaluation of the cervix, vaginal wall and forni-

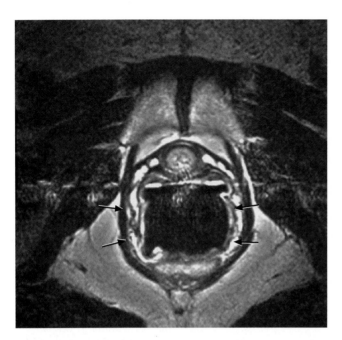

Fig. 10-20. Transaxial fast spin echo T2-weighted image (TR 4500, effective TE 120, 4 Nex, 16 echo train) acquired using endovaginal coil. Note peripheral increased signal intensity surrounding the muscular wall of the vagina *(arrows)*, representing the perivaginal venous plexus.

ces, pelvic side walls and parametria as compared with standard body coil images.[7,63] They are useful for evaluating subtle parametrial invasion in patients with cervical carcinoma or for depicting tumors involving the vagina or uretha. They also allow for visualization of tissue planes separating tumor from surrounding structures, which may not be evident on body coil images. However, the coil may displace the cervix laterally or superiorly, causing it to move beyond the sensitive range of the coil. Similarly, large tumors may extend beyond the sensitive range of the coil.[68] Images must be supplemented by body coil images to evaluate for lymphadenopathy.

In patients with cervical carcinoma, standard transaxial images should be supplemented with those obtained in the coronal plane for evaluation of parametrial invasion and with sagittal images for evaluation of invasion into the bladder, rectum, and uterine corpus.[26] Oblique scans, prescribed perpendicular to the true axis of the cervix, may be even more useful than images oriented orthogonal to the magnet bore.[8]

A combination of T1- and T2-weighted spin echo sequences is usually employed in the evaluation of patients with cervical cancer. T1-weighted images allow for excellent depiction of gross morphology and provide good definition of tissue planes and lymph nodes. However, in the absence of significant morphologic abnormality, cervical carcinoma is poorly visualized on T1-weighted

images because of isointensity of tumor with normal cervix, parametria, and other surrounding structures.[68]

Fast spin echo (i.e., RARE) sequences have recently become widely available and provide excellent image quality, with improved efficiency for acquisition of T2-weighted images. However, fat appears intense on these images, as compared with conventional T2-weighted images, and they may also provide suboptimal tissue contrast for evaluation of some types of female pelvic pathology.[34] Furthermore, fast spin echo images are subject to blurring, particularly when long echo trains or short echo times are used.

Although gradient echo images are useful for vascular depiction and for acquiring dynamic contrast enhanced images, unenhanced gradient echo images often result in suboptimal tissue contrast for staging of cervical cancer and other gynecologic malignancies.[72] Accentuation of susceptibility artifacts related to surgical clips and bowel gas can also obscure portions of the relevant anatomy on gradient echo images.

Contrast material

As noted previously, T1-weighted images are generally less useful than T2-weighted images for staging of cervical carcinoma. However, with the addition of paramagnetic contrast material, some studies indicate that T1-weighted images yield similar information as T2-weighted images.[29] Following gadopentetate dimeglumine administration, the cervical stroma undergoes variably intense contrast enhancement.[37] The use of contrast material may assist in detecting subtle tumor invasion of the parametria and vaginal wall. However, other investigators report that distinction between tumor and adjacent cervical stroma and determination of the depth of cervical stromal or parametrial invasion continue to be most accurately depicted on T2-weighted images.[78] Stromal, parametrial, vaginal, and bladder wall invasion can be overestimated on contrast enhanced images.[85] For all of the above reasons, standard contrast enhanced imaging has not played a major role in the evaluation of patients with cervical carcinoma.

Improvement in distinction between cervical carcinoma and surrounding cervical stroma has been achieved with use of dynamic contrast enhanced imaging. This technique has compared favorably with T2-weighted or delayed contrast enhanced T1-weighted images, in terms of tumor delineation and parametrial invasion.[25,100] The cervical stroma usually enhances less intensely than myometrium on dynamic contrast enhanced images.[31] However, in some patients, equivalent enhancement of the cervix and myometrium may be observed.[34]

Staging accuracy

The accuracy of MR for providing locoregional staging of cervical carcinoma and its efficacy as compared with clinical examination have been a source of some debate in the literature. Most reports indicate that the accuracy provided by MR staging far exceeds that achieved using clinical staging alone.[70,76] On the other hand, several studies have come to the opposing conclusion. In one small study, for example, MR accurately staged only three of eleven patients, whereas clinical staging was correct in eight patients.[80] Similar trends have been evident in other studies.[10,94]

Information regarding parametrial spread of cervical carcinoma is of clinical importance. However, this determination can be difficult on MR images. In one study of 41 patients, sensitivity for determination of extension of cervical cancer to involve the uterine corpus, parametria, vagina, bladder, and lymph nodes was 63%, 38%, 43%, 67%, and 38%, respectively.[81] In a later study involving 169 patients, the positive predictive value of MR for determination of parametrial tumor invasion was only 43%.[53] The major limitation of MR has been a relatively high number of false positive results based on observation of nonmalignant abnormal parametrial signal intensity. For example, parametrial tumor extension can be simulated by normal or engorged vascular structures, inflammatory changes related to pelvic infection,[76] or radiation therapy.

Tumor invasion into the vagina may be difficult to visualize, particularly when low-resolution techniques are used.[73]

Lymph nodes

Lymph node signal intensity patterns have not proved useful in distinguishing benign from malignant nodes. Thus lymph node size is the only useful criterion for determination of malignant lymphadenopathy in the pelvis. Pelvic lymph nodes measuring greater than 1 cm in diameter are usually regarded as suspicious for malignant involvement. However, 1 cm is an arbitrary cutoff; nonenlarged nodes may harbor malignancy, and, conversely, reactive nodes may be substantially larger than 1 cm. In a study involving 136 patients with cervical carcinoma, Kim et al[50] found that measurement of the minimum axial diameter of pelvic lymph nodes provides greater accuracy than the maximum axial diameter. Using 1 cm minimum axial diameter as the criterion for malignant lymphadenopathy yielded 62% sensitivity and 98% specificity, with overall accuracy of 93%. In addition to enlarged nodes, clusters of nonenlarged nodes should also be considered suspicious for malignant involvement.[73] Gadolinium chelate contrast material has not proved useful for differentiation of enlarged lymph nodes caused by metastatic cervical cancer and reactive lymph nodes.[50]

Indirect information regarding the likelihood of nodal tumor can also be acquired using MR. The incidence of nodal metastasis in patients with cervical carcinoma is increased significantly when tumor size is greater than 4 cm or when parametrial or bladder invasion is present.[38]

Postradiation changes

Decreased signal intensity of cervical carcinoma can be observed on T2-weighted images following administration of chemotherapy or radiotherapy.[75] Reduction in lesion signal intensity is usually observed 3 to 6 months following completion of radiation therapy, and it is accompanied by a decrease in tumor size.[24] Documentation of progressive decline in T1 relaxation values has been used as a quantitative index of response to radiation therapy.[71]

The hallmark of successful radiation therapy is eradication of the cervical mass as well as any associated abnormal increased cervical signal intensity on T2-weighted images. However, residual abnormal signal intensity may be observed in many patients despite tumor eradication.[20] These foci of increased signal intensity probably reflect immature fibrosis (i.e., granulation tissue).[23] Some authors have indicated that immature fibrosis can result in high signal intensity for up to 12 months following completion of radiation therapy.[19] Heavily T2-weighted images are useful for increasing the distinction in signal intensity between residual/recurrent tumor and posttreatment fibrosis.

Isolated abnormal signal intensity following radiotherapy should not be used as evidence of a residual tumor, although abnormal signal intensity observed in conjunction with a mass indicates that a residual tumor is likely. In patients with a residual tumor demonstrating decreasing signal intensity 6 months following treatment, complete tumor response ultimately occurs.[24] This pattern most often occurs in patients with large tumors. The absence of any signal intensity alteration by 6 months, however, suggests nonresponse to treatment.

VAGINA
Anatomic Variations

Mullerian duct anomalies, which can affect the vagina, were discussed previously. These abnormalities may result in absence or duplication of the vagina.[9] Although the hymen itself is not directly visualized, in patients with imperforate hymen hematometrocolpos may be observed.

Normal Appearance

High signal intensity on T2-weighted images is observed centrally, caused by glandular tissue and mucus and secretions within the vaginal canal. This is surrounded by the relatively low signal intensity muscular wall of the vagina. Vaginal mucus and related glands are of increased prominence during the early follicular and late secretory phases of the menstrual cycle; the resultant high signal intensity serves to improve contrast between the vaginal canal and its surrounding muscular wall.[36,60] A prominent venous plexus lies peripheral to

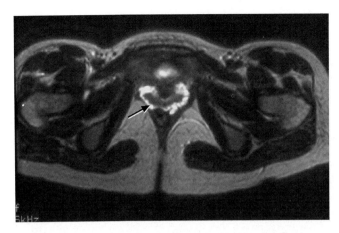

Fig. 10-21. A prominent perivaginal venous plexus is demonstrated on transaxial fast spin echo T2-weighted image (TR 4000, effective TE 120, 2 Nex, 16 echo train) (arrow).

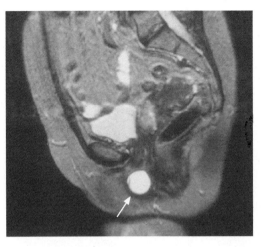

Fig. 10-22. Sagittal T2-weighted image (TR 2500, TE 90, 2 Nex) in patient with cervical carcinoma demonstrates 3 cm rounded hyperintense structure in the perivaginal region (arrow), representing a Bartholin gland cyst.

the vaginal wall, demonstrating increased signal intensity on T2-weighted images as a result of slow flow (Figs. 10-20 and 10-21).[60] Prominent enhancement of the perivaginal tissues is observed on contrast enhanced images.

Paravaginal Cysts

Paravaginal cysts are frequently asymptomatic and are encountered as incidental findings.[67] Paravaginal cysts include Bartholin gland cysts, keratinous or epithelial inclusion cysts, paraurethral mucous cysts, mesonephric (wolffian duct) cysts, and cysts of the canal of Nuck. Bartholin gland cysts, which are the most common, are usually observed posterolateral to the vaginal orifice, are round or oval, have well-defined margins, and may be several cm in size (Fig. 10-22).

The signal intensity of these cysts varies with their internal contents. Serous cysts appear hypointense on T1-weighted and markedly hyperintense on T2-weighted images, whereas increased signal intensity on T1-weighted images is observed in cysts with high proteinaceous content. Other cysts may contain hemorrhagic contents, which can exhibit a variety of signal patterns depending on the oxidation state of the blood breakdown products.

Observation of solid components within these cysts should raise suspicion for underlying malignancy. However, because of their small size, such solid components may be difficult to appreciate. Conversely, debris caused by infection may result in overlapping findings.

Posttreatment Appearance

In patients who have undergone previous hysterectomy, the vaginal cuff usually has a linear, smooth appearance, though portions of the cuff may be poorly visualized because of adjacent surgical clips.[12] However, in some patients, the vagina appears nodular, simulating a vaginal mass (Figs. 10-23 A and B). This appearance

is particularly worrisome when hysterectomy was performed for treatment of malignant neoplasm. T2-weighted images are useful in distinguishing between posthysterectomy nodularity and tumor recurrence. Postoperative changes retain the normal signal intensity of the vagina on T2-weighted images (i.e., low signal intensity muscular layer with surrounding high signal intensity). However, in patients with recurrent tumor, the vaginal muscularis shows increased signal intensity.

In patients who have received pelvic radiation, the vagina may demonstrate increased signal intensity on T2-weighted images.[68] Other findings observed in these patients include increased bone marrow signal intensity on T1- and T2-weighted images, increased or decreased signal intensity of fat, increased signal intensity of muscle and fascial planes on T2-weighted images, decreased size and signal intensity of ovaries and uterus on T2-weighted images, and thickening of the bladder wall with variable signal intensity on T2-weighted images.[68] Enterovaginal and vesicovaginal fistulas may also be observed.

Tumor Involvement

A normal appearance of the vagina on MR images is generally reliable for excluding tumor involvement.[15] However, false positive results are more frequently encountered. For example, morphologic and/or signal intensity alterations resulting from vaginal inflammation or congestion can closely simulate tumor invasion.

OVARIES/ADNEXAE
Anatomic and Other Variations

The ovaries are most frequently identified along the pelvic sidewall, though their position is quite variable,

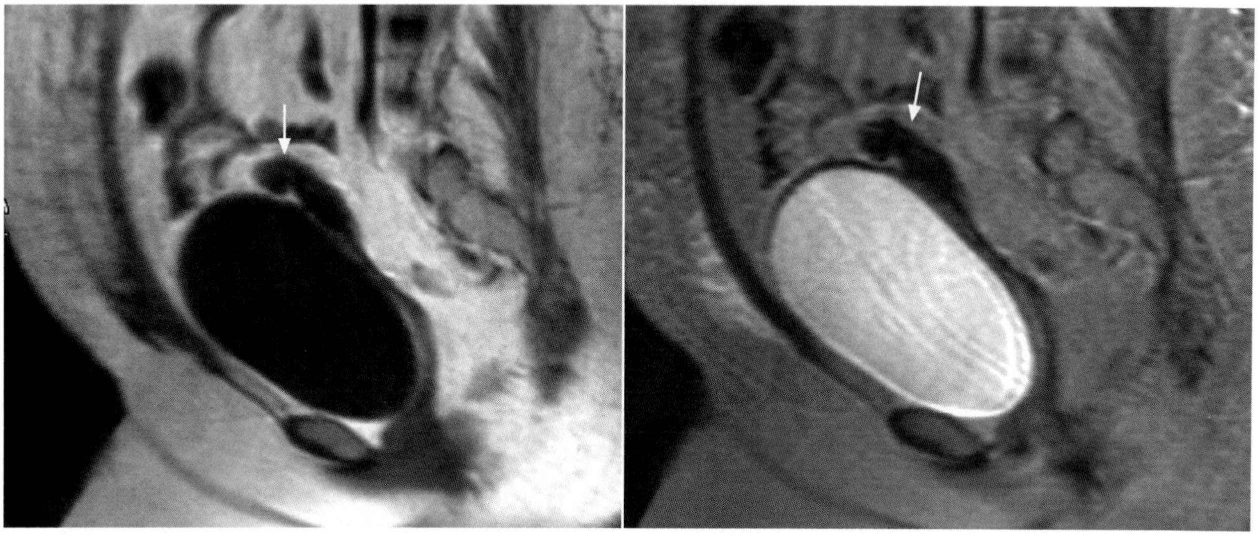

Fig. 10-23. Midsagittal T1-weighted **(A)** (TR 500, TE 13, 4 Nex) and fast spin echo T2-weighted **(B)** (TR 4000, effective TE 100, 2 Nex, 12 echo train length) images in patient following total abdominal hysterectomy. The vaginal cuff demonstrates a nodular appearance on both images *(arrows)*, with maintenance of uniform decreased signal intensity on the T2-weighted image.

particularly in multiparous women.[60] Uterine enlargement may result in their displacement into the upper pelvis or low abdomen. The ovaries can also be found along the course of the psoas muscle, extending into the inguinal canal or into the labium majorus,[9] or located within the pelvic cul-de-sac.

In reproductive age patients undergoing pelvic radiation therapy—usually for treatment of cervical cancer—the ovaries may be removed from the radiation port to preserve their function. The transposed ovaries are identified on MR images along the paracolic gutters, where they may produce mass effect on the bowel.[48] Unless one is aware of the expected location of such transposed ovaries, physiologic cysts arising from them may be interpreted as evidence of tumor recurrence or other pathology.

More than the usual two ovaries are present in 2% to 4% of females; rarely one or both ovaries may be absent.[9] The ovaries are also subject to variations in configuration, including elongated, triangular, crescentic, flattened, or irregular shapes instead of the usual smooth oval shape.[9]

The ovaries may be isointense with surrounding fat on moderately T2-weighted images, rendering them difficult to identify. They may also be isointense with pelvic bowel loops, likewise confounding their identification. In the latter situation, orally administered contrast material can be used to increase (positive contrast agents) or decrease (negative contrast agents) the gastrointestinal tract lumen, allowing for improved visualization of the ovaries (Figs. 10-24, *A* and *B*). Visualization of follicles, which appear as small hyperintense foci on T2-weighted images, is important for identification of the ovaries. Such follicles may not be evident when images are insufficiently T2 weighted, when they are of inadequate signal-to-noise ratio or inadequate spatial resolution, or when image quality is limited due to motion artifacts.[79] Another cause for failure to observe follicles is use of inappropriate photographic techniques (i.e., window and level settings).[60]

Ovarian volume in reproductive age women is 6 ml, as compared with 1 ml in premenarchal and 2.5 ml in postmenopausal females.[60] Because of their small size and usual absence of cysts, the ovaries may be difficult to identify in the latter groups.

One or both fallopian tubes may be absent or hypoplastic, and partial or complete duplication may also occur.[9] The fallopian tubes may also demonstrate a convoluted appearance as a result of retained fetal tortuosity.[9] A small volume of fluid may be observed within the pelvic cul-de-sac in normal subjects.

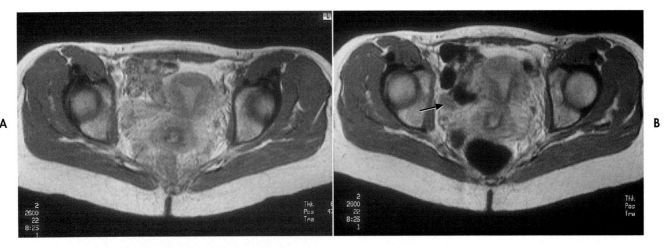

Fig. 10-24. Transaxial proton density–weighted images (TR 2600, TE 22, 2 Nex) obtained before **(A)** and after **(B)** oral administration of perfluorooctylbromide. Distinction between bowel loops and adnexal structures is difficult on the precontrast image because of the isointensity of these structures. However, with negative enhancement of the bowel lumen, the right ovary *(arrow)* is easily identified.

Ovarian Masses
Functional cysts

Simple ovarian cysts are very commonly observed as incidental findings on MR images (Figs. 10-25 and 10-26).[65] They appear round or oval, without soft tissue components or wall thickening, and with fluid-like signal intensity on all sequences. They are most apparent when high-resolution, heavily T2-weighted images are obtained.

Follicular cysts arise when ovarian follicles enlarge without rupture, and corpus luteum cysts occur following their rupture.[65] Theca lutein cysts result from ovarian stimulation by endogenous or exogenous hormones and are often multiple and bilateral. Although follicular and luteal cysts are often indistinguishable from one another, hemorrhage is more common with corpus luteum cysts.

Physiologic ovarian cysts are usually observed in women of reproductive age, though they can also occur in postmenopausal women. Consequently, a cystic ovarian mass in a postmenopausal woman does not necessarily indicate malignancy. In one study, simple adnexal cysts were observed in 17% of 184 asymptomatic postmenopausal women.[52] There was no correlation between the presence of such cysts and hormonal therapy. The authors of this study advise that when small (<3 cm) cysts are observed in postmenopausal women, they may be followed nonsurgically if they demonstrate no evidence of nodularity or septations.[52]

Functional ovarian cysts typically demonstrate uniform decreased and increased signal intensity on T1- and T2-weighted images. However, their signal intensity may vary according to their internal contents. For example, cysts containing hemorrhagic or proteinaceous contents appear hyperintense on T1-weighted images and relatively hypointense on T2-weighted images. The presence of hemorrhagic components, in particular, may appear to represent soft tissue nodularity, thereby causing confusion for ovarian neoplasm.

Lesion characterization

Distinction between benign cysts and cystic tumors is not always possible. Benign cystic lesions, such as simple, follicular, and luteal cysts, as well as mucinous and serous cystadenomas, may have a similar appearance (Fig. 10-27).[59] However, findings suggestive of neoplasm include soft tissue nodularity or septations, as well as large size.

Even when the presence of soft tissue components indicates a cystic neoplasm, characterization remains difficult, since similar findings are often observed with benign and malignant epithelial tumors of the ovary.[68] The observation of prominent solid components, thick septations, or ancillary findings such as ascites, enlarged lymph nodes, peritoneal nodules, or omental thickening raise strong suspicion for ovarian carcinoma. However, these signs are also not definitive. Some septations or other solid lesion components may not be evident on MR images. Acquisition of images in at least two planes is useful for detecting small nodules within ovarian lesions.[59] Similarly, peritoneal tumor spread may be microscopic and also poorly visualized. In the evaluation for peritoneal disease, the use of glucagon is particularly

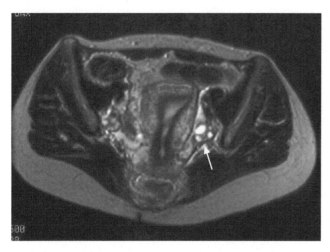

Fig. 10-25. A cluster of physiologic cysts is demonstrated within the left ovary *(arrow)* on transaxial fast spin echo T2-weighted image (TR 4500, effective TE 120, 4 Nex, 16 echo train). The uterus is anteverted.

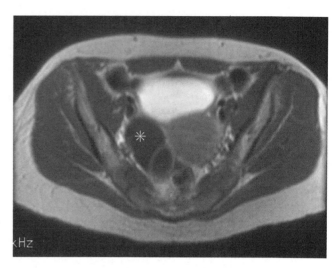

Fig. 10-27. Transaxial T1-weighted image (TR 500, TE 11, 4 Nex) demonstrates septated cyst *(asterisk)* involving right ovary in 47-year-old female.

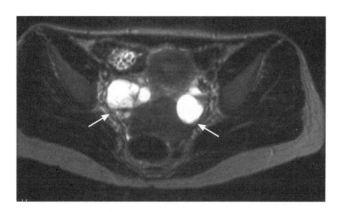

Fig. 10-26. Simple adnexal cysts are demonstrated bilaterally *(arrows)* in 24-year-old female on transaxial fast spin echo T2-weighted image (TR 4000, effective TE 120, 2 Nex, 16 echo train).

important. Ascites is a relatively nonspecific finding and does not correlate strongly with the presence of peritoneal metastases.[68] The presence of calcification is another finding that may increase suspicion of malignancy. However, standard spin echo MR images are inherently insensitive to depiction of calcifications.[92] When calcifications are suspected, gradient echo images should be acquired.

Highly variable signal intensity may be observed within cystic ovarian tumors, corresponding to mucinous or hemorrhagic components and tissue debris; these changes can obscure underlying soft tissue components and complicate distinction of benign and malignant lesions.[68] When hemorrhage is observed within a cystic

ovarian mass, the lesion must be closely evaluated for signs of malignancy. When a benign hemorrhagic cyst is suspected, ultrasound may be used to document its ultimate resolution.[65] In some situations, use of contrast material can be useful for separating cystic and solid components. When contrast material is given, unenhanced T1-weighted images must first be acquired.[34] Some ovarian lesions, such as those containing hemorrhage or fat, may be hyperintense on unenhanced T1-weighted images, simulating the appearance of lesion enhancement. Most adnexal masses demonstrate a nonspecific contrast enhancement pattern, so that contrast material does not usually improve lesion characterization.[85]

Hemorrhagic ovarian lesions may appear indistinguishable from those containing fat (i.e., dermoid), since both appear hyperintense on T1-weighted images (Figs. 10-28, *A* and *B*). This is a relatively frequent situation, since hemorrhagic ovarian lesions are common, and dermoid cyst (i.e., cystic teratoma) is the most common ovarian tumor. Both types of lesions may be isointense with subcutaneous fat on T1- and T2-weighted images. Another less frequent mass with high signal intensity on T1-weighted images is lymphocele, which may be present in patients who have undergone previous lymphadenectomy.

Observation of chemical shift misregistration artifacts along the frequency encoded direction of the image can be used to indicate the presence of a fat-fluid interface.[65] However, fat- and hemorrhage-containing lesions are most definitively distinguished using fat suppression techniques. Fat saturation involves delivery of radiofrequency pulses at the resonant frequency of fat, resulting in selective suppression of fat signal intensity. Con-

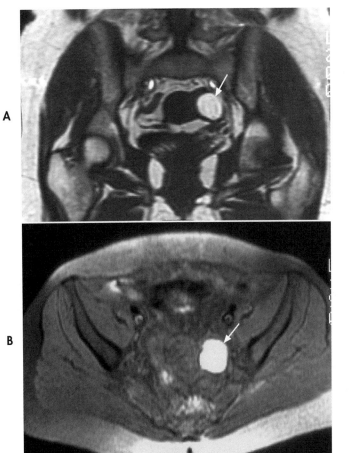

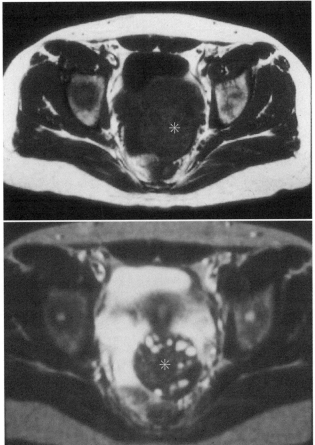

Fig. 10-28. A, Coronal T1-weighted image (TR 300, TE 20, 1 Nex) demonstrates 2 cm left adnexal mass *(arrow)* with signal intensity characteristics similar to those of fat. **B,** Transaxial T1-weighted image with fat suppression reveals persistent hyperintensity, indicating absence of fat, with signal characteristics likely caused by hemorrhage within ovarian cyst.

Fig. 10-29. Transaxial T1-weighted **(A)** and T2-weighted **(B)** images demonstrate marked enlargement of the left ovary *(asterisk)* with prominence of follicles along its periphery in patient with acute ovarian torsion.

versely, water saturation pulses can be used to reduce the signal intensity of hemorrhagic fluid.[49] The short tau inversion recovery (STIR) method also results in fat suppression. However, such suppression is based on the short T1 relaxation of fat, not on its specific resonant frequency. Consequently, other short T1 tissues, such as hemorrhage or contrast enhancing tissues, may be potentially suppressed on STIR images. One report indicates that endometriomas may occasionally demonstrate suppression on STIR images.[59]

Endometriomas may appear similar to hemorrhagic ovarian cysts, though features that suggest the former diagnosis include multiplicity, alteration in morphology, and nonuniform signal intensity on T2-weighted images.[65] The presence of multiple sites of hemorrhage of different ages is also characteristic. Fibrous implants and

adhesions resulting from endometriosis are not reliably depicted on MR images.[65]

Even when it can be determined that a given ovarian mass is solid, this does not indicate that ovarian carcinoma is the necessary diagnosis. For example, metastases to the ovaries can occur, particularly from gastrointestinal tract tumors (i.e., Krukenberg tumor).[83] Struma ovarii can also present as an ovarian mass with both cystic and solid components. The associated calcifications are relatively inconspicuous on spin echo MR images.[58]

Ovarian torsion may occur in patients with ovarian masses. In patients with ovarian torsion, findings consist of dilatation of adnexal vasculature, deviation of the uterus toward the affected side, edema within the surrounding fat, and mild ascites (Figs. 10-29, *A* and *B*).[51] These findings are nonspecific and can occur with a variety of ovarian abnormalities. When torsion progresses to hemorrhagic ovarian infarction, more characteristic findings are observed, including masslike protrusion of the affected ovary, which is surrounded by engorged vessels, hematoma, and absence of ovarian enhancement with contrast material. Another finding indicating hemorrhagic infarction is peripheral high signal intensity of the involved ovary on T1-weighted images.[45] Intermittent or partial torsion of its vascular pedicle can lead to "massive ovarian edema," which can simulate an ovarian neoplasm.[27]

Patients with polycystic ovary syndrome often demonstrate enlarged ovaries because of hypertrophied stroma, though large cysts are not a feature of this condition.[65] Diagnosis should be based on clinical and laboratory findings, since MR findings may overlap with those of normal ovaries.

Decreased signal intensity on T2-weighted images can be observed with Brenner tumor, as well as fibrothecomas (Fig. 10-10).[59] Pedunculated leiomyoma may simulate a solid low signal intensity ovarian mass.[95] Unusually large nabothian cysts can simulate a cystic adnexal mass.[90]

REFERENCES

1. Apicella P, Mirowitz SA: Interactive multiplanar interpolation of two-dimensional MR images, Clin Imaging 19(4):287-290, 1995.
2. Arrive L, Chang YCF, Hricak H et al: Radiation-induced uterine changes: MR imaging, Radiology 170:55-58, 1989.
3. Arrive L, Hricak H, Martin MC: Pelvic endometriosis: MR imaging, Radiology 171:687-692, 1989.
4. Ascher SM, Arnold LL, Patt RH et al: Adenomyosis: prospective comparison of MR imaging and transvaginal sonography, Radiology 190:803-806, 1994.
5. Ascher SM, Scoutt LM, McCarthy SM et al: Uterine changes after dilatation and curettage: MR imaging findings, Radiology 180:433-435, 1991.
6. Barton JW, McCarthy SM, Kohorn EI et al: Pelvic MR imaging findings in gestational trophoblastic disease, incomplete abortion, and ectopic pregnancy: are they specific? Radiology 186:163-168, 1993.
7. Baudouin CJ, Soutter WP, Gilderdale DJ et al: Magnetic resonance imaging of the uterine cervix using an intravaginal coil, Magn Reson Med 24:196-203, 1992.
8. Baumgartner BR, Bernardino ME: MR imaging of the cervix: off-axis scan to improve visualization of zonal anatomy, Am J Roentgenol 153:1001-1002, 1989.
9. Bergman RA, Thompson SA, Afifi AK et al: Compendium of human anatomic variation: text, atlas, and world literature, Baltimore, 1988, Urban & Schwarzenberg.
10. Brodman M, Friedman F Jr, Dottino P et al: A comparative study of computerized tomography, magnetic resonance imaging, and clinical staging for the detection of early cervix cancer, Gynecol Oncol 36:409-412, 1990.
11. Brown HK, Stoll BS, Nicosia SV et al: Uterine junctional zone: correlation between histologic findings and MR imaging, Radiology 179:409-413, 1991.
12. Brown JJ, Gutierrez ED, Lee JKT: MR appearance of the normal and abnormal vagina after hysterectomy, Am J Roentgenol 158:95-99, 1992.
13. Brown JJ, Thurnher S, Hricak H: MR imaging of the uterus: low-signal-intensity abnormalities of the endometrium and endometrial cavity, Magn Reson Imaging 8:309-313, 1990.
14. Carrington BM, Hricak H, Nuruddin RN et al: Mullerian duct anomalies: MR imaging evaluation, Radiology 176:715-720, 1990.
15. Chang YC, Hricak H, Thurnher S et al: Vagina: evaluation with MR imaging. Part II. Neoplasms, Radiology 169:175-179, 1988.
16. Dang HT, Terk MR, Colletti PM et al: Primary lymphoma of the cervix: MRI findings with gadolinium, Magn Reson Imaging 9:941-944, 1991.
17. Demas BE, Hricak H, Jaffe RB: Uterine MR imaging: effects of hormonal stimulation, Radiology 159:123-126, 1986.
18. Dudiak CM, Turner DA, Patel SK et al: Uterine leiomyomas in the infertile patient: preoperative localization with MR imaging versus US and hysterosalpingography, Radiology 167:627-630, 1988.
19. Ebner F, Kressel HY, Mintz MC et al: Tumor recurrence versus fibrosis in the female pelvis: differentiation with MR imaging at 1.5 T, Radiology 166:333-340, 1988.
20. Egashira K, Nakamura K, Terashima H et al: MR imaging in uterine cervical cancer after radiotherapy, Radiat Med 10:117-122, 1992.
21. Fedele L, Dorta M, Brioschi D et al: Magnetic resonance evaluation of double uteri, Obstet Gynecol 74:844-847, 1989.
22. Fedele L, Dorta M, Brioschi D et al: Magnetic resonance imaging in Mayer-Rokitansky-Kuster-Hauser syndrome, Obstet Gynecol 76:593-596, 1990.
23. Fluckiger F, Ebner F, Poschauko H et al: Value of magnetic resonance tomography after primary irradiation of carcinoma of the cervix uteri: evaluation of therapeutic success and follow-up, Strahlentherapie Onkol 167:152-157, 1991.
24. Flueckiger F, Ebner F, Poschauko H et al: Cervical cancer: serial MR imaging before and after primary radiation therapy—a 2 year follow-up study, Radiology 184:89-93, 1992.
25. Fujita T, Ito K, Choji T et al: Usefulness of 2D FLASH multislice dynamic MR imaging for evaluation of parametrial invasion in cervical carcinoma, Nippon Igaku Hoshasen Gakkai Zasshi 53:472-474, 1993.
26. Goto M, Okamura S, Ueki M et al: Evaluation of magnetic resonance imaging in the diagnosis of extension in uterine cervical cancer cases with special attention to imaging planes, Nippon Sanka Fujinka Gakkai Zasshi—Acta Obstet Gynaecol Jpn 42:1627-1633, 1990.
27. Hall BP, Printz DA, Roth J: Massive ovarian edema: ultrasound and MR characteristics, J Comput Assist Tomogr 17:477-479, 1993.
28. Hamlin DJ, Pettersson H, Fitzsimmons J et al: MR imaging of uterine leiomyomas and their complications, J Comput Assist Tomogr 9:902-907, 1985.

29. Hanabayashi T, Imai A, Itoh N et al: Enhanced magnetic resonance imaging evaluation for spread of cervical carcinoma, Int J Gynaecol Obstet 43:297-304, 1993.

30. Hawes DR, Hemann LS, Cornell AE et al: Hemangioma of the uterine cervix: sonographic and MR diagnosis, J Comput Assist Tomogr 15:152-154, 1991.

31. Hirano Y, Kubo K, Hirai Y et al: Preliminary experience with gadolinium-enhanced dynamic MR imaging for uterine neoplasms, RadioGraphics 12:243-256, 1992.

32. Hoeffner EG, Soulen RL, Christensen CW: Gelatin sponge mimicking a pelvic neoplasm on MR imaging, Am J Roentgenol 157:1227-1228, 1991.

33. Hricak H: Postoperative and postradiation changes in the pelvis, Magn Reson Q 6:276-297, 1990.

34. Hricak H: Current trends in MR imaging of the female pelvis, RadioGraphics 13:913-919, 1993.

35. Hricak H, Chang YCF, Cann CE et al: Cervical incompetence: preliminary evaluation with MR imaging, Radiology 174:821-826, 1990.

36. Hricak H, Chang YC, Thurnher S: Vagina: evaluation with MR imaging. Part I. Normal anatomy and congenital anomalies, Radiology 169:169-174, 1988.

37. Hricak H, Hamm B, Semelka RC et al: Carcinoma of the uterus: use of gadopentetate dimeglumine in MR imaging, Radiology 181:95-106, 1991.

38. Hricak H, Quivey JM, Campos Z et al: Carcinoma of the cervix: predictive value of clinical and magnetic resonance (MR) imaging assessment of prognostic factors, Int J Radiat Oncol Biol Phys 27:791-801, 1993.

39. Hricak H, Stern JL, Fisher MR et al: Endometrial carcinoma staging by MR imaging, Radiology 162:297-305, 1987.

40. Hricak H, Tscholakoff D, Heinrichs L et al: Uterine leiomyomas: correlation of MR, histopathologic findings, and symptoms, Radiology 158:385-391, 1986.

41. Janus CL, Bateman B, Wiczyk H et al: Evaluation of the stimulated menstrual cycle by magnetic resonance imaging, Fertil Steril 54:1017-1020, 1990.

42. Janus CL, Mendelson DS, Moore S et al: Staging of cervical carcinoma: accuracy of magnetic resonance imaging and computed tomography, Clin Imaging 13:114-116, 1989.

43. Janus CL, Wiczyk HP, Laufer N: Magnetic resonance imaging of the menstrual cycle, Magn Reson Imaging 6:669-674, 1988.

44. Karasick S, Lev-Toaff AS, Toaff ME: Imaging of uterine leiomyomas, Am J Roentgenol 158:799-805, 1992.

45. Kawakami K, Murata K, Kawaguchi N et al: Hemorrhagic infarction of the diseased ovary: a common MR finding in two cases, Magn Reson Imaging 11:595-597, 1993.

46. Kawakami S, Togashi K, Sagoh T et al: Uterine deformity caused by surgery during pregnancy, J Comput Assist Tomogr 18:272-274, 1994.

47. Kier R: Nonovarian gynecologic cysts: MR imaging findings, Am J Roentgenol 158:1265-1269, 1992.

48. Kier R, Chambers SK: Surgical transposition of the ovaries: imaging findings in 14 patients, Am J Roentgenol 153:1003-1006, 1989.

49. Kier R, Smith RC, McCarthy SM: Value of lipid- and water-suppression MR images in distinguishing between blood and lipid within ovarian masses, Am J Roentgenol 158:321-325, 1992.

50. Kim SH, Kim SC, Choi BI et al: Uterine cervical carcinoma: evaluation of pelvic lymph node metastasis with MR imaging, Radiology 190:807-811, 1994.

51. Kimura I, Togashi K, Kawakami S et al: Ovarian torsion: CT and MR imaging appearances, Radiology 190:337-341, 1994.

52. Levine D, Gosink BB, Wolf SI et al: Simple adnexal cysts: the natural history in postmenopausal women, Radiology 184:653-659, 1992.

53. Lien HH, Blomlie V, Iversen T et al: Clinical stage I carcinoma of the cervix: value of MR imaging in determining invasion into the parametrium, Acta Radiol 34:130-132, 1993.

54. Lien HH, Blomlie V, Kjorstad K et al: Clinical stage I carcinoma of the cervix: value of MR imaging in determining degree of invasiveness, Am J Roentgenol 156:1191-1194, 1991.

55. Lubich LM, Alderman MG, Ros PR: Magnetic resonance imaging of leiomyomata uteri: assessing therapy with the gonadotropin-releasing hormone agonist leuprolide, Magn Reson Imaging 9:331-334, 1991.

56. Mark AS, Hricak H: Intrauterine contraceptive devices: MR imaging, Radiology 162:311-314, 1987.

57. Mark AS, Hricak H, Heinrichs LW et al: Adenomyosis and leiomyoma: differential diagnosis with MR imaging, Radiology 163:527-529, 1987.

58. Matsumoto F, Yoshioka H, Hamada T et al: Struma ovarii: CT and MR findings, J Comput Assist Tomogr 14:310-312, 1990.

59. Mawhinney RR, Powell MC, Worthington BS, et al: Magnetic resonance imaging of benign ovarian masses, Br J Radiol 61:179-186, 1988.

60. McCarthy S: Magnetic resonance imaging of the normal female pelvis, Radiol Clin North Am 30:769-775, 1992.

61. McCarthy S, Scott G, Majumdar S et al: Uterine junctional zone: MR study of water content and relaxation properties, Radiology 171:241-243, 1989.

62. McCarthy SM, Tauber C, Gore J: Female pelvic anatomy: MR assessment of variations during the menstrual cycle and with use of oral contraceptives, Radiology 160:119-123, 1986.

63. Milestone BN, Schnall MD, Lenkinski RE et al: Cervical carcinoma: MR imaging with an endorectal surface coil, Radiology 180:91-95, 1991.

64. Mintz MC, Thickman DI, Gussman D et al: MR evaluation of uterine anomalies, Am J Roentgenol 148:287-290, 1987.

65. Mitchell DG: Benign disease of the uterus and ovaries: applications of magnetic resonance imaging, Radiol Clin North Am 30:777-787, 1992.

66. Mitchell DG, Schonholz L, Hipert PL et al: Zones of the uterus: discrepancy between US and MR images, Radiology 174:827-831, 1990.

67. Mouloupoulos LA, Varma DG, Charnsangavej C et al: Magnetic resonance imaging and computed tomography appearance of asymptomatic paravaginal cysts, Clin Imaging 17:126-132, 1993.

68. Outwater E, Kressel HY: Evaluation of gynecologic malignancy by magnetic resonance imaging, Radiol Clin North Am 30:789-806, 1992.

69. Pellerito JS, McCarthy SM, Doyle MB et al: Diagnosis of uterine anomalies: relative accuracy of MR imaging, endo-

vaginal sonography, and hysterosalpingograph, Radiology 183:795-800, 1992.

70. Rubens D, Thornbury JR, Angel C et al: Stage IB cervical carcinoma: comparison of clinical, MR, and pathologic staging, Am J Roentgenol 150:135-138, 1988.

71. Santoni R, Bucciolini M, Chiostrini C et al: Quantitative magnetic resonance imaging in cervical carcinoma: a report on 30 cases, Br J Radiol 64:498-504, 1991.

72. Schmidt B, Kolbel G, Kuper K et al: T2-weighted MR images of gynecologic tumors with the FLASH sequence: the initial experiences at 1.5 T, Rofo Fortschr Geb Rontgenstr Neuen Bildgeb Verfahr 151:306-310, 1989.

73. Schnall MD: Magnetic resonance evaluation of uterine malignancies, Semin Ultrasound, CT MRI 15:27-37, 1994.

74. Scoutt LM, Flynn SD, Luthringer DJ et al: Junctional zone of the uterus: correlation of MR imaging and histologic examination of hysterectomy specimens, Radiology 179:403-407, 1991.

75. Sironi S, Belloni C, Taccagni G et al: Invasive cervical carcinoma: MR imaging after preoperative chemotherapy, Radiology 180:719-722, 1991.

76. Sironi S, Belloni C, Taccagni GL et al: Carcinoma of the cervix: value of MR imaging in detecting parametrial involvement, Am J Roentgenol 156:753-756, 1991.

77. Sironi S, Colombo E, Villa G et al: Myometrial invasion by endometrial carcinoma: assessment with plain and gadolinium-enhanced MR imaging, Radiology 185:207-212, 1992.

78. Sironi S, De Cobelli F, Scarfone G et al: Carcinoma of the cervix: value of plain and gadolinium-enhanced MR imaging in assessing degree of invasiveness, Radiology 188:797-801, 1993.

79. Smith RC, Reinhold C, McCauley TR et al: Multicoil high-resolution fast spin-echo MR imaging of the female pelvis, Radiology 184:671-675, 1992.

80. Soeters RP, Beningfield SJ, Dehaeck K et al: The value of magnetic resonance imaging in patients with carcinoma of the cervix (a pilot study), Eur J Surg Oncol 17:119-124, 1991.

81. Soyer P, Rigaud C, Masselot J et al: Evaluation of the role of MRI at 1.5 T in the staging of the initial extension of cancer of the uterine cervix, J Belge Radiol 74:85-90, 1991.

82. Stehling MK, Mansfield P, Ordidge RJ et al: Echo-planar imaging of the human fetus in utero, Magn Reson Med 13:314-318, 1990.

83. Takemori M, Nishimura R, Obayashi C et al: Magnetic resonance imaging of Krukenberg tumor from gastric cancer, Eur J Obstet Gynecol Reprod Biol 47:161-163, 1992.

84. Takemori M, Nishimura R, Sugimura K: Magnetic resonance imaging of uterine leiomyosarcoma, Arch Gynecol Obstet 251:215-218, 1992.

85. Thurner SA: MR imaging of pelvic masses in women: contrast-enhanced vs unenhanced images, Am J Roentgenol 159:1243-1250, 1992.

86. Togashi K, Kawakami S, Kimura I et al: Uterine contrac-

87. Togashi K, Kawakami S, Kimura I et al: Sustained uterine contractions: a cause of hypointense myometrial bulging, Radiology 187:707-710, 1993.

88. Togashi K, Nishimura K, Itoh K et al: Uterine cervical cancer: assessment with high-field MR imaging, Radiology 160:431-435, 1986.

89. Togashi K, Nishimura K, Itoh K et al: Adenomyosis: diagnosis with MR imaging, Radiology 166:111-114, 1988.

90. Togashi K, Noma S, Ozasa H: CT and MR demonstration of nabothian cysts mimicking a cystic adnexal mass, J Comput Assist Tomogr 11:1091-1092, 1987.

91. Togashi K, Ozasa H, Konishi I et al: Enlarged uterus: differentiation between adenomyosis and leiomyoma with MR imaging, Radiology 171:531-534, 1989.

92. Tsuruda JS, Bradley WG: MR detection of intracranial calcification: a phantom study, Am J Neuroradiol 8:1049-1055, 1987.

93. van Gils APG, Tham RTOTA, Falke THM et al: Abnormalities of the uterus and cervix after diethylstilbesterol exposure: correlation of findings on MR and hysterosalpingography, Am J Roentgenol 153:1235-1238, 1989.

94. Waggenspack GA, Amparo EG, Hannigan EV: MR imaging of uterine cervical carcinoma, J Comput Assist Tomogr 12:409-414, 1988.

95. Weinreb JC, Barkoff ND, Megibow A et al: The value of MR imaging in distinguishing leiomyomas from other solid pelvic masses when sonography is indeterminate, Am J Roentgenol 154:295-299, 1990.

96. Woo GM, Twickler DM, Stettler RW et al: The pelvis after cesarean section and vaginal delivery: normal MR findings, Am J Roentgenol 161:1249-1252, 1993.

97. Woodward PJ, Wagner BJ, Farley TE: MR imaging in the evaluation of female infertility, RadioGraphics 13:293-310, 1993.

98. Yamashita Y, Harada M, Sawada T et al: Normal uterus and FIGO stage I endometrial carcinoma: dynamic gadolinium-enhanced MR imaging, Radiology 186:495-501, 1993.

99. Yamashita Y, Takahashi M, Katabuchi H et al: Adenoma malignum: MR appearances mimicking nabothian cysts, Am J Roentgenol 162:649-650, 1994.

100. Yamashita Y, Takahashi M, Sawada T et al: Carcinoma of the cervix: dynamic MR imaging, Radiology 182:643-648, 1992.

101. Yamashita Y, Torashima M, Takahashi M et al: Hyperintense uterine leiomyoma at T2-weighted MR imaging: differentiation with dynamic enhanced MR imaging and clinical implications, Radiology 189:721-725, 1993.

102. Yoder IC: Diagnosis of uterine anomalies: relative accuracy of MR imaging, endovaginal sonography and hysterosalpingography, Radiology 185:343, 1992.

103. Zawin M, McCarthy S, Scoutt LM et al: High-field MRI and US evaluation of the pelvis in women with leiomyomas, Magn Reson Imaging 8:371-376, 1990.

tions: possible diagnostic pitfall at MR imaging, J Magn Reson Imaging 3:889-893, 1993.

Section Four

MUSCULOSKELETAL SYSTEM

11

Knee

MENISCI

The most frequent indication for magnetic resonance (MR) imaging of the knee is a suspected meniscal tear. MR is highly sensitive for detection of meniscal tears. However, many pitfalls can lead to false-positive or false-negative diagnoses.

Anatomic variations

The menisci are subject to anatomic variations in their size, shape, and position. The menisci typically have a triangular configuration on coronal or sagittal images. Peripheral sagittal images through the meniscus depict a "bow-tie" configuration corresponding to the body of the meniscus. Enlargement and globular configuration of the meniscus are manifestations of a discoid meniscus.[95] This congenital variation is more common with the lateral meniscus than with the medial meniscus and predisposes to meniscal degeneration and tears. Visualization of a "bow-tie" configuration on three or more successive sagittal images has been used as an indication of discoid meniscus (Figs. 11-1 and 11-2). However, patient

---

ENTITIES THAT MAY SIMULATE MENISCAL ABNORMALITY

- Intrameniscal degenerative changes
- Narrow window display
- Gradient-echo imaging
- Vascular pedicle
- Exercise
- Calcification
- Partial volume averaging of free edge/middle third
- Meniscofemoral ligaments
- Lateral geniculate artery
- Popliteus tendon/sheath
- Transverse intermeniscal ligament
- Truncation artifact
- Motion artifact
- Chemical shift misregistration artifact
- Fibrofatty tissue at meniscocapsular junction
- Postoperative changes
- Susceptibility artifact

---

size, slice thickness, and intersection gap must be considered when applying this criterion. For example, a meniscus seen on three consecutive 3 mm thick images may be visualized on only two images of 5 mm thickness. Discoid meniscus is not an "all-or-none" phenomenon; rather, variable degrees of discoid change may be manifested.

Reduced size of the meniscus or a portion of a meniscus (e.g., the anterior horn of the lateral meniscus) may also be encountered as an anatomic variant. Patients with juvenile rheumatoid arthritis can also demonstrate hypoplastic or atrophic menisci.[88] Meniscal shortening can be simulated when the knee is placed in an exces-

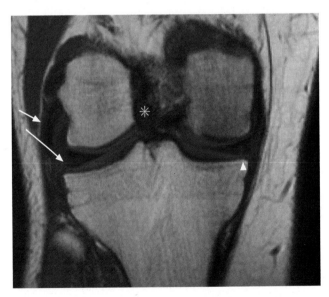

Fig. 11-1. Coronal T1-weighted image (TR 550, TE 20, 2 Nex) demonstrates discoid lateral meniscus *(arrow)*. The height of the lateral meniscus is considerably increased as compared with that of the medial meniscus, which demonstrates a tear in its midportion *(arrowhead)*. Also note partial visualization of the fibular collateral ligament *(small arrow)*. The remainder of the ligament could be identified on a more posterior section. There is also evidence of anterior cruciate ligament tear *(asterisk)* and reduced signal intensity within the medial femoral condyle caused by marrow contusion.

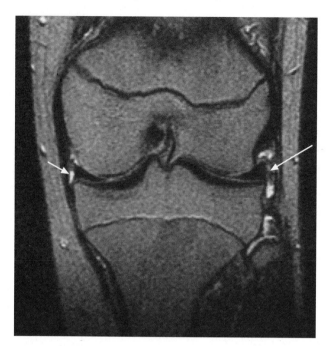

Fig. 11-2. Coronal T2-weighted image (TR 2250, TE 75, 1 Nex) in skeletally immature knee demonstrates unfused femoral and tibial physes, with increased signal intensity adjacent to the physis caused by chemical shift misregistration artifact. Also note relative increased size of the lateral meniscus *(arrow)*, indicating mild discoid morphology. There is fluid within a prominent meniscosynovial recess along the medial aspect of the knee *(small arrow)*, which may simulate meniscocapsular separation.

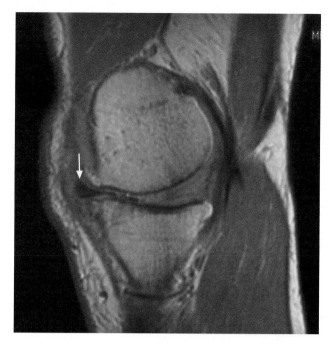

Fig. 11-3. Sagittal proton density–weighted image (TR 2250, TE 16, 1 Nex) demonstrates anterior subluxation of the anterior horn of the medial meniscus *(arrow)*. There is associated degenerative joint disease manifested by hyaline cartilage thinning and anterior femoral condyle osteophyte formation. Note extensive tear involving the posterior horn of the medial meniscus.

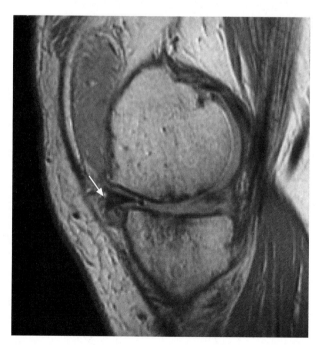

Fig. 11-4. Anterior subluxation of the anterior horn of the medial meniscus *(arrow)* is demonstrated on sagittal proton density–weighted image (TR 2250, TE 16, 1 Nex). The meniscus shows degenerative signal changes anteriorly and an extensive degenerative-type tear posteriorly. A joint effusion is also present.

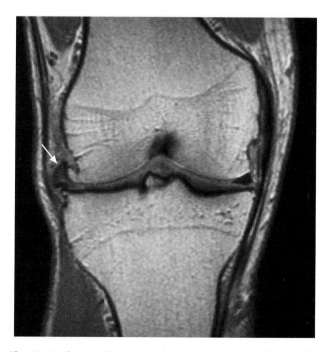

Fig. 11-5. The medial meniscus *(arrow)* is subluxed medially on this coronal proton density–weighted image (TR 2250, TE 16, 1 Nex). Extensive signal is noted throughout the medial meniscus, indicating a degenerative-type tear, and marked medial compartment degenerative joint disease is seen as well. Note linear structures within distal femur and proximal tibia, which represent penetrating vessels.

sive external rotation. Correlation with coronal and transaxial images is helpful in making this determination.

Alterations in meniscal position most frequently relate to displacement of torn meniscal fragments. However, subluxation of an intact meniscus can also occur. This most frequently involves the anterior horns, which sublux forward relative to the anterior tibial plateau (Figs. 11-3 to 11-5). This is associated with degenerative joint disease, though it is unclear whether meniscal subluxation occurs secondary to joint space narrowing or whether it could be a primary factor in the development of degenerative changes.

Simulation of Meniscal Tear
Intrameniscal degenerative changes

A meniscal tear is usually diagnosed on MR images when linear intrameniscal signal intensity is seen extending to an articular surface (i.e., grade III signal alterations). Numerous entities can simulate a meniscal tear. Globular (grade I) or linear (grade II) intrameniscal signal intensity abnormalities usually indicate mucoid and eosinophilic meniscal degeneration.[46] Grade I signal changes are easily distinguished from a meniscal tear. However, distinction from grade II changes may be difficult, particularly when the linear abnormal signal intensity approaches the articular surface (Fig. 11-6). When contact of abnormal meniscal signal intensity with the articular surface is questionable, an arthroscopically identifiable meniscal tear is usually not present.[24] Brightening of the signal alteration as it approaches the articular surface indicates a meniscal tear, whereas meniscal degeneration usually exhibits reduced signal intensity as the articular surface is approached.[49,100,103]

Grade II signal alterations have been subdivided into IIA (a linear increased signal that fails to extend to an articular surface on any image), IIB (extends to an articular surface on only one image and in only one view), and IIC (wedge-shaped signal that does not contact surface).[29] In the series by Dillon et al, grade IIB signal abnormalities were usually seen in the meniscal body and demonstrated apparent articular extension on a single coronal image. These findings did not correlate with an arthroscopically visible meniscal tear, whereas tears were seen in half of the patients with grade IIC signal abnormalities. The likelihood of an arthroscopically identifiable meniscal tear increases in proportion to the number of images on which contact between meniscal signal intensity and the articular surface is demonstrated, though for some tears such contact may be evident on only a single image.[24]

Meniscal degeneration increases with patient age and can lead to grade III signal alterations or diffuse meniscal signal alterations.[46] This likely contributes to decreased accuracy of MR imaging for diagnosis of meniscal tear in elderly patients.[46]

When intrameniscal degenerative changes are present,

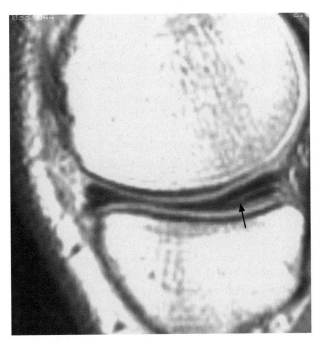

Fig. 11-6. Sagittal proton density–weighted image (TR 2250, TE 16, 1 Nex) photographed with "meniscal window" settings demonstrates linear increased signal intensity *(arrow)* within the substance of the posterior horn of the medial meniscus. This abnormal signal intensity approaches but does not appear to extend to the inferior articular surface, indicating type II signal pattern.

the meniscal surface will appear intact to the arthroscopist, and the MR will be considered to have yielded a false-positive result. While MR may indeed overstage some meniscal abnormalities, the limitations of arthroscopy as a "gold standard" have been recognized.[78] When extensive meniscal signal changes are noted on MR images, it is highly likely that the involved meniscus is abnormal, even though it may demonstrate a normal surface appearance, since arthroscopy does not permit evaluation of the meniscal substance. Arthroscopy may also provide for limited evaluation of some inaccessible portions of the menisci, such as the posterior periphery of the medial meniscus.

Visualization of meniscal signal abnormalities—including those indicative of a tear—does not necessarily correlate to patient symptomatology; these changes can be encountered in asymptomatic patients.[15,55] Close correlation between imaging findings, patient history, and a physical examination is therefore necessary to provide meaningful assessment of the significance of MR observations.

Image display factors

Image display factors including window and level settings affect the ability to accurately characterize meniscal signal abnormalities. Whereas high contrast narrow window settings are routinely used in some centers to increase the conspicuousness of abnormal meniscal signal intensity, these images can potentially overaccentuate the extent of an abnormal signal. In such cases, it is possible that intrameniscal degenerative changes will be misinterpreted as a meniscal tear. No significant improvement in detection of meniscal tears has been found when meniscal window images are used.[16] It is important that image display factors be consistent among different patients at a given site, so that such errors are avoided.

Imaging plane

The menisci are usually evaluated using sagittal images, though oblique sagittal gradient echo images acquired about the meniscus (i.e., radial imaging) has been advocated as a means of improving depiction of the meniscus and related abnormalities. This technique yields images similar to those obtained during arthrography, in that the meniscus is segmentally profiled. In a series of 259 arthroscopically proven cases, however, it was found that radial images provide no significant improvement as compared with standard orthogonal views.[79] To the contrary, radial images were found to have several limitations. For example, the meniscocapsular junction can be hyperintense on such images, obscuring peripheral meniscal tears. Saturation effects occur where images overlap one another in the central knee, causing artifactual signal loss.

Pulse sequence parameters

Gradient echo pulse sequences can also cause intrameniscal signal alterations to become accentuated, causing tears to become obscured or overestimated.[43] Selection of pulse sequence parameters (i.e., TR, TE, flip angle) should be based on controlled optimization studies. Furthermore, clinical experience should provide a template for the range of expected meniscal signal alterations using a given set of imaging parameters.

Vascular pedicle

There are causes for meniscal signal alterations other than degeneration or tear. In children and early adolescents, prominent intrameniscal signal intensity is often visualized within the posterior horns extending from the meniscocapsular junction (Figs. 11-7 to 11-8, A-C). This is related to the vascular pedicle of the meniscus, which undergoes subsequent regression in the adult.[88] These findings become less prominent during the early teen years.

Exercise/calcification

Increased meniscal signal intensity can also reflect a transient reaction to recent stress, rather than a permanent alteration in meniscal structure. Increased intrameniscal signal intensity can be observed in patients following recent or prolonged exercise such as running, during which the menisci are subjected to significant impaction forces.[57,83,89] An additional cause for increased meniscal signal intensity is scarring or reactive change related to meniscal calcifications.[46] These findings can simulate a meniscal tear.

Partial volume effects

Volume averaging of the meniscus with adjacent anatomic structures can also simulate a meniscal tear. Sagittal images acquired through the periphery of the meniscus frequently demonstrate horizontally oriented meniscal signal alterations. These findings are due to partial volume averaging of the meniscal body with adjacent fat[42] and can appear to represent meniscal degeneration or a tear. These partial volume effects can also render tears involving the free edge or middle third of the menisci difficult to visualize.[68,78] Tears involving these portions of the meniscus may be more easily detected on coronal rather than sagittal images. Some vertical meniscal tears may also be missed on sagittal images, though they are easily identified in the coronal plane. Thin section transaxial images have been used to identify meniscal tears.[5] However, such tears are rarely evident on routine transaxial spin echo or gradient echo images.

The midportion of the meniscus is visualized on pe-

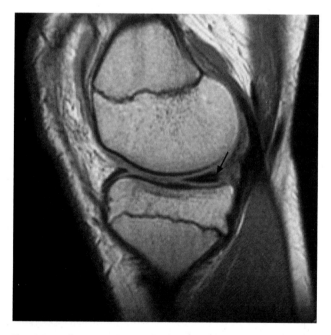

Fig. 11-7. There is a linear focus of relative increased signal intensity *(arrow)* noted within the posterior horn of the medial meniscus on this sagittal proton density–weighted image (TR 2250, TE 16, 1 Nex). This represents the meniscal vascular pedicle in this skeletally immature knee. Also note unfused femoral and tibial physes.

ripheral sagittal images, where a "bow-tie" configuration is seen. The "bow-tie" appearance of the meniscal body is normally evident on at least one sagittal image.[100] When the meniscal body is not visualized, a tear should be suspected (Figs. 11-9, *A* and *B* and 11-10, *A* and *B*).

Meniscofemoral ligaments/Geniculate artery

Fibrofatty tissue is interposed between the meniscofemoral ligaments (i.e., ligaments of Humphry and Wrisberg) and the medial aspects of the menisci. Relative increased signal intensity associated with fibrofatty tissue can simulate a meniscal tear[19,99,106,110] (Fig. 11-11, *A* and *B*). The oblique orientation of the apparent tear is atypical for a meniscal injury, and coronal images will depict the meniscus as normal. Along the lateral aspect of the knee, the lateral geniculate artery can also contribute to simulation of a meniscal tear.[42]

Popliteus tendon

Fibrofatty tissue located between the low signal intensity posterior horn of the lateral meniscus and the adjacent popliteus tendon can also simulate a meniscal tear on T1- or proton density–weighted images[42,110] (Figs. 11-12 to 11-16, *B*). Fluid located within the popliteus tendon sheath can present a similar pitfall on T2-weighted images. Conversely, an actual tear involving the posterior horn of the lateral meniscus may be overlooked when the fragment is assumed to represent the normal popliteus tendon.

Transverse ligament

The transverse intermeniscal ligament unites the anterior horns of the medial and lateral menisci (Fig. 11-17). This low signal intensity structure is closely apposed to the anterior meniscal horns and is surrounded by fi-

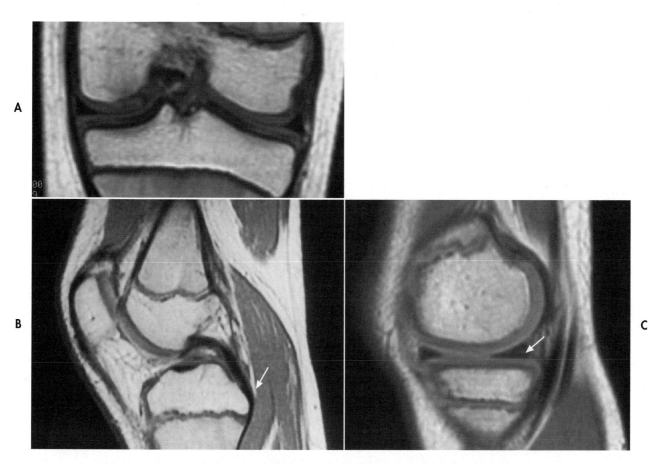

Fig. 11-8. A, Coronal T1-weighted image (TR 500, TE 20, 2 Nex) in 11-year-old female demonstrates relatively thick hyaline articular cartilage. A thin linear focus of decreased signal intensity separates the two cartilaginous laminae. **B** and **C,** Sagittal proton density–weighted images (TR 2250, TE 16, 1 Nex) demonstrate a relatively low insertion of posterior cruciate ligament *(arrow).* There is also relatively increased signal intensity noted within the posterior horn of the medial meniscus *(arrow),* representing the meniscal vascular pedicle.

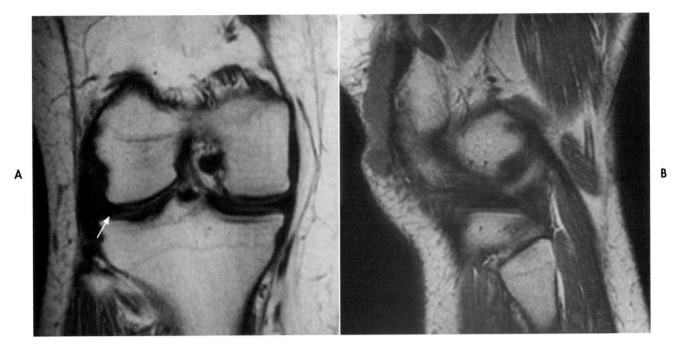

Fig. 11-9. A, An obliquely oriented tear *(arrow)* involving the midportion of the lateral meniscus is identified on coronal T1-weighted image (TR 500, TE 20, 2 Nex). The tear extends into a parameniscal cyst laterally. **B,** Tear is poorly visualized on sagittal proton density–weighted image (TR 2250, TE 16, 1 Nex) acquired through the midportion of the meniscus or on adjacent images.

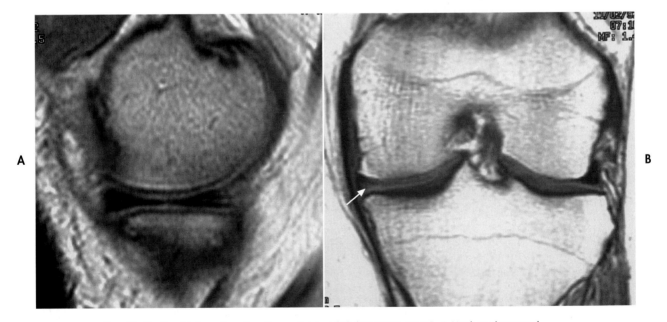

Fig. 11-10. Sagittal proton density–weighted **(A)** (TR 2250, TE 16, 1 Nex) and coronal T1-weighted **(B)** (TR 500, TE 20, 2 Nex) images of the knee, filmed using "meniscal window" settings. The sagittal image acquired through the periphery of the medial meniscus fails to demonstrate the expected "bow-tie" configuration. This is due to a tear involving the meniscal body *(arrow)*, as confirmed on coronal image.

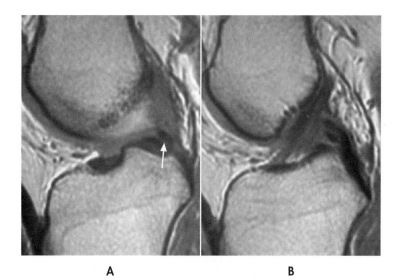

Fig. 11-11. A, A linear oblique focus of relative increased signal intensity *(arrow)* simulates the appearance of a meniscal tear on sagittal proton density–weighted image (TR 2250, TE 16, 1 Nex). The apparent tear is due to fibrofatty tissue interposed between the anterior meniscofemoral ligament and the posterior horn of the lateral meniscus, as verified on adjacent image **(B).**

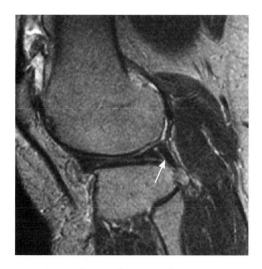

Fig. 11-12. A linear focus of increased signal intensity *(arrow)* extends through the posterior horn of the lateral meniscus, simulating meniscal tear on sagittal T2-weighted image (TR 2250, TE 70, 1 Nex). This represents fluid within the popliteus tendon sheath, with the dark structure located dorsal to the sheath representing the tendon itself. Note globular foci of decreased signal intensity within the distended suprapatellar bursa *(asterisk),* caused by blood clot. This may simulate hyperplastic synovium (pannus), osteochondral bodies, or tumor.

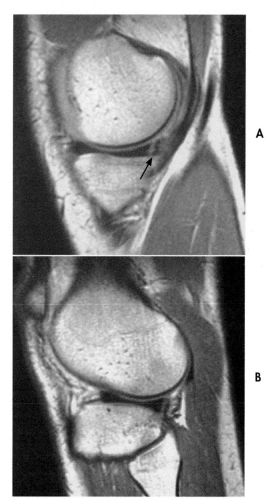

Fig. 11-13. A, Parasagittal proton density–weighted image (TR 2250, TE 16, 1 Nex) along medial aspect of knee demonstrates vertical increased signal intensity *(arrow)* caused by peripheral tear of posterior horn of medial meniscus. This tear has a similar appearance to normal popliteus tendon sheath, as depicted on a lateral image in same patient **(B).**

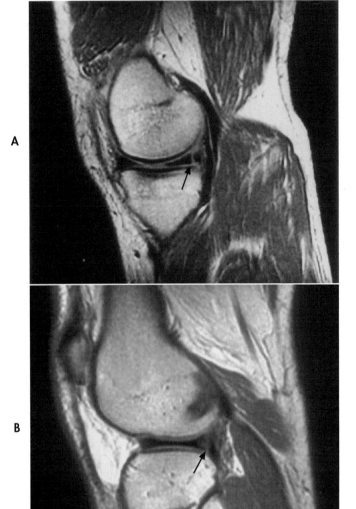

A

B

Fig. 11-14. Sagittal proton density–weighted images (TR 2250, TE 16, 1 Nex) demonstrate vertical linear foci *(arrows)* of increased signal intensity extending through the posterior knee medially **(A)** and laterally **(B)**. On the lateral side, this represents fibrofatty tissue surrounding the popliteus tendon, whereas similar finding medially indicates a peripheral meniscal tear.

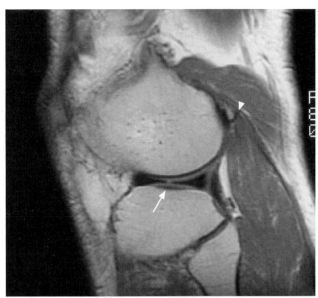

Fig. 11-15. Sagittal proton density–weighted image (TR 2200, TE 20, 1 Nex) through the lateral meniscus demonstrates small rounded focus of intrameniscal signal *(arrow)* representing a radial tear. A linear focus of increased signal intensity along the posterior aspect of the meniscus represents the popliteus tendon sheath, which may simulate meniscal tear. The fabella is visualized within the lateral head of the gastrocnemius muscle *(arrowhead)*.

brofatty tissue that can simulate a meniscal tear[42,110] (Figs. 11-18 and 11-19). This pitfall most frequently involves the anterior horn of the lateral meniscus. Close inspection will show the rounded transverse ligament to be present on successive sagittal images, allowing for its recognition and distinction from a meniscal tear.

Each of these causes for simulated meniscal tears can be easily recognized. Exclusion of a meniscal tear can be confirmed by comparison of sagittal images with those acquired in other planes, particularly the coronal plane. When an apparent meniscal tear cannot be identified in both the sagittal and the coronal images, the possibility of a pseudotear should be considered.

Truncation artifact

Truncation artifacts reflect the limited ability of the Fourier transform to accurately depict sharp transitions in image contrast. These artifacts are manifested as a series of alternating high and low signal intensity lines paralleling a high-contrast interface. A truncation artifact is most apparent when a rectangular (e.g., 128×256) matrix is used and is usually seen along the phase-encoding direction of the image. The low signal intensity meniscus is bordered by high signal intensity hyaline cartilage and subjacent marrow fat; this presents a high contrast interface where truncation artifacts arise.

The phase-encoding direction is usually assigned along the anteroposterior axis of the knee by default. However, reorientation of phase encoding along the superior-inferior axis can be performed to redirect popliteal artery pulsation artifacts away from the cruciate ligaments. In this situation, truncation artifacts may appear as curvilinear increased signal intensity correspond-

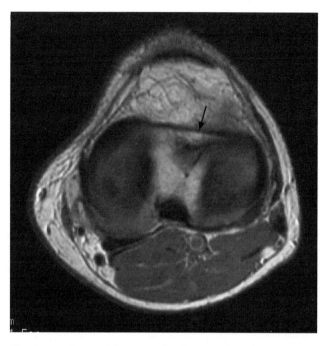

Fig. 11-17. Transaxial proton density–weighted image demonstrates the transverse intermeniscal ligament of the knee *(arrow).*

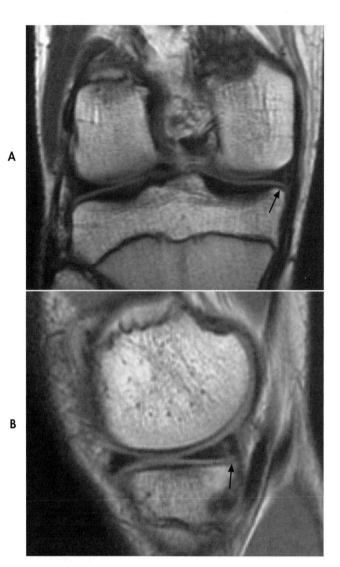

Fig. 11-16. A, Coronal T1-weighted image (TR 550, TE 20, 2 Nex) demonstrates vertical focus of increased signal intensity near the medial meniscocapsular attachment *(arrow).* **B,** Sagittal proton density–weighted image (TR 2250, TE 16, 1 Nex) demonstrates a vertical peripheral tear of the medial meniscus *(arrow).* The portion of meniscus located between the tear and the meniscocapsular attachment simulates the appearance of the normal popliteus tendon.

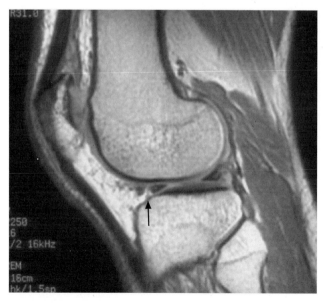

Fig. 11-18. Sagittal proton density–weighted image (TR 2250, TE 16, 1 Nex) demonstrates apparent tear *(arrow)* involving anterior horn of lateral meniscus. This is due to fibrofatty tissue interposed between the meniscus and the adjacent transverse intermeniscal ligament.

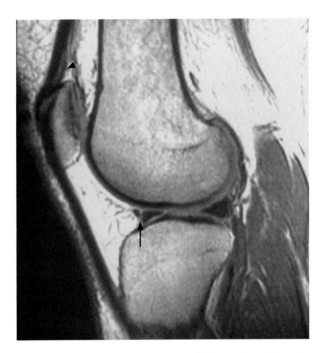

Fig. 11-19. There is an apparent vertical tear involving the anterior horn of the lateral meniscus *(arrow)* on sagittal proton density–weighted image (TR 2250, TE 16, 1 Nex). This is due to fibrofatty tissue surrounding the transverse intermeniscal ligament where it is apposed to the normal anterior lateral meniscus. Also note linear focus of relative increased signal intensity within the distal quadriceps tendon *(arrowhead)* caused by fibrofatty tissue between the tendinous laminae.

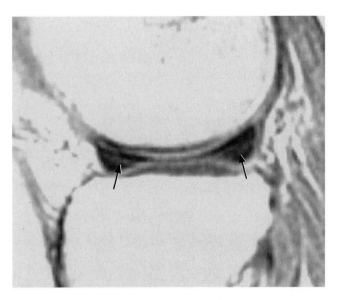

Fig. 11-20. A series of curvilinear foci of increased signal intensity *(arrows)* parallel the femoral condyle and overlie the lateral meniscus on sagittal proton density–weighted image (TR 2250, TE 16, 1 Nex) photographed using "meniscal window" settings. These represent truncation artifacts originating from high-contrast interface between marrow fat/hyaline cartilage and meniscus.

ing to the configuration of the femoral condyle. These artifacts can traverse the menisci, simulating a meniscal tear[105] (Fig. 11-20).

There are several options for reducing truncation artifacts. First, a moderate (e.g., 192 × 256) or high (e.g., 256 × 256) resolution imaging matrix will render these artifacts less prominent. Truncation artifacts are usually not evident on high-resolution images. Second, phase encoding may be oriented along the anteroposterior axis of the knee, so that truncation artifacts are redirected and less likely to simulate a meniscal tear. Third, filtering methods can be used to decrease the prominence of truncation artifacts.

Motion artifact

Reorientation of phase encoding along the superior-inferior axis of the knee can simulate a meniscal tear through another mechanism. When motion occurs during image acquisition, partial or complete replications of the moving structure (i.e., ghost artifacts) occur and propagate along the phase-encoding direction of the image. Motion of the knee can therefore lead to high signal intensity replications of the femoral condyles. These

artifacts traverse the menisci, where they can closely simulate the appearance of a meniscal tear[69] (Figs. 11-21, *A* and *B* to 11-24). Such artifacts can arise from even subtle knee motion. To distinguish motion artifacts from actual tears, the image should be closely inspected for additional evidence of patient motion. This can be manifested as generalized blurring or as ghosting artifacts elsewhere in the image. When uncertainty persists, images should be reacquired after implementing methods to diminish the likelihood of patient motion. These methods can include reassurance, application of physical restraints about the knee, or use of analgesics or sedatives for patients who are particularly uncomfortable or anxious. Another option is to repeat the sequence with the phase-encoded direction oriented along the anteroposterior axis of the knee, so that motion artifacts will be displaced away from the menisci.

Chemical shift misregistration artifact

A chemical shift misregistration artifact refers to artifactual displacement of signal intensity at fat-water interfaces. They are manifested as artifactual decreased signal intensities at one fat-water border, with corresponding increased signal intensity at the opposite fat-water border. These artifacts occur along the frequency-encoded direction of the image and reflect the difference in precessional frequency between fat and water protons. When frequency encoding is oriented along the superior-

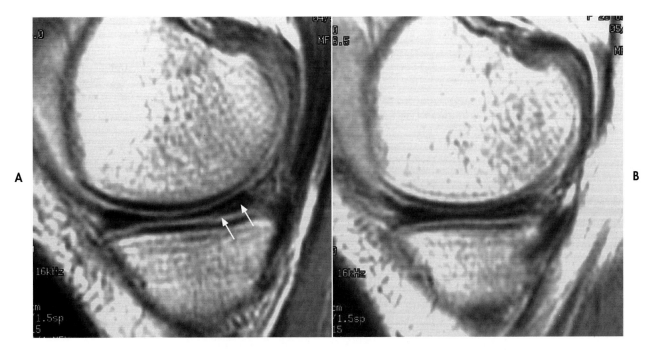

Fig. 11-21. A, Curvilinear signal *(arrows)* extends through the posterior horn of the medial meniscus and appears to communicate with the inferior articular surface, on sagittal proton density–weighted image (TR 2250, TE 16, 1 Nex). **B,** However, same sequence acquired 5 days later demonstrates no evidence of meniscal tear. Previous findings are due to subtle motion of the knee during image acquisition.

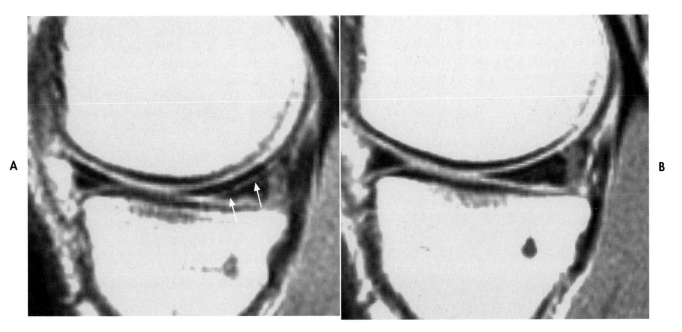

Fig. 11-22. A, Linear increased signal intensity *(arrows)* is observed within the lateral meniscus, with apparent extension to the inferior articular surface on sagittal proton density-weighted image (TR 2250, TE 16, 1 Nex). While these findings are suggestive of meniscal tear, repeat image using identical parameters **(B)** demonstrates the meniscus to be normal.

inferior axis of the knee, the high signal intensity component of these artifacts can tranverse the meniscus, simulating a tear. Chemical shift misregistration effects are reduced when a broad receiver bandwidth is used, though this reduces the signal-to-noise ratio of the image. Chemical shift effects are also reduced when images are acquired on a low field strength unit and when small voxel sizes are used. Fat suppression techniques represent another means for reducing chemical shift artifacts. Finally, gradient reorientation will redirect such artifacts away from the menisci.

Meniscocapsular separation

Meniscocapsular separation is a specific type of tear in which the meniscus is torn peripherally near its attachment at the joint capsule. This type of tear may be difficult to visualize arthroscopically. It is also unique in that it can undergo spontaneous healing because of its proximity to vascular supply. Meniscocapsular separation is diagnosed on MR images when a vertically oriented fluid collection is visualized along the meniscocapsular junction (Figs. 11-23 to 11-24).

Diagnosis of meniscocapsular separation is associated with several pitfalls. Prominent fibrofatty tissue may be present at the meniscocapsular junction; this can simulate the appearance of separation on T1- or proton density–weighted images. T2-weighted images must be used to confirm that high-signal intensity in this location represents fluid rather than fat. Fat suppression techniques can be useful in this determination. Another cause for a false-positive diagnosis is fluid within the meniscosynovial recesses (Figs. 11-2, 11-25, and 11-26). These recesses are located along the superior and inferior margins of the meniscocapsular junction and can be distended with synovial fluid. In some patients, the superior and inferior meniscosynovial recesses approach one another and appear to represent a continuous linear fluid collection. Close inspection will usually reveal these recesses to have an angular tip and to be separate rather than continuous.

High signal intensity within the meniscus may persist in patients who have sustained previous meniscal tears.[25] Therefore MR images do not necessarily indicate an acute meniscal injury, and correlation with clinical information is again important.

Posttherapy changes

Meniscal signal intensity alterations also persist following primary repair of a meniscal tear.[25,34] While these signal alterations frequently resemble linear degenerative (type II) changes, they can be indistinguishable from meniscal tears. These findings can be evident for at least 1 year after surgery and do indicate a retear.[51]

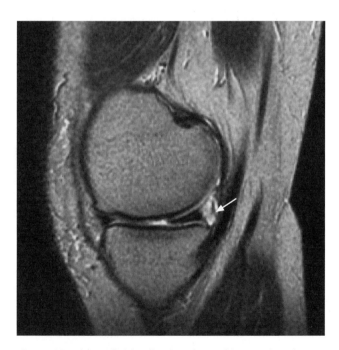

Fig. 11-23. Linear fluid collection *(arrow)* is noted at the meniscocapsular junction, indicating separation on sagittal T2-weighted image (TR 2250, TE 70, 1 Nex). The signal intensity of this abnormality was similar to that of fat on the first echo image.

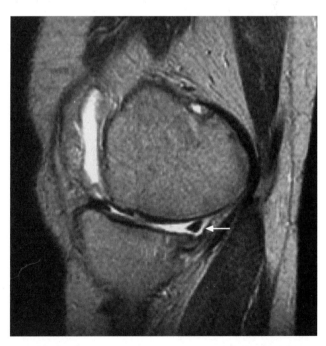

Fig. 11-24. A continuous linear fluid collection *(arrow)* is demonstrated along the posterior aspect of the posterior horn of the medial meniscus on sagittal T2-weighted image (TR 2250, TE 70, 1 Nex). This represents a meniscocapsular separation and is to be distinguished from fluid within prominent meniscosynovial recesses, which do not form a continuous appearance as seen here.

The menisci can be difficult to evaluate in patients who have undergone previous partial meniscectomy. Considerable meniscal deformity and abnormal intrameniscal signal intensity can be observed in such patients. In those patients in whom the meniscal remnant is well defined and without diffuse amorphous signal alterations, the remnant can be evaluated for tears using standard MR criteria. However, when the meniscal remnant appears significantly deformed or even fragmented and contains diffuse linear and/or globular signal alterations, these postoperative changes can either simulate or obscure meniscal tears.[34,78,98] Blunting of the meniscal tip can be a normal finding following a previous meniscectomy.[26]

Observation of fluid tracking into a tear involving the meniscal remnant on T2-weighted images is very specific for a retear. However, most tears do not demonstrate this finding, thus T2-weighted imaging is very insensitive.[4] MR arthrography, using intraarticular contrast material, can improve the accuracy of MR imaging for detection of tears involving the meniscal remnant. In one series, accuracy for standard MR was 66%, whereas MR arthrography yielded an 88% accuracy.[4]

Susceptibility artifact

Intraarticular metal, hemorrhage, or air can result in susceptibility artifacts. These artifacts appear as foci of signal void that can be surrounded by irregular increased signal intensity. The high-signal intensity component can overlie the meniscus, simulating a meniscal tear[94] (Figs. 11-27, A and B). Susceptibilty artifacts can also result in anatomic distortion in a localized region of the image. These artifacts are less prominent when imaging is performed using low field strength systems, short echo times, a high-resolution matrix, and spin echo rather than gradient echo pulse sequences. Susceptibility artifacts are also more prominent on images acquired using fat saturation (Figs. 11-28, A and B). Small signal void foci are frequently observed in and around the knee joint in patients who have undergone a previous arthroscopy. These represent metallic microfragments related to instrumentation, and they are usually not evident on plain radiographs.

Pulse sequence parameters

The detection of meniscal tears requires images that have adequate signal-to-noise ratio. The combined effect of long TR and short TE on proton density–weighted spin echo images is advantageous in this regard and allows for identification of most meniscal tears. Although T1-weighted images can be acquired more rapidly, they may display suboptimal signal-to-noise ratios, particularly when low-field strength systems and single-data excitations are used. Use of a dedicated extremity coil improves the signal-to-noise ratio considerably, and quadrature coils or multicoil arrays are especially advantageous.

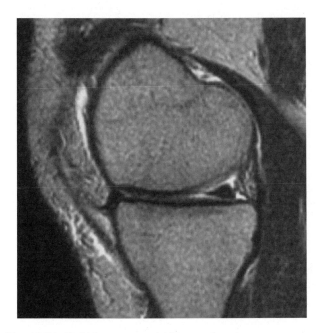

Fig. 11-25. Fluid is present within prominent meniscosynovial recesses on sagittal T2-weighted image (TR 2250, TE 70, 1 Nex). This appearance simulates a meniscocapsular separation.

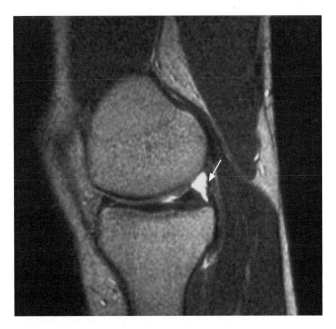

Fig. 11-26. Sagittal T2-weighted image (TR 2250, TE 70, 1 Nex) demonstrates fluid within prominent superior meniscosynovial recess *(arrow)*, simulating a meniscocapsular separation.

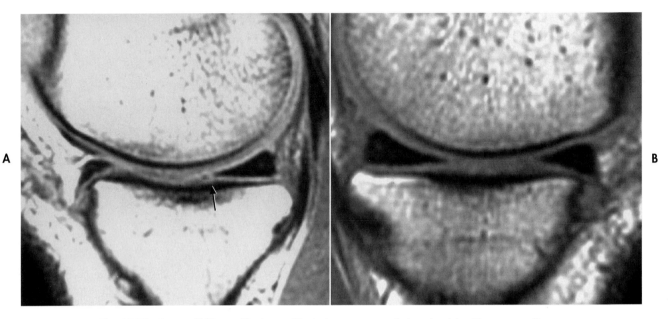

Fig. 11-27. Susceptibility artifact, manifested as an area of signal void with surrounding hyperintensity *(arrow)*, simulates a tear of the posterior horn of the medial meniscus in this patient with intra-articular air related to previous arthrocentesis **(A)**. Repeat MR examination performed at a later date demonstrates the medial meniscus to have a normal appearance **(B)**.

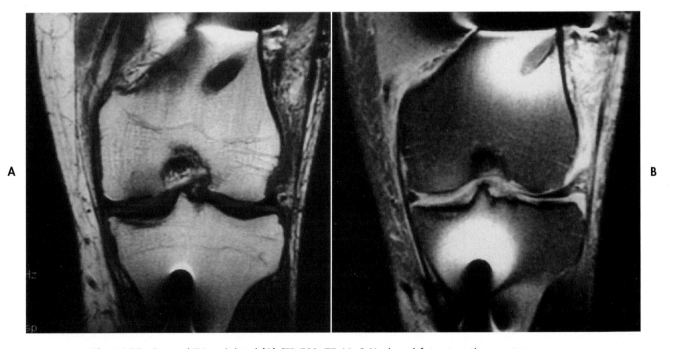

Fig. 11-28. Coronal T1-weighted **(A)** (TR 500, TE 11, 2 Nex) and fat saturation proton density–weighted **(B)** (TR 2250, TE 16, 1 Nex) images in patient who underwent anterior cruciate ligament reconstruction. There are foci of artifactual signal loss surrounded by increased signal intensity, with the latter findings markedly accentuated on fat suppressed image. High signal intensity within the marrow space on fat suppressed image may simulate bone marrow edema.

Although T2-weighted images are acquired in most centers, these images cannot be relied on for demonstrating meniscal tears. Most tears depicted on proton density–weighted images are not be visualized on corresponding T2-weighted images[68] because of the reduced signal-to-noise ratio on T2-weighted images and the lack of contained fluid within most tears. T2-weighted images are most useful for evaluating abnormalities of the intraarticular space and juxtaarticular soft tissues.

Adequate spatial resolution is also necessary for detecting small meniscal tears. Knee imaging should be performed using a restricted field-of-view (e.g., 16 cm), moderate resolution imaging matrix (e.g., 192 × 256), and relatively thin slices (e.g., 3 to 4 mm) with minimal interslice gaps (e.g., 0.5 mm).[100] These parameters result in small voxel sizes, which place even greater emphasis on the need for high signal-to-noise ratio.

One subtle and often overlooked sign of meniscal tear is the "notch sign."[23] This appears as a subtle irregularity of the meniscal surface, often in the absence of abnormal intrameniscal signal intensity (Fig. 11-29). Radial meniscal tears appear as small foci of abnormal signal intensity within the substance of the meniscus. They are often rounded rather than having the linear oblique configuration typical of most tears (Figs. 11-16, *A* and *B*). Radial meniscal tears can be difficult to visualize on MR images, particularly when they involve the posterior horn of the lateral meniscus.[30] Three-dimensional reconstructions of standard two-dimensional data can be useful in improving the depiction of these and other tears.[30]

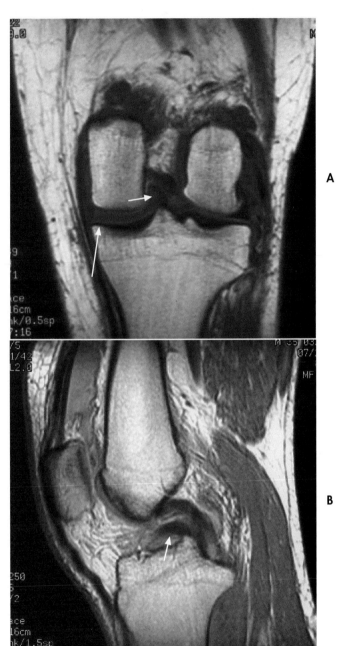

A

B

Fig. 11-30. A, Increased signal intensity and shortening of the medial meniscus *(arrow)* are demonstrated on coronal T1-weighted image (TR 550, TE 20, 2 Nex). A large meniscal fragment *(small arrow)* is displaced into the intercondylar notch, lodged beneath the posterior cruciate ligament. This is also depicted on sagittal proton density-weighted image **(B)** (TR 2250, TE 16, 1 Nex). A large joint effusion is present.

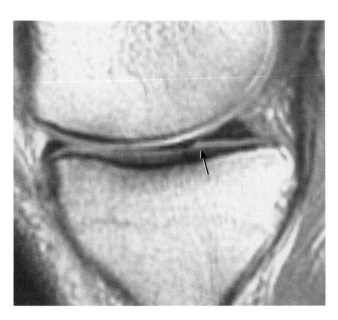

Fig. 11-29. A small notch *(arrow)* along the undersurface of the posterior horn of the medial meniscus is the only indication of a meniscal tear on this sagittal proton density–weighted image (TR 2250, TE 16, 1 Nex).

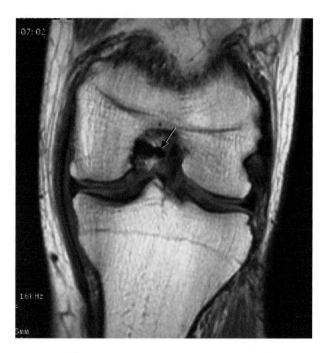

Fig. 11-31. There is apparent duplication of the posterior cruciate ligament on this coronal T1-weighted image (TR 550, TE 20, 2 Nex). The medial structure *(arrow)* represents a meniscal fragment that has been displaced into the intercondylar notch because of a bucket-handle type of tear.

Decreased meniscal size is another indication of a tear, even when intramensical signal abnormalities are not observed. The posterior horn of the medial meniscus—a frequent site of tear—should be approximately twice as long as the corresponding anterior horn. This is in distinction to the lateral meniscus, where the anterior and posterior horns are of similar size. When the medial meniscus does not demonstrate this normal disparity in size between its anterior and posterior horns, a displaced (i.e., bucket handle) tear of the posterior medial meniscus should be suspected (Figs. 11-30, *A* and *B*).

Identification of displaced meniscal fragments can be difficult. These fragments frequently migrate into the intercondylar notch where they can appear to represent the posterior cruciate or meniscofemoral ligaments[37,96,111] (Fig. 11-31).

CRUCIATE LIGAMENTS
Anatomic variations

Anatomic variants include congenital absence or accessory slips of a cruciate ligament.[10] A relatively low tibial insertion of the posterior cruciate ligament can be observed in children[88] (Figs. 11-32, *A* and *B* and 11-33).

ENTITIES THAT MAY SIMULATE CRUCIATE LIGAMENT ABNORMALITIES

- Relative hyperintensity anterior cruciate ligament
- Eosinophilic degeneration
- Fluid along synovial reflection
- Partial volume averaging with adjacent fat/fluid/femoral condyle
- Incorrect patient positioning/imaging axis
- Popliteal artery pulsation artifacts
- Postoperative changes

Signal intensity characteristics

The normal posterior cruciate ligament appears of uniformly low signal intensity on all pulse sequences. This differs from the anterior cruciate ligament, which is mildly hyperintense on both T1- and T2-weighted sequences.[47,60] The anterior cruciate ligament is also somewhat less defined than the posterior cruciate ligament. These findings reflect the composition of the anterior cruciate ligament, which consists of small fascicles of collagenous fibers surrounded by and intertwined with fibrofatty tissues.[47] The posterior cruciate ligament, by contrast, consists of closely packed parallel fascicles. Despite these differences in overall composition, individual fibers of the anterior and posterior cruciate ligaments are histologically similar.[47] The relative hyperintensity of the normal anterior cruciate ligament should not be misconstrued as evidence of hemorrhage and/or edema related to injury.

Localized or diffuse foci of relative increased signal intensity can be observed within both cruciate ligaments because of eosinophilic degeneration.[104] These findings are most prevalent in elderly patients and can simulate partial thickness cruciate ligament tears.[47]

Fluid can be seen tracking along the synovial reflection anterior to the anterior cruciate ligament in patients with joint effusions (Fig. 11-34). This does not imply injury to the ligament itself.

The anterior cruciate ligament courses lateral to the posterior cruciate ligament, so both structures are frequently not identified on a single midsagittal image. The anterior cruciate ligament is usually more difficult to evaluate than the posterior cruciate ligament because of the fanlike morphology of the anterior cruciate ligament and its more oblique course through the intercondylar notch. Because of these features, the entire length of the anterior cruciate ligament often cannot be visualized on a single sagittal image (Fig. 11-39). In such cases, the anterior cruciate ligament must be evaluated segmentally over two or three adjacent sections. The posterior cruciate ligament is thicker and more cordlike and is more closely aligned along the sagittal plane.

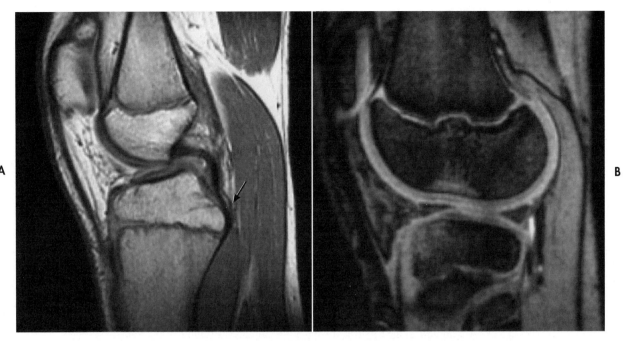

Fig. 11-32. A, Sagittal proton density–weighted image (TR 2250, TE 20, 1 Nex) in 13-year-old male demonstrates relatively low insertion of the posterior cruciate ligament *(arrow).* **B,** Sagittal oblique gradient echo image (TR 400, TE 12, 20-degree flip angle, 2 Nex) demonstrates prominent hyaline cartilage with low signal intensity line separating cartilaginous laminae. An unfused physeal plate is also demonstrated. Note marrow edema within the subchondral femoral condyle caused by trabecular bone injury.

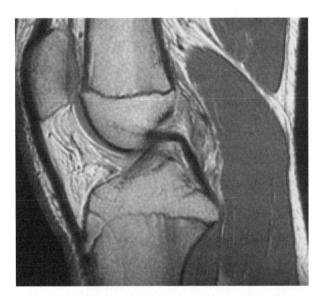

Fig. 11-33. Midsagittal proton density–weighted image (TR 2250, TE 16, 1 Nex) demonstrates relatively low insertion of the posterior cruciate ligament in skeletally immature knee. Also note that the anterior cruciate ligament can only be partially visualized on this image. Incomplete fusion of the physeal plate is also demonstrated.

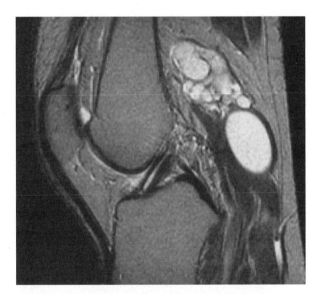

Fig. 11-34. A large popliteal cyst is present within the gastrocnemius-semimembranosus bursa. This cyst contains multiple loculations of varying size caused by intervening septae. There is partial visualization of the anterior cruciate ligament, despite the absence of abnormality of this structure. Also note fluid extending along the synovial reflection ventral to the anterior cruciate ligament.

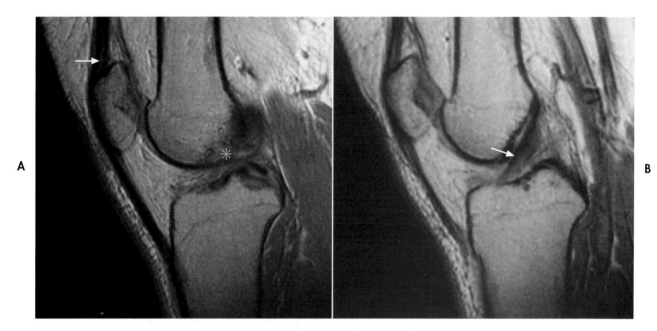

Fig. 11-35. A, Midsagittal proton density–weighted image (TR 2250, TE 16, 1 Nex) demonstrates apparent rupture of the anterior cruciate ligament *(asterisk).* This is due to partial volume averaging of the ligament with adjacent fat in the intercondylar notch. **B,** The adjacent image demonstrates the ligament *(arrow)* to be intact. Also noted on **A** are linear foci of relative increased signal intensity extending throughout the quadriceps tendon *(arrow).* While these findings may simulate inflammatory and/or posttraumatic process, they represent fibrofatty tissue interposed between the laminae of the tendon complex.

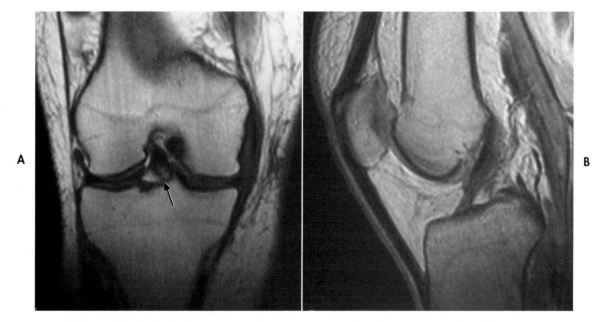

Fig. 11-36. A, There is an apparent hematoma related to the anterior cruciate ligament *(arrow)* on coronal T1-weighted image (TR 500, TE 20, 2 Nex). This is due to partial volume averaging of the ligament with adjacent fat. The anterior cruciate ligament is normal, as verified on sagittal proton density-weighted image **(B)** (TR 2250, TE 16, 1 Nex).

Partial volume effects

Because the cruciate ligaments course obliquely through the intercondylar notch, sagittal images may display partial volume averaging between the cruciate ligaments and adjacent fat.[68] Apparent focal thickening or relative increased signal intensity of the cruciate ligaments can result. Partial volume averaging of the anterior cruciate ligament with the lateral femoral condyle can also occur on sagittal images, again simulating tear of the former structure.[104,108] The anterior cruciate ligament can undergo volume averaging with synovial fluid in patients with joint effusion, which can also simulate a tear.[108] Because the midportion of the anterior cruciate ligament is somewhat thinner than that of the posterior cruciate ligament, it is more vulnerable to partial volume effects.[47] Waviness and ill definition of the cruciate ligaments—particularly the anterior cruciate ligament—can also be observed in the absence of injury.[107] These findings can simulate partial or full thickness tear (Figs. 11-35, A and B).

Imaging planes

Alignment of the anterior cruciate ligament along the sagittal plane is improved when the knee in positioned in approximately 15 degrees of external rotation.[68,82] When this is unsuccessful or cannot be achieved because of patient discomfort, an oblique imaging plane can be prescribed parallel to the course of the anterior cruciate ligament, as shown on an initial coronal sequence.[16] Careful inspection of coronal images for evidence of cruciate ligament injury can also be instrumental as an adjunct to sagittal images, since they are often less vulnerable to partial volume effects.[36] However, partial volume averaging of the anterior cruciate ligament with adjacent fat can occur on coronal images, simulating ligamentous injury (Figs. 11-36, A and B).

Partial volume effects can be reduced with use of thin imaging slices (e.g., 3 mm) and small interslice gaps (<0.5 mm). Three-dimensional Fourier transform sequences provide contiguous images that can be reformatted in any orthogonal or oblique imaging plane. Multiplanar reformation of images acquired using isotropic voxels (voxels with equal cubic dimensions) are of equivalent spatial resolution to the original data set (Figs. 11-37, A-C to 11-38, A-C). However, some loss of resolution occurs when anisotropic images are reformatted. The major limitation of three-dimensional Fourier imaging is significant prolongation of image acquisition time, since phase encoding is performed along both the conventional phase encode and the slice select directions. Acquisition time is increased proportional to the number of partitions (phase encoded steps in the slice-select di-

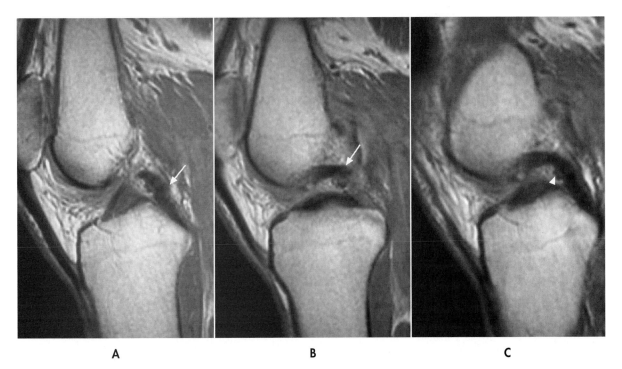

A   B   C

Fig. 11-37. A and **B,** Two contiguous sagittal proton density–weighted images (TR 2250, TE 16, 1 Nex) demonstrate segmental visualization of posterior cruciate ligament *(arrows),* making its evaluation difficult. **C,** Reformatted image from same data set shows the ligament in continuity, verifying that it is intact. The ligament of Humphrey *(arrowhead)* can also be visualized.

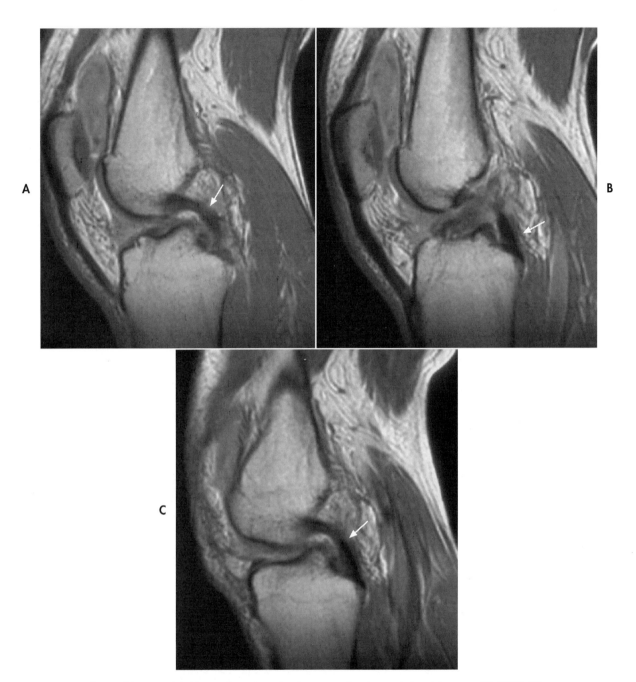

Fig. 11-38. A and **B,** Two adjacent sagittal proton density–weighted images (TR 2250, TE 16, 1 Nex) provide segmental visualization of the posterior cruciate ligament *(arrow),* making its evaluation difficult. **C,** Reformatted image from same data set demonstrates entire ligament *(arrow)* on single image, verifying that it is normal. The anterior cruciate ligament is torn.

rection) acquired. Because 32 to 64 partitions are usually necessary to provide adequate spatial resolution and coverage, three-dimensional imaging is impractical using standard spin-echo sequences. However, gradient-echo sequences can be used to provide reasonable acquisition times. Imaging parameters including TR, TE, and flip angle should be optimized to provide adequate

signal-to-noise ratio and tissue contrast for visualization of cruciate ligament as well as other knee pathology.

A tricubic interpolation or other similar algorithms can be used to retrospectively reformat standard two-dimensional Fourier transform spin-echo images along the course of the cruciate ligaments or other structures of interest.[3] While this technique can be very useful, some degradation of image quality is incurred.

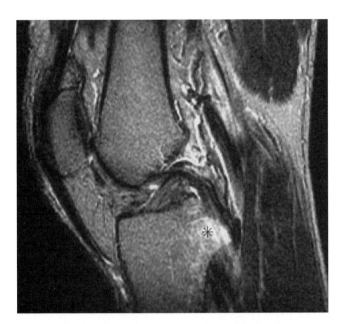

Fig. 11-39. Popliteal artery pulsation artifact obscures visualization of the cruciate ligaments on sagittal T2-weighted image (TR 2250, TE 70, 1 Nex), and results in artifactual increased signal intensity within the distal posterior cruciate ligament. There is also an apparent high signal intensity lesion within the posterior tibia, *(asterisk)* likewise related to vascular pulsation artifact.

Pulsation artifacts

Pulsation of the popliteal artery results in a series of high and low signal intensity artifacts that propagate along the phase-encoding direction (i.e., usually antero-posterior) of the image. Cruciate ligament tears can be either simulated or obscured by these artifacts (Fig. 11-45). There are several approaches for reducing the effects of a vascular pulsation artifact on the cruciate ligaments. First, spatial presaturation radiofrequency pulses applied above and below the imaging slice will reduce the signal intensity of flowing blood, and hence the artifacts generated as a result of their motion. Gradient moment nulling involves implementation of additional gradient lobes to rephase the signal of flowing spins. This method requires a nominally long echo time and is useful primarily on T2-weighted sequences.

Gradient reorientation offers yet another complementary approach to the problem of vascular pulsation artifacts. This technique involves reassignment of the phase-encoded gradient along the superior-inferior rather than anterior-posterior axis of the knee. While this does not eliminate vascular pulsation artifacts, it does redirect them away from the cruciate ligaments. Because tissue extending outside the field-of-view in the phase-encoded direction will lead to aliasing (i.e., wraparound) artifacts, an oversampling technique such as no-phase wrap should be used.

Indirect signs of cruciate ligament injury

Laxity of the cruciate ligaments is a secondary indication of a tear. However, laxity of these ligaments can be observed in the absence of tears.[60] Cruciate ligament laxity can occur when the knee is not positioned in full extension. In addition, laxity of one cruciate ligament can occur secondary to disruption of its counterpart. For example, forward subluxation of the tibia in patients with anterior cruciate ligament tears can cause laxity and redundancy of the posterior cruciate ligament. In this situation, one must recognize that the observed laxity does not imply primary injury to the posterior cruciate ligament. In one study, the anterior cruciate ligament was consistently torn whenever 7 mm or more of anterior subluxation of the tibia was observed, and tibial subluxation of 5 mm was highly suggestive of such tear.[108] The anterior horn of the lateral meniscus may appear uncovered as a result of anterior tibial subluxation in patients with anterior cruciate ligament injury.[50,104]

Inferences regarding the status of the cruciate ligaments can be made by other indirect observations as well. For example, a line drawn parallel to the posterior margin of the distal posterior cruciate ligament should intersect the medullary cavity of the femur. When it does not, this indicates anterior cruciate ligament injury.[86] Another sign used to diagnose anterior cruciate ligament tears is increased depth (>1.5 mm) of the lateral condylopatellar sulcus, which is caused by an impaction injury.[22] Other abnormalities that may be found in association with cruciate ligament tears include cartilaginous defects, localized fluid collections, and trabecular or cortical bone injuries, particularly those involving the lateral femoral condyle and lateral tibial plateau.[50] In one study, trabecular bone injury involving the lateral compartment of the knee was observed in 40% of patients with evidence of an anterior cruciate ligament tear.[104]

In some patients it may be difficult to determine the acuity of a cruciate ligament injury.[107] The presence of granulation tissue in a subacute injury may appear similar to acute edema and hemorrhage on T2-weighted images. With chronic cruciate ligament tears, edema and hemorrhage are ultimately replaced by fibrotic tissue. As a result, abnormal increased signal intensity is no longer observed. In such cases, one must rely on alterations in morphology of the cruciate ligaments for diagnosis. Complete absence of the anterior cruciate ligament may occur in some patients with chronic tears of this structure. In other patients, fibrous strands span the intercondylar notch along the expected course of the anterior cruciate ligament and can simulate the appearance of an intact ligament.[107]

Postoperative changes

Reconstructed anterior cruciate ligaments can demonstrate a variety of appearances on MR images[6,21,26,72,114]

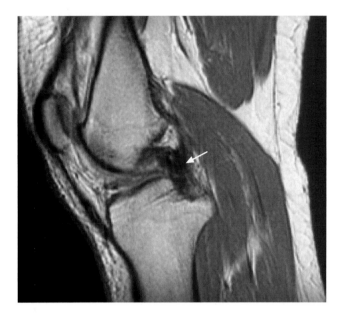

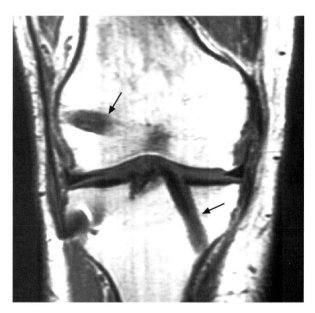

Fig. 11-40. Sagittal proton density–weighted image (TR 2250, TE 16, 1 Nex) demonstrates apparent thickening, irregularity, and increased signal intensity related to the posterior cruciate ligament *(arrow)* caused by previous surgical repair of this structure.

Fig. 11-41. Coronal T1-weighted image (TR 800, TE 25, 2 Nex) in patient with anterior cruciate ligament reconstruction demonstrates graft extending through the medial tibial plateau and lateral femoral condyle *(arrows)*. A metal artifact caused by surgical clip is present along the lateral tibial plateau.

(Figs. 11-40 and 11-41). Foci of relative increased signal intensity, ill definition, a wavy contour, or even nonvisualization can be found, even with intact neoligaments. In one series, the graft was not discernible in 11 of 27 examinations.[72] Therefore criteria used to evaluate native cruciate ligaments cannot necessarily be applied following ligament reconstruction.

Metallic implants placed during cruciate ligament reconstruction can result in signal void (i.e., susceptibility) artifacts. However, many implants are made of titanium, which is nonferromagnetic; these implants result in localized signal void artifacts that do not seriously impair diagnostic accuracy of MR.[90] One exception is the Perfex stainless steel interference screw, which is ferromagnetic and leads to a significant geometric distortion of the image.[90]

OTHER LIGAMENTS AND TENDONS
Collateral Ligaments

The collateral ligaments of the knee may be torn during injuries involving extreme valgus or varus stress. Injury to the collateral ligaments is often associated with damage to the menisci and anterior cruciate ligaments. The medial collateral ligament is injured far more frequently than the lateral collateral ligament. Injury is di-

agnosed by visualization of edema surrounding the ligament (grade I), focal signal alteration within the substance of the ligament (grade II), or frank disruption or detachment of the ligament (grade III).

The collateral ligaments are not adequately evaluated on sagittal images. Improved anatomic depiction is provided on images acquired in the coronal plane, though transaxial images may also be used. The course of the lateral collateral ligament is somewhat oblique with reference to the coronal plane. Therefore the entire extent of the lateral collateral ligament is usually not visualized on a single coronal image (see Fig. 11-1). Rather, the ligament is visualized segmentally over several adjacent images.

T1-weighted images are not reliable for demonstrating collateral ligament injuries. These images should be supplemented with coronal and/or transaxial T2-weighted images. Improved depiction of the collateral ligaments and associated injuries is achieved when fat suppression is used in conjunction with proton density– and T2-weighted images[70] (Figs. 11-42, *A* and *B*).

Visualization of edema or fluid medial to the collateral ligaments should not be interpreted as evidence of injury to these structures, since these findings may represent intraarticular joint fluid. Diagnosis of collateral ligament injury will result in abnormal signal intensity along the nonarticular side of the ligament as well.

Fibrofatty tissue interposed between the joint capsule

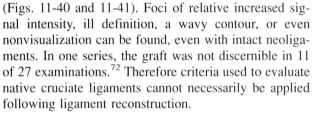

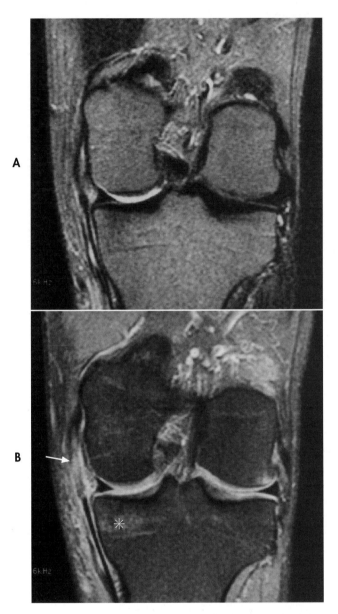

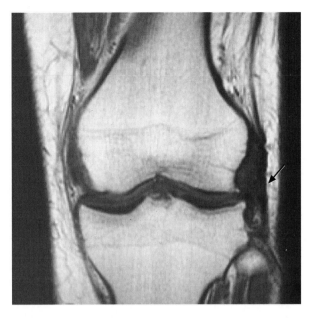

Fig. 11-43. Coronal T1-weighted image (TR 550, TE 20, 2 Nex) in patient who underwent previous lateral collateral ligament reconstruction. Thickening of the lateral collateral ligament is noted *(arrow)*, as well as subtle metallic artifact along its superior aspect where it is fused with the iliotibial band.

Fig. 11-42. Conventional T2-weighted **(A)** (TR 2250, TE 75, 1 Nex) and fat suppressed proton density–weighted **(B)** (TR 2250, TE 16, 1 Nex) images. There is markedly improved conspicuousness of bone marrow edema *(asterisk)* related to trabecular bone injury, as well as improved depiction of medial collateral ligament injury *(arrow)* on the fat suppressed image. Also noted is relative increased signal intensity of hyaline cartilage with fat suppression.

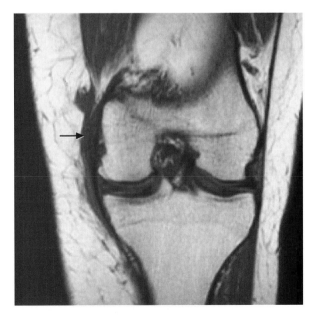

Fig. 11-44. Thickening and ill definition of the medial collateral ligament *(arrow)* are seen on coronal T1-weighted image (TR 500, TE 20, 2 Nex), a result of previous surgical repair of this structure.

and the collateral ligaments can also simulate collateral ligament injury.[110] In addition, bursal fluid collections can occur along the course of the collateral ligaments, representing another cause for simulation of collateral ligament injury.[59] Ossification within the proximal medial collateral ligament (Pelligrini-Stieda disease) can simulate subacute ligamentous hemorrhage on T1-weighted images. Fat suppression techniques can be used to provide distinction.

Thickening of the collateral ligaments, with associated abnormal signal intensity on proton density– and T2-weighted images, is frequently observed following surgical reconstruction (Figs. 11-43 and 11-44). Small foci of signal void are also present, representing susceptibility artifacts caused by the presence of metal.

Transverse intermeniscal and meniscofemoral ligaments

Accessory ligaments of the knee include the transverse intermeniscal ligament and the anterior (Humphrey) and posterior (Wrisberg) meniscofemoral ligaments. The transverse ligament extends between the anterior horns of the medial and lateral menisci. The meniscofemoral ligaments course between the lateral meniscus and the lateral aspect of the medial femoral condyle (Fig. 11-45). These structures provide ancillary stabilization of the menisci. Their primary significance on MR images is in potential simulation of meniscal tears, as previously discussed.

These accessory ligaments are variably present and when present can be of variable prominence.[38,110] A meniscofemoral ligament is present in approximately 71% of individuals.[10] In most individuals, either the anterior or the posterior ligament is present, with only approximately 6% having both ligaments.[10] The presence of these ligaments is often not bilaterally symmetric.

Quadriceps and patellar tendons

As with other ligaments and tendons, diagnosis of injury to the quadriceps and patellar tendons is based on abnormal morphology (e.g., thickening, irregularity, disruption) and/or abnormal signal intensity characteristics. Inflammatory changes (i.e., tendinitis) can result in findings such as focal thickening and increased signal intensity that simulate partial thickness tears.[12]

The patellar tendon usually has a taut appearance in normal individuals. Careful inspection of the entire extensor mechanism should be carried out when laxity of the patellar tendon is encountered. The patellar tendon can assume a corrugated appearance in patients with quadriceps tendon rupture, patellar fracture, or patellectomy.[11]

The normal patellar tendon increases in diameter slightly as it progresses from proximal to distal.[33] This mild gradual thickening should not be interpreted as evidence of tendinitis or a partial tear. The normal patellar tendon is generally less than 7 mm in diameter.[33]

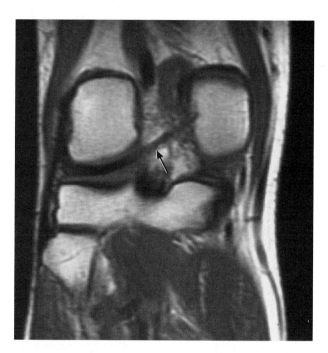

Fig. 11-45. The posterior meniscofemoral ligament of Wrisberg is seen coursing from the lateral meniscus *(arrow)* to the medial femoral condyle on this coronal T1-weighted (TR 800, TE 25, 2 Nex) image.

Foci of relative increased signal intensity can be observed within the distal quadriceps and proximal patellar tendons in normal individuals (Figs. 11-19, 11-35, A and B, and 11-46). These findings are caused by fibrofatty tissue interposed between the tendinous laminae and can simulate tendinitis or a partial tear.[77,81,117] The quadriceps tendon normally has three laminae, but occasionally two or four layers may be present.[117] A thin zone of relatively increased signal intensity is also frequently present posterior to the proximal patellar tendon.[33] These signal intensity alterations can be of variable prominence; their consistent location and the lack of associated focal tendinous enlargement allow distinction from pathology.

Foci of ossification can occur within the quadriceps and patellar tendons, resulting in relative increased signal intensity and enlargement (Fig. 11-47). Fat suppressed T1-weighted images will allow for distinction of marrow fat (as in ossification) from edema or hemorrhage. Partial volume averaging of these tendons with adjacent fat is another cause for apparent quadriceps or patellar tendon signal intensity alterations (Fig. 11-48). Correlation of images acquired in multiple planes will allow the normal character of the tendon to be confirmed.

Following surgical repair, the extensor mechanism tendons can demonstrate focal thickening and signal in-

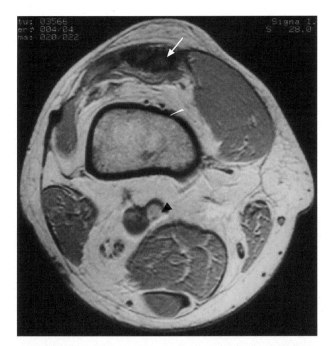

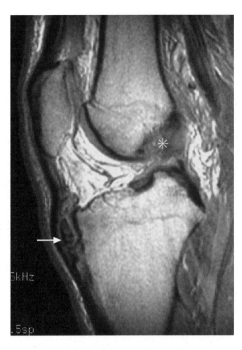

Fig. 11-46. Transaxial gradient echo image (TR 450, TE 5, 90-degree flip angle, 2 Nex) depicts foci of relatively increased signal intensity *(arrow)* within the quadriceps tendon. These represent fibrofatty tissue interposed between the laminae of the vastus tendons. Note relatively increased signal intensity within the popliteal artery *(arrowhead)* as compared with the adjacent vein. This is due to accentuated flow-related enhancement caused by increased flow velocity, with greater saturation of more slowly flowing venous blood.

Fig. 11-47. A focus of ossification *(arrow)* is present within the distal patellar tendon on midsagittal proton density–weighted image (TR 2250, TE 16, 1 Nex). Also note torn anterior cruciate ligament *(asterisk)*, joint effusion, and patellofemoral degenerative joint disease.

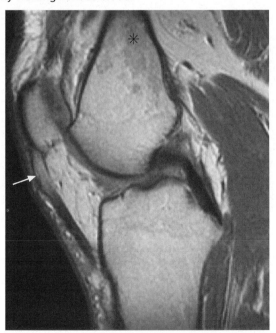

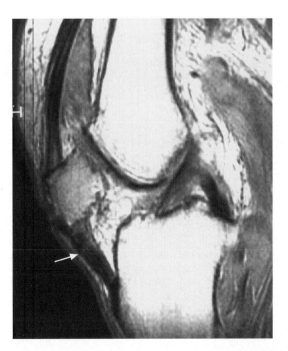

Fig. 11-48. There is an apparent tear *(arrow)* involving the proximal patellar tendon on sagittal proton density–weighted image (TR 2250, TE 16, 1 Nex). This is due to partial volume averaging of the tendon with adjacent fat within the infrapatellar fat pad. Note hematopoietic marrow elements *(asterisk)* within the distal femoral metaphysis as well as patellofemoral compartment degenerative joint disease.

Fig. 11-49. Midsagittal proton density–weighted image (TR 2250, TE 16, 1 Nex) demonstrates patellar tendon graft *(arrow)*. The neotendon is short, resulting in inferior position of the patella. There is mild globular increased signal intensity within the proximal portion of the graft. A joint effusion is also noted, and there is irregularity of the margins of the patella.

tensity alterations (Fig. 11-49). Ancillary findings that serve as clues to previous surgery include edema or scarring in the adjacent soft tissues, small foci of signal void caused by micrometallic fragments or larger foci corresponding to surgical clips, and possibly altered position of the patella.

JOINT SPACE

Synovial fluid

A small amount of synovial fluid can be observed within the knee joint space of normal individuals.[9] Such fluid is usually located immediately behind the patella and may extend into the suprapatellar bursa. However, it does not result in distention of the bursa or joint capsule. The "saddle-bag" appearance of joint fluid along the lateral aspects of the joint space on coronal images indicates significant joint effusion.

Schweitzer et al found that a 1 ml collection of joint fluid is generally detectable on MR images.[87] Small amounts of fluid initially collect between the femoral condyles and the infrapatellar fat pad, as well as surrounding the medial meniscus. With accumulation of a slightly larger volume of fluid (e.g., 3 ml), the fluid distributes into the suprapatellar bursa and posteromedial to the posterior cruciate ligament. Still larger volumes of

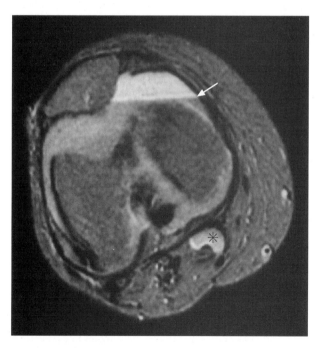

Fig. 11-50. A fluid-fluid level *(arrow)* is demonstrated within the knee joint on transaxial T2-weighted image (TR 2250, TE 70, 1 Nex). This is due to hemarthrosis related to acute fracture of the medial femoral condyle. A small popliteal cyst *(asterisk)* is also noted in the region of the gastrocnemius-semimembranosus bursa.

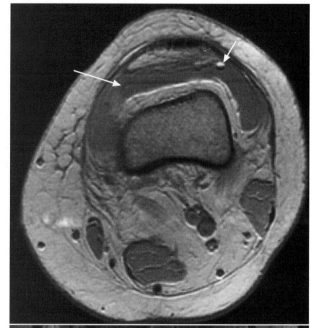

A

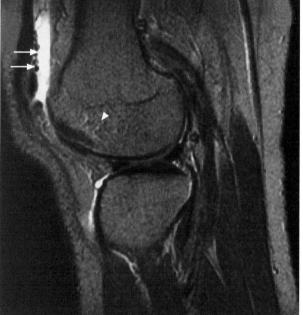

B

Fig. 11-51. A, Transaxial T1-weighted gradient echo image (TR 450, TE 5, 90-degree flip angle, 2 Nex) demonstrates fluid-fluid level in the knee joint of patient who underwent recent trauma. The presence of lipomatous components within the joint space is verified by observation of chemical shift misregistration artifact *(arrow)*. A focal droplet of high signal intensity also manifests evidence of chemical shift misregistration *(small arrow)*. Additional images demonstrated a radiographically occult femur fracture. **B,** Sagittal T2-weighted image (TR 2250, TE 70, 1 Nex) demonstrates intraarticular lipid droplets *(arrows)* that are of low signal intensity and that could potentially simulate osteochondral bodies. The fracture site *(arrowhead)* is also depicted on this image.

fluid collect within the meniscosynovial recesses and popliteus tendon sheath.

Hemorrhage

Hemorrhage within the joint space may be present in patients who have sustained a recent knee injury. In patients with hemarthrosis, a fluid-fluid level can be observed within the distended joint space on sagittal or transaxial images (Fig. 11-50). Generally, the dependent component is of reduced signal intensity relative to the nondependent component on T2-weighted images. Increased signal intensity may also be present on T1-weighted images as a result of hemorrhage. Such signal intensity alterations can simulate the appearance of intraarticular fat (i.e., lipohemarthrosis), which indicates an underlying fracture.[52] Distinction between simple hemarthrosis and lipohemarthrosis can be made with fat suppression images. When such images are not available, the fluid-fluid interface should be closely evaluated for a chemical shift misregistration artifact. This is manifested as a parallel line of artifactual increased or decreased signal intensity along the frequency encoding direction (Figs. 11-51, *A* and *B* to 11-53). This artifact arises at fat-water interfaces, such as occurs with lipohemarthrosis. Four discrete signal intensity layers are often noted within the joint space in patients with lipohemarthrosis. These represent fat, a chemical shift misregistration ar-

tifact, serum, and red blood cells as they progress from nondependent to dependent levels.[52]

In some patients, lipohemarthrosis presents as high signal intensity fat droplets within the joint space, rather than as a discrete fat-fluid level. In such cases, the fat droplets can simulate intraarticular loose bodies on T2-weighted images, where they display relative reduced signal intensity compared with surrounding joint fluid or hemorrhage (Fig. 11-57) Because osteochondral bodies also contain marrow fat, fat suppression sequences or observation of chemical shift effects may not be useful. Correlation with plain radiographs and direct evaluation of the underlying bony structures will usually allow for distinction.

Chemical shift misregistration artifacts originating at the interface between joint fluid within the suprapatellar bursa and adjacent retropatellar fat can simulate the appearance of fluid-fluid levels on transaxial images (Fig. 11-54). In questionable cases, chemical shift artifacts can be verified on the basis of their displacement with gradient reorientation or their elimination when fat suppression methods are used.

Another common manifestation of hemarthrosis is an intraarticular clot. A clot appears as discrete rounded or-irregularly shaped foci within the distended joint space (Figs. 11-12 and 11-55). The T2-shortening effects of iron result in reduced signal intensity on T2-weighted

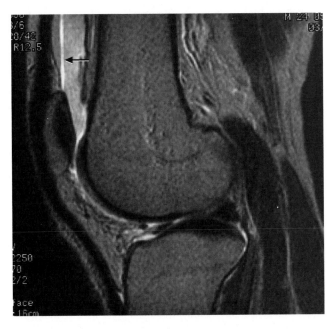

Fig. 11-52. Sagittal T2-weighted image (TR 2250, TE 70, 1 Nex) depicts lipohemarthrosis in patient who sustained recent femoral condyle fracture. The presence of fat is verified by differential signal intensity within the suprapatellar bursa, as well as by chemical shift misregistration artifact *(arrow)* at the fat-fluid interface.

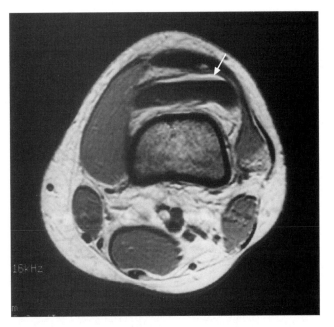

Fig. 11-53. High signal intensity representing fat is visualized along the nondependent portion of the suprapatellar bursa on this transaxial T1-weighted gradient echo image (TR 400, TE 5, 90-degree flip angle, 2 Nex). Chemical shift misregistration artifact is present at the fat-fluid interface. A fracture of the tibial plateau was evident on additional images.

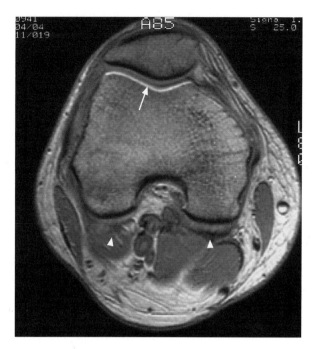

Fig. 11-54. A band of increased signal intensity *(arrow)* paralleling the margin of the anterior femoral condyles is evident on transaxial T1-weighted gradient echo image (TR 400, TE 5, 90-degree flip angle, 2 Nex). This is due to chemical shift misregistration artifact along the frequency encode direction of the image. Vascular pulsation artifact *(arrowheads)* related to the popliteal artery is present along the phase encode direction of the image. Also note intermediate intraluminal signal intensity within the popliteal vessels that makes patency of these vessels difficult to determine. This is due to counteracting effects of relatively high flip angle leading to saturation of flowing spins and inherent flow-related enhancement of gradient echo technique.

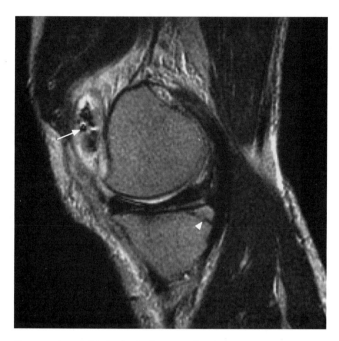

Fig. 11-55. Multiple foci of markedly decreased signal intensity *(arrow)* are present within the suprapatellar joint space on sagittal T2-weighted image (TR 2250, TE 70, 1 Nex). These represent clot related to acute fracture of the tibial plateau *(arrowhead)*, which is partially visualized on this image.

and gradient-echo images, while variable signal characteristics are observed on T1-weighted images.

The above findings are not specific for an intraarticular clot. Intraarticular osteochondral bodies and intraarticular masses can present a similar appearance. In particular, synovial hyperplasia and pigmented villonodular synovitis contain hemosiderin, which also results in T2 shortening (Figs. 11-56 and 11-57). Plain radiographs can be evaluated for evidence of radioopaque osteochondral bodies or for erosive changes caused by villonodular synovitis, and clinical history and analysis of joint fluid may also be helpful. Paramagnetic contrast agents such as gadopentetate dimeglumine prominently enhance hyperplastic synovial tissue, assisting in distinction from intraarticular clot.[1,8,44,54,56]

MR images may not show evidence of intraarticular blood in some individuals with proven hemorrhagic joint effusion caused by isointensity of blood products with surrounding joint fluid. The bathing of extravasated red blood cells in oxygen-rich synovial fluid may decrease the conspicuousness of signal intensity alterations because of blood breakdown products, in a manner analogous to that which occurs with intracranial subarachnoid hemorrhage.

Synovial tissue

Standard T1- and T2-weighted images provide poor distinction between synovial fluid and prominent synovial tissue. Therefore synovitis or synovial hyperplasia can be difficult to detect. In some patients, prominent synovial tissue can appear slightly higher in signal intensity than joint fluid on T1-weighted images and slightly lower in signal intensity on T2-weighted images.[97] Images acquired immediately after intravenous administration of paramagnetic contrast material show enhancement of abnormal synovial tissue, whereas normal synovium and joint fluid do not enhance significantly. This improves detection of synovial lesions in patients with painful joint swelling.[112] Images acquired immediately after intravenous contrast material administration can show rimlike enhancement around the joint space, which reflects early diffusion of contrast material through the synovium.[113] This should not be interpreted as evidence of synovial inflammation.

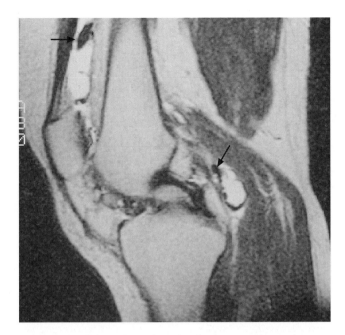

Fig. 11-56. Nodular foci of markedly decreased signal intensity *(arrows)* are observed within the knee joint space on sagittal T2-weighted image (TR 2000, TE 80, 1 Nex). These reflect hemosiderin in patient with pigmented villonodular synovitis. These foci can simulate hemorrhagic products (i.e., clot), synovial hyperplasia, or osteochondral bodies. Accentuation of signal loss was present on corresponding gradient echo images.

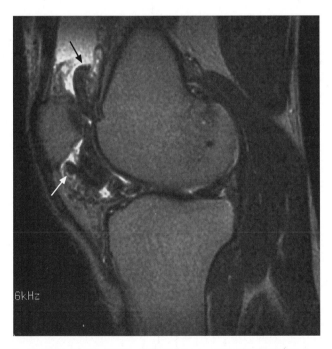

Fig. 11-57. Sagittal T2-weighted image (TR 2250, TE 70, 1 Nex) demonstrates multiple hypointense filling defects *(arrows)* throughout the knee joint space. Although these are suggestive of osteochondral bodies, corresponding plain radiograph showed no apparent calcifications. Findings are due to synovial hyperplasia/neoplasia.

Contrast enhancement patterns

Paramagnetic contrast agents also result in mild enhancement of normal joint fluid on delayed images obtained following intravenous administration; the intensity of such enhancement increases after exercise.[32,57,113] Enhancement of joint fluid can obscure visualization of abnormal synovial enhancement. In addition, considerable heterogeneity may be observed within the joint space because of poor mixing of enhanced and unenhanced joint fluid; this can simulate intraarticular pathology.[113] The arthrographic effect produced on delayed contrast enhanced images can improve detection of meniscal tears that are equivocal on standard unenhanced images.[32]

Simulation of intraarticular masses

In addition to blood clot, other entities can simulate intraarticular masses. Intraarticular air can result from a previous intervention, such as joint aspiration, or can arise as a result of the "vacuum phenomenon." In either case, intraarticular foci of marked decreased signal intensity with possible surrounding hyperintensity are observed.[94] These findings are accentuated on images acquired using gradient-echo or fat-saturation techniques. Similar susceptibility artifacts can also result from metallic fragments or clips related to previous surgery. Partial volume averaging of joint fluid with retropatellar fat can also simulate the appearance of an intraarticular mass, particularly on transaxial images. Reactive synovial hyperplasia (i.e., pannus) can also appear to represent a tumor within the joint space.

Synovial plicae

Synovial plicae, embryologic remnants of strandlike fibrous tissue, appear as thin curvilinear foci of decreased signal intensity outlined by surrounding joint fluid (Fig. 11-58). Plicae are most frequently observed in the suprapatellar bursa but can occur elsewhere throughout the knee. In most instances, these plicae are regarded as incidental findings of little or no clinical significance. However, mediopatellar plicae have been associated with patellar subluxation and related symptoms.[74]

Osteochondral joint bodies

Osteochondral joint bodies can be difficult to detect on MR images. When these bodies are not directly visualized because of their isointensity with surrounding structures, the presence of a small localized fluid collection may serve as a secondary indicator of their presence. The search for osteochondral bodies is particularly difficult in the absence of joint effusion. In such cases, introduction of saline or paramagnetic contrast material solution into the joint space can improve depiction of the intraarticular space. Osteochondral bodies should also be searched for in atypical locations. such as within synovial recesses, joint extensions such as popliteal cysts, me-

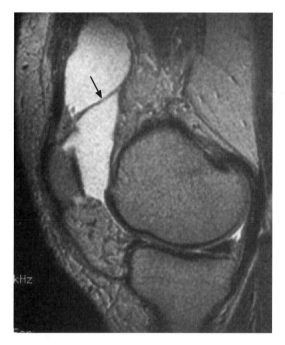

Fig. 11-58. Sagittal T2-weighted image (TR 2250, TE 70, 1 Nex) depicts plica *(arrow)* coursing through the suprapatellar bursa in patient with large joint effusion.

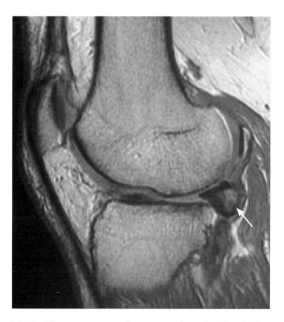

Fig. 11-59. The presence of an osteochondral body *(arrow)* within a meniscectomy defect simulates an in situ meniscus with globular degenerative change on this sagittal proton density-weighted (TR 2250, TE 16, 1 Nex) image.

niscectomy defects, and juxtaarticular soft tissues such as the infrapatellar fat pad (Fig. 11-59).

The meniscofemoral ligament (of Wrisberg) can appear to represent an osteochondral fragment within the posterior knee on sagittal images.[19] On close inspection, the ligament can be traced over several adjacent images, and it can also be identified on coronal images.

HYALINE CARTILAGE
Chemical shift misregistration artifacts

The junction between marrow fat and hyaline cartilage represents a fat-water interface, which can give rise to chemical shift misregistration artifacts. These artifacts result in artifactual linear increased and decreased signal intensities that can alter the apparent thickness of hyaline cartilage. Reorientation of the phase and frequency-encoding gradients can permit more accurate determination of cartilage thickness. The use of a wide receiver bandwidth, decreased voxel size, and decreased magnetic field strength will all contribute to decreasing the prominence of chemical shift misregistration effects. In addition, such effects are less prominent on T1- rather than T2-weighted sequences and on sequences employing fat suppression.

Hyaline cartilage thickness

Hyaline cartilage thickness can be difficult to determine when it is isointense with joint fluid, as occurs on standard proton density– and T2-weighted images.[20] Other pulse sequences often allow better differentiation between these tissues. T1-weighted images, for example, depict hyaline cartilage as moderately hyperintense relative to joint fluid, whereas on heavily T2-weighted images cartilage is hypointense as compared with fluid. The flexible contrast scale of gradient echo sequences is frequently used to distinguish hyaline cartilage and fluid,[53] though imaging parameters (i.e., TR, TE, flip angle) must be optimized for this application[116] (Figs. 11-60*A* and *B* and 11-61*A-C*). Three-dimensional gradient echo sequences can assist in determining cartilage thickness, particularly when spoiled gradient-echo sequences are used.[2] Fat suppression results in marked hyperintensity of hyaline cartilage and can also improve its depiction[53,102] (Fig. 11-62). The use of fat suppressed gradient-echo images has also been found advantageous for determining cartilage thickness.[80] Even when the above techniques are used, however, depiction of early cartilage degeneration has remained difficult.

Signal intensity variations

Hyaline cartilage is relatively thick in skeletally immature patients and demonstrates a trilaminar appearance[88] (Fig. 11-37). While a trilaminar appearance can

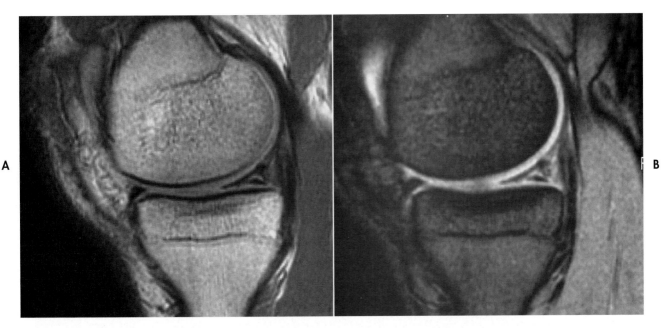

Fig. 11-60. Sagittal proton density–weighted spin echo **(A)** (TR 2250, TE 20, 1 Nex) and gradient echo **(B)** (TR 400, TE 12, 20-degree flip angle, 2 Nex) images depict tear of posterior horn medial meniscus. Relative increased signal intensity of hyaline cartilage overlying the femoral and tibial articular surfaces is noted on gradient echo image.

also be visible in adults, it is less conspicuous because of reduced cartilage thickness.[41,62] Recht et al have observed this trilaminar appearance more consistently using fat suppressed, gradient-echo images.[80] They speculated that lack of visualization of the most superficial layer could serve as an indicator for mild cartilage loss. Heterogeneous signal intensity is frequently visible within the hyaline cartilage overlying the medial tibial plateau in the absence of documented cartilage abnormalities, particularly on fat suppressed images (Fig. 11-63). This may reflect structural alterations related to weight bearing.

Artifactual heterogeneous signal intensity can be seen within the patellar articular cartilage on gradient-echo images, simulating the appearance of chondromalacia patellae.[48] Gross patient motion, vascular pulsation artifacts, or susceptibility artifacts caused by air or metallic substances are other causes for artifactual heterogeneous signal intensity related to cartilage.[94]

The magic angle phenomenon is usually associated with artifactually increased signal intensity of tendons when they are oriented at approximately 55 degrees relative to the magnetic field. This phenomenon can also affect hyaline cartilage when its collagen bundles are oriented at a similar angle.[84] This represents another cause for artifactual increased or heterogeneous cartilaginous signal intensity.

Areas of hypointensity within hyaline cartilage can in-

dicate chondrocalcinosis. However, chondrocalcinosis is often not depicted on MR images, because of the relative insensitivity of MR to calcification.

Chondromalacia patellae is also frequently not detectable on MR images in its earliest stages.[41] With early chondromalacia, the patellar articular cartilage can appear paradoxically increased rather than decreased in thickness, as a result of swelling and blistering. Another unexpected phenomenon may be observed in patients who have undergone previous meniscectomy. These patients are subject to development of accelerated degenerative joint disease, which is typically associated with loss of hyaline cartilage. However, the hyaline cartilage overlying the resected meniscus can appear paradoxically increased rather than decreased in thickness in some patients (Fig. 11-64A and B). Increased thickness of hyaline cartilage has also been observed following transection of the anterior cruciate ligament.[13]

OSSEOUS STRUCTURES
Pulse sequences

The juxtaarticular osseous structures should be carefully evaluated on MR images in patients with knee pain. Diagnosis of bone marrow lesions in the knee, as elsewhere, is usually based on visualization of focal or diffuse abnormal reduced marrow signal intensity on T1-

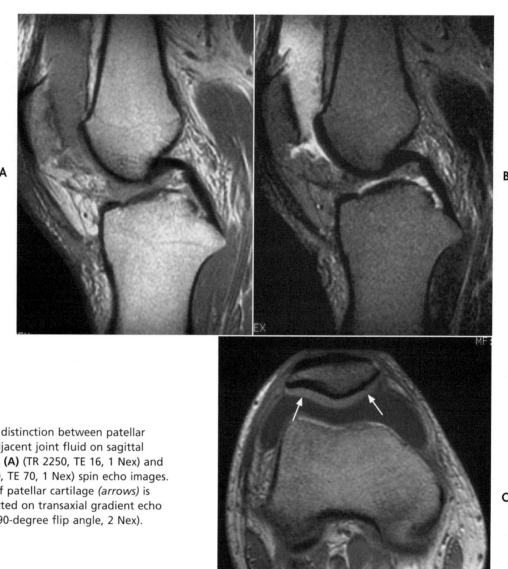

Fig. 11-61. There is poor distinction between patellar articular cartilage and adjacent joint fluid on sagittal proton density–weighted **(A)** (TR 2250, TE 16, 1 Nex) and T2-weighted **(B)** (TR 2250, TE 70, 1 Nex) spin echo images. However, the thickness of patellar cartilage *(arrows)* is considerably better depicted on transaxial gradient echo image **(C)** (TR 400, TE 5, 90-degree flip angle, 2 Nex).

weighted images. While abnormal increased marrow signal intensity may also be present on conventional T2-weighted images, findings are generally more conspicuous on T1-weighted images or on specialized sequences such as short tau inversion recovery (STIR) or fat suppressed T2-weighted imaging (Fig. 11-48).

Hematopoietic marrow

Residual or reconverted hematopoietic marrow displays relatively reduced signal intensity on T1-weighted images and can appear to represent marrow neoplasms or other lesions (Figs. 11-48 and 11-65). Prominent he-

matopoietic marrow is routinely observed throughout the distal femoral and proximal tibial metaphyses in children.[31,109] Reconversion of fatty to hematopoietic marrow can occur in these locations in adults as a result of anemia or marrow infiltration. Prominent red marrow is frequently observed about the knee in females of reproductive age, reflective of physiologic anemia.[27,85] These findings are particularly prominent in overweight females and in those who smoke cigarettes.

In the presence of hematopoietic marrow, abnormal signal intensity should be limited to the metaphyseal region. The epiphyses of the knee are not believed to ac-

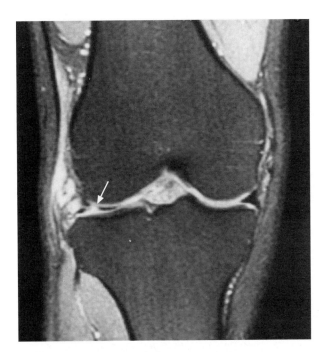

Fig. 11-62. Coronal fat suppressed proton density–weighted image (TR 2250, TE 16, 1 Nex) depicts tear involving midportion of lateral meniscus *(arrow)*. The tear communicates with a fluid collection, representing a parameniscal cyst, along the lateral joint line. Relative hyperintensity of hyaline articular cartilage is also noted with the use of fat suppression.

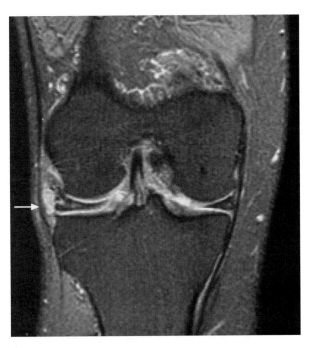

Fig. 11-63. Coronal proton density–weighted fat suppressed image (TR 2250, TE 10, 1 Nex) demonstrates linear tear of lateral meniscus, which extends into a parameniscal cyst *(arrow)*. Note heterogeneous signal intensity of hyaline articular cartilage overlying medial tibial plateau.

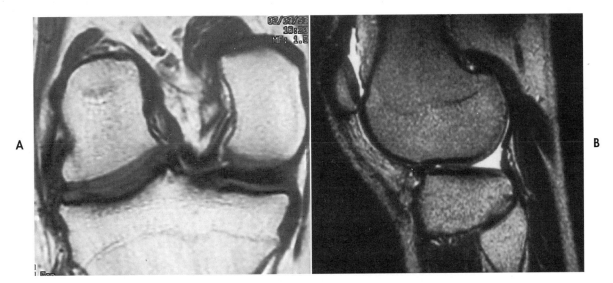

Fig. 11-64. A, Relatively increased thickness of hyaline cartilage along the lateral femoral and tibial articular surfaces is noted on coronal T1-weighted image (TR 500, TE 19, 2 Nex) in patient who underwent previous lateral meniscectomy. **B,** Sagittal T2-weighted image (TR 2250, TE 70, 1 Nex) depicts fluid filling the meniscectomy defect.

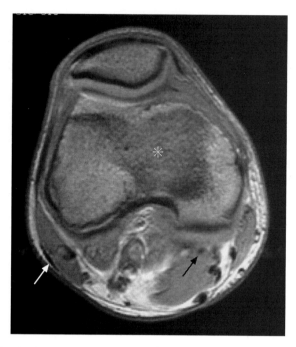

Fig. 11-65. Transaxial gradient echo image (TR 400, TE 5, 90-degree flip angle, 2 Nex) demonstrates apparent marrow lesion within the proximal tibial metaphysis (asterisk). This low signal intensity represents hematopoietic marrow in skeletally immature knee. Note popliteal artery pulsation artifact *(arrows)* projecting along the phase encode direction of the image.

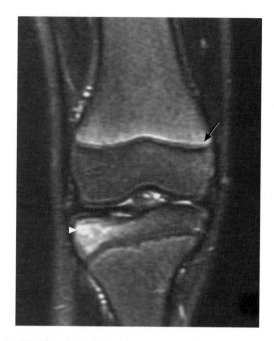

Fig. 11-66. There is relative hyperintensity within the distal femoral metaphysis on coronal fast spin echo fat suppressed T2-weighted image (TR 4000, effective TE 96, 2 Nex, 16 echo train). These findings represent residual hematopoietic marrow in 11-year-old female. A linear zone of increased signal intensity *(arrow)* proximal to the femoral physis is due to chemical shift misregistration artifact. Also noted is hyperintensity resulting from bone marrow contusion *(arrowhead)* involving the lateral tibial epiphysis related to recent trauma.

tively participate in hematopoiesis in adults. Hematopoietic marrow elements should not display significant hyperintensity on T2-weighted images, as can be observed with some neoplasms. Hematopoietic marrow is usually less intense than surrounding yellow marrow on T2-weighted images. However, relative hyperintensity of hematopoietic marrow is observed on fat suppressed pulse images, which can further simulate infiltrative marrow disorders (Figs. 11-66 and 11-67). The patella routinely demonstrates mild hyperintensity as compared with adjacent bony structures on fat suppressed T2-weighted images, presumably because of hematopoietic elements. Another feature used to distinguish hematopoietic marrow from tumor, infection, or other marrow lesions is the usual bilateral symmetry of hematopoietic marrow. Body coil images that display both knees simultaneously may be obtained to evaluate for symmetry in problematic cases.

Physis

The physis is unfused in skeletally immature patients[40,88] (Figs. 11-7, 11-8, and 11-32). Hyaline cartilage of the physis is located adjacent to marrow fat, presenting a fat-water interface where chemical shift misregistration artifacts can arise. Such artifacts can re-

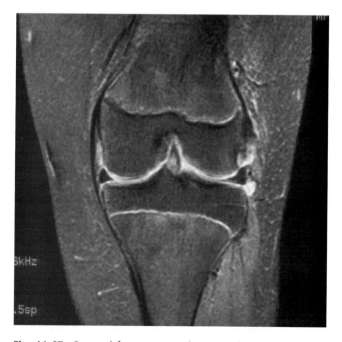

Fig. 11-67. Coronal fat suppressed proton density–weighted image (TR 2250, TE 16, 1 Nex) demonstrates relative hyperintensity of marrow within distal femur and proximal tibia. These findings are due to residual hematopoietic marrow in 14-year-old female. Also note linear hyperintensity related to physeal plates.

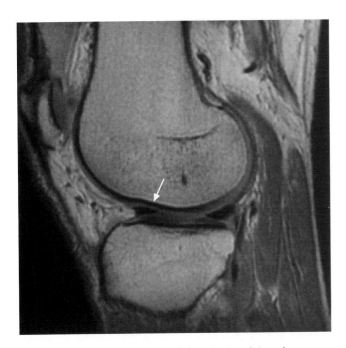

Fig. 11-68. There is apparent deformity involving the anterior inferior lateral femoral condyle *(arrow)* on sagittal proton density–weighted image (TR 2250, TE 16, 1 Nex). This finding represents the normal patellocondylar notch. Also noted is physeal scar within posterior distal femur and subjacent small bone island.

sult in artifactual increased signal intensity within adjacent marrow, simulating marrow edema or infiltration (Figs. 11-2, 11-66, and 11-67). Following physeal closure, a linear zone of decreased marrow signal intensity is seen representing fibrous scar (Figs. 11-68 and 11-69).

Signal intensity variations

Bony trabeculae. Regional variations in trabecular bone structure can also result in apparent marrow signal abnormalities about the knee. Horizontal linear decreased signal intensity is frequently observed in the subchondral region of the medial tibial plateau as a result of reinforced weight-bearing trabeculae. Similar findings can be observed in the lateral tibial plateau in some patients. The distal femur and, less commonly, the proximal tibia have a striated marrow pattern in some patients. Vertically oriented linear foci of relatively decreased signal intensity result in a pattern similar to that produced on plain radiographs in patients with osteopathia striata. This MR pattern should be regarded as a normal variation.

Penetrating vessels. The juxtaarticular portions of the distal femur and proximal tibia frequently demonstrate punctate foci of relatively decreased signal intensity on T1- and T2-weighted images (Fig. 11-5). These represent penetrating vessels, and they appear hyperintense on fat suppressed T2-weighted images. Rounded foci of decreased marrow signal intensity on all images

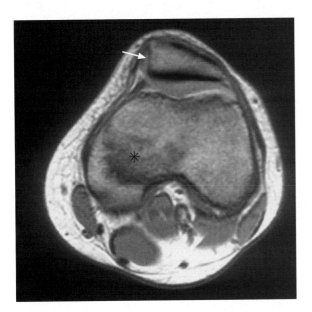

Fig. 11-69. Transaxial gradient echo image (TR 400, TE 5, 90-degree flip angle, 2 Nex) depicts a vertically oriented medial patellar facet *(arrow)*. Heterogeneity within the marrow space of the femur *(asterisk)* is due to cartilage in incompletely fused physis in 14-year-old female.

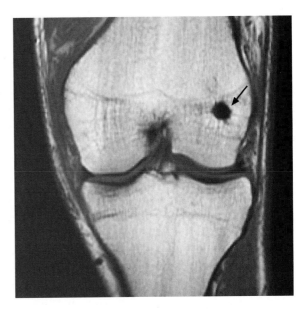

Fig. 11-70. A focus of markedly decreased signal intensity *(arrow)* is noted within the marrow space of the lateral femoral condyle on coronal T1-weighted image (TR 550, TE 20, 2 Nex), representing an incidental bone island.

are commonly observed, usually representing condensations of cortical bone (i.e., bone islands) (Figs. 11-68 and 11-70). Fibrous defects and enchondromas are other common causes for focal marrow signal alterations about the knee. These benign lesions demonstrate variable signal characteristics on T2-weighted images. Cortical desmoids may be observed along the posterior medial femoral condyle, usually in adolescents, and also must be distinguished from aggressive lesions.

Marrow edema. Localized abnormal bone marrow signal intensity is frequently evident on MR images in patients who have sustained recent knee trauma, paticularly valgus injury, rotational injury, or direct trauma.[67,101,115] These findings represent bone marrow edema related to trabecular bone injury and appear hypointense on T1-weighted and hyperintense on T2-weighted images relative to surrounding fatty marrow (Fig. 11-72). These findings are usually observed in the subcortical regions and can simulate neoplasm or other infiltrative marrow disorders. Plain radiographs usually demonstrate no correlate to this finding, though increased radiopharmaceutical uptake may be present on scintigraphic examination.

Trabecular injury frequently occurs in association with a meniscal or ligamentous tear but can present as an isolated finding.[101] In indeterminate cases, a follow-up MR examination may be necessary to document interval resolution of abnormal marrow signal intensity. When marrow edema demonstrates a linear configuration and approaches a cortical surface, an underlying cortical fracture should be suspected.[63]

Reactive marrow edema may also result from nontraumatic causes such as infarct and infection. Extensive marrow edema can obscure a small underlying focus of osteochondritis (Fig. 11-71). In patients with osteochondral lesions, a rim of fluid surrounding the lesion indicates that loosening has occurred. However, peripheral hyperintensity can also result from a chemical shift misregistration artifact.[66] Cystic changes, which may represent intraosseous ganglia, are frequently noted within the marrow space near the attachments of the anterior and posterior cruciate ligaments and can be associated with marrow edema.[64] These findings may simulate an aggressive osseous lesion.

Vascular pulsation artifact. Pulsation of the popliteal artery can lead to artifactual foci of increased or decreased signal intensity that simulate marrow lesions (Figs. 11-39, 11-65, and 11-72). Methods for reducing such artifacts have been previously discussed and include spatial presaturation, gradient moment nulling, and gradient reorientation.

Partial volume averaging. Transaxial images acquired through the physis can appear to depict a fracture or aggressive marrow lesion (Fig. 11-73). Partial volume averaging of marrow with adjacent soft tissues can also

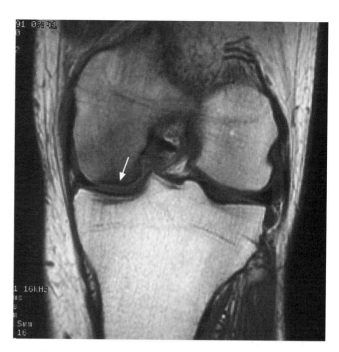

Fig. 11-71. Reduced signal intensity is observed throughout the medial femoral condyle on coronal T1-weighted image (TR 550, TE 20, 2 Nex). This is due to extensive reactive marrow edema secondary to acute osteonecrosis. The small osteonecrotic nidus *(arrow)* can be seen along the weight-bearing surface of the femoral condyle.

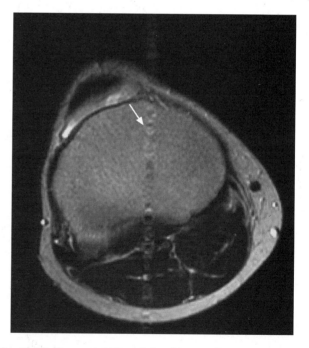

Fig. 11-72. Transaxial T2-weighted image (TR 2000, TE 80, 1 Nex) demonstrates a series of alternating high and low signal intensity artifacts *(arrows)* that propagate along the phase encode direction of the image. These are related to pulsatile blood flow within the popliteal artery.

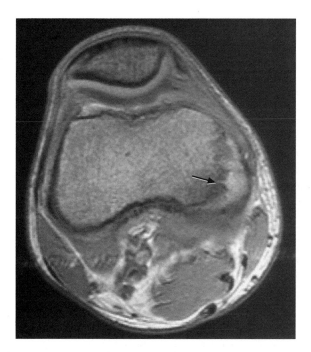

Fig. 11-73. Transaxial gradient echo image (TR 400, TE 5, 90-degree flip angle, 2 Nex) depicts an apparent fracture *(arrow)* through the medial aspect of the proximal tibia. This represents the unfused tibial physis.

simulate marrow lesions. These findings are resolved through correlation with images acquired in alternate imaging planes. Partial volume averaging of the medial aspects of the femoral condyles with fat and other structures within the intercondylar notch can simulate osteochondral lesions and other marrow lesions on sagittal images (Figs. 11-74*A* and *B* to 11-76*A* and *B*).

Susceptibility artifacts. Susceptibility artifacts related to metal can either simulate or obscure marrow lesions. These artifacts can preclude adequate evaluation of the knee in patients with knee prostheses.[58,65]

Shading artifacts. Shading artifacts can result from patient contact with the coil, eccentric positioning of the patient within the coil, or acquisition of images near the periphery of the coil.[75] Shading artifacts can also occur on body coil images when a surface coil is located within the field-of-view (Fig. 11-77). These artifacts can also arise from hardware problems relating to radiofrequency transmission. Shading artifacts are manifested as relatively decreased signal intensity within a portion of the image, usually near its periphery. When this affects the extremities, decreased marrow signal intensity can simulate marrow replacement or edema.

Anatomic variations. The tibia can be of variable length, and the tibia, fibula, or patella may be congenitally absent.[10] The patella may have a bipartite configu-

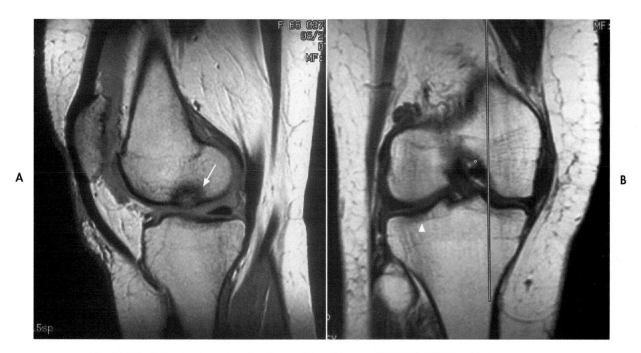

Fig. 11-74. A, Sagittal proton density–weighted image (TR 2250, TE 16, 1 Nex) suggests osteochondral lesion involving medial femoral condyle *(arrow)*. This is due to partial volume averaging of the condyle with the adjacent intercondylar notch, as confirmed on coronal T1-weighted **(B)** (TR 500, TE 20, 2 Nex) in which the position of **A** is marked. Reduced marrow signal intensity within the medial tibial plateau is also evident, representing reinforced stress trabeculae *(arrowhead)*.

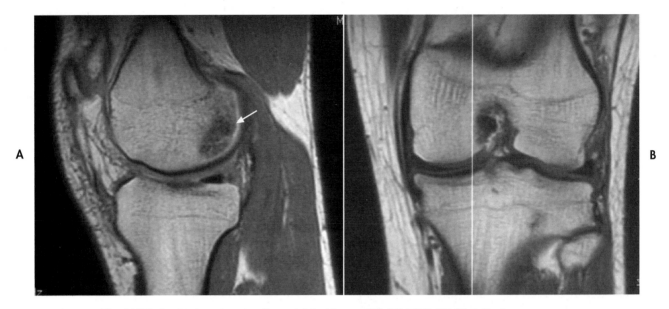

Fig. 11-75. Sagittal proton density-weighted image **(A)** (TR 2250, TE 16, 1 Nex) demonstrates apparent low signal intensity marrow abnormality within posterior femur *(arrow)*. This represents partial volume averaging of marrow with bone cortex located along the concavity of the femoral condyle. Coronal T1-weighted (TR 500, TE 19, 2 Nex) image **(B)** verifies normal marrow signal intensity, and depicts plane along which image **(A)** was acquired.

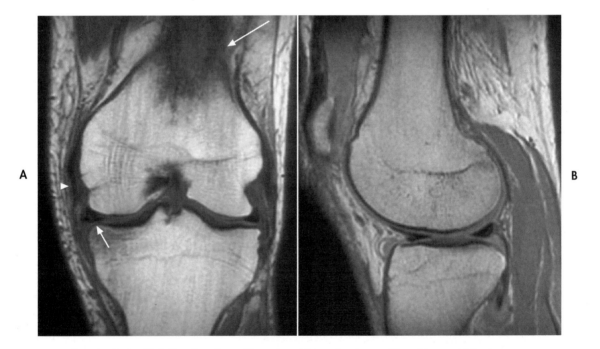

Fig. 11-76. An ill-defined region of low signal intensity *(arrow)* is evident within the distal femoral metaphysis on coronal T1-weighted (TR 550, TE 19, 2 Nex) image **(A)**. This represents partial volume averaging of marrow fat with adjacent bone cortex, as verified by normal marrow appearance on corresponding sagittal image **(B)**. A torn medial collateral ligament *(arrowhead)* and medial meniscus *(small arrow)* are also evident in figure **(A)**.

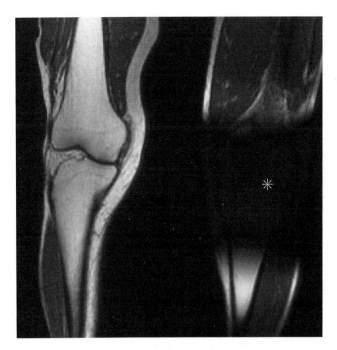

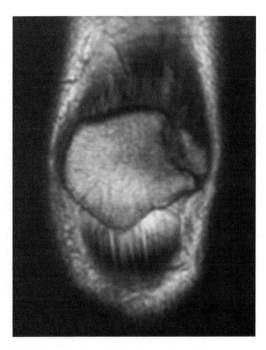

Fig. 11-77. Coronal T1-weighted image (TR 550, TE 20, 2 Nex) obtained using the body coil demonstrates severe shading artifact *(asterisk)* that obscures visualization of the left knee. These artifacts were caused by the presence of a local (knee) coil within the field of view.

Fig. 11-78. Bipartite patella is demonstrated on this coronal T1-weighted image (TR 550, TE 20, 2 Nex).

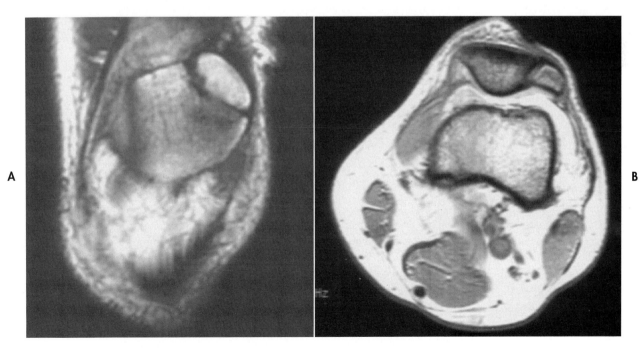

A

B

Fig. 11-79. Coronal T1-weighted **(A)** (TR 500, TE 20, 2 Nex) and transaxial gradient echo **(B)** (TR 450, TE 5, 90-degree flip angle, 2 Nex) images demonstrate bipartite patella, which may be mistaken for a patellar fracture.

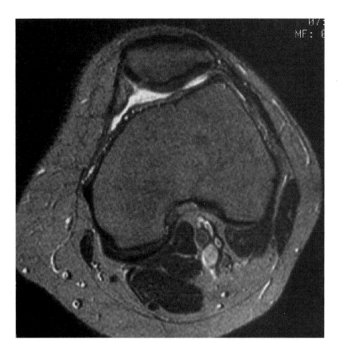

Fig. 11-80. Congenital deformity of the femoral trochlear groove is depicted on transaxial T2-weighted image (TR 3000, TE 70, 1 Nex). There is flattening of the anterior aspect of the medial femoral condyle. A joint effusion and thinning of the patellar articular cartilage are also noted.

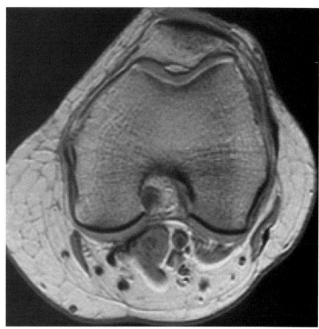

Fig. 11-81. Transaxial gradient echo image (TR 400, TE 5, 90-degree flip angle, 2 Nex) demonstrates apparent abnormality of the patella. This appearance is due to partial volume averaging of the patella with retropatellar fat.

ration, which can simulate a fracture (Figs. 11-78 to 11-79A and B). The medial and lateral patellar facets vary in their configuration; these variations can predispose to patellar subluxation. The trochlear groove of the femur is subject to congenital deformity, which may also predispose to patellar subluxation (Fig. 11-80).

A dorsal defect of the patella represents an ingrowth of fibrous tissue with associated sclerosis and is of no clinical significance.[45,76] This appears as a well-defined focus of heterogeneous or decreased signal intensity within the superior lateral aspect of the patella and can simulate other bone lesions.[45]

Patellar subluxation

Patellar subluxation may not be apparent on conventional MR images acquired with the knee in neutral position. When patellar subluxation is suspected, a patellar tracking (i.e., kinematic) study can be performed by acquiring images rapidly with the knee in variable degrees of flexion and extension.[91] Kinematic examinations of the knee should be performed with the patient supine, since pressure exerted on the knee in the prone position can displace the patella and simulate subluxation.[92] Use of rapid-gradient echo or echo-planar sequences can allow imaging to be performed during active rather than passive motion of the knee joint, permitting more accurate evaluation.[14,92] In addition, loading of the patellofemoral joint with external weight can improve evaluation for patella alignment and tracking.[93] Lateralization and tilting of the patella has been observed in normal subjects.[14]

A patellar fracture can be simulated when the patella undergoes partial volume averaging with retropatellar fat on transaxial images (Fig. 11-81).

A subtle depression in the contour of the anterior aspect of the lateral femoral condyle represents the condylopatellar sulcus; this can simulate an impaction type of osteochondral fracture (Figs. 11-68 and 11-82). This sulcus is generally less than 1.2 mm deep in normal individuals.[22] Cortical irregularity can be observed along the posterior aspect of the femoral condyles in normal individuals[73] as well as in the region of the tibial tubercle. These findings must be distinguished from osteochondritis and Osgood-Schlatter disease, respectively.

SOFT TISSUES
Cystic lesions

Several types of benign cystic masses commonly occur in the juxtaarticular soft tissues of the knee. While some of these entities can be associated with knee pain,

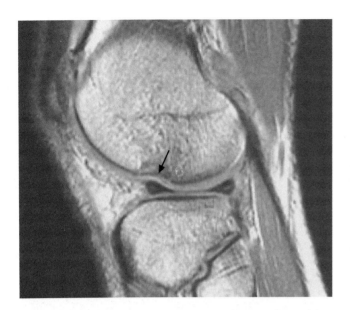

Fig. 11-82. An osteochondral impaction fracture *(arrow)* is present along the anterior lateral femoral condyle on sagittal proton density–weighted image (TR 2250, TE 16, 1 Nex). This is distinguished from the normal patellocondylar notch by its accentuated concavity and underlying marrow signal abnormality representing marrow edema.

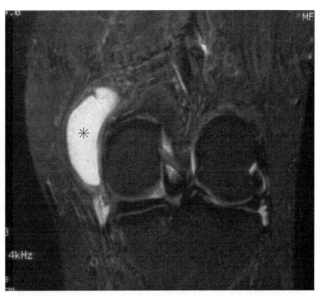

Fig. 11-83. Coronal fat suppressed T2-weighted image (TR 2250, TR 75, 1 Nex) depicts fluid collection *(asterisk)* extending superior to knee joint medially, representing an atypical synovial cyst.

their major significance is distinction from soft tissue neoplasms.

Synovial cysts are fluid-filled extensions of the joint space. In one series of more than 1000 consecutive MR examinations, popliteal cysts occurred in approximately 5% of patients.[35] Popliteal cysts are more frequent in patients with internal derangement of the knee, such as tears of the posterior horn of the medial meniscus and of the anterior cruciate ligament.[35]

Synovial cysts can occur in various locations about the knee, with the posterior upper calf most frequent. The neck of the cyst communicates with the joint space via a hiatus between the medial head of the gastrocnemius muscle and the semimembranosus tendon. Popliteal cysts can dissect through the soft tissues of the calf and can rupture, causing acute pain simulating that of thrombophlebitis. In the latter situation, fluid is often observed throughout the fascial planes of the proximal calf.

Synovial cysts can occur in atypical locations, and their communication with the joint space may be difficult to visualize (Figs. 11-83 and 11-84). T2-weighted images can demonstrate such communication when fluid is present within the cyst neck. When such fluid cannot be identified, intraarticular injection of air, saline, or contrast material can allow communication with the joint space to be confirmed. Most synovial cysts have smooth margins and uniform signal characteristics identical to those of fluid. In some patients, synovial cysts demon-

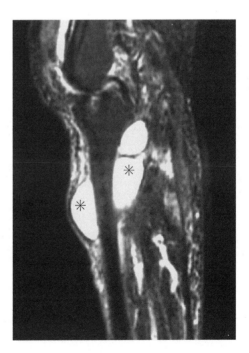

Fig. 11-84. Sagittal T2-weighted fat suppressed image (TR 2800, TE 80, 1 Nex) demonstrates an atypical synovial cyst *(asterisks)* with septated fluid components located anterior as well as posterior to the proximal tibia. Diffuse soft tissue edema throughout the posterior calf is also present.

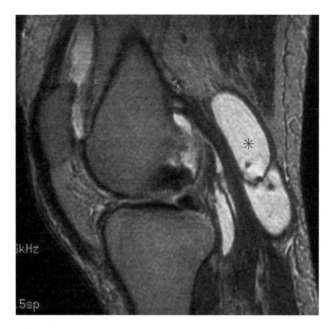

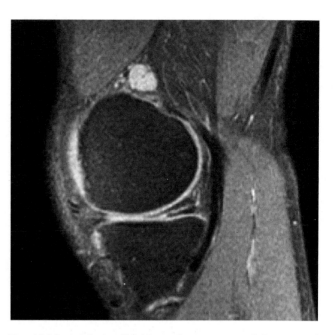

Fig. 11-85. Sagittal T2-weighted image (TR 2250, TE 70, 1 Nex) demonstrates large popliteal cyst *(asterisk)* containing several small filling defects. While these could represent loose osteochondral bodies, findings in this patient were due to hemorrhagic products (i.e., clot).

Fig. 11-86. A lobular fluid intensity mass containing several septations is noted superior to the medial femoral condyle on sagittal proton density–weighted fat suppressed image (TR 2500, TE 20, 1 Nex). This represents an incidental ganglion cyst. Note linear tear involving the posterior horn of medial meniscus. Hyperintensity of hyaline cartilage and moderately increased intensity of muscle are also observed, due to use of fat suppression.

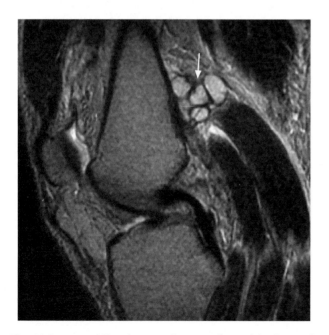

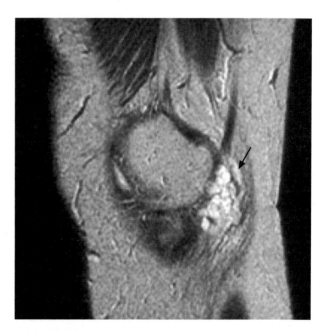

Fig. 11-87. A multilocular ganglion cyst *(arrow)* is observed posterior to the distal femoral metaphysis on sagittal T2-weighted image (TR 2250, TE 70, 1 Nex).

Fig. 11-88. Sagittal T2-weighted image (TR 2250, TE 70, 1 Nex) demonstrates multilobular high signal intensity lesion (arrow) posterior to the medial femoral condyle. This represents fluid in the pes anserine bursa caused by bursitis.

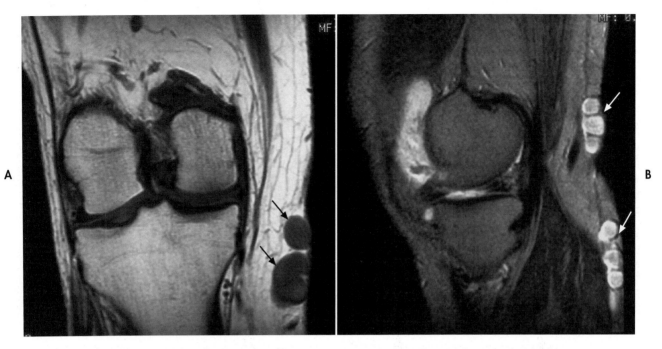

Fig. 11-89. Coronal T1-weighted **(A)** (TR 550, TE 20, 2 Nex) and sagittal T2-weighted **(B)** (TR 2250, TE 70, 1 Nex) images demonstrate multiple nodular lesions *(arrows)* with apparent cystic characteristics in the superficial soft tissues of the knee. These represent large venous varicosities.

strate a multilocular appearance with internal septations (Fig. 11-39) or filling defects representing synovial hyperplasia, osteochondral bodies, or hemorrhagic products, which can be difficult to distinguish from one another on MR images (Fig. 11-85).

Ganglion cysts are also commonly encountered about the knee; these do not communicate with the joint space. They typically demonstrate uniform hyperintensity, though they are frequently multilocular[18] (Figs. 11-86 and 11-87). Bursal fluid collections are another cause of cystic lesions that may be found in various locations about the knee.[39,61] Among the most common is the pes anserine bursa, located along the medial knee joint (Fig. 11-88). Meniscal cysts arise in relation to meniscal tears. They can appear as a focus of intrameniscal cystic degeneration or, more commonly, as a parameniscal cystic mass[18] (Figs. 11-62 and 11-63). An unusual cause for a cystic soft tissue mass is cystic degeneration of the popliteal artery. Large venous varicosities can be observed within the soft tissues of the knee, appearing hyperintense on flow compensated T2-weighted or gradient-echo images (Fig. 11-89*A* and *B*). Varicosities are identified on the basis of their serpentine configuration. Pulsation artifacts related to the popliteal artery may simulate soft tissue lesions as they traverse the image along the phase-encoding direction (Fig. 11-60).

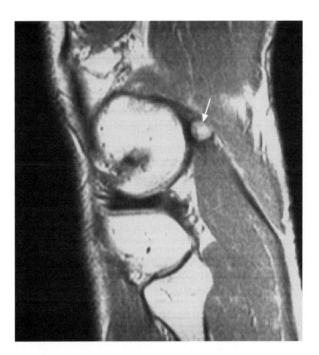

Fig. 11-90. Sagittal proton density–weighted image (TR 2250, TE 20, 1 Nex) demonstrates rounded focus of relatively increased signal intensity *(arrow)* within the lateral head of the gastrocnemius muscle, representing the fabella.

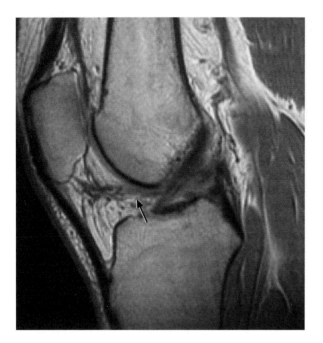

Fig. 11-91. A linear region of decreased signal intensity *(arrow)* extends through the infrapatellar fat pad on sagittal proton density–weighted image (TR 2250, TE 16, 1 Nex). This represents scarring along the course of an arthroscopic tract.

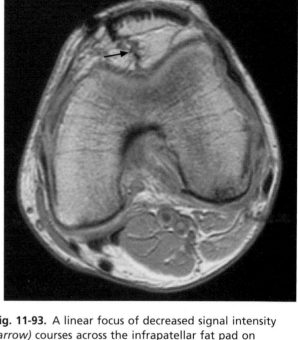

Fig. 11-93. A linear focus of decreased signal intensity *(arrow)* courses across the infrapatellar fat pad on transaxial gradient echo image (TR 450, TE 5, 90-degree flip angle, 2 Nex). This marks an arthroscopic tract, with low signal intensity caused by metallic microfragments.

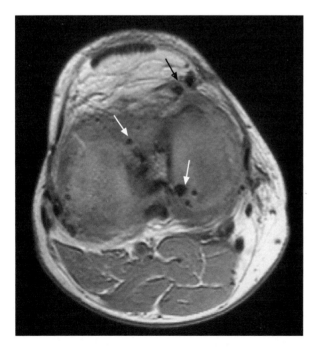

Fig. 11-92. Multiple small signal void foci *(arrows)* are seen throughout the knee on transaxial gradient echo image (TR 450, TE 5, 90-degree flip angle, 2 Nex). These represent metallic microfragments resulting from previous arthroscopy and meniscectomy.

Fabella

The fabella appears relatively intense on T1-weighted images, because of its marrow fat, and can be mistaken for a soft tissue lesion (Figs. 11-15 and 11-90). The location of this structure within the lateral head of the gastrocnemius muscle is characteristic.

Postoperative changes

In patients who have undergone previous arthroscopy, linear abnormal signal intensity is observed within the infrapatellar fat pad, corresponding to the scope tract[98] (Fig. 11-91). Tiny foci of marked decreased intensity are also frequently observed within the soft tissues of the knee on gradient echo images, as a result of deposited metallic microfragments (Figs. 11-92 and 11-93). Irregular signal intensity within the infrapatellar fat pad can also reflect inflammatory changes resulting from synovitis.[88] Scalloping or truncation of the fat pads about the knee is also a specific, although relatively insensitive, indicator of synovial proliferation.[87]

REFERENCES

1. Adam G, Dammer M, Bohndorf K et al: Rheumatoid arthritis of the knee: value of gadopentate dimeglumine-enhanced MR imaging, Am J Roentgenol 156:125-129, 1991.

2. Adam G, Nolte-Ernsting C, Prescher A et al: Experimental hyaline cartilage lesions: two-dimensional spin-echo versus three-dimensional gradient-echo MR imaging, J Magn Reson Imaging 1:665-672, 1991.

3. Apicella P, Mirowitz SA: Interactive multiplanar interpolation of two-dimensional MR images, Clin Imaging, in press.

4. Applegate GR, Flannigan BD, Tolin BS et al: MR diagnosis of recurrent tears in the knee: value of intraarticular contrast material, Am J Roentgenol 161:821-825, 1993.

5. Araki Y, Ootani F, Tsukaguchi I et al: MR diagnosis of meniscal tears of the knee: value of axial three-dimensional Fourier transformation GRASS images, Am J Roentgenol 158:587-590, 1992.

6. Autz G, Goodwin C, Singson RD: Magnetic resonance evaluation of anterior cruciate ligament repair using the patellar tendon double bone block technique, Skeletal Radiol 20:585-588, 1991.

7. Barnett MJ: MR diagnosis of internal derangements of the knee: effect of field strength on efficacy, Am J Roentgenol 161:115-118, 1993.

8. Beltran J, Caudill JL, Herman LA et al: Rheumatoid arthritis: MR imaging manifestations, Radiology 165:153-157, 1987.

9. Beltran J, Noto AM, Herman LJ et al: Joint effusions: MR imaging, Radiology 158:133-137, 1986.

10. Bergman RA, Thompson SA, Afifi AK et al: Compendium of human anatomic variation: text, atlas, and world literature, Baltimore, 1988, Urban & Schwarzenberg.

11. Berlin RC, Levinsohn EM, Chrisman H: The wrinkled patellar tendon: an indication of abnormality in the extensor mechanism of the knee, Skeletal Radiol 20:181-185, 1991.

12. Bodne D, Quinn SF, Murray WT et al: Magnetic resonance images of chronic patellar tendinitis, Skeletal Radiol 17:24-28, 1988.

13. Braunstein EM, Brandt KD, Albrecht M: MRI demonstration of hypertrophic articular cartilage repair in osteoarthritis, Skeletal Radiol 19:335-339, 1990.

14. Brossmann J, Muhle C, Schroder C et al: Patellar tracking patterns during active and passive knee extension: evaluation with motion-triggered cine MR imaging, Radiology 187:205-212, 1993.

15. Brunner MC, Flower SP, Evancho AM et al: MRI of the athletic knee. Findings in aysmptomatic professional basketball and collegiate football players, Invest Radiol 24:72-75, 1989.

16. Buckwalter KA, Braunstein EM, Janizek DB et al: MR imaging of meniscal tears: narrow versus conventional window width photography, Radiology 187:827-830, 1993.

17. Buckwalter KA, Pennes DR: Anterior cruciate ligament: oblique sagittal MR imaging, Radiology 175:276-277, 1990.

18. Burk DL Jr, Dalinka MK, Kanal E et al: Meniscal and ganglion cysts of the knee: MR evaluation, Am J Roentgenol 150:331-336, 1988.

19. Carpenter WA: Meniscofemoral ligament simulating tear of the lateral meniscus: MR features, J Comput Assist Tomogr 14:1033-1034, 1990.

20. Chandnani VP, Ho C, Chu P et al: Knee hyaline cartilage evaluated with MR imaging: a cadaveric study involving multiple imaging sequences and intraarticular injection of gadolinium and saline solution, Radiology 178:557-561, 1991.

21. Cheung Y, Magee TH, Rosenberg ZS et al: MRI of anterior cruciate ligament reconstruction, J Comput Assist Tomogr 16:134-137, 1992.

22. Cobby MJ, Schweitzer ME, Resnick D: The deep lateral femoral notch: an indirect sign of a torn anterior cruciate ligament, Radiology 184:855-858, 1992.

23. Davis SJ, Teresi LM, Bradley WG et al: The "notch" sign: meniscal contour deformities as indicators of tear in MR imaging of the knee, J Comput Assist Tomogr 14:975-980, 1990.

24. De Smet AA, Norris MA, Yandow DR et al: MR diagnosis of meniscal tears of the knee: importance of high signal in the meniscus that extends to the surface, Am J Roentgenol 161:101-107, 1993.

25. Deutsch AL, Mink JH, Fox JM et al: Peripheral meniscal tears: MR findings after conservative treatment or arthroscopic repair, Radiology 176:485-488, 1990.

26. Deutsch AL, Mink JH, Fox JM et al: The postoperative knee, Magn Reson Q 8:23-54, 1992.

27. Deutsch AL, Mink JH, Rosenfelt FP et al: Incidental detection of hematopoietic hyperplasia on routine knee MR imaging, Am J Roentgenol 152:333-336, 1989.

28. Di Cesare E, Simonetti C, Morettini G et al: Popliteal artery entrapment: MR findings, J Comput Assist Tomogr 16:295-297, 1992.

29. Dillon EH, Pope CF, Jokl P et al: The clinical significance of stage 2 meniscal abnormalities on magnetic resonance knee images, Magn Reson Imaging 8:411-415, 1990.

30. Disler DG, Kattapuram SV, Chew FS et al: Meniscal tears of the knee: preliminary comparison of three-dimensional MR reconstruction with two-dimensional MR imaging and arthroscopy, Am J Roentgenol 160:343-345, 1993.

31. Dooms GC, Fisher MR, Hricak H et al: Bone marrow imaging: magnetic resonance studies related to age and sex, Radiology 155:429-432, 1985.

32. Drapé J-L, Thelen P, Gay-Depassier P et al: Intraarticular diffusion of Gd-DOTA after intravenous injection in the knee: MR imaging evaluation, Radiology 188:227-234, 1993.

33. El-Khoury GY, Wira RL, Berbaum KS et al: MR imaging of patellar tendinitis, Radiology 184:849-854, 1992.

34. Farley TE, Howell SM, Love KF et al: Meniscal tears: MR and arthrographic findings after arthroscopic repair, Radiology 180:517-522, 1991.

35. Fielding JR, Franklin PD, Kustan J: Popliteal cysts: a reassessment using magnetic resonance imaging, Skeletal Radiol 20:433-435, 1991.

36. Fitzgerald SW, Remer EM, Friedman H et al: MR evaluation of the anterior cruciate ligament: value of supplementing sagittal images with coronal and axial images, Am J Roentgenol 160:1233-1237, 1993.

37. Fritz RC, Helms CA: Visualization of meniscofemoral ligaments on coronal MR of the knee (letter), Am J Roentgenol 157:1126-1127, 1991.

38. Grover JS, Bassett LW, Gross ML et al: Posterior cruciate ligament: MR imaging, Radiology 174:527-530, 1990.

39. Hall FM, Joffe N: CT imaging of the anserine bursa, Am J Roentgenol 150:1107-1108, 1988.

40. Harcke HT, Synder M, Caro PA et al: Growth plate of the normal knee: evaluation with MR imaging, Radiology 183:119-123, 1992.

41. Hayes CW, Sawyer RW, Conway WF: Patellar cartilage le-

sions: in vitro detection and staging with MR imaging and pathologic correlation, Radiology 176:479-483, 1990.

42. Herman LJ, Beltran J: Pitfalls in MR imaging of the knee, Radiology 167:775-781, 1988.

43. Heron CW, Calvert PT: Three-dimensional gradient-echo MR imaging of the knee: comparison with arthroscopy in 100 cases, Radiology 183:839-844, 1992.

44. Herve-Somma CMP, Sebag GH, Prieur A-M et al: Juvenile rheumatoid arthritis of the knee: MR evaluation with Gd-DOTA, Radiology 182:93-98, 1992.

45. Ho VB, Kransdorf MJ, Jelinek JS et al: Dorsal defect of the patella: MR features, J Comput Assist Tomogr 15:474-476, 1991.

46. Hodler J, Haghighi P, Pathria MN et al: Meniscal changes in the elderly: correlation of MR imaging and histologic findings, Radiology 184:221-225, 1992.

47. Hodler J, Haghighi P, Trudell D et al: The cruciate ligaments of the knee: correlation between MR appearance and gross and histologic findings in cadaveric specimens, Am J Roentgenol 159:357-360, 1992.

48. Hodler J, Resnick D: Chondromalacia patellae, Am J Roentgenol 158:106-107, 1992.

49. Kaplan PA, Nelson NL, Garvin KL et al: MR of the knee: the significance of high signal in the meniscus that does not clearly extend to the surface, Am J Roentgenol 156:333-336, 1991.

50. Kaye JJ: Ligament and tendon tears: secondary signs, Radiology 188:616-617, 1993.

51. Kent RH, Pope CF, Lynch JK et al: Magnetic resonance imaging of the surgically repaired meniscus: six-month follow-up, Magn Reson Imaging 9:335-341, 1991.

52. Kier R, McCarthy SM: Lipohemarthrosis of the knee: MR imaging, J Comput Assist Tomogr 14:395-396, 1990.

53. Konig H, Sauter R, Deimling M et al: Cartilage disorders: comparison of spin-echo, CHESS, and FLASH sequence MR images, Radiology 164:753-758, 1987.

54. Konig H, Sieper J, Wolf K-J: Rheumatoid arthritis: evaluation of hypervascular and fibrous pannus with dynamic MR imaging enhanced with Gd-DTPA, Radiology 176:473-477, 1990.

55. Kornick J, Trefelner E, McCarthy S et al: Meniscal abnormalities in the asymptomatic population at MR imaging, Radiology 177:463-465, 1990.

56. Kursunoglu-Brahme S, Riccio T, Weisman MH et al: Rheumatoid knee: role of gadopentetate-enhanced MR imaging, Radiology 176:831-835, 1990.

57. Kursunoglu-Brahme S, Schwaighofer B, Gundry C et al: Jogging causes acute changes in the knee joint: an MR study in normal volunteers, Am J Roentgenol 154:1233-1235, 1990.

58. Laakman RW, Kaufman B, Han JS et al: MR imaging in patients with metallic implants, Radiology 157:711-714, 1985.

59. Lee JK, Yao L: Tibial collateral ligament bursa: MR imaging, Radiology 178:855-857, 1991.

60. Lee JK, Yao L, Phelps CT et al: Anterior cruciate ligament tears: MR imaging compared with arthroscopy and clinical tests, Radiology 166:861-864, 1988.

61. Lee KR, Cox GG, Neff JR et al: Cystic masses of the knee: arthrographic and CT evaluation, Am J Roentgenol 148:329-334, 1987.

62. Lehner KB, Rechl HP, Gmeinseser JK et al: Structure, func-

tion, and degeneration of bovine hyaline cartilage: assessment with MR imaging in vitro, Radiology 170:495-499, 1989.

63. Lynch TCP, Crues JV III, Morgan FW et al: Bone abnormalities of the knee: prevalence and significance at MR imaging, Radiology 171:761-766, 1989.

64. McLaren DB, Buckwalter KA, Vahey TN: The prevalence and significance of cyst-like changes at the cruciate ligament attachments in the knee, Skeletal Radiol 21:365-369, 1992.

65. Mechlin M, Thickman D, Kressel HY et al: Magnetic resonance imaging of postoperative patients with metallic implants, Am J Roentgenol 143:1281-1284, 1984.

66. Mesgarzadeh M, Sapega AA, Bonakdarpour A et al: Osteochondritis dissecans: analysis of mechanical stability with radiography, scintigraphy, and MR imaging, Radiology 165:775-780, 1987.

67. Mink JH, Deutsch AL: Occult cartilage and bone injuries of the knee: detection, classification, and assessment with MR imaging, Radiology 170:823-829, 1989.

68. Mink JH, Levy T, Crues JV III: Tears of the anterior cruciate ligament and menisci of the knee: MR imaging evaluation, Radiology 167:769-774, 1988.

69. Mirowitz SA: Motion artifact as a pitfall in diagnosis of meniscal tear on gradient reoriented MRI of the knee, J Comput Assist Tomogr 18:279-282, 1994.

70. Mirowitz SA, Shu HH: MR evaluation of knee collateral ligaments and related injuries: comparison of T1-weighted, T2-weighted and fat suppressed T2-weighted sequences with correlation to clinical examination, J Magn Reson Imaging, in press.

71. Modl JM, Sether LA, Haughton VM et al: Articular cartilage: correlation of histologic zones with signal intensity at MR imaging, Radiology 181:853-855, 1991.

72. Moeser P, Bechtold RE, Clark T et al: MR imaging of anterior cruciate ligament repair, J Comput Assist Tomogr 13:105-109, 1989.

73. Moore SG, Bisset GS III, Siegel MJ: Pediatric musculoskeletal MR imaging, Radiology 179:345-360, 1991.

74. Nakanishi K, Inoue M, Murakami T et al: MRI evaluation of plica synovialis mediopatellaris, SMRM Book of Abstracts 1992, p 2632.

75. Narayana PA, Brey WW, Kulkarni MV et al: Compensation for surface coil sensitivity variation in magnetic resonance imaging, Magn Reson Imaging 6:271-274, 1988.

76. Owsley DW, Mann RW: Bilateral dorsal defect of the patella (letter), Am J Roentgenol 154:1347-1348, 1990.

77. Pope CF, Bula V, Heinz W et al: Patellar tendonitis: significance of signal increase on gradient-echo and fat-saturation spin-echo sequences, SMRM Book of Abstracts 1992, p 2605.

78. Quinn SF, Brown TF: Meniscal tears diagnosed with MR imaging versus arthroscopy: how reliable a standard is arthroscopy? Radiology 181:843-847, 1991.

79. Quinn SF, Brown TR, Szumowski J: Menisci of the knee: radial MR imaging correlated with arthroscopy in 259 patients, Radiology 185:577-580, 1992.

80. Recht MP, Kramer J, Marcelis S et al: Abnormalities of articular cartilage in the knee: analysis of available MR techniques, Radiology 187:473-478, 1993.

81. Reicher MA, Hartzman S, Bassett LW et al: MR imaging of the knee. Part I. Traumatic disorders, Radiology 162:547-551, 1987.

82. Reicher MA, Hartzman S, Duckwiler GR et al: Meniscal injuries: detection using MR imaging, Radiology 159:753-757, 1986.

83. Reinig JW, McDevitt ER, Ove PN: Progression of meniscal degenerative changes in college football players: evaluation with MR imaging, Radiology 181:255-257, 1991.

84. Rubenstein JD, Kim JK, Morava-Protzner I et al: Effects of collagen orientation on MR imaging characteristics of bovine articular cartilage, Radiology 188:219-226, 1993.

85. Schuck JE, Czarnecki DJ: MR detection of probable hematopoietic hyperplasia involving the knees, proximal femurs, and pelvis (letter), Am J Roentgenol 153:655-656, 1989.

86. Schweitzer ME, Cervilla V, Kursunoglu-Brahme S et al: The PCL line: an indirect sign of anterior cruciate ligament injury, Clin Imaging 16:43-48, 1992.

87. Schweitzer ME, Falk A, Pathria M et al: MR imaging of the knee: can changes in the intracapsular fat pads be used as a sign of synovial proliferation in the presence of an effusion? Am J Roentgenol 160:823-826, 1993.

88. Semac MO Jr., Deutsch D, Bernstein BH et al: MR imaging in juvenile rheumatoid arthritis, Am J Roentgenol 150:873-878, 1988.

89. Shellock FG, Mink JH: Knees of trained long-distance runners: MR imaging before and after competition, Radiology 179:635-637, 1991.

90. Shellock FG, Mink J, Curtin S et al: MR imaging and metallic implants for anterior cruciate ligament reconstruction: assessment of ferromagnetism and artifact, J Magn Reson Imaging 2:225-228, 1992.

91. Shellock FG, Mink JH, Deutsch AL et al: Patellar tracking abnormalities: clinical experience with kinematic MR imaging in 130 patients, Radiology 172:799-804, 1989.

92. Shellock FG, Mink JH, Deutsch AL et al: Kinematic MR imaging of the patellofemoral joint: comparison of passive positioning and active movement techniques, Radiology 184:574-577, 1992.

93. Shellock FG, Mink JH, Deutsch AL et al: Patellofemoral joint: identification of abnormalities with active-movement, "unloaded" versus "loaded" kinematic MR imaging techniques, Radiology 188:575-578, 1993.

94. Shogry MEC, Pope TL Jr: Vacuum phenomenon simulating meniscal or cartilaginous injury of the knee at MR imaging, Radiology 180:513-515, 1991.

95. Silverman JM, Mink JH, Deutsch AL: Discoid menisci of the knee: MR imaging appearance, Radiology 173:351-354, 1989.

96. Singson RD, Feldman F, Staron R et al: MR imaging of displaced bucket-handle tear of the medial meniscus, Am J Roentgenol 156:121-124, 1991.

97. Singson RD, Zalduondo FM: Value of unenhanced spin-echo MR imaging in distinguishing between synovitis and effusion of the knee, Am J Roentgenol 159:569-571, 1992.

98. Smith DK, Totty WG: The knee after partial meniscectomy: MR imaging features, Radiology 176:141-144, 1990.

99. Spritzer CE, Vogler JB, Martinez S et al: MR imaging of the knee: preliminary results with a 3DFT GRASS pulse sequence, Am J Roentgenol 150:597-603, 1988.

100. Stoller DW, Martin C, Crues JV III et al: Meniscal tears: pathologic correlation with MR imaging, Radiology 163:731-735, 1987.

101. Tervonen O, Snoep G, Stuart MJ et al: Traumatic trabecular lesions observed on MR imaging of the knee, Acta Radiol 32:389-392, 1991.

102. Totterman S, Weiss SL, Szumowski J et al: MR fat suppression technique in the evaluation of normal structures of the knee, J Comput Assist Tomogr 13:473-479, 1989.

103. Traughber PD, Murray WT: Lateral meniscal pseudotear of "Line of Murray" (letter), Am J Roentgenol 157:649-650, 1991.

104. Tung GA, Davis LM, Wiggins ME et al: Tears of the anterior cruciate ligament: primary and secondary signs at MR imaging, Radiology 188:661-667, 1993.

105. Turner DA, Rapoport MI, Erwin WD et al: Truncation artifact: a potential pitfall in MR imaging of the menisci of the knee, Radiology 179:629-633, 1991.

106. Vahey TN, Bennett HT, Arrington LE et al: MR imaging of the knee: pseudotear of the lateral meniscus caused by the meniscofemoral ligament, Am J Roentgenol 154:1237-1239, 1990.

107. Vahey TN, Broome DR, Kayes KJ et al: Acute and chronic tears of the anterior cruciate ligament: differential features at MR imaging, Radiology 181:251-253, 1991.

108. Vahey TN, Hunt JE, Shelbourne KD: Anterior translation of the tibia at MR imaging: a secondary sign of anterior cruciate ligament tear, Radiology 187:817-819, 1993.

109. Vogler JB III, Murphy WA: Bone marrow imaging, Radiology 168:679-693, 1988.

110. Watanabe AT, Carter BC, Teitelbaum GP et al: Normal variations in MR imaging of the knee: appearance and frequency, Am J Roentgenol 153:341-344, 1989.

111. Weiss KL, Morehouse HT, Levy IM: Sagittal MR images of the knee: a low-signal band parallel to the posterior cruciate ligament caused by a displaced bucket-handle tear, Am J Roentgenol 156:117-119, 1991.

112. Whitten CG, Moore TE, Yuh WT et al: The use of intravenous gadopentetate dimeglumine in magnetic resonance imaging of synovial lesions, Skeletal Radiol 21:215-218, 1992.

113. Winalsi CS, Aliabadi P, Wright RJ et al: Enhancement of joint fluid with intravenously administered gadopentetate dimeglumine: technique, rationale, and implications, Radiology 187:179-185, 1993.

114. Yamato M, Yamagishi T: MRI of patellar tendon anterior cruciate ligament autografts, J Comput Assist Tomogr 16:604-607, 1992.

115. Yao L, Lee JK: Occult intraosseous fracture: detection with MR imaging, Radiology 167:749-751, 1988.

116. Yao L, Sinha S, Seeger LL: MR imaging of joints: analytic optimization of GRE techniques at 1.5 T, Am J Roentgenol 158:339-345, 1992.

117. Zeiss J, Saddemi SR, Ebraheim NA: MR imaging of the quadriceps tendon: normal layered configuration and its importance in cases of tendon rupture, Am J Roentgenol 159:1031-1034, 1992.

12

Shoulder*

ROTATOR CUFF

Imaging Techniques

Conventional spin echo

Investigations documenting the value of shoulder MR have primarily utilized conventional spin echo pulse sequences. These sequences continue to be the most widely used method for performing shoulder MR imaging. This is due to their established efficacy, universal availability, and the widespread familiarity with their contrast scale and imaging parameters.

Pulse sequence parameters. A combination of T1-weighted, proton density–weighted, and T2-weighted sequences is required for evaluation of the shoulder. Imaging parameters are selected in an effort to maximize signal-to-noise ratio, tissue contrast, spatial resolution, and artifact control while maintaining reasonable imaging times. T1-weighted images are acquired using repetition time (TR) 500 to 800 msec, echo time (TE) 12 to 20 msec, and two to four excitations. These images are necessary for evaluation of the marrow space and periarticular fat planes. In addition, they often render the highest quality anatomic depiction for evaluation of bone and soft tissue structures.

Proton density/T2-weighted images are acquired using TR 2200 to 3000 msec, TE 20 to 30 msec (first echo)/70 to 80 msec (second echo), and one or two excitations. Proton density–weighted images provide maximal signal-to-noise ratio because of their use of long TR and short TE, and they are often the most sensitive sequence for depicting signal intensity alterations within the rotator cuff. In spite of their relatively poor signal-to-noise ratio, T2-weighted images are essential for detecting soft tissue edema or fluid collections and for characterizing signal alterations within the rotator cuff. A slice thickness of 3 to 4 mm with 0.5 to 1 mm interslice gap is used, in combination with an imaging ma-

trix consisting of 128 to 192 (phase) $\times$ 256 (frequency) and a 14- to 18-cm field-of-view.

Artifact suppression methods. A number of imaging options can be useful for suppressing artifacts. Respiratory ordered phase encoding is useful for decreasing respiratory motion artifacts without prolonging imaging time. Spatial presaturation radiofrequency pulses reduce the signal intensity of inflowing protons, thereby decreasing vascular pulsation artifacts. Gradient moment nulling can be used with T2-weighted sequences to rephase moving spins and thus decrease respiratory motion and vascular pulsation artifacts. Oversampling techniques such as no-phase wrap are useful for eliminating aliasing artifacts caused by tissue extending beyond the prescribed field-of-view.

Other pulse sequences

Fast spin echo sequences. In addition to conventional spin echo sequences, several newer methods are available for shoulder MR imaging. The fast spin echo technique is based on the rapid acquisition relaxation enhanced (RARE) sequence originally described by Hen-

---

```
┌─────────────────────────────────────────────┐
│   ENTITIES THAT MAY SIMULATE ROTATOR CUFF    │
│                ABNORMALITY                    │
├─────────────────────────────────────────────┤
```

- Motion artifact
- Peribursal fat simulating contrast extravasation
- Critical zone signal variation
- "Magic angle" phenomenon
- Interposition/overlap of muscular fibers
- Internal rotation arm
- Partial volume averaging with fat/fluid
- Hyaline cartilage overlying humeral head
- Chemical shift misregistration artifact
- Postoperative changes
- Focal tendinopathy simulating tear
- Incomplete peribursal fat plane
- Apparent retraction of musculotendinous junction
- Fluid in the subacromial bursa

---

*Portions of this chapter were previously published in Mirowitz SA: Imaging techniques, normal variations, and diagnostic pitfalls in shoulder magnetic resonance imaging, MRI Clin North Am 1:19-36, 1993.

ENTITIES THAT MAY OBSCURE ROTATOR CUFF ABNORMALITY

- Suboptimal pulse sequence parameters
- Motion artifact
- Susceptibility artifact
- Gradient echo/fast spin echo sequences
- Contrast extravasation simulating peribursal fat
- Inadequate anteroposterior coverage
- Poor signal-to-noise ratio (absence of surface coil)
- Ingrowth of granulation/fibrotic tissue into tear
- Small partial thickness tears

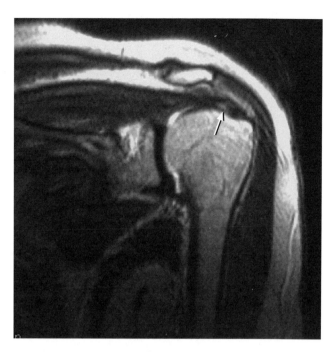

Fig. 12-1. Coronal oblique fast spin echo proton density–weighted image (TR 3000, effective TE 23, 2 Nex, 8 echo train) demonstrates diffuse blurring involving all anatomic structures. A focus of abnormal signal intensity *(arrow)* is present within the distal supraspinatus tendon.

nig.[20] With this method, a series of 180-degree radiofrequency refocusing pulses is applied following an initial 90-degree excitation pulse. Each of the echoes generated is separately phase encoded. As a result, imaging time is reduced proportional to the echo train length (usually 4 to 16 echoes). The resultant time savings can be used to decrease examination time or to improve signal-to-noise ratio, spatial resolution, and T2 weighting by prescribing longer TR, TE, number of excitations, and a higher resolution matrix than would be practical using conventional spin echo imaging.

Studies that have evaluated fast spin echo imaging of the brain, spine, and pelvis indicate that it generally provides high-quality images while maintaining tissue contrast equivalent to that of conventional T2-weighted spin echo images.[24,50] Reported differences in tissue contrast relate to the relatively increased signal intensity of fat on fast spin echo images and reduced sensitivity to depiction of susceptibility effects generated by hemorrhagic breakdown products. Some implementations of T2-weighted fast spin echo imaging can result in significant alterations in tissue contrast, which compromise lesion detection.[5] However, the sensitivity of fast spin echo images to depiction of fluid is extremely high. These images are subject to blurring, particularly when a relatively short TE or long echo train is used (Fig. 12-1).

In our experience thus far, fast spin echo provides high-quality images of the shoulder and seems to be capable of demonstrating fluid within full thickness rotator cuff tears. However, its efficacy for depicting more subtle signal alterations, such as those related to tendinitis or partial thickness tears, is unproven at this time.

Gradient echo sequences. Gradient echo sequences use relatively short TR, TE, and reduced flip angle and substitute gradient refocusing for the 180-degree RF refocusing pulse used in spin echo imaging. This allows the imaging time to be reduced while preserving an adequate signal-to-noise ratio. Tissue contrast on gradient echo images varies with alterations in TR, TE, and flip angle. Generally, a decreased flip angle and increased TE contribute to increased T2 weighting on short TR gradient echo images. One or many images can be acquired during a single TR. Multislice sequences provide increased signal-to-noise ratio and relatively proton density weighted tissue contrast.[8]

Multislice steady state gradient echo images have been used for evaluation of the rotator cuff.[45] Typical imaging parameters include TR 400 msec, TE 15 msec, and 15-degree flip angle. There is, however, sparse data regarding the sensitivity of gradient echo imaging relative to conventional spin echo imaging for detection of rotator cuff tears. It should not be assumed that the criteria developed using spin echo imaging will necessarily apply to interpretation of gradient echo images, since gradient echo images display substantially different tissue contrast. It is anticipated that relatively proton density–weighted sequences will not permit detection of small amounts of fluid or high signal intensity edema/granulation tissue related to rotator cuff tears that would be seen on T2-weighted spin echo images.

Magnetic susceptibility artifacts are accentuated on gradient echo images because of the absence of a 180-degree refocusing radio frequency pulse. These are manifested as foci of artifactual signal void that can have peripheral hyperintensity. Such artifacts occur in the presence of metal, air, or calcium and are more promi-

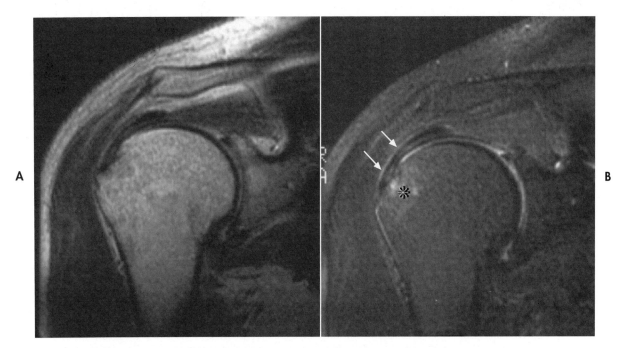

Fig. 12-2. A, It is difficult to distinguish the signal intensity of fat from that of fluid on coronal oblique T2-weighted image (TR 2200, TE 70, 1 Nex). **B,** This distinction is facilitated with the use of fat suppression that highlights a small amount of fluid within the subacromial bursa *(arrows)*. There is also improved conspicuousness of marrow edema within the lateral humeral head *(asterisk)* on the fat-suppressed image and relative hyperintensity of hyaline cartilage. Linear increased signal intensity is present within the rotator cuff tendon. There is heterogeneous suppression of subcutaneous fat adjacent to the surface coils.

nent on images acquired at high field strength, using relatively long echo times or large voxel sizes.

Fat suppression

Several fat-suppression methods are available. These include radiofrequency presaturation of the lipid peak (fat saturation), phase contrast methods in which echo sampling is performed when fat and water protons are out of phase with one another (Dixon method), and short tau inversion recovery (STIR) imaging in which suppression of fat is based on its short T1 relaxation time.[49] Other methods and combinations of these methods are also available.

Advantages of fat suppression include improved depiction of bone marrow abnormalities,[19,36] improved distinction between fat and fluid on T2-weighted images (Figs. 12-2, *A* and *B*), increased conspicuousness of signal intensity abnormalities as a result of improved dynamic range characteristics, reduced artifacts related to respiratory motion, and elimination of chemical shift misregistration artifacts.[34]

Disadvantages of some fat-suppression techniques include a reduced number of imaging slices per unit time,

increased sensitivity to susceptibility artifacts, presentation of unfamiliar tissue contrast, reduced effectiveness of fat suppression using low to mid field strength systems, lack of universal availability, and sensitivity to magnetic-field nonuniformity (Figs. 12-2, *A* and *B*).

The use of fat suppression improves the depiction of small amounts of fluid within small full thickness and partial thickness rotator cuff tears.[37,53] Data continue to be accumulated, but it appears that fat saturation improves sensitivity for evaluation of rotator cuff pathology (Figs. 12-3, *A* and *B*).

MR arthrography

MR arthrography has been used to evaluate the rotator cuff and the labral-capsular complex[14] (Figs. 12-4, 12-5). This technique requires injection of 12 to 20 ml of paramagnetic contrast material solution (1 ml gadopentetate dimeglumine in 250 ml saline) into the glenohumeral joint, followed by acquisition of T1-weighted images.[14,22] The use of a fluoroscopy room is usually required, since a test dose of iodinated contrast material is given to verify intraarticular needle position before injection of the paramagnetic contrast solution. An alter-

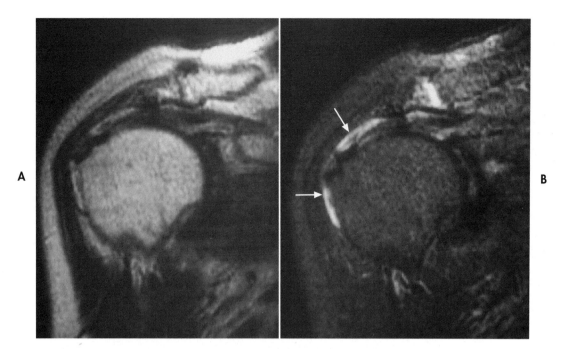

Fig. 12-3. Coronal oblique T2-weighted image **(A)** (TR 2200, TE 70, 1 Nex) and corresponding fat-suppressed image obtained using identical parameters **(B).** The fat-suppressed image provides improved distinction between fluid within the subacromial bursa *(arrows)* and peribursal fat, and results in improved conspicuousness of full thickness rotator cuff tear.

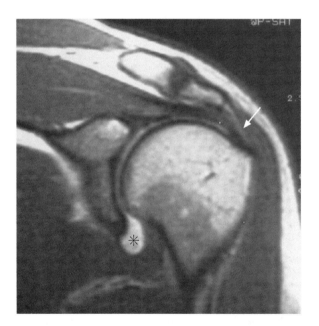

Fig. 12-4. Coronal oblique T1-weighted image (TR 660, TE 25) obtained following intraarticular administration of gadopentetate dimeglumine solution. The joint space is distended and opacified by the paramagnetic contrast agent *(asterisk).* There is no extravasation of contrast material into or through the rotator cuff in this patient. Note that the signal intensity of the contrast material is similar to that of fat within the peribursal fat plane *(arrow)* and subcutaneous tissues. (From Mirowitz SA: MRI Clin North Am 1:19-36, 1993.)

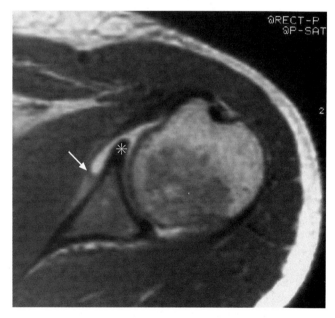

Fig. 12-5. Transaxial T1-weighted image (TR 600, TE 25) from MR arthrogram. The paramagnetic contrast material solution allows for excellent delineation of the normal fibrocartilaginous glenoid labrum *(asterisk)* and for determination of the site of capsular insertion *(arrow).* (From Mirowitz SA: MRI Clin North Am 1:19-36, 1993.)

native method involves injection of saline instead of paramagnetic contrast material, with subsequent acquisition of T2-weighted rather than T1-weighted images.

The diagnosis of a rotator cuff tear on MR arthrography is based on the observation of contrast material leakage outside the joint capsule and either into (partial tear) or through (full thickness tear) the rotator cuff tendons. The contrast material solution distends the joint capsule and outlines the contour of the glenoid labrum.

Pitfalls of MR arthrography. Although some encouraging results have been achieved with the use of MR arthrography, several important drawbacks have been recognized. For example, MR arthrography is associated with increased cost for MR examination of the shoulder and increased discomfort for the patient, and it carries a remote chance of complications. Moreover, MR arthrography alone cannot be used to detect bursal surface partial thickness tears, intrasubstance tears, or rotator cuff tendinitis. For all of these reasons, it seems unlikely that MR arthrography will become established as a routine screening method. Instead, it will probably be reserved as a problem-solving technique for selected patients in whom initial MR examination yields equivocal results.

It should be emphasized that T1-weighted images must be acquired before the installation of contrast material into the joint space. Despite the added time that this entails, false positive results may be obtained when baseline imaging is omitted. These errors relate to confusion of high signal intensity peribursal fat for contrast material extravasation into the subacromial-subdeltoid bursa.[22] This has led to overestimation of partial tears as full thickness tears. Conversely, false negative results can occur when extravasated contrast material is presumed to represent normal peribursal fat tissue. Fat-suppressed T1-weighted images can provide distinction between paramagnetic contrast material and fatty tissue so that preinjection images are not mandatory.[15] The use of fat suppression also increases the conspicuousness of extravasated contrast material. In tendons with friable margins, imhibition of contrast material into the tendon can be observed on fat-suppressed images.[41]

Imaging planes

A series of coronal gradient echo or short TR spin echo images is initially acquired using the body coil. Using these images for localization, a series of transaxial images is then prescribed. The field-of-view is off-centered laterally to encompass the shoulder, and images are acquired using either a spin echo or a gradient echo technique from below the bony glenoid inferiorly to the top of the shoulder superiorly. These transaxial images are useful for evaluating the labral-capsular complex.

Transaxial images also serve as localizer images for the prescription of coronal oblique images, which are of primary importance for evaluating the rotator cuff. Co-

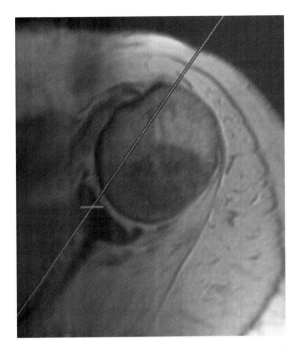

Fig. 12-6. Transaxial gradient echo image at the level of the bony glenoid. A ray has been placed along the axis of the supraspinatus tendon. This demonstrates the slight divergence in angulation between the supraspinatus tendon and bony glenoid, which is an important consideration in orientation of coronal oblique images for evaluation of the rotator cuff. (From Mirowitz SA: MRI Clin North Am 1:19-36, 1993.)

ronal oblique images are prescribed along the course of the supraspinatus tendon, which is identified on transaxial images acquired near the superior aspect of the shoulder. Coronal oblique images should not be prescribed using the bony glenoid for reference, because its orientation varies slightly from that of the supraspinatus tendon (Fig. 12-6). Hence, the rotator cuff demonstrates increased partial volume effects on images obtained using the bony glenoid for reference. Once the angle of the supraspinatus tendon has been determined, the bony glenoid can be used to indicate appropriate anterior-posterior coverage for image acquisition. Coverage should be adequate to visualize the subscapularis tendons anteriorly and the majority of the infraspinatus/teres minor muscles posteriorly. In addition to its primary importance for evaluation of the rotator cuff, coronal or coronal oblique images are also useful for assessing the superior and inferior portions of the fibrocartilaginous glenoid labrum.[29,58]

Sagittal oblique images are often used to supplement coronal oblique images for evaluation of the rotator cuff. T1-weighted sagittal oblique images help to detect acromial deformity and subacromial spurs, which contribute to rotator cuff impingement. Proton density–weighted/

T2-weighted sagittal oblique images are useful for defining and localizing some small rotator cuff tears.

Patient positioning

Imaging should be performed with the patient in a supine position, with the head directed toward the bore of the imager. A few moments should be taken at the outset of the examination to ensure the patient's comfort; this minimizes motion throughout the examination. Many patients are more comfortable with their legs slightly elevated to relieve back pressure. Measures to counteract anxiety and claustrophobia should also be considered when appropriate.

The upper extremity should be placed in a neutral to slightly externally rotated position, with the thumb pointing up slightly laterally. Although it is desirable to image the shoulder with the arm in mild external rotation, this may be uncomfortable for many patients; discomfort may be reduced by providing support beneath the elbow.[7] The arm should be placed at the patient's side;

placement of the arm on the abdomen can result in movement of the arm with respiration.

Surface coils

A surface coil must be used to achieve an adequate signal-to-noise ratio in conjunction with the relatively small field-of-view, the thin slices, and the high-resolution matrices that result in good spatial resolution. A variety of surface-coil configurations are available for shoulder imaging. Among the most frequently used coils are single-loop coils, which have a curved configuration. Placement of a surface coil in a coronal oblique position over the top of the shoulder rather than in a strict anterior or posterior position allows for improvement in the signal-to-noise ratio for evaluation of the rotator cuff.[16] It is important to use retaining straps with these coils to prevent their movement during the examination. A pair of separated, flat, circular surface coils can be used as a Helmholtz pair; the shoulder is positioned between these

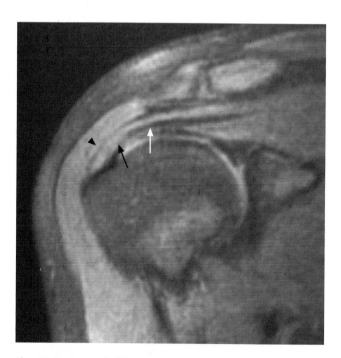

Fig. 12-7. Coronal oblique fat-suppressed proton density–weighted image (TR 2500, TE 20, 1 Nex) in normal subject. A well-defined focus of moderately increased signal intensity *(black arrow)* is present within the substance of the distal supraspinatus tendon, in the region of the critical zone. This focus is isointense with skeletal muscle. Relative increased signal intensity is also present, caused by muscular components of the cuff that are interposed between the undersurface of the supraspinatus tendon and the joint capsule *(white arrow)* and that overlie the supraspinatus tendon and extend to the greater tuberosity *(arrowhead)*. (From Mirowitz SA: MRI Clin North Am 1:19-36, 1993.)

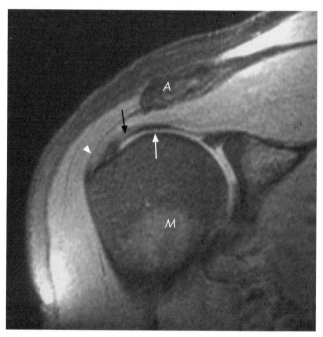

Fig. 12-8. Coronal oblique fat-suppressed proton density–weighted image (TR 2500, TE 20, 1 Nex) in normal subject. A focus of moderate increased signal intensity (isointense with skeletal muscle) is present within the supraspinatus tendon, in the region of the critical zone *(black arrow)*. Muscular fibers of the rotator cuff extend along the superolateral aspect of the supraspinatus tendon near its insertion into the greater humeral tuberosity *(arrowhead)*. Hyaline cartilage along the humeral head demonstrates marked hyperintensity *(white arrow)* and hematopoietic marrow within the proximal humeral metaphysis *(M)* is moderately hyperintense as a result of the use of fat suppression. Mild inferior sloping of the lateral acromion process *(A)* is also present. (From Mirowitz SA: MRI Clin North Am 1:19-36, 1993.)

two coils. Although most shoulder coils used in the past were linear, coils that use quadrature technology and multicoil arrays are now available and further improve the signal-to-noise ratio.

The size of the surface coil should be concordant with the size of the shoulder being examined. Because the sensitive range of the coil is proportional to its diameter, a large coil should be used for large patients. The signal intensity of tissues located close to the surface coil (e.g., subcutaneous fat) is considerably higher than that of deeper tissues. This occasionally causes difficulty in characterizing these tissues. For example, fat located next to the coil can appear relatively hyperintense on T2-weighted images, thus simulating fluid. Software algorithms that provide linear correction of signal intensity are available, so coil burnout is minimized and signal uniformity is improved throughout the field-of-view.

Pitfalls and Variations
Signal intensity variations of the rotator cuff

Most tendons appear uniformly hypointense on all pulse sequences, with signal intensity equivalent to that of cortical bone. Consequently, the presence of any focus of relatively increased signal intensity within the rotator cuff tendons has been regarded as abnor-

mal.[23,26,33,60,61] However, foci of relatively increased signal intensity can be observed within the tendinous cuff in asymptomatic subjects and do not necessarily indicate pathology.

Anterior rotator cuff. Within the anterior rotator cuff, a focus of relatively increased signal intensity is often observed in the distal supraspinatus tendon.[25,30,34,55] This focus is located approximately 1 cm proximal to the insertion of this tendon into the greater tuberosity of the humerus and measures approximately 1 cm in length[25,34] (Figs. 12-7, 12-8). It exhibits a round to oval configuration and has well-defined margins. It is most prominent on proton density–weighted images, particularly those acquired using fat suppression,[34] and may also appear prominent on gradient echo images.[25]

This focus is isointense with skeletal muscle on all pulse sequences. Since muscle is considerably hypointense on T2-weighted images, this focus is difficult to discern on T2-weighted images (Figs. 12-9, *A* and *B*). It is important to verify that this normal signal variation does not demonstrate signal intensity on T2-weighted images, which approaches that of fluid; this indicates the presence of a rotator cuff tear (partial, interstitial, or full thickness). Furthermore, this signal variation should not be associated with any morphologic alterations of the ro-

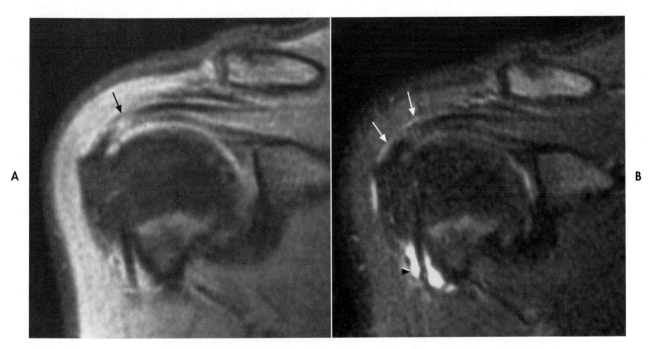

Fig. 12-9. Coronal oblique fat-suppressed proton density–weighted **(A)** (TR 2500, TE 20, 1 Nex) and T2-weighted **(B)** (TR 2500, TE 70) images in a normal subject. Moderately increased signal intensity is present in the region of the critical zone of the supraspinatus tendon *(black arrow)*. This focus maintains isointensity with skeletal muscle on both short and long echo time images. T2-weighted image demonstrates markedly increased signal intensity because of fluid within the subacromial-subdeltoid bursa *(white arrows)* and biceps tendon sheath *(arrowhead)*. (From Mirowitz SA: MRI Clin North Am 1:19-36, 1993.)

tator cuff tendons, such as thinning, irregularity, or discontinuity.[25,34]

The location and configuration of this focus of relatively increased signal intensity is concordant with the critical zone of the supraspinatus tendon. The critical zone is characterized by aberrant microvascularity; it is, in essence, a microvascular watershed zone. The critical zone is predisposed to developing ischemic changes and is a site subjected to repeated physical trauma from impingement between the humeral head and the coracoacromial arch. Because of these factors, the critical zone is a dominant site of development for rotator cuff pathologic conditions. The aberrant vascularity of the critical zone may account for the signal alterations observed on MR images in this location; it is also possible that subclinical degenerative alterations can be present in asymptomatic subjects in this location, accounting for its altered signal intensity.[34]

Another hypothesis of the basis for signal variations in this location relates to the "magic angle" theory. Collagenous fibers oriented at 55 degrees relative to the main magnetic field exhibit artifactual increased signal intensity on MR images.[10,13] The "magic angle" phenomenon may contribute to the focus of relatively increased signal intensity within the anterior supraspinatus tendon, since the tendon deviates anteriorly at or near this position.[25]

Posterior rotator cuff. Another focus of relatively increased signal intensity is observed in a slightly more posterior location within the rotator cuff (Fig. 12-10). This focus has a linear or trapezoidal configuration and appears to be related to interposition of muscle fibers between the distal tendinous components of the supraspinatus and infraspinatus/teres minor portions of the cuff[7,34,54] (Figs. 12-7, 12-8, and 12-11). Overlap between muscular and tendinous components of the rotator cuff complex is accentuated when images are acquired with the patient's arm in internal rotation (Figs. 12-12, *A* and *B*). In this position the infraspinatus tendon is located superior and lateral to the supraspinatus.[7] This orientation also occurs sometimes with the patient's arm in a neutral position and can result in apparent discontinuity of the supraspinatus tendon.[7] Muscle fibers also extend distally along the inferior aspect of the cuff tendons and are interposed between these tendons superiorly and the joint capsule inferiorly[34] (Fig. 12-7).

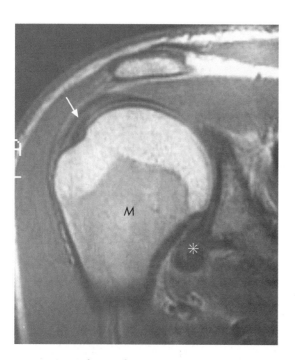

Fig. 12-10. Linear focus of moderately increased signal intensity *(arrow)* is identified within the substance of the posterior rotator cuff tendons on coronal oblique proton density–weighted image (TR 2200, TE 20, 1 Nex). This is due to interposition of muscular elements with cuff tendons. Also noted is reduced signal intensity throughout the humeral metaphysis *(M)*, corresponding to hematopoietic marrow. There is also a masslike focus of low signal intensity located inferior to the glenoid *(asterisk)*, which is due to redundancy of the axillary recess of the joint capsule.

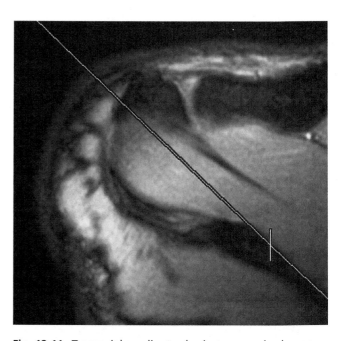

Fig. 12-11. Transaxial gradient echo image acquired near the superior aspect of the shoulder. A ray has been placed along the axis of the infraspinatus tendon, which was visualized on an adjacent image. This demonstrates the divergence in angulation between the tendinous components of the supraspinatus and infraspinatus muscles and the presence of muscular components of the cuff interposed between these two structures. (From Mirowitz SA: MRI Clin North Am 1:19-36, 1993.)

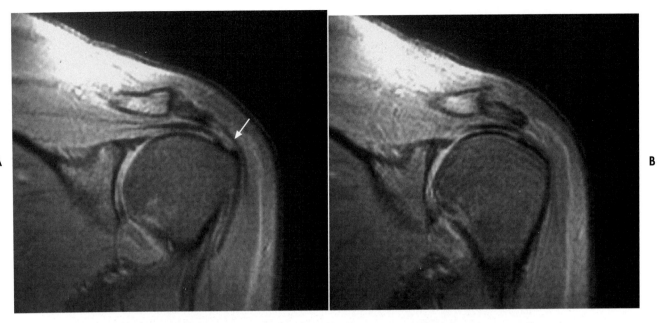

A   B

Fig. 12-12. Coronal oblique proton density–weighted images (TR 2200, TE 20, 1 Nex) obtained using fat saturation. Images were acquired with the patient's arm in internal **(A)** and external **(B)** rotation. There is relatively increased signal intensity noted *(arrow)* along the superior aspect of the distal supraspinatus tendon because of the overlapping muscle fibers on the internally rotated image.

It should be reemphasized that each of the signal variations described above should maintain isointensity with skeletal muscle on all pulse sequences and should not approach the signal intensity of fluid on T2-weighted images. This criterion and familiarity with the location and morphology of these signal variations facilitates their recognition and helps to distinguish them from significant pathologic conditions.

Partial volume effects. Another potential cause of artifactual increased signal intensity within the rotator cuff is partial volume averaging of the supraspinatus tendon with fat that is anterior to the tendon (Figs. 12-13, 12-14, *A* and *B*). This finding can simulate a rotator cuff tear[54]; it should not be apparent on fat-suppressed images. Fluid within the subacromial-subdeltoid bursa can also undergo partial volume averaging with the supraspinatus tendon, simulating a tear.[40] With the arm in external rotation, fluid in the biceps tendon sheath can also be averaged with the supraspinatus tendon, simulating a tear.[7]

Hyaline cartilage overlying the humeral head can appear to represent diffuse moderate signal intensity within the supraspinatus tendon, which is suggestive of tendinitis.[54]

Artifacts. Motion artifacts resulting from gross motion, vascular pulsation, or respiratory motion generate high signal intensity ghosting artifacts that can overlie the rotator cuff tendons and simulate a pathologic con-

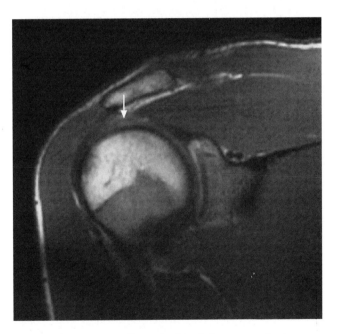

Fig. 12-13. Apparent discontinuity of the supraspinatus tendon *(arrow)* is evident on this coronal oblique T1-weighted image (TR 650, TE 18, 2 Nex). This is due to partial volume averaging of the tendon with fat located anterior to it. Also noted is reduced signal intensity secondary to prominent hematopoietic marrow within the humeral neck and bony glenoid.

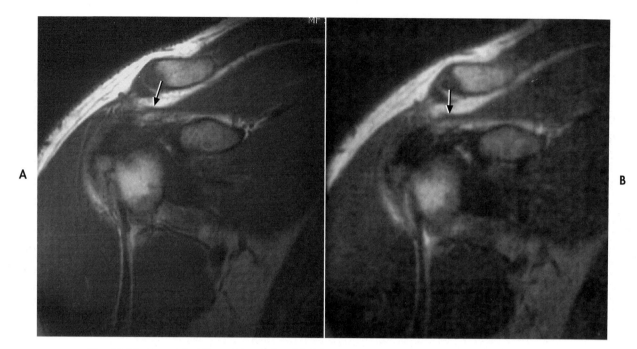

Fig. 12-14. Coronal oblique T1-weighted **(A)** (TR 400, TE 18, 2 Nex) and T2-weighted **(B)** (TR 2200, TE 70, 1 Nex) images demonstrate apparent discontinuity of supraspinatus tendon *(arrows),* caused by partial volume averaging with adjacent fat.

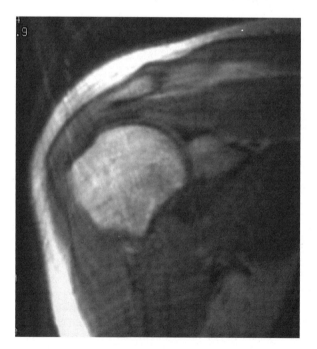

Fig. 12-15. Coronal oblique proton density–weighted image (TR 2200, TE 20, 1 Nex) in normal subject demonstrates a series of curvilinear increased signal intensity that overlie the rotator cuff. These artifacts are due to motion of the shoulder during image acquisition and may either simulate or obscure rotator cuff abnormalities.

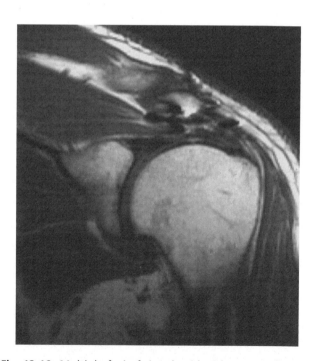

Fig. 12-16. Multiple foci of signal void with surrounding hyperintensity are noted in the region of the rotator cuff on coronal oblique T1-weighted image (TR 650, TE 18, 2 Nex) in a patient who underwent previous surgical rotator cuff repair. Visualization of the underlying soft tissues is obscured by these findings. Resection of the acromion process is also evident.

dition (Fig. 12-15). Chemical shift misregistration artifacts arising at the interface between the rotator cuff and the peribursal fat plane can also lead to artifactually increased signal intensity.

Postoperative changes

Abnormal increased signal intensity on all pulse sequences can be observed in patients who have received a recent injection of corticosteroids or other medications into muscle or tendons of the shoulder. Patients who have undergone previous rotator cuff repair often show extensive signal intensity and morphologic alterations that complicate the evaluation of a recurrent tear (Figs. 12-16, 12-17). Altered signal intensity of bony structures can also be present, and prominent metallic artifacts may obscure visualization of important anatomic structures (Figs. 12-18, *A* and *B*). Following primary repair of the rotator cuff, intermediate to high signal intensity can be observed within the cuff on T2-weighted images in addition to tendinous irregularity. These alterations of signal intensity and morphology may be indistinguishable from a partial thickness tear.[40]

Limitations in the detection of rotator cuff tears

Although observation of hyperintensity on T2-weighted images within the rotator cuff is the primary

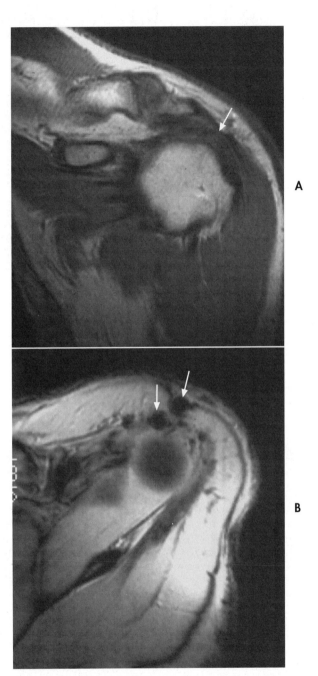

Fig. 12-18. A, Coronal oblique proton density–weighted image (TR 2200, TE 20, 1 Nex) in patient who underwent previous rotator cuff repair and acromioplasty. There is absence of the acromion process, with susceptibility artifact from metallic shavings. There is also diffuse moderate increased signal intensity throughout the supraspinatus tendon *(arrow).* **B,** Accentuation of susceptibility effects *(arrows)* is present on transaxial gradient echo image (TR 300, TE 15, 30-degree flip angle, 2 Nex) in region of rotator cuff.

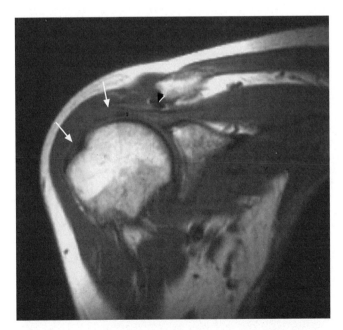

Fig. 12-17. Coronal oblique T1-weighted image (TR 650, TE 18, 2 Nex) in a patient who underwent previous rotator cuff repair. There is diffuse globular increased signal intensity throughout the supraspinatus tendon *(arrows),* with metal artifact located along the bursal surface of the tendon near the musculotendinous junction *(arrowhead).* The acromion process has been resected.

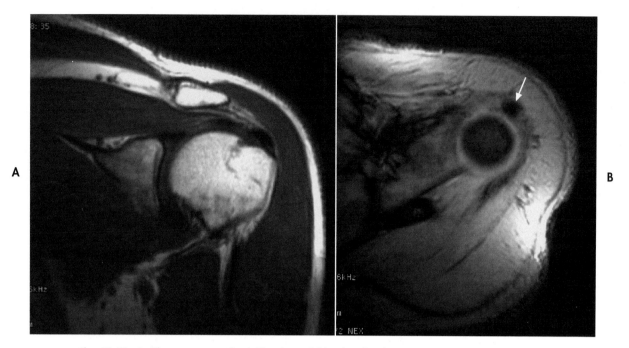

Fig. 12-19. A, The presence of calcification within the distal supraspinatus tendon is poorly visualized on coronal oblique T1-weighted image (TR 650, TE 18, 2 Nex). **B,** Calcification is more sensitively depicted on transaxial gradient echo image (TR 300, TE 15, 30-degree flip angle, 2 Nex), where it produces a focal signal void *(arrow).*

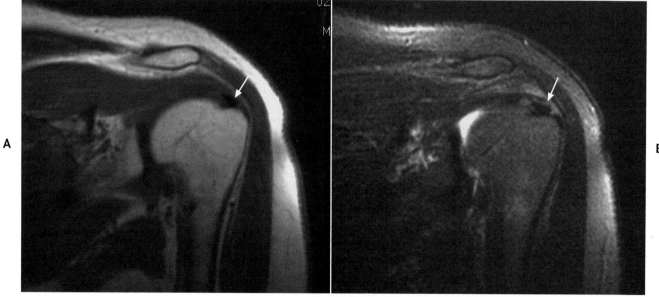

Fig. 12-20. Coronal oblique T1-weighted **(A)** (TR 650, TE 18, 2 Nex) and fast spin echo fat-suppressed T2-weighted **(B)** (TR 3000, effective TE 90, 2 Nex, 16 echo train) images demonstrate a subtle focus of relatively decreased signal intensity within the distal supraspinatus tendon *(arrow).* These findings are due to calcific tendinitis, as verified on plain radiograph **(C)** *(arrow).*

criterion for diagnosing a rotator cuff tear, some tears (partial and full thickness) do not demonstrate these findings[44] and can be recognized only through alterations of tendon morphology. These aberrant signal characteristics are probably the result of the ingrowth of granulation tissue and/or fibrotic tissue into the tear site. This tissue often appears relatively hypointense on T2-weighted images and prevents fluid from extending into the cuff defect.[44]

MR has not been highly sensitive for detecting partial thickness rotator cuff tears.[37,44,47,53] This is perhaps related to insufficient amounts of high signal intensity fluid within the tear site or to limitations in spatial resolution. We have found that fat-suppressed T2-weighted images can help to identify partial thickness cuff tears, but that many such tears remain difficult to detect.

Limitations in characterizing rotator cuff injury

Distinction of the various grades of rotator cuff injury can be difficult in some cases. For example, inflammatory and/or degenerative alterations within the cuff (i.e., tendinitis) can appear to be similar to partial thickness intrasubstance tendinous tears[44,52] (Fig. 12-2). Similarly, extensive partial thickness cuff tears can be difficult to distinguish from small, full thickness tears.[27,52,54,58,59]

Calcification within the rotator cuff tendons is characteristic of calcific tendinitis. Although focal or diffuse signal alterations can be observed within the cuff because of associated inflammatory changes, calcifications themselves are usually inapparent on spin echo MR images.

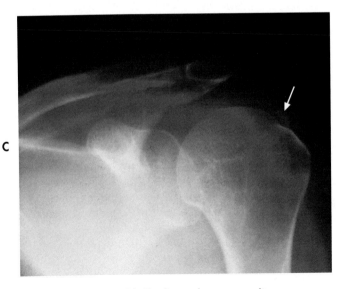

Fig. 12-20, cont'd. For legend, see opposite page.

When calcific tendinitis is suspected, gradient echo images can result in improved depiction of calcifications as foci of signal void (Figs. 12-19, *A* and *B*, 12-20, *A* to *C*).

Ancillary Signs of Rotator Cuff Injury
Musculotendinous junction

The musculotendinous junction of the supraspinatus is usually located over the apex of the humeral head. Proximal retraction of the musculotendinous junction is indirect evidence of a full thickness tear of the supraspinatus tendon. The precise location of the musculotendinous junction can be difficult to determine, since there is not a complete and distinct transition from purely muscular to purely tendinous fibers at this point. Rather, there is a transition from primarily muscular to primarily tendinous fibers that may be somewhat gradual.[34] There are variations in the position of the musculotendinous junction among individuals. However, the musculotendinous junction is usually located not more than 15 degrees medial to the 12 o'clock position.[38]

Retraction of the musculotendinous junction does not occur in patients with partial thickness rotator cuff tears. Similarly, many patients with small full thickness tears do not manifest this finding.[44] Therefore, although retraction of the musculotendinous junction can be a useful ancillary sign of moderate to large full thickness rotator cuff tears, one must be aware of the limitations of this sign.

Peribursal fat plane

The subacromial-subdeltoid bursa has an associated fat plane (peribursal fat plane) that demonstrates increased signal intensity on T1-weighted images. Focal or generalized discontinuity of the peribursal fat plane has been used as an ancillary sign of rotator cuff pathology,[61] with the apparent discontinuity presumed to be the result of reactive inflammatory edema. However, portions of the peribursal fat plane may not be evident in some asymptomatic subjects. Apparent absence of the peribursal fat plane is most frequent on sections acquired through the anterior supraspinatus tendon[30,34] (Fig. 12-21). Apparent discontinuity of the peribursal fat plane was observed at the level of the supraspinatus tendon in 12 of 15 asymptomatic subjects[34] and in 17 of 30 subjects[25] in two studies. Other investigators have also noted the absence of the peribursal fat plane, but with reduced prevalence.[6,38] Although the fat plane may be anatomically intact in these subjects, the lack of visualization of portions of this structure may be related to limitations in spatial resolution.

Subacromial-subdeltoid bursa

The presence of fluid within the subacromial-subdeltoid bursa has also been proposed as an ancillary

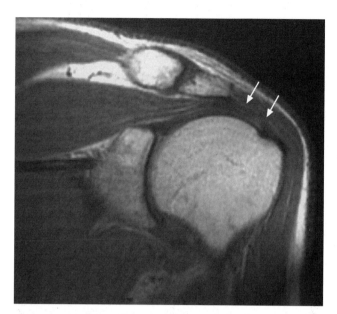

Fig. 12-21. Coronal oblique proton density–weighted image (TR 2500, TE 20, 1 Nex) in normal subject demonstrates mild hypertrophy of the acromioclavicular joint and slight impression on the underlying rotator cuff. Portions of the peribursal fat plane *(arrows)* cannot be visualized on this image, which was acquired through the anterior aspect of the shoulder. (From Mirowitz SA: MRI Clin North Am 1:19-36, 1993.)

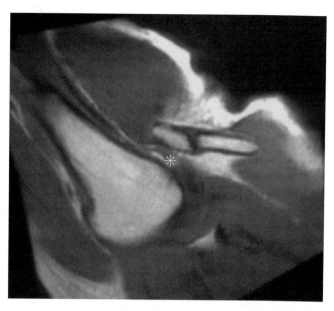

Fig. 12-22. Coronal oblique T1-weighted image (TR 650, TE 18, 2 Nex) in a normal subject was acquired with the subject's arm positioned above his head. The acromiohumeral space *(asterisk)* has become relatively narrow, resulting in some apparent impingement of the underlying musculotendinous rotator cuff.

sign of rotator cuff tear. In patients with glenohumeral joint effusions, joint fluid can escape through a defect in the rotator cuff to enter this bursa. However, a small amount of fluid can also be visualized in the subacromial bursa in many normal subjects.[34,38] Bursal fluid is most frequently observed on fat-suppressed T2-weighted images[34] (Fig. 12-9). The presence of small amounts of bursal fluid is usually not apparent on conventional T2-weighted images because of the similar signal intensity of fluid and fat.[6,25,34] Only a thin film of fluid is observed in normal subjects; a significant volume of fluid is considered to be abnormal. However, significant bursal fluid collections are not specific for rotator cuff tear, because they may also be found in association with subacromial bursitis. Fluid may also be observed within the subacromial bursa following rotator cuff repair.[40]

Impingement

One advantage of MR for shoulder imaging is that it allows direct visualization of rotator cuff impingement. Impingement can be the result of hypertrophic degenerative changes of the acromio-clavicular joint, subacromial osteophytes, and a low-lying or abnormally shaped ac-

romion process.[47] Prominence of the acromio-clavicular joint and acromio-clavicular osteophytes can be observed in asymptomatic individuals, in addition to a mild apparent impression on the underlying musculotendinous cuff[6,30,34,38] (Figs. 12-19, *A* and *B*). Such minor degrees of apparent impingement should not be considered significant. Conversely, one must recognize that the presence of significant impingement may not be visible on images acquired with the arm at the patient's side. Impingement usually occurs or is most severe with the arm abducted and lifted above the patient's head (Fig. 12-22). In selected patients, a coronal oblique sequence can be acquired with the arm placed over the patient's head. However, space restrictions within the bore of the magnet may be a limiting factor for many patients.

An apparent spur can be observed along the undersurface of the mid-to-lateral aspect of the acromion process (Figs. 12-23, 12-24). This pseudospur projects inferolaterally on coronal oblique images and represents an inferior tendon slip of the deltoid muscle.[25] A true osteophyte usually demonstrates some internal hyperintensity on T1-weighted images because of the presence of marrow fat, whereas hyperintensity is absent in the pseudospur.

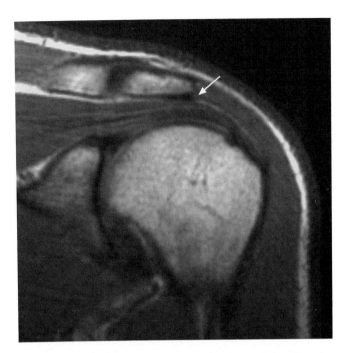

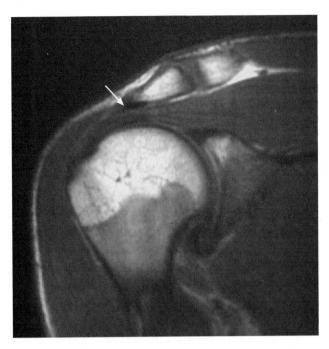

Fig. 12-23. Coronal oblique proton density–weighted image (TR 2200, TE 20, 1 Nex) in normal subject. An angular focus of uniform decreased signal intensity *(arrow)* projects laterally from the undersurface of the acromion process. This finding represents a tendinous slip of the deltoid muscle and may simulate the appearance of a subacromial osteophyte. (From Mirowitz SA: MRI Clin North Am 1:19-36, 1993.)

Fig. 12-24. Coronal oblique T1-weighted image (TR 400, TE 18, 2 Nex) demonstrates apparent spur projecting from inferolateral acromion process *(arrow)*. However, this finding represents a tendinous slip of deltoid muscle insertion.

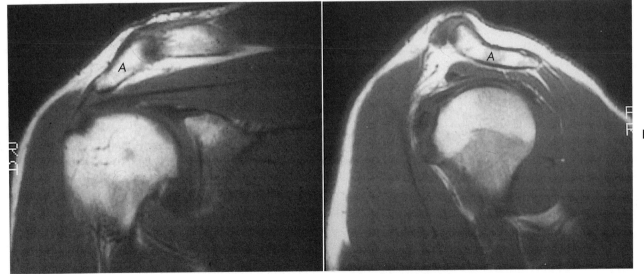

Fig. 12-25. Coronal oblique **(A)** and sagittal oblique **(B)** T1-weighted images depict hooked (Type III) acromion process *(A)*.

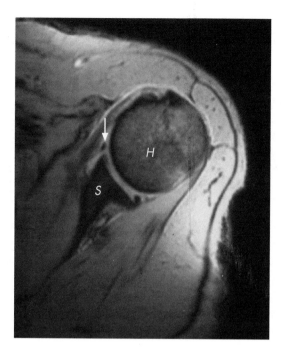

Fig. 12-26. Transaxial gradient echo image (TR 300, TE 15, 30-degree flip angle, 2 Nex) demonstrates relatively decreased signal intensity of the scapula *(S)* as compared with the adjacent humeral head *(H)*. These findings are due to relative increased percentage of hematopoietic marrow within the scapula. Dark lines outline fascial planes on this image. These findings represent chemical shift phase cancellation artifact and correspond to pixels containing both fat and water protons on this opposed phase image. The proximity of the low signal intensity middle glenohumeral ligament *(arrow)* to the anterior glenoid labrum simulates a labral tear.

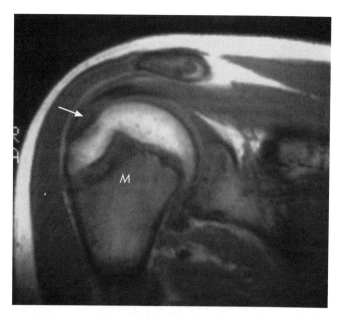

Fig. 12-27. There is decreased signal intensity corresponding to prominent hematopoietic marrow within the humeral metaphysis *(M)* on this coronal oblique T1-weighted image (TR 650, TE 18, 2 Nex). An unfused humeral physis is also noted. Motion artifacts that propagate across the phase-encoding direction of the image overlie the tendinous rotator cuff, simulating pathology *(arrow)*.

The shape of the acromion process can influence the development of impingement syndrome in some patients. The acromion is classified according to whether it has a flat, curved, or hooked undersurface.[9,52] This determination is best made with sagittal oblique images. A hooked acromion process has been observed more frequently in patients with impingement syndrome and with rotator cuff tear[9] (Figs. 12-25, *A* and *B*).

Osseous structures

The osseous structures about the shoulder joint should be routinely evaluated for evidence of bone-related causes of shoulder pain. Although hematopoietic marrow throughout most of the appendicular skeleton has undergone conversion to fatty marrow in adults, the proximal humeral metaphysis is a frequent exception (Figs. 12-2, 12-12, and 12-13). T1-weighted images frequently reveal foci of relatively decreased signal intensity within the proximal humeral metaphysis, scapula, and distal clavicle of normal adults (Fig. 12-26). Hematopoietic marrow is particularly prominent in children and adoles-

cents who have not yet undergone complete marrow conversion (Fig. 12-27). Hematopoietic marrow can also be prominent in patients with anemia or diffuse marrow replacement as a result of reconversion of fatty marrow to hematopoietic marrow.

Distinction between residual or reconverted hematopoietic marrow and marrow lesions is based on the lack of medullary cavity expansion, cortical destruction, and juxtacortical soft tissue mass with hematopoietic marrow. In addition, hematopoietic marrow maintains relative hypointensity on T2-weighted images, whereas many marrow lesions demonstrate variable regions of hyperintensity. Hematopoietic marrow usually involves both extremities in a relatively symmetric fashion.

It has been indicated that hematopoietic marrow is not present within the epiphyses beyond infancy.[51,56] Therefore, the presence of epiphyseal signal intensity alterations has been regarded as evidence of marrow pathology. However, we have observed that signal intensity alterations compatible with residual hematopoietic marrow are frequently observed within the proximal humeral epiphysis in normal adults[35] (Figs. 12-10, 12-28, 12-29). These findings most frequently manifest as curvilinear foci of relatively decreased signal intensity along the subcortical region of the medial humeral head (Fig. 12-30). Hematopoietic marrow can be observed throughout the humeral heads in patients who have undergone re-

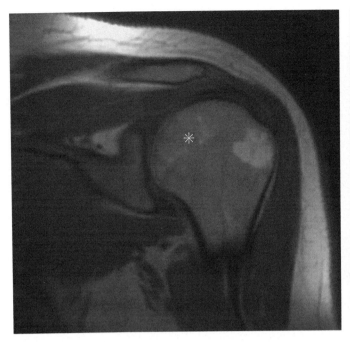

Fig. 12-28. Coronal oblique T1-weighted image (TR 650, TE 18, 2 Nex) in 30-year-old female demonstrates extensive hematopoietic marrow throughout most of the proximal humeral epiphysis *(asterisk).*

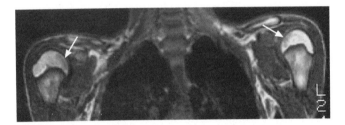

Fig. 12-29. Heterogeneous decreased signal intensity within the marrow space of the humeral epiphyses *(arrows)* and proximal metaphyses is noted on coronal T1-weighted image (TR 400, TE 16, 1 Nex). This is due to residual hematopoietic marrow in 11-year-old male.

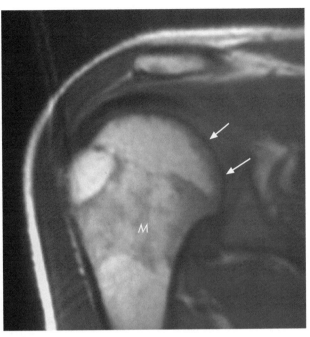

Fig. 12-30. Coronal oblique T1-weighted image (TR 650, TE 18, 2 Nex) in normal subject demonstrates foci of relatively decreased signal intensity within the proximal humeral metaphysis *(M)* representing hematopoietic marrow. Curvilinear extension of hematopoietic marrow along the medial aspect of the humeral epiphysis is also demonstrated *(arrows).* (From Mirowitz SA: MRI Clin North Am 1:19-36, 1993.)

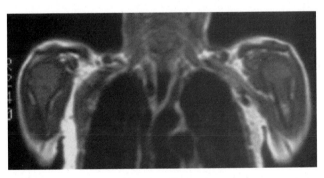

Fig. 12-31. Coronal T1-weighted image (TR 550, TE 11, 4 Nex) demonstrates symmetric reduced signal intensity within both humeral heads in a patient with severe anemia caused by gastrointestinal tract bleeding. This represents reconverted hematopoietic marrow.

conversion because of severe anemia (Fig. 12-31). Hematopoietic marrow can appear hyperintense relative to surrounding fatty marrow on fat-saturation T2-weighted or STIR images; this can contribute further to the simulation of neoplasm or other types of pathology (Figs. 12-32, *A* and *B*).

Transaxial images obtained through the humeral head may demonstrate a focus of relatively decreased signal intensity that can simulate an aggressive lesion. This is due to partial volume averaging with hematopoietic marrow within the humeral metaphysis. Similarly, the physis can appear as an irregular focus of relatively

decreased signal intensity that suggests a fracture or neoplasm (Figs. 12-27, 12-33).

Focal regions of abnormal signal intensity on both T1-weighted and T2-weighted images are also frequently observed within the proximal humerus of patients undergoing shoulder MR examination. These findings are

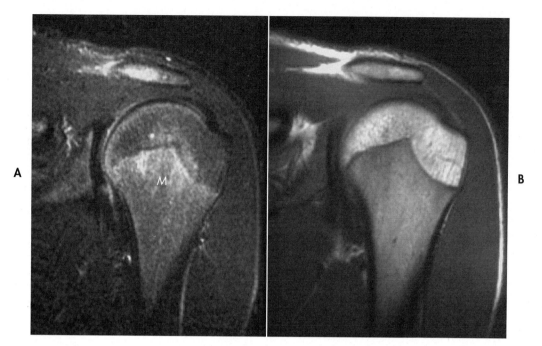

Fig. 12-32. A, Coronal oblique fat-suppressed T2-weighted image (TR 2200, TE 70, 1 Nex) demonstrates relative hyperintensity in marrow space of proximal humeral metaphysis *(M)*. This is caused by normal residual hematopoietic marrow, as demonstrated on the corresponding T1-weighted image **(B)** (TR 400, TE 18, 2 Nex).

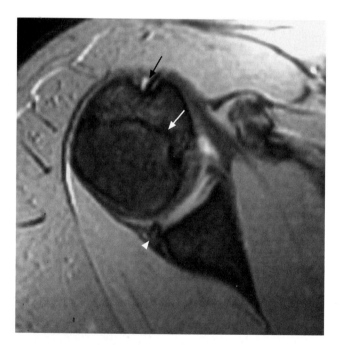

Fig. 12-33. The incompletely fused physis demonstrates curvilinear decreased signal intensity *(white arrow)* on this transaxial gradient echo image (TR 300, TE 15, 30-degree flip angle, 2 Nex). A linear focus of increased signal intensity within the substance of the posterior glenoid labrum is also demonstrated *(arrowhead)*, who has no history of glenohumeral dislocation. This is a normal finding that may simulate the appearance of a labral tear. Also note the focus of increased signal intensity within the bicipital groove *(black arrow)*, representing a branch of the circumflex humeral artery.

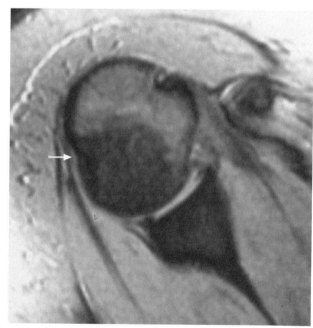

Fig. 12-34. Transaxial gradient echo image (TR 300, TE 15, 30-degree flip angle, 2 Nex) demonstrates normal flattening of the posterolateral humeral head *(arrow)*. This finding can simulate a Hill-Sachs deformity.

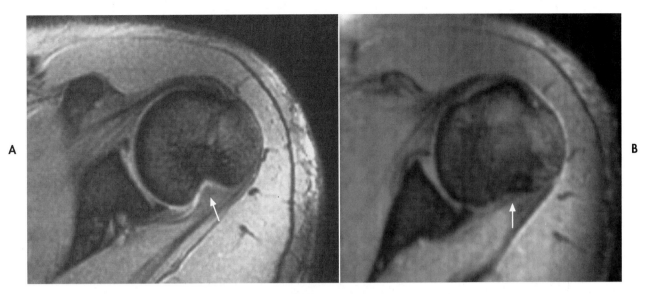

Fig. 12-35. Transaxial gradient echo images (TR 300, TE 15, 30-degree flip angle, 2 Nex) in patient with recurrent glenohumeral dislocation. A bony (Hill-Sachs) defect is demonstrated within the superior posterolateral humeral head in **A** *(arrow)*. This is to be distinguished from normal flattening of the posterolateral humeral head, which is also demonstrated at a slightly lower level **(B)** *(arrow)*.

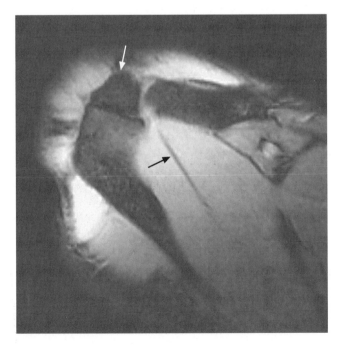

Fig. 12-36. A low signal intensity structure is noted adjacent to the acromion process on transaxial gradient echo image (TR 300, TE 15, 30-degree flip angle, 2 Nex), corresponding to an os acromiale *(white arrow)*. Linear decreased signal intensity within the supraspinatus muscle represents a tendinous slip *(black arrow)*.

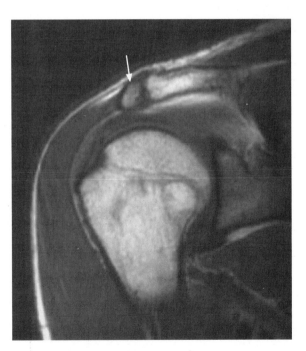

Fig. 12-37. Coronal oblique T1-weighted image (TR 650, TE 18, 2 Nex) demonstrates an os acromiale *(arrow)*, which can simulate the appearance of the acromioclavicular joint.

often the result of benign entities that are encountered incidentally, such as bone islands, fibroosseous defects, and subchondral cysts. Cystic changes arising near the greater tuberosity are frequently present in patients with rotator cuff pathology, but they can also be observed in asymptomatic individuals.[3,34] Ill-defined abnormal signal intensity can reflect marrow edema in patients who have sustained recent shoulder trauma. High signal intensity within the distal clavicle on T2-weighted images has been described in association with posttraumatic osteolysis.[12] The above entities should not be misinterpreted as more serious marrow pathologic conditions that might warrant intervention, such as neoplasm, infection, or infiltrative marrow diseases.

The posterolateral humeral head demonstrates a region of normal flattening on transaxial images (Figs. 12-34, 12-35, A and B). This finding could be misinterpreted as evidence of a Hill-Sachs lesion, particularly in a patient with a history of glenohumeral dislocation. However, normal humeral flattening occurs near the inferior aspect of the humeral head, whereas a true Hill-Sachs lesion is found in a more cephalad location.[57] In addition, a Hill-Sachs defect can be associated with abnormal marrow signal intensity as the result of marrow edema.

Bone marrow displays an appearance on gradient echo images that differs from that on spin echo images.[46] Gradient echo images depict the marrow space as relatively hypointense. This is due to susceptibility effects generated at the many interfaces between bony trabeculae and intervening marrow fat and cellular marrow elements.

An os acromion is present in approximately 5% of individuals and represents the failure of the acromion process to join with the scapula[2] (Figs. 12-36, 12-37). The coracoid process can be discontinuous with the remainder of the scapula. The humeral head is rarely completely absent.[2]

Soft tissues

In the presence of intrinsic or extrinsic magnetic field inhomogeneities, incomplete suppression of fat signal intensity can result in signal intensity alterations that simulate soft tissue pathology.[1] Heterogeneous signal intensity can occur on fat-suppressed images, particularly in the vicinity of the surface coil, as a result of alterations in the local magnetic field (Fig. 12-2).

Curvilinear foci of decreased signal intensity are often observed on gradient echo images along fascial planes. These are chemical shift phase cancellation artifacts and occur in voxels containing both fat and water protons. They occur when gradient echo images are acquired using an echo time at which the phase of fat and water protons are opposed, resulting in cancellation of their signal intensities.

Foci of markedly decreased signal intensity can be observed within the soft tissues of the shoulder following rotator cuff surgery.[40] These reflect tiny metal fragments and are most evident on gradient echo images. Abnormal marrow signal intensity can also be observed postoperatively in patients who have undergone resection of the distal acromion process.[40]

Elastofibroma is a common benign soft tissue mass of the shoulder. This fibroelastic lesion is usually found between the inferior scapula and the posterior chest wall. It is usually less than 3 cm in diameter and can be bilateral.[28] It occurs predominantly in older adults and more often in women. Elastofibromas typically demonstrate signal characteristics similar to those of skeletal muscle on all pulse sequences, but they can have foci of relatively increased signal intensity similar to that of fat.[17,28] This appearance can simulate a variety of soft tissue neoplasms, such as desmoid tumor, liposarcoma, hemangioma, hemorrhagic primary or secondary malignancy, and others.[28]

The supraspinatus muscle belly can have two divisions.[6] The infraspinatus and teres minor muscles may be inseparable, and the teres minor muscle is occasionally absent.[2] The subscapularis can have an associated secondary muscle, termed the subscapularis minor.[2]

Glenohumeral joint space

A small amount of synovial fluid can be observed within the glenohumeral joint space and its associated recesses (principally the subcoracoid recess) under physiologic conditions.[6,34] The estimated volume of physiologic joint fluid is less than 5 ml and is usually approximately 1 to 2 ml.[6]

There are various bursae that may be present about the shoulder joint. When distended by fluid, these bursae can simulate cystic soft tissue masses. The superior subscapularis bursa is the most frequent and is present in up to 90% of the population[61] (Fig. 12-38). This bursa is of variable size and communicates with the glenohumeral joint between the superior and middle glenohumeral ligaments.[43,61] Folds of capsular tissue and the superior glenohumeral ligament within the superior aspect of the bursa can simulate a pathologic condition.[61] Other bursae in the region of the shoulder are located in the subacromial-subdeltoid region, ventral to the subscapularis tendon, and between the infraspinatus tendon and the joint capsule.[43]

Redundancy of synovium within the axillary recess of the joint space can be observed on coronal oblique images, simulating a soft tissue mass (Fig. 12-10). The joint capsule can appear redundant on transaxial images within the arm in external rotation.

Biceps tendon

The long head of the biceps tendon should be routinely evaluated on shoulder MR examinations. A small amount of synovial fluid is frequently present within the

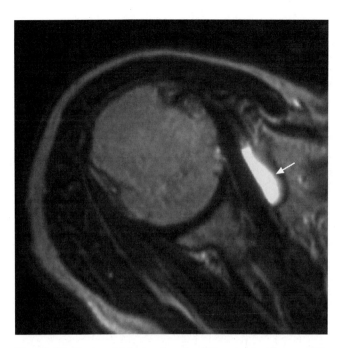

Fig. 12-38. Transaxial fast spin echo T2-weighted image (TR 4000, effective TE 95, 2 Nex, 16 echo train) demonstrates fluid collection within the subscapularis bursa *(arrow)*.

biceps tendon sheath in asymptomatic subjects[25,34,38] (Fig. 12-9). Such fluid is usually present along the dependent aspect of the tendon sheath and does not completely encircle the biceps tendon. Additional fluid may be present in patients with glenohumeral joint effusion as a result of communication between the biceps tendon sheath and the glenohumeral joint space[25] (Fig. 12-39).

A rounded focus of increased signal intensity is frequently observed along the lateral aspect of the bicipital groove (Figs. 12-33, 12-40). This represents branches of the anterior circumflex humeral artery and vein.[25] Hyperintensity of this structure on gradient echo images is due to flow-related enhancement and can simulate a focal fluid collection.

A focus of relatively increased signal intensity may be observed within the substance of the long head biceps tendon as a result of the magic angle phenomenon.[11] This finding can simulate bicipital tendinitis or a partial thickness tear.

The biceps muscle has a third head in approximately 12% of individuals.[2] The long head of the biceps muscle may be absent, with the bicipital tendon arising within its respective groove.[2]

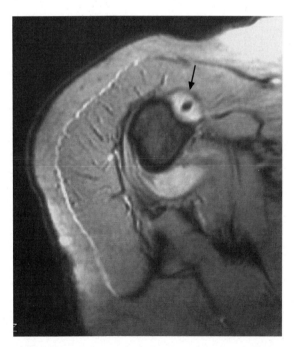

Fig. 12-39. Transaxial gradient echo image (TR 300, TE 15, 30-degree flip angle, 2 Nex) depicts a large volume of fluid within the bicipital tendon sheath *(arrow)*. This is due to communication with glenohumeral joint, which contains large effusion (seen posteriorly), rather than an intrinsic pathologic condition involving the biceps tendon.

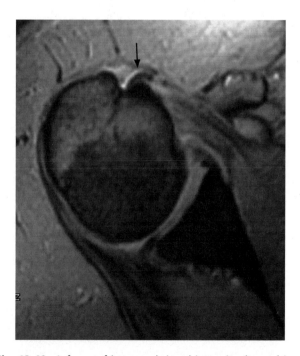

Fig. 12-40. A focus of increased signal intensity *(arrow)* is present along the proximal long head biceps tendon on this transaxial gradient echo image (TR 300, TE 15, 30-degree flip angle, 2 Nex). Although this suggests a focal fluid collection, it represents flow-related enhancement within a branch of the circumflex humeral artery.

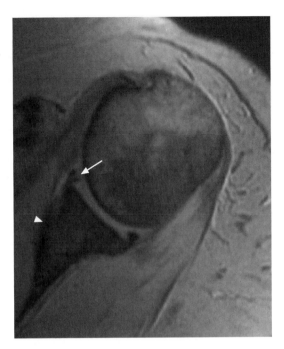

Fig. 12-41. Transaxial gradient echo image (TR 300, TE 15, 30-degree flip angle, 2 Nex) in normal subject demonstrates a cleft anterior glenoid labrum *(arrow).* The anterior labrum is slightly smaller in size than the posterior labrum. The glenohumeral joint capsule inserts somewhat medially in this subject, representing a type II capsular insertion *(arrowhead).* (From Mirowitz SA: MRI Clin North Am 1:19-36, 1993.)

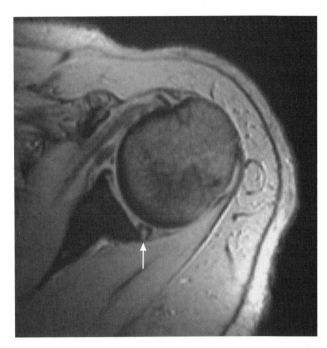

Fig. 12-42. Transaxial gradient echo image (TR 300, TE 15, 30-degree flip angle, 2 Nex) in patient without glenohumeral instability. The anterior glenoid labrum is small and appears somewhat blunted. The posterior labrum is larger and also demonstrates a blunted configuration. There is a globular focus of increased signal intensity within the substance of the posterior labrum *(arrow).* (From Mirowitz SA: MRI Clin North Am 1:19-36, 1993.)

GLENOID LABRUM-CAPSULAR COMPLEX

The fibrocartilaginous glenoid labrum varies considerably in morphology,[39] and the variations can simulate labral pathology. The labrum typically has a smooth, triangular shape. Common variations of labral shape include blunted, rounded, irregular, cleaved, and notched configurations[30,32] (Figs. 12-41 through 12-45). In one study of asymptomatic subjects, the anterior labrum demonstrated a classic triangular shape in only 45% of subjects, and the posterior labrum was triangular in 78% of subjects.[39] The anterior and posterior labra appeared rounded in 19% and 12% of subjects, respectively. Cleaved and notched configurations were less common. It has been suggested that a cleaved labral configuration may actually be the result of the inferior glenohumeral ligament in proximity to the anterior labrum.[30] Labral configuration frequently is not symmetric bilaterally.[39] These morphologic alterations are assumed to represent anatomic variations, but it has been suggested that they may increase in prominence with age and therefore could be reflective of a degenerative process.[42]

In addition to its variable morphology, the labrum also varies considerably in size. The labrum can be uniformly or focally extremely small in the absence of a tear[31,32,39] (Figs. 12-46 through 12-48). However, complete absence of the labrum or visualization of labral separation from the bony glenoid indicates a tear.[31] The posterior labrum is often slightly smaller than the anterior labrum.[25]

An unusually large labrum can also be seen in asymptomatic subjects[32,39] (Fig. 12-49). This appearance must be distinguished from the rounded and expanded appearance of the anterior labrum, which has been described in association with a tear. This finding, which is termed the glenoid labrum ovoid mass (GLOM) sign, represents a torn labrum that has retracted superiorly.[29] The inferior labrum can appear somewhat globular in normal subjects because of redundancy of the adjacent joint capsule.[29]

Gradient echo images (particularly multislice steady state gradient echo images) are often used for evaluation of the glenoid labrum. Typical imaging parameters include TR 700 to 900 msec, TE 10 to 12 msec, flip angle 20 degrees, field-of-view 14 to 18 cm, imaging matrix 128 × 256, and two excitations.[31]

Gradient echo images generally depict the fibrocartilaginous labrum as a hypointense structure (Fig. 12-48).

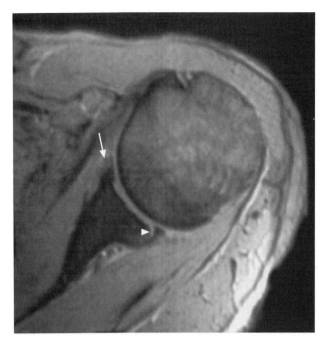

Fig. 12-43. Transaxial gradient echo image (TR 300, TE 15, 30-degree flip angle, 2 Nex) in normal subject demonstrates cleft anterior glenoid labrum *(arrow)*. Hyaline articular cartilage undercuts the posterior labrum, which may potentially simulate the appearance of a tear *(arrowhead)*. (From Mirowitz SA: MRI Clin North Am 1:19-36, 1993.)

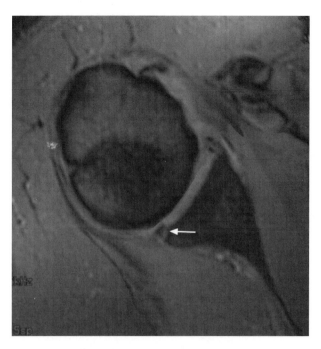

Fig. 12-44. Transaxial gradient echo image (TR 300, TE 15, 30-degree flip angle, 2 Nex) demonstrates a cleft appearance of the anterior fibrocartilaginous glenoid labrum. Also note undercutting of posterior labrum by high signal intensity hyaline cartilage *(arrow)*, which can simulate a tear.

ENTITIES THAT MAY SIMULATE LABRAL ABNORMALITIES

- Variations in labral shape
- Labral asymmetry
- Increased or decreased labral size
- Undercutting by hyaline cartilage
- Increased labral signal intensity
- Separation of superior labrum
- Glenohumeral ligaments
- Subscapularis tendon
- Joint capsule
- Intraarticular air

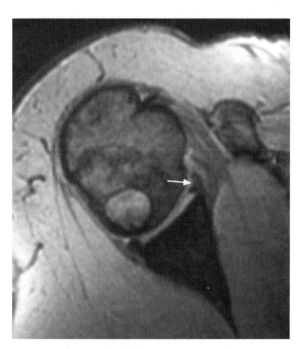

Fig. 12-45. Transaxial gradient echo image (TR 300, TE 15, 30-degree flip angle, 2 Nex) demonstrates cleft configuration of the anterior glenoid labrum *(arrow)*.

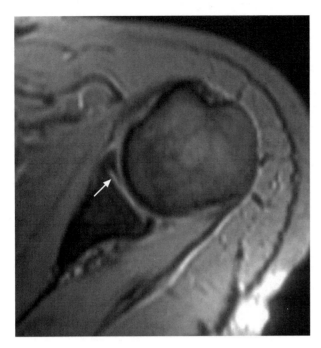

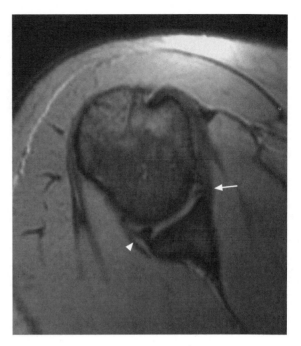

Fig. 12-46. Transaxial gradient echo image (TR 300, TE 15, 30-degree flip angle, 2 Nex) in patient without glenohumeral instability. There is marked asymmetry in the size of the glenoid labra, with the anterior labrum substantially larger than the posterior labrum. The posterior labrum demonstrates a blunted configuration, while the anterior labrum has a more typical triangular shape. The labra are devoid of internal signal intensity in this patient. Note undercutting of the anterior labrum by hyaline cartilage, which has a relative increased signal intensity *(arrow)*. (From Mirowitz SA: MRI Clin North Am 1:19-36, 1993.)

Fig. 12-47. Transaxial gradient echo image (TR 300, TE 15, 30-degree flip angle, 2 Nex) in normal subject demonstrates the anterior glenoid labrum *(arrow)* to be considerably smaller than the posterior labrum *(arrowhead)*. Linear increased signal intensity related to hyaline cartilage along the articular surface of the bony glenoid is present subjacent to the fibrocartilaginous labrum. The glenohumeral joint capsule inserts close to the anterior labrum in this subject representing a type I capsular insertion. (From Mirowitz SA: MRI Clin North Am 1:19-36, 1993.)

However, hyaline cartilage along the articular surface of the bony glenoid is hyperintense. The high signal intensity of hyaline cartilage subjacent to the fibrocartilaginous labrum can simulate the appearance of a tear at the labral base (Figs. 12-45, 12-46, 12-48, 12-49, and 12-50). Hyaline cartilage appears smooth and continuous, parallels the bony glenoid, is of uniform thickness, and does not extend through the labrum.[25,29,31] These criteria are useful in differentiating hyaline articular cartilage from most labral tears.

Whereas the labrum is often devoid of internal signal intensity, foci of increased signal intensity can be observed within the labrum in the absence of a tear[6,18,31,39] (Figs. 12-47 and 12-35). Such hyperintense foci are usually located near the base of the labrum and can have a linear or globular configuration. Although it is possible that these findings represent degenerative alterations rather than normal variations,[21,31,38] such findings have been observed in children as well as in adults.[18] When such foci of increased signal intensity are observed in a labrum that has a normal morphology, a tear is unlikely.[6]

Linear high signal intensity extending through the labrum to involve both of its surfaces has been used as a sign of labral tear.[18,29] However, this appearance has also been observed in asymptomatic subjects. In one study, these findings were observed in 7 of 26 presumably normal labra.[31]

Separation of a portion of the superior labrum and bony glenoid can be observed as a normal variant[4] with a small amount of fluid extending into the base of the superior labrum. This finding is more frequently observed in older patients[21] and can simulate a superior labrum, anterior and posterior (SLAP) injury that occurs near the insertion of the long head biceps tendon. Variations exist in the prominence and configuration of the superior glenohumeral ligament and the superior fibrocartilaginous glenoid labrum.[4] A linear focus of relatively increased signal intensity can also be observed between the superior labrum and proximal bicipital tendon in normal subjects.[4] These findings can also contribute to simulation of a SLAP lesion.

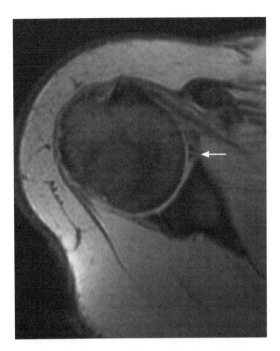

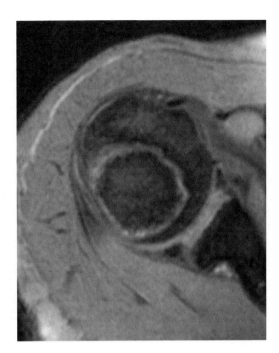

Fig. 12-48. Transaxial gradient echo image (TR 300, TE 15, 30-degree flip angle, 2 Nex) in patient without glenohumeral instability. Linear increased signal intensity located between the anterior labrum and the adjacent glenohumeral ligament *(arrow)* may appear to represent a tear. (From Mirowitz SA: MRI Clin North Am 1:19-36, 1993.)

Fig. 12-49. Transaxial gradient echo image (TR 300, TE 15, 30-degree flip angle, 2 Nex) demonstrates prominent anterior and posterior cartilaginous glenoid labrum in a 14-year-old male. There is also a circular high signal intensity area within the humeral head due to hyaline cartilage within the unfused humeral physis.

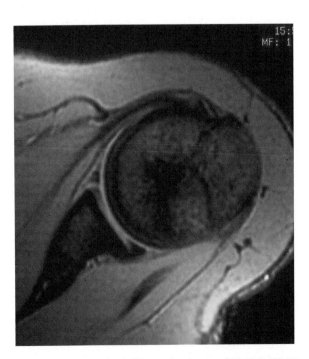

Fig. 12-50. Transaxial gradient echo image (TR 300, TE 15, 30-degree flip angle, 2 Nex) demonstrates undercutting of the fibrocartilaginous anterior labrum by high signal intensity hyaline cartilage.

The glenohumeral joint capsule or its specialized thickenings, the glenohumeral ligaments, can simulate a labral tear when they are closely applied to the labrum[25,29,30] (Figs. 12-26, 12-48, and 12-51). When this occurs, these structures appear to represent avulsed labral fragments, with the space between the ligament/capsule and the surface of the labrum representing the apparent tear[54] (Figs. 12-45 and 12-48). Similarly, the subscapularis tendon can appear to represent an avulsed fragment arising from the anterior labrum.[32] The middle glenohumeral ligament can attach directly to the labrum, which can cause the labrum to appear elongated or redundant.[42] The glenohumeral ligaments are variable in their presence and in their attachment to the glenoid, with the middle glenohumeral ligament subject to the greatest variation.[43] In one study, the middle and inferior glenohumeral ligaments were not identified in 15% of shoulders, presumably because they were absent.[30] The superior glenohumeral ligament is the most difficult to visualize and is infrequently identified on MR images.[30]

Another entity that can simulate a labral tear is the presence of intraarticular air. Intraarticular air can be related to joint aspiration, arthrography, or the vacuum phenomenon. Such air can lead to artifacts on gradient echo images that are characterized by a central signal void

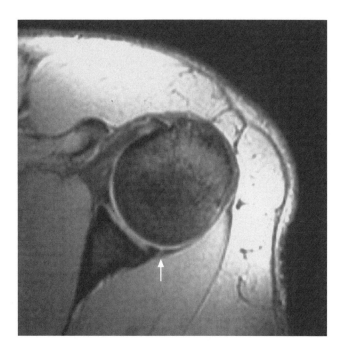

Fig. 12-51. Transaxial gradient echo image (TR 300, TE 15, 30-degree flip angle, 2 Nex) demonstrates fibrofatty tissue interposed between the posterior glenoid labrum and the posterior joint capsule *(arrow)*. This finding simulates a tear involving the posterior labrum.

with surrounding hyperintensity. These findings can simulate cartilaginous surface irregularity or discrete cartilaginous defects.[48]

Success in diagnosing labral tears varies considerably according to the site of the tear. The greatest sensitivity has been in detecting anterior labral tears, followed by superior labral tears. Results have been very poor for tears involving the posterior or inferior labrum.[29] Fraying of the cartilaginous glenoid labrum is usually not visible on MR images, including those obtained after intraarticular contrast material injection.[21]

Positioning of the arm affects the ability to detect labral abnormalities. The posterior labrum is best visualized with the arm in external rotation. However, this can impair visualization of abnormalities related to the anterior labrum. Consequently, it is recommended that labral imaging be performed initially with the arm in a neutral position;[42] additional images may be obtained with the arm in external rotation if a posterior labral lesion is suspected.[42]

The insertion site of the anterior glenohumeral joint capsule is subject to variation. A type I capsule inserts in close proximity to the glenoid labrum, whereas types II and III represent progressively more medial sites of insertion toward the scapular neck[43,59] (Figs. 12-41 and 12-47). Each of these capsular insertion types can be encountered in asymptomatic subjects[39] and may simulate

capsular stripping. The posterior joint capsule consistently inserts along the glenoid rim.[39,43]

REFERENCES

1. Anzai Y, Lufkin RB, Jabour BA et al: Fat-suppression failure artifacts simulating pathology on frequency-selective fat-suppression MR images of the head and neck, AJNR 1992; 13:879-884, 1992.
2. Bergman RA, Thompson SA, Afifi AK et al: Compendium of human anatomic variation: text, atlas, and world literature. Baltimore, 1988, Urban & Schwarzenberg.
3. Burk DL Jr, Torres JL, Marone PJ et al: MR imaging of shoulder injuries in professional baseball players, Magn Reson Imaging 1:385-389, 1991.
4. Cartland JP, Crues JV III, Stauffer A et al: MR imaging in the evaluation of SLAP injuries of the shoulder: findings in 10 patients, AJR 159:787-792, 1992.
5. Catasca J, Mirowitz SA: Fast spin echo T_2-weighted MR imaging of the abdomen, Radiology 185(P):234, 1992.
6. Chandnani V, Ho C, Gerharter J et al: MR findings in asymptomatic shoulders: a blind analysis using symptomatic shoulders as controls, Clin Imaging 16:25-30, 1992.
7. Davis SJ, Teresi LM, Bradley WG et al: Effect of arm rotation on MR imaging of the rotator cuff, Radiology 181:265-268, 1991.
8. Elster AD: Gradient-echo MR imaging: techniques and acronyms, Radiology 186:1-8, 1993.
9. Epstein RE, Schweitzer ME, Frieman BG et al: Hooked acromion: prevalence on MR images of painful shoulders, Radiology 187:479-481, 1993.
10. Erickson SJ, Cox IH, Hyde JS et al: Effect of tendon orientation on MR imaging signal intensity: a manifestation of the "magic angle" phenomenon, Radiology 181:389-392, 1991.
11. Erickson SJ, Fitzgerald SW, Quinn SF et al: Long bicipital tendon of the shoulder: normal anatomy and pathologic findings on MR imaging, AJR 158:1091-1096, 1992.
12. Erickson SJ, Kneeland JB, Komorowski RA et al: Post-traumatic osteolysis of the clavicle: MR features, J Comput Assist Tomogr 14:835-837, 1990.
13. Erickson SJ, Prost RW, Timins ME: The "magic angle" effect: background physics and clinical relevance, Radiology 188:23-25, 1993.
14. Flannigan B, Kurunoglu-Brahme S, Snyder S et al: MR arthrography of the shoulder: comparison with conventional MR imaging, AJR 155:829-832, 1990.
15. Fritz RC, Stoller DW: Fat-suppression MR arthrography of the shoulder [letter], Radiology 185:614-615, 1992.
16. Glickstein MF: MR imaging of the shoulder: optimizing surface-coil positioning [letter], AJR 153:431-432, 1989.
17. Gould ES, Javors BR, Morrison J et al: MR appearance of bilateral periscapular elastofibromas, J Comput Assist Tomogr 13:701-703, 1989.
18. Gudinchet F, Naggar L, Ginalski JM et al: Magnetic resonance imaging of nontraumatic shoulder instability in children, Skeletal Radiol 21:19-21, 1992.
19. Harned EM, Mitchell DG, Burk DL Jr et al: Bone marrow findings on magnetic resonance images of the knee: accentuation by fat suppression, Magn Reson Imaging 8:27-31, 1990.

20. Hennig J, Naureth A, Friedburg H: RARE imaging: a fast imaging method for clinical MR, Magn Reson Med 3:823-833, 1986.

21. Hodler J, Kursunoglu-Brahme S, Flannigan B et al: Injuries involving the superior portion of the glenoid labrum involving the insertion of the biceps tendon: MR imaging findings in nine cases, AJR 159:565-568, 1992.

22. Hodler J, Kursunoglu-Brahme S, Snyder SJ et al: Rotator cuff disease: assessment with MR arthrography versus standard MR imaging in 36 patients with arthroscopic confirmation, Radiology 182:431-436, 1992.

23. Iannotti JP, Zlatkin MB, Esterhai JL et al: Magnetic resonance imaging of the shoulder. Sensitivity, specificity, and predictive value, J Bone Joint Surg [Am] 73:17-29, 1991.

24. Jones KM, Mulkern RV, Schwartz RB et al: Fast spin-echo MR imaging of the brain and spine: current concepts, AJR 158:1313-1320, 1992.

25. Kaplan PA, Bryans KC, Davick JP et al: MR imaging of the normal shoulder: variants and pitfalls, Radiology 184:519-524, 1992.

26. Kieft GJ, Bloem JL, Obermann WR et al: Normal shoulder: MR imaging, Radiology 159:741-745, 1986.

27. Kneeland JB, Middleton WD, Carrera GF et al: MR imaging of the shoulder: diagnosis of rotator cuff tears, AJR 149:333-337, 1987.

28. Kransdorf MJ, Meis JM, Montgomery E: Elastofibroma: MR and CT appearance with radiologic-pathologic correlation, AJR 159:575-579, 1992.

29. Legan JM, Burkhard TK, Goff WB II et al: Tears of the glenoid labrum: MR imaging of 88 arthroscopically confirmed cases, Radiology 179:241-246, 1991.

30. Liou JTS, Wilson AJ, Totty WG et al: The normal shoulder: common variations that simulate pathologic conditions at MR imaging, Radiology 186:435-441, 1993.

31. McCauley TR, Pope CF, Jokl P: Normal and abnormal glenoid labrum: assessment with multiplanar gradient-echo MR imaging, Radiology 183:35-37, 1992.

32. McNiesh LM, Callaghan JJ: CT arthrography of the shoulder: variations of the glenoid labrum, AJR 149:963-966, 1987.

33. Middleton WD, Kneeland JB, Carrera GF, et al: High-resolution MR imaging of the normal rotator cuff, AJR 148:559-564, 1987.

34. Mirowitz SA: Normal rotator cuff: MR imaging with conventional and fat-suppression techniques, Radiology 180:735-740, 1991.

35. Mirowitz SA: Hematopoietic bone marrow within the proximal humeral epiphysis in normal adults: investigation with MR imaging, Radiology 188:689-693, 1993.

36. Mirowitz SA, Reinus W: Relative conspicuity of bone marrow lesions on MR: comparison of conventional and fat suppressed spin echo and inversion recovery pulse sequences, Magn Reson Imaging 2(P):47, 1992.

37. Mirowitz SA, Shady K, Reinus WR: Diagnostic performance of fat suppression MR imaging for detection of rotator cuff pathology, Radiology 181(P):247, 1991.

38. Neumann CH, Holt RG, Steinbach LS, et al: MR imaging of the shoulder: appearance of the supraspinatus tendon in asymptomatic volunteers, AJR 158:1281-1287, 1992.

39. Neumann CH, Petersen SA, Jahnke AH: MR imaging of the labral-capsular complex: normal variations, AJR 157:1015-1021, 1991.

40. Owen RS, Iannotti JP, Kneeland JB et al: Shoulder after surgery: MR imaging with surgical validation, Radiology 186:443-447, 1993.

41. Palmer WE, Brown JH, Rosenthal DI: Rotator cuff: evaluation with fat-suppressed MR arthrography, Radiology 188:683-687, 1993.

42. Rafii M, Forooznia H: Variations of normal glenoid labrum [letter], AJR 152:201-202, 1989.

43. Rafii M, Firooznia H, Golimbu C et al: CT arthrography of capsular structures of the shoulder, AJR 146:361-367, 1986.

44. Rafii M, Firooznia H, Sherman O et al: Rotator cuff lesions: signal patterns at MR imaging, Radiology 177:817-823, 1990.

45. Resendes M, Helms CA, Eddy R et al: Double-echo MPGR imaging of the rotator cuff, J Comput Assist Tomogr 15:1077-1079, 1991.

46. Sebag GH, Moore SG: Effect of trabecular bone on the appearance of marrow in gradient-echo imaging of the appendicular skeleton, Radiology 174:855-859, 1990.

47. Seeger LL, Gold RH, Bassett LW et al: Shoulder impingement syndrome: MR findings in 53 shoulders, AJR 150:343-347, 1988.

48. Shogry MEC, Pope TL Jr: Vacuum phenomenon simulating meniscal or cartilaginous injury of the knee at MR imaging, Radiology 180:513-515, 1991.

49. Simon JH, Szumowski J: Proton (fat/water) chemical shift imaging in medical magnetic resonance imaging. Current status, Invest Radiol 27:865-874, 1992.

50. Smith RC, Reinhold C, Lange RC et al: Fast spin-echo MR imaging of the female pelvis. Part I. Use of a whole-volume coil, Radiology 184:665-669, 1992.

51. Steiner RM, Mitchell DG, Rao VM et al: Magnetic resonance imaging of bone marrow: diagnostic value in diffuse hematologic disorders, Magn Reson Q 6:17-34, 1990.

52. Stiles RG, Otte MT: Imaging of the shoulder, Radiology 188:603-613, 1993.

53. Traughber PD, Goodwin TE: Shoulder MRI: arthroscopic correlation with emphasis on partial tears, J Comput Assist Tomogr 16:129-133, 1992.

54. Tsai JC, Zlatkin MB: Magnetic resonance imaging of the shoulder, Radiol Clin North Am 28:279-291, 1990.

55. Vahlensieck M, Pollack M, Lang P et al: Two segments of the supraspinous muscle: cause of high signal intensity at MR imaging? Radiology 186:449-454, 1993.

56. Vogler III JB, Murphy WA: Bone marrow imaging, Radiology 168:679-693, 1988.

57. Workman TL, Burkhard TK, Resnick D et al: Hill-Sachs lesion: comparison of detection with MR imaging, radiography, and arthroscopy, Radiology 185:847-852, 1992.

58. Zlatkin MB, Bjorkengren AG, Gylys-Morin V et al: Cross-sectional imaging of the capsular mechanism of the glenohumeral joint, AJR 150:151-158, 1988.

59. Zlatkin MB, Dalinka MK, Kressel HY: Magnetic resonance imaging of the shoulder, Magn Reson Q 5:3-22, 1989.

60. Zlatkin MB, Iannotti JP, Roberts MC, et al: Rotator cuff tears: diagnostic performance of MR imaging, Radiology 172:223-229, 1989.

61. Zlatkin MB, Reicher MA, Kellerhouse LE et al: The painful shoulder: MR imaging of the glenohumeral joint, J Comput Assist Tomogr 12:995-1001, 1988.

13

Hips and Small Joints

HIP
Anatomic Variations

Anatomic variations that may involve the bony pelvis and hip include absence of the acetabular notch, failure of the pubic and ischial rami to unify, division of the greater sciatic foramen by an accessory ischial spine, and prominence of the gluteal tuberosity of the femur resulting in a so-called third trochanter.[6]

Soft tissue variations include complete independence of the iliacus and psoas muscles; variable presence, origin, and prominence of the psoas minor muscle; and longitudinal division of the iliopsoas, piriformis, or tensor fascia lata muscles.[6] On T1-weighted images, the tensor fascia lata muscle often appears hyperintense relative to surrounding muscles because of fat interposed between individual muscle fascicles.

Signal Intensity Variations

The femoral capital epiphysis is usually of uniform increased signal intensity on T1-weighted images because of the presence of predominantly fatty marrow. Within the proximal femoral metaphysis, however, residual hematopoietic marrow is frequently present, resulting in multifocal or confluent regions of relatively decreased signal intensity (Figs. 13-1 and 13-2).[18,105] On T1-weighted images these findings can simulate marrow infiltration, although their bilateral symmetry and relative reduced intensity on T2-weighted images should allow for differentiation. Of course, hematopoietic marrow within the femoral neck and elsewhere may become

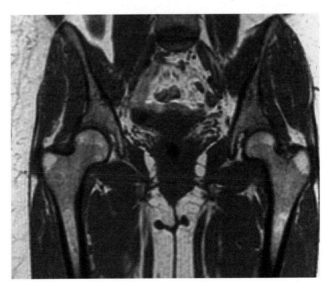

Fig. 13-2. There is relatively decreased signal intensity throughout the femoral necks and proximal shafts bilaterally on this coronal T1-weighted image (TR 400, TE 12, 2 Nex). Similar findings are present throughout the bony pelvis, with all of the above representing hematopoietic marrow in a 32-year-old female. There is decreased hematopoietic marrow within the femoral epiphyses, greater trochanters, and the midshaft of both femurs, resulting in their relative hyperintensity.

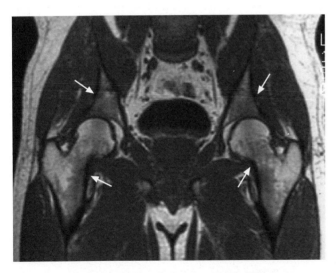

Fig. 13-1. Ill-defined foci of relatively decreased signal intensity are noted within the marrow space of both femoral necks and acetabulae (arrows) on this coronal T1-weighted image (TR 400, TE 12, 2 Nex) representing normal hematopoietic marrow elements.

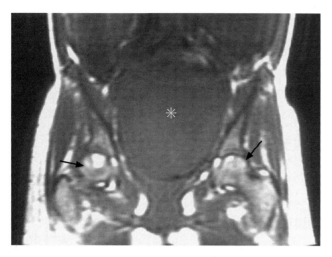

Fig. 13-3. Coronal T1-weighted image (TR 300, TE 12, 2 Nex) in a 37-year-old female with a large uterine mass *(asterisk)* and related chronic anemia. There is low signal intensity as a result of hematopoietic marrow reconversion involving the majority of both femoral epiphyses *(arrows)*.

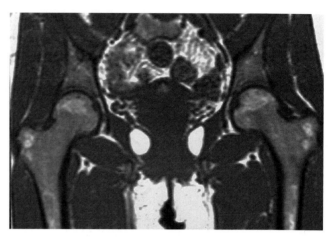

Fig. 13-5. Relatively decreased signal intensity is noted on this coronal T1-weighted image (TR 470, TE 12, 2 Nex) within the femoral metaphyses bilaterally and involving portions of the femoral heads and greater trochanters. These findings are the result of reconverted hematopoietic marrow in a menstrual-age female.

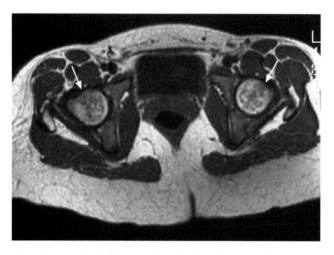

Fig. 13-4. Transaxial T1-weighted image (TR 500, TE 12, 2 Nex) demonstrates mottled heterogeneous signal intensity *(arrrows)* with symmetric involvement of both femoral heads representing residual foci of hematopoietic marrow in a menstrual-age female.

more prominent in patients with anemia or marrow replacement because of the reconversion of fatty marrow to hematopoietic marrow. In the femoral neck, local conversion of hematopoietic marrow to fatty marrow elements also occurs in patients with avascular necrosis of the femoral head.[65,90]

Hematopoietic marrow is usually not observed within the epiphyses of adults. However, in patients with severe anemia epiphyseal marrow can also undergo reconversion (Figs. 13-3, 13-4, and 13-5). Although this is most frequently observed within the humeral heads, the femoral heads can also be involved.[61] Hematopoietic marrow within the femoral heads can simulate avascular necrosis or other abnormalities such as tumor, infection, or posttraumatic marrow edema. Hematopoietic marrow can appear mildly hyperintense on fat-suppressed spin echo or inversion-recovery images, which can further the confusion for pathology (Figs. 13-6, *A* and *B*). The greater and lesser trochanters are epiphyseal equivalents and thus, usually do not demonstrate hematopoietic marrow in normal subjects. This can cause them to appear hyperintense on T1-weighted images relative to marrow within the adjacent femoral neck.

Obliquely oriented, linear foci of relatively decreased signal intensity are frequently observed within the femoral neck (Fig. 13-7). These represent bony trabeculae that are reinforced as a result of weight-bearing stresses.[51] A horizontally oriented, linear focus of decreased intensity in the femoral head corresponds to the physis in children and to the physeal scar in adults (Fig. 13-8).[51] A stress fracture of the femoral neck also demonstrates a linear configuration, although it can be easily distinguished from the physeal scar by its more caudal location and its lack of continuity across the entire femoral neck (Figs. 13-9, *A* and *B*).

Bone islands are frequently encountered in the proximal femurs; they are of uniform decreased signal intensity on all pulse sequences, concordant with cortical bone (Figs. 13-10, *A* and *B*). Heterogeneous fat suppression can result in focal or diffuse areas of relatively increased marrow signal intensity that can simulate a pathologic condition (Figs. 13-11, *A* and *B*). Such heterogeneity is

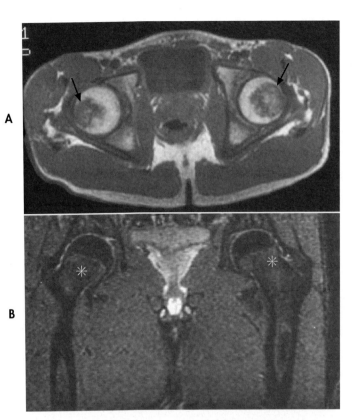

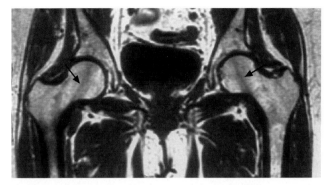

Fig. 13-7. Obliquely oriented linear foci *(arrows)* of relatively decreased signal intensity are observed on coronal T1-weighted image (TR 470, TE 12, 2 Nex) within both proximal femora. These findings are the result of reinforced trabeculae from weight-bearing stress.

Fig. 13-6. Transaxial T1-weighted image **(A)** (TR 450, TE 12, 2 Nex) demonstrates foci of low signal intensity within both femoral heads *(arrows)*, suggestive of avascular necrosis. However, these findings are the result of partial volume averaging of fatty marrow of the femoral head with hematopoietic marrow within the proximal femoral neck in a 14-year-old patient. The coronal STIR image **(B)** (TR 2900, TE 20, 1 Nex, inversion time 160) demonstrates relative hyperintensity of red marrow within the femoral necks and proximal shafts *(asterisks)* that may be mistaken for pathologic involvement. Also note relative hyperintensity of hyaline cartilage overlying the femoral heads and at the physeal plate.

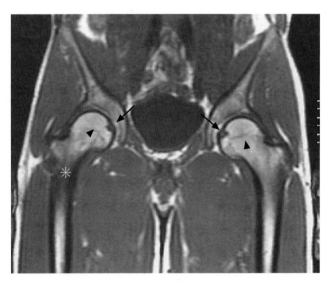

Fig. 13-8. The normal fovea are demonstrated as small, rounded foci of relatively decreased signal intensity *(arrows)* within the femoral capital epiphyses on this coronal T1-weighted image (TR 400, TE 12, 4 Nex). A linear focus of decreased intensity corresponds to the physeal scar *(arrowheads)*. There is apparent decreased signal intensity within the marrow space of the proximal right femoral shaft *(asterisk)*. This latter finding is due to partial volume averaging with adjacent musculature of the anterior thigh.

more commonly observed with use of fat saturation than with short tau inversion recovery (STIR) images.

Avascular Necrosis
Simulation of avascular necrosis

The most frequent indication for MR evaluation of the hips is suspected avascular necrosis of the femoral head. This entity leads to discrete curvilinear abnormal signal intensity within the superior aspect of the femoral head. Another characteristic feature is the double-line sign, which refers to parallel high-signal and low-signal intensity rims along the periphery of a focus of avascular necrosis on T2-weighted images. This latter finding relates to inflammatory changes that occur along the reactive interface between necrotic and viable marrow, which are

in turn surrounded by sclerotic bone. However, alteration of the double-line sign has been observed following gradient reorientation, suggesting that chemical shift misregistration artifact may play a role in some situations.[96]

The diagnosis of avascular necrosis is usually straightforward, particularly when a characteristic MR appear-

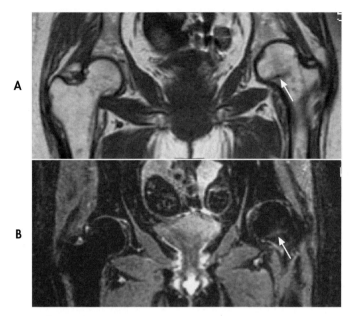

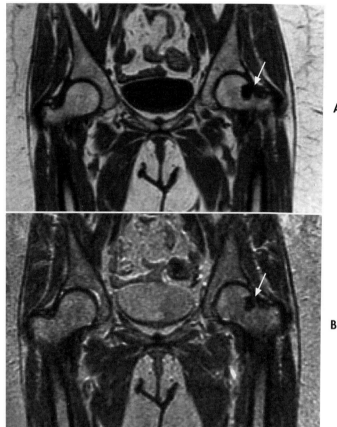

Fig. 13-9. Coronal T1-weighted image **(A)** (TR 400, TE 12, 2 Nex) demonstrates horizontally oriented focus of relatively decreased signal intensity *(arrow)* involving the proximal left femoral neck. This abnormality, which represents a stress fracture, is broader and located inferiorly to the physeal scar. It also demonstrates corresponding hyperintensity on STIR image **(B)** (TR 2500, TE 20, 1 Nex, inversion time 160).

Fig. 13-10. A rounded focus of decreased signal intensity *(arrow)* is observed within the left hip on coronal T1-weighted **(A)** (TR 400, TE 12, 2 Nex) and T2-weighted **(B)** (TR 2500, TE 70, 1 Nex) images, representing an incidental bone island.

ance is noted in the proper clinical setting. However, the appearance of avascular necrosis can be similar to that of other conditions. For example, in the early stages of avascular necrosis, ill-defined signal abnormalities are observed, reflecting reactive marrow edema (Figs. 13-12, A and B).[63,102] This can simulate osteomyelitis, transient osteoporosis, posttraumatic marrow edema, or neoplasm.[9,29,66] Even in its later stages, with the development of more discrete signal alterations, avascular focus can assume a variety of atypical configurations, potentially leading to diagnostic difficulty.

One sign that is apparently specific to avascular necrosis is the observation of preserved marrow fat within a region enclosed by abnormal marrow signal intensity. This sign is not observed with other abnormalities involving the femoral head, including osteoarthritis, transient osteoporosis, and rheumatoid arthritis.[46] Despite its specificity, however, this sign is relatively insensitive, having been observed in only 47% of 133 femoral heads with avascular necrosis.[46] In children with Legg-Calvé-Perthes disease, abnormal signal intensity resembling cystic changes has been observed within the anterior femoral metaphysis.[37] The pathologic basis for these observations is not known.

The fovea capitis can simulate a small focus of avascular necrosis of the femoral head (Figs. 13-8, 13-13, and

13-14).[51] However, it can usually be recognized on the basis of its small size, typical location, and bilateral symmetry. Partial volume averaging can also result in apparent marrow lesions in the hip, including avascular necrosis (Figs. 13-5, 13-6, and 13-8). For example, on transaxial images, fatty marrow within the femoral head can be averaged with red marrow of the femoral neck. Coronal images are subject to partial volume averaging of fatty marrow with cortical bone of the anterior femur. In both situations, evaluation of images acquired in alternate planes helps to distinguish partial volume effects from actual pathologic conditions (Figs. 13-15, A and B).

In the femoral neck, a herniation pit appears as a small, well-defined focus of abnormally increased signal intensity on long TR images (Fig. 13-16, A and B). This normal variant is related to the ingrowth of fibrous

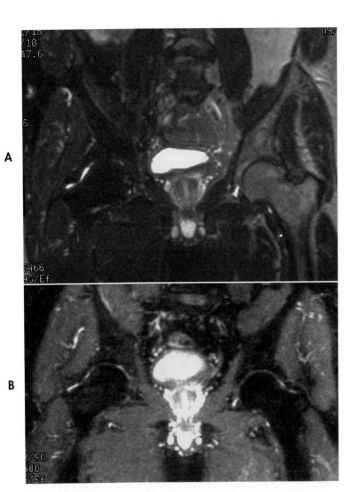

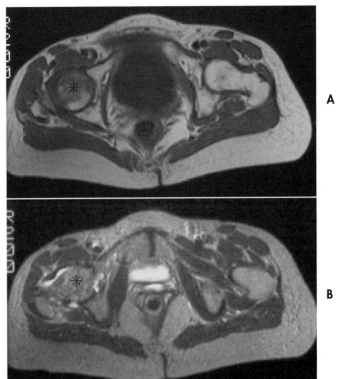

Fig. 13-12. Corresponding transaxial T1-weighted **(A)** (TR 600, TE 10, 2 Nex) and T2-weighted **(B)** (TR 3500, TE 90, 1 Nex) images demonstrate relatively ill-defined focus of abnormal signal intensity *(asterisk)* involving the right femoral head in a patient with subacute avascular necrosis. An associated hip-joint effusion is also demonstrated.

Fig. 13-11. Coronal fat-saturated fast spin echo T2-weighted image **(A)** (TR 5500, effective TE 100, 4 Nex, 16 echo train) demonstrates marked asymmetry of marrow bilaterally. There is apparent relatively increased signal intensity involving the marrow space of the left femoral head and neck and of the left bony pelvis compared with the right. These findings are the result of inhomogeneous fat saturation, verified by symmetric homogeneous suppression of signal intensity throughout these areas bilaterally on corresponding fast spin echo STIR image **(B)** (TR 2500, effective TE 16, 2 Nex, inversion time 160, 8 echo train).

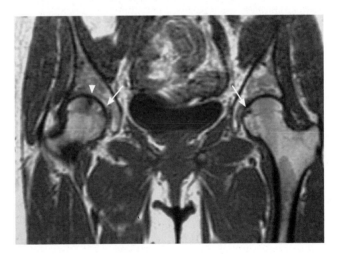

Fig. 13-13. Coronal T1-weighted image (TR 470, TE 12, 2 Nex) demonstrates small, well-defined foci of relatively decreased signal intensity *(arrows)* corresponding to the normal fovea capitis bilaterally. This must be distinguished from a somewhat larger and more ill-defined focus of abnormally decreased signal intensity *(arrowhead)* within the superior pole of the right femoral head, corresponding to a site of avascular necrosis.

and cartilaginous tissues into the femoral cortex.[17,72] Femoral herniation pits usually demonstrate signal characteristics similar to those of fluid and can occasionally undergo rapid enlargement.[17]

Detection of avascular necrosis

Avascular necrosis may not be evident on MR images that are acquired soon after its onset. At this early stage, when intervention could be particularly beneficial, signal intensity alterations are not observed on T1-weighted and T2-weighted spin echo or STIR images. However,

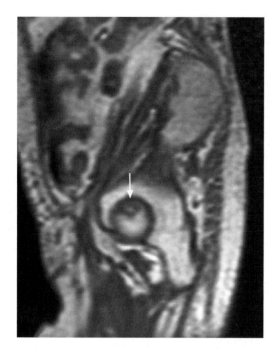

Fig. 13-14. Sagittal T1-weighted image (TR 500, TE 10, 2 Nex) of the femoral head demonstrates rounded focus of relatively decreased signal intensity *(arrow)* corresponding to the fovea capitis. These findings may simulate avascular necrosis of the femoral head.

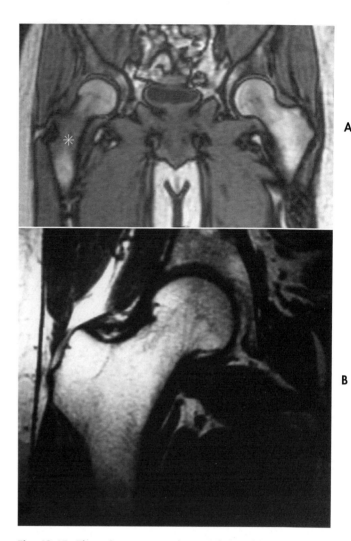

Fig. 13-15. There is apparent abnormal signal intensity *(asterisk)* involving the right femoral neck on body coil coronal T1-weighted gradient echo image **(A)** (TR 110, TE 2, 1 Nex, 90-degree flip angle). These findings are the result of partial volume averaging of marrow with femoral cortex and surrounding soft tissues, as is documented on the corresponding T1-weighted image **(B)** (TR 600, TE 11, 2 Nex), obtained using a surface coil and reduced slice thickness.

dynamic gadolinium chelate–enhanced gradient echo images do allow for detection of avascular necrosis at this very early stage.[70] Using this technique, normal marrow undergoes prominent early contrast enhancement, whereas ischemic marrow does not. Images acquired 1 week after onset of ischemia depict a prominently enhancing rim that surrounds the central nonenhancing ischemic focus. This pattern can also be observed on equilibrium phase contrast-enhanced fat-suppressed T1-weighted images.[52] Another pattern that may be observed is contrast enhancement diffusely involving the femoral head and neck and extending into the proximal femoral shaft. The two patterns described above may be concomitant in some patients.

Fat-suppressed images, obtained using either fat saturation T2-weighted or STIR sequences, usually result in maximal conspicuousness of marrow lesions. However, osteonecrosis of the femoral head is an exception, because conventional T1-weighted images are often superior to fat-suppressed images for lesion detection and definition.[60]

Follow-up/posttherapy evaluation

Patients with intracapsular hip fractures are at risk of developing avascular necrosis. However, when MR is performed in the immediate postfracture period, it is generally not of value in predicting which patients will subsequently develop avascular necrosis.[3]

The signal intensity characteristics of avascular necrosis do not correlate with the likelihood of secondary complications and do not contribute to the prediction of which patients will benefit from core decompression.[13,49] However, measurements of the lesion's size and of the percentage of weight-bearing femoral cortex involved with the osteonecrotic lesion help to determine which lesions will progress to femoral head collapse and may help to select patients for core decompression.

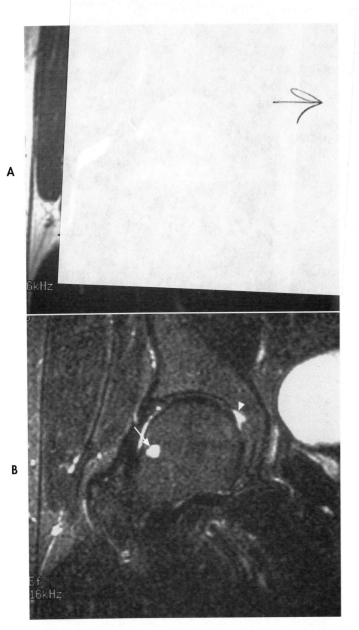

A

B

Fig. 13-16. Coronal T1-weighted **(A)** (TR 600, TE 11, 2 Nex) and fat-saturated fast-spin echo T2-weighted **(B)** (TR 3200, effective TE 100, 2 Nex, 12 echo train) images depict rounded focus of fluidlike signal intensity *(arrow)* involving lateral femoral neck, representing a herniation pit. A physiologic volume of fluid *(arrowhead)* is present within the hip joint.

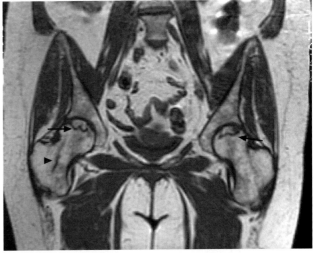

Fig. 13-17. Coronal T1-weighted image (TR 400, TE 12, 2 Nex) demonstrates avascular necrosis of both femoral heads *(arrows)*. A linear focus of decreased signal intensity *(arrowhead)* is noted within the right femoral neck, corresponding to a core decompression tract.

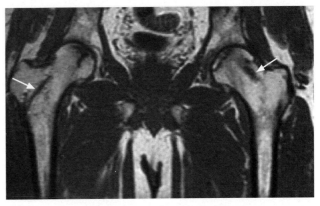

Fig. 13-18. There are linear foci of decreased signal intensity *(arrows)* extending through the femoral necks bilaterally on this coronal T1-weighted image (TR 450, TE 12, 2 Nex). These findings are the result of core decompression tracts that were performed for treatment of bilateral avascular necrosis of the femoral heads.

Core decompression is performed in some centers in cases of early avascular necrosis. The core tract appears as a linear area of abnormal signal intensity extending through the femoral neck and head (Figs. 13-17 and 13-18).[26] Fluid is often present within the tract. A decrease in the extent of avascular necrosis is rarely observed during the first year after performance of core decompres-sion, although some small lesions may decrease in size.[13] Furthermore, there is usually no alteration in the signal intensity pattern of such lesions during this time. In some patients who do not undergo core decompression, the sig-nal alterations of avascular necrosis may be inapparent on follow-up MR examinations, indicating spontaneous revascularization.[47]

Transient Osteoporosis/Bone Marrow Edema Syndrome

Transient osteoporosis appears as an ill-defined focus of abnormally decreased and increased signal intensity on T1-weighted and T2-weighted images, respectively, within the femoral head (Figs. 13-19, A and B). These findings are usually distinguished easily from the more discrete signal abnormalities of avascular necrosis, although the latter condition can be ill defined in its early stages.[103] Conversely, although diffuse signal abnormalities are most commonly observed in patients with transient osteoporosis, a focal pattern can also occur.[30] In atypical cases, the signal abnormalities of transient osteoporosis can extend beyond the femoral head and into the femoral neck.[77] Joint effusion is commonly observed in patients with transient osteoporosis, although this also

may accompany avascular necrosis and many other entities.[98] In equivocal cases, gadolinium chelate–enhanced T1-weighted images can be used to demonstrate decreased enhancement within ischemic marrow, which should not occur in cases of transient osteoporosis.

Bone marrow edema involving the femoral head can be observed in a variety of conditions other than transient osteoporosis. These entities, which can have an identical MR appearance, include infection, marrow contusion or fracture, and infiltrative neoplasms, in addition to early osteonecrosis (Figs. 13-20, A and B).[34]

Some authors distinguish transient osteoporosis from transient bone marrow edema syndromes, but these are probably related entities.[34] In the former syndrome, radiographic osteopenia is visible within 8 weeks of the onset of pain, whereas radiographic changes are not evident in the latter syndrome. For patients with transient osteoporosis, abnormal marrow signal intensity generally

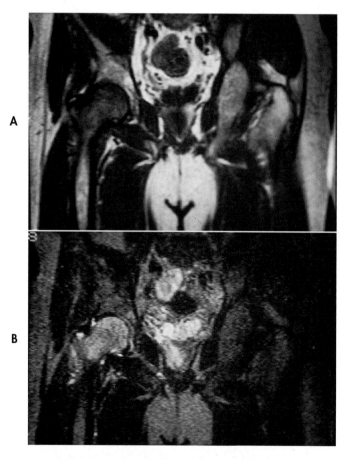

Fig. 13-19. Coronal T1-weighted image **(A)** and T2-weighted image **(B)** demonstrate diffuse abnormal signal intensity throughout the right femoral head in a patient with transient osteoporosis of the hip.

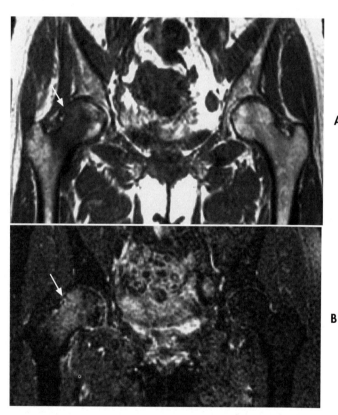

Fig. 13-20. Coronal T1-weighted image **(A)** (TR 400, TE 12, 2 Nex) and fat-suppressed T2-weighted image **(B)** (TR 2500, TE 70, 1 Nex) demonstrate ill-defined focus of abnormal signal intensity involving the right femoral head and proximal neck *(arrow)*. These findings are the result of metastatic disease in a patient with lung cancer and widespread osseous metastases, although they may simulate early avascular necrosis or transient bone marrow edema.

normalizes within 1 year following the onset of symptoms without intervention. Increased intraosseous pressure has been documented, and pain relief has been achieved with core decompression.[38] For these patients, signal intensity of the femoral head returns to normal within approximately 3 months after decompression. Clinical response and histologic findings indicate that bone marrow edema syndrome could represent an early, reversible phase of avascular necrosis. A transient bone marrow edema pattern has also been observed in children with hip pain.[74] Anterior-to-posterior progression of signal abnormalities within the femoral head and neck has been observed in some patients with transient osteoporosis, with resolution of the abnormal signal following the same pattern.[33]

Fluid Collections/Soft Tissues

A small amount of fluid is often present in normal hip joints; this does not represent a significant joint effusion (Fig. 13-21).[5,64]

The iliopsoas bursa is present in most individuals, with an average size of 6 × 3 cm, making it the largest synovial bursa in the body.[55,104] This bursa is located between the iliopsoas muscle/tendon and the hip-joint capsule, lateral to the femoral vessels, and can extend into the pelvis. The bursa communicates with the hip joint in 15% of individuals. Distention of the iliopsoas bursa may occur in a number of conditions, including rheumatoid arthritis, synovial chondromatosis, gout, infection, pigmented villonodular synovitis, osteoarthritis, trauma, and avascular necrosis.[104] Fluid within the iliopsoas bursa can simulate a cystic or necrotic soft tissue mass about the hip.[55,78,104] Specifically, a distended iliopsoas bursa may be confused with an inguinal or femoral hernia, psoas abscess, femoral aneurysm, hematoma, arteriovenous fistula, neoplasm, lymphadenopathy, or undescended testis.[104] Most of these entities are distinguished from a distended bursa by their lack of fluid signal intensity on T2-weighted images. A pseudobursa can form adjacent to a hip prosthesis and likewise can simulate a soft tissue mass.

A focus of increased signal intensity, representing fibrofatty tissue, may be observed surrounding the central tendon of the iliopsoas muscle, particularly on T1-weighted images (Fig. 13-22). Fibrofatty tissue can also be interposed between the semimembranosus and semitendinosus components of the conjoined hamstring tendon, resulting in apparent intratendinous signal intensity that can simulate tendinitis or a partial thickness tear (Fig. 13-23). Fibrofatty tissue interposed between the fascicles of the tensor fascia lata muscles can result in marked heterogeneity of these muscles (Fig. 13-24).

Cartilage thickness

A variety of techniques have been used to define the thickness and integrity of hyaline cartilage at the hip joint. Major challenges in this effort have included isointensity between cartilage and joint fluid or other surrounding structures and the lack of sufficient spatial resolution. Fat-suppressed spin-echo sequences depict cartilage as hyperintense and have shown promise for de-

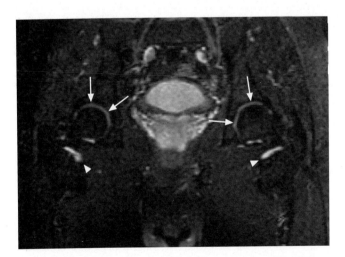

Fig. 13-21. Coronal fat-suppressed T2-weighted image (TR 2500, TE 70, 1 Nex) demonstrates relative hyperintensity of hyaline cartilage overlying both femoral heads *(arrows)*. Also noted is a physiologic volume of fluid within both hip joints *(arrowheads)*.

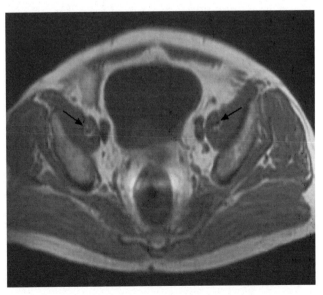

Fig. 13-22. Symmetric foci of relatively increased signal intensity *(arrows)* are observed on this transaxial T1-weighted image (TR 500, TE 12, 2 Nex) within the iliopsoas muscles bilaterally. These findings represent fat surrounding the central iliopsoas tendon.

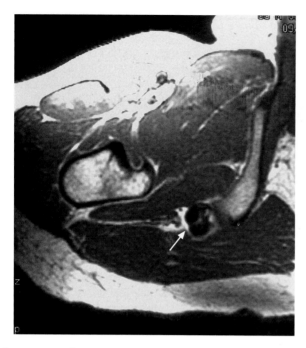

Fig. 13-23. A focus of relatively increased signal intensity *(arrow)* is noted within the conjoined hamstring tendon near its insertion on this transaxial T1-weighted image (TR 400, TE 11, 2 Nex). These findings represent fibrofatty tissue interposed between the semimembranosis and semitendinosis tendons and may simulate tendinitis or a partial tear.

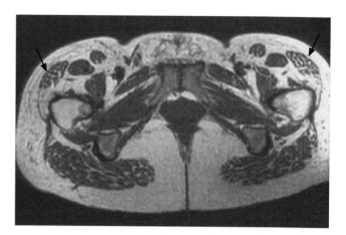

Fig. 13-24. Transaxial T1-weighted image (TR 470, TE 12, 2 Nex) demonstrates a speckled appearance of the tensor fascia lata muscles bilaterally *(arrows)* as a result of the normal fatty tissue within these muscle groups.

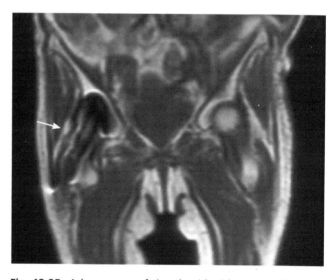

Fig. 13-25. A large area of signal void with surrounding hyperintensity *(arrow)* is observed in the region of the right hip on this coronal T1-weighted image (TR 500, TE 12, 4 Nex). These findings are the result of an intertrochanteric metallic fixation device and obscure visualization of the femoral head and neck. Also note anatomic distortion involving the acetabular region that is also related to susceptibility artifact.

termining cartilage thickness (Figs. 13-6 and 13-21). However, a study of cadaver hips concluded that the accuracy of measurements obtained using even these optimized sequences is currently insufficient to be clinically meaningful.[36] Distinction between adjacent femoral and acetabular cartilage is difficult, and, even when such distinction is possible, measurements of acetabular cartilage thickness are often misleading. Foci of heterogeneous signal intensity may be observed within the cartilage of patients with degenerative joint disease.[10]

Because of the difference in resonant frequency of fat and water protons, chemical shift misregistration artifacts may also obscure portions of the hyaline cartilage and render its measurement inaccurate. These artifacts are expressed along the frequency encode direction of the image, and they are accentuated on high field strength systems and when large voxel sizes or narrow receiver bandwidths are used.

Postoperative Changes

Metallic fixation pins, compression devices, or prostheses in the femoral neck or head produce signal void because of susceptibility artifact (Fig. 13-25).[48] Peripheral hyperintensity may surround the central signal void. These artifacts can obscure visualization of the hip and

surrounding soft tissues. Decreased signal intensity related to these artifacts can also simulate marrow lesions on T1-weighted images, and the high signal intensity component may simulate marrow or soft tissue lesions on T2-weighted images.

The severity of susceptibility artifacts partially depends on the constituent material of the orthopedic device. For example, titanium and other relatively nonfer-

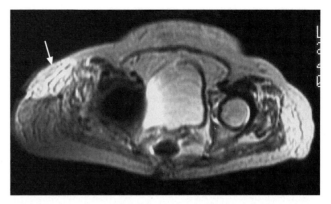

Fig. 13-27. A large area of signal void is present within the region of the right femoral head on this transaxial T2-weighted image (TR 2200, TE 70, 2 Nex). This obscures visualization of the femoral head and the immediate surrounding soft tissue structures. Considerable edema throughout the soft tissues of the lateral hip is noted *(arrow)* as a result of placement of the prosthesis 2 days before imaging.

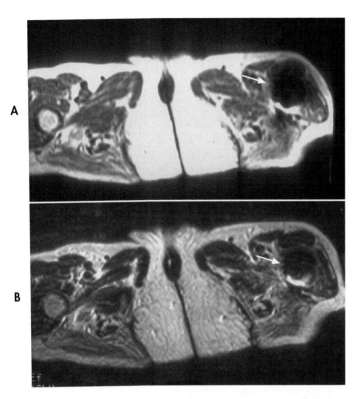

Fig. 13-26. Transaxial T1-weighted spin echo image **(A)** (TR 500, TE 11, 4 Nex) and fast-spin echo T2-weighted image **(B)** (TR 4000, effective TE 120, 4 Nex, 16 echo train) of a patient with a left femoral head prosthesis. The signal void artifact related to this prosthesis *(arrow)* is noticeably reduced on the fast spin echo image, despite the use of a considerably longer echo time.

rous implants produce significantly less artifacts than do stainless steel devices.[20] Optimization of imaging parameters can also affect the prominence of susceptibility artifacts. These artifacts are minimized with relatively short echo times and small voxel sizes (i.e., reduced field-of-view and slice thickness and high-resolution matrix). Gradient echo sequences accentuate susceptibility artifacts because of the absence of a 180-degree refocusing radiofrequency pulse, whereas the multiplicity of such refocusing pulses on fast spin echo (i.e., RARE) sequences reduces their prominence (Figs. 13-26, *A* and *B*). Local magnetic-field nonuniformity in the vicinity of ferromagnetic items can also lead to inhomogeneous fat suppression.

In patients who have undergone recent placement of orthopedic implants, abnormal marrow signal intensity attributable to postsurgical edema can simulate or obscure lesions in and around the hip and can mimic postoperative soft tissue infection (Fig. 13-27).[27]

Bone grafting is performed on some patients who undergo total hip replacement. Autologous bone grafts demonstrate relatively increased signal intensity on T1-weighted images, consistent with fatty marrow. However, homologous grafts typically show relatively reduced signal intensity following transplantation, persisting for up to 2 years.

Neoplasms

For patients with neoplasms involving the hip, as elsewhere, tumor calcification and ossification may be better depicted on CT than on MR images.[50] Similarly, subtle periosteal reaction can be more easily identified on CT images. Benign cystic soft tissue lesions, such as ganglia and synovial cysts, although more frequently encountered about the knee, can also present in the hip and should not be mistaken for malignancy. Whereas MR sensitively depicts most osseous and soft tissue neoplasms, these lesions often display nonspecific features, which are discussed in Chapters 14 and 15.

ANKLE/FOOT

Osseous Structures

Anatomic variations

There are a number of bony anatomic variations that occur about the ankle joint and foot. The tibia can vary in length, and morphology may be absent in some patients.[6] The fibula can also be absent. The calcaneus, navicular, and other tarsal bones may be congenitally fused by osseous, cartilaginous, or fibrous tissue; talocalcaneal and calcaneonavicular coalition are most common.[45]

The tarsal bones, metatarsals, and phalanges can vary

in number, size, and configuration.[6] Sesamoid bones and ossicles occur in multiple locations, and can simulate osteochondral fragments (Fig. 13-28).[73] Sesamoid bones, such as the os peroneum, are embedded within ankle tendons. Secondary ossification centers, such as the os trigonum, are also common about the ankle; there are approximately 30 accessory tarsal ossicles.[6] Sesamoid

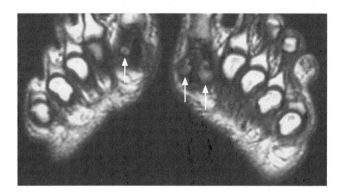

Fig. 13-28. Transaxial T1-weighted image (TR 500, TE 20, 2 Nex) demonstrates multiple sesamoid bones *(arrows)* along the plantar aspect of both feet and near the first metatarsophalangeal joints.

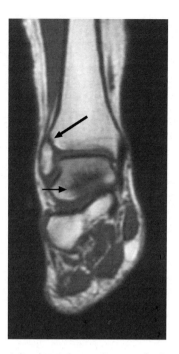

Fig. 13-29. Partial volume averaging results in an ill-defined area of apparent abnormally decreased signal intensity involving the talus *(arrow)* on coronal T1-weighted image (TR 450, TE 11, 2 Nex). In addition, there is an apparent fracture line involving the lateral malleolus *(large arrow)*, which actually represents the cortex of the lateral aspect of the tibia.

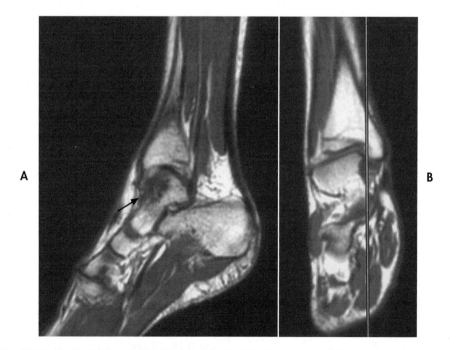

Fig. 13-30. Sagittal T1-weighted image **(A)** (TR 500, TE 11, 2 Nex) demonstrates apparent focus of osteonecrosis involving the talar dome *(arrow)*. However, these findings are the result of partial volume averaging of the talus with adjacent soft tissues, as is verified on coronal T1-weighted image **(B)** (TR 500, TE 11, 2 Nex), in which the position of *A* is annotated.

bones and ossicles have the potential to simulate other abnormalities. In addition, the presence of an accessory navicular bone has been associated with tears of the posterior tibial tendon.[44]

Osseous lesions

Partial volume averaging may give rise to apparent marrow lesions, including tumor, infection, and post-traumatic marrow edema (Figs. 13-29 and 13-30, *A* and *B*). For example, apparent marrow abnormalities of the distal tibia may be caused by volume averaging with cartilage overlying the tibial plafond or with fluid within the tibiotalar joint. An intraarticular low signal intensity line has been noted within the ankle joint, which can simulate a chondral fragment.[19] The calcaneus may contain prominent focal deposits of fat within its marrow space. Heterogeneous signal intensity may be observed throughout portions of the ankle on fat-suppressed images (Fig. 13-31). This is due to local magnetic-field inhomogeneities, particularly at tissue-air interfaces, that are accentuated by the curved anatomy of the ankle. Improved homogeneity of fat suppression may be achieved with the placement of bags of fluid around the ankle.

Cortical irregularity can be observed along the posterior aspect of the tibiotalar joint on sagittal images.[73] Thickening of the cortical surface of the talus can also

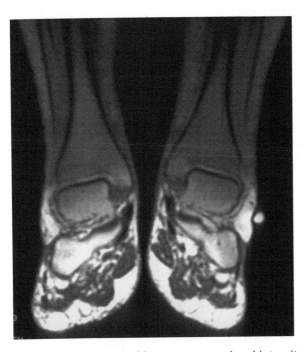

Fig. 13-31. There is marked heterogeneous signal intensity throughout both ankles on this coronal fat-saturated T1-weighted image (TR 500, TE 11, 2 Nex). These findings are the result of nonuniformity of the local magnetic field, causing heterogeneous fat saturation.

be seen and can simulate osteonecrosis. Similar findings may be observed along the insertion site of the posterior tibial tendon on the navicular bone and near the insertion of the Achilles tendon on the calcaneus.[73,82]

MR is exquisitely sensitive to marrow edema following ankle injury. However, its relative insensitivity to small cortical fragments limits its use in the evaluation of patients who have had an ankle trauma.[108] There are also other subtle bone abnormalities, such as periostitis and subtalar osteoarthritis, that may be better depicted on CT than on MR images.[82] Although thin section gradient echo images are useful for defining ankle ligaments, these images may not reliably depict marrow abnormalities.[45]

Signal intensity alterations within the marrow space of the ankle are often nonspecific. For example, in a patient with diabetes, neuropathic arthropathy and osteomyelitis may have a similar appearance.[68] Marrow edema resulting from infection can also be indistinguishable from that caused by trauma.[45] Abnormal marrow signal intensity can be observed deep to a site of soft tissue infection as a result of reactive hyperemia; this can simulate osteomyelitis.[45] Avascular necrosis of the tarsal bones may appear as relatively ill-defined foci of abnormal signal intensity that can simulate osteomyelitis, bone contusion, reflex sympathetic dystrophy, or osteochondral injury.[88]

Synovial osteochondromatosis results in a multiplicity of loose bodies within the ankle joint. The signal intensity of such loose bodies is highly variable on T1-weighted and T2-weighted images, although central high signal intensity from marrow fat with peripheral hypointensity from cortical bone is most frequently observed.[8]

Cartilage

High-resolution images may allow discrimination of the layers of hyaline cartilage in the ankle and other sites.[67] The differential signal intensity of these layers corresponds to variations in collagen density and orientation and in cartilage composition. A trilaminar appearance is usually observed, consisting of two low signal intensity layers encompassing a middle layer of relatively increased signal intensity.

Soft Tissues
Anatomic variations

Accessory muscles can occur about the ankle; the most common is a peroneus quartus muscle, present in approximately 20% of the population. It extends from the peroneus brevis muscle to the peroneal tubercle of the calcaneus.[54] The accessory soleus muscle is another important anatomic variant (Figs. 13-32 and 13-33). This muscle is located between the Achilles tendon and the flexor hallucis longus muscle,[6] where it may simulate a

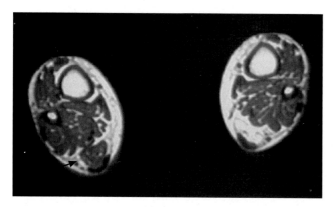

Fig. 13-32. Transaxial T1-weighted image (TR 470, TE 20, 2 Nex) demonstrates an accessory soleus muscle *(arrow)* of the right ankle. Although this asymmetric soft tissue mass may simulate a neoplasm or other abnormality, close inspection reveals architectural characteristics similar to those exhibited by skeletal muscle elsewhere throughout the ankles.

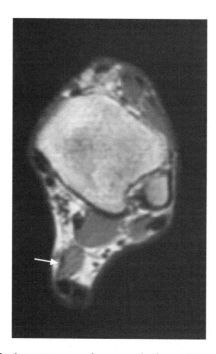

Fig. 13-33. An accessory soleus muscle *(arrow)* is demonstrated deep to the Achilles tendon on this transaxial proton density–weighted image (TR 2500, TE 20, 1 Nex).

soft tissue mass. However, isointensity of these accessory muscles with other muscles on all pulse sequences should allow distinction.[21] In addition, close inspection of such pseudomasses reveals architectural features typical of muscle, such as fine streaks of fibrofatty tissue. Accessory soleus muscles may have additional clinical significance; they can cause ankle discomfort, necessi-

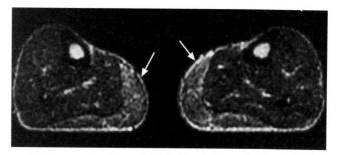

Fig. 13-34. Transaxial T2-weighted image (TR 2600, TE 80, 1 Nex) demonstrates relatively increased signal intensity within the gastrocnemius muscles *(arrows)* bilaterally compared with the surrounding musculature of both calf regions.

tating fasciectomy or muscle resection. Bilateral accessory soleus muscles have been observed.[76] Compression of the posterior tibial nerve by anomalous muscle tissue occasionally results in tarsal tunnel syndrome. One report describes an accessory flexor digitorum longus muscle as a causative factor in this syndrome.[35]

Mild apparent thickening of the plantar fascia is observed near its insertion into the calcaneus; this should not suggest plantar fasciitis.[88] Mildly increased signal intensity on T2-weighted images may be encountered within the medial head of the gastrocnemius muscle in normal subjects (Fig. 13-34).

Imaging technique

Image acquisition using the body coil or head coil permits simultaneous evaluation of both ankles, allowing the assessment of symmetry and improving the ability to distinguish anatomic variants from pathologic conditions. However, use of these coils may compromise spatial resolution, since a relatively large field-of-view is also generally used.[54] Use of a small coil, such as a saddle coil or a Helmholtz coil, is advised for ankle imaging to maximize the signal-to-noise ratio and spatial resolution.[65] It is important to limit movement of the ankle by taping it in position and/or buttressing it with padding material within the coil.[45]

Soft tissue masses

Morton's neuroma, which originates from an interdigital plantar nerve, usually demonstrates relatively low signal intensity on T1-weighted images and is approximately isointense with fat on T2-weighted images (Figs. 13-35, *A* and *B*).[45] The conspicuousness of such lesions may be improved on fat-suppressed images.

Most masses encountered about the ankle have a relatively nonspecific appearance on MR images, consisting of relatively decreased signal intensity on T1-weighted

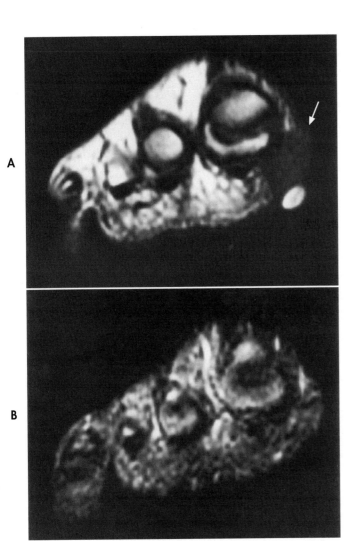

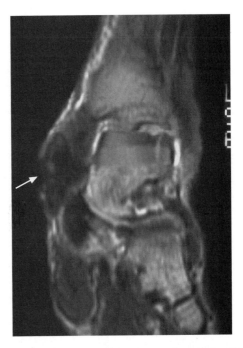

Fig. 13-36. Coronal T2-weighted image (TR 2200, TE 80, 1 Nex) demonstrates large, lobular, soft tissue mass *(arrow)* with homogeneously decreased signal intensity involving the medial aspect of the left ankle, representing a fibromatous tendon sheath tumor.

Fig. 13-35. Coronal T1-weighted image **(A)** (TR 410, TE 11, 2 Nex) and T2-weighted image **(B)** (TR 3200, TE 80, 1 Nex) demonstrate presumed Morton's neuroma *(arrow)* along the plantar aspect of the right foot. Note that the lesion is inconspicuous on the T2-weighted image because of its isointensity with surrounding fat and other structures.

images and moderately increased intensity on T2-weighted images.[45] Departure from this typical signal intensity pattern allows for improved specificity. For example, some masses may appear markedly hyperintense on T2-weighted images, similar to fluid. Synovial cysts and ganglion cysts may have a similar appearance, although the latter have no connection with the joint space.[88] The appearance of a synovial sarcoma can be similar to that of a synovial cyst, but the former usually shows more irregular morphology.[88] Bursal fluid collections can simulate a cystic soft tissue mass about the ankle. Masses with reduced signal intensity on T2-weighted images include pigmented villonodular syno-

vitis, giant cell tumor of the tendon sheath, hemophilic arthropathy, rheumatoid arthritis, fibromatosis, and osteochondromatosis (Fig. 13-36).[45,88]

A small amount of fluid is often present within the ankle and subtalar joint spaces of normal individuals, and mild distention of the posterior joint recess may also be seen (Fig. 13-37).[87,88] However, distention of the anterior joint recess by fluid is considered abnormal. The retrocalcaneal bursa is located between the Achilles tendon and the calcaneus; a small amount of fluid seen within this bursa is normal.[11,88] Inflammation in this region can be observed in patients with Achilles tendon injury.[45] In the foot, fluid may be present in the intermetatarsal bursae.

Ligaments
Imaging technique

Because of their small size and oblique course, complete visualization of ankle ligaments requires relatively thin sections with minimal intersection gaps combined with a small field-of-view to optimize spatial resolution. Maintenance of an adequate signal-to-noise ratio requires a small, high-quality local coil.

Optimal depiction of the ankle ligaments also highly depends on obtaining images in the appropriate plane. Many ankle ligaments are not adequately visualized on at least one of the three orthogonal imaging planes. Using 3-mm spin echo sagittal images, Kier et al. identi-

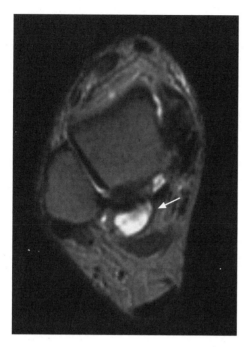

Fig. 13-37. Fluid is seen within the ankle joint space and distending the posterior joint recess *(arrow)* on this transaxial T2-weighted image (TR 3100, TE 80, 1 Nex).

fied the majority (70%) of only 20% of ankle ligaments, whereas coronal images depicted 50% of ligaments, and transaxial images depicted 40%.[42] The combination of all three orthogonal planes resulted in visualization of all ligaments, with the exception of the tibionavicular ligament. Thus, unless clinical information clearly implicates a single ligament, images should generally be acquired in all three orthogonal planes for patients with suspected ligamentous ankle injuries.[42]

Visualization of ankle ligaments is also assisted by proper positioning of the foot during imaging. In a typical resting position, the foot assumes approximately 20 degrees of plantar flexion.[84] This position is not conducive to complete depiction of the lateral collateral ligaments of the ankle. Instead, it is recommended that the foot be taped in full dorsiflexion for improved visualization of the inferior tibiofibular and anterior and posterior fibulotalar ligaments, the deltoid ligament, and the spring ligament.[84] Conversely, the entire length of the fibulocalcaneal, tibionavicular, and tibiotalar ligaments is best visualized with the foot in full plantar flexion. If the foot must be imaged in a neutral position because of the patient's discomfort or for other reasons, then oblique imaging planes can be used to provide optimal depiction of these ligaments.

Schneck et al. found that transaxial images provided the best depiction of the anterior, posterior, and inferior tibiofibular ligaments and the anterior and posterior fibu-

lotalar ligaments when the foot was dorsiflexed.[84] The spring, tibiocalcaneal, and posterior tibiotalar portions of the deltoid ligament were most completely visualized on coronal images obtained with the foot dorsiflexed. When the foot was plantar flexed, the fibulocalcaneal ligament and the tibionavicular and anterior tibiotalar portions of the deltoid ligament were best seen on transaxial images; the sagittal plane resulted in superior depiction of the spring ligament.

The use of three-dimensional Fourier transform gradient echo imaging can be very useful, since images can be retrospectively reformatted along the course of ankle ligaments.[43]

Acquisition of MR images following intraarticular contrast material injection (i.e., MR arthrography) may reveal ligamentous tears, such as those involving the anterior talofibular ligament, that are not evident on conventional MR images.[14,56]

Ligament injury

The primary criterion for diagnosing ligamentous tears is discontinuity or absence of the involved ligament; focal areas of abnormal signal intensity or morphologic irregularity can also be observed.[12] However, some intact ankle ligaments may not be visualized in their entirety, and some demonstrate focal or diffuse areas of relatively increased signal intensity. Both of these findings can simulate ligamentous tear.

Some components of the medial collateral (deltoid) ligament, such as the tibiocalcaneal and tibionavicular ligaments, are of variable thickness in normal subjects. Whereas most components of the deltoid ligament are consistently visualized, the anterior tibiotalar ligament may not be seen in all subjects, even when using three-dimensional Fourier transform gradient echo images.[43] The deltoid ligament can also be of heterogeneous signal intensity, particularly on coronal images. This appearance can appear to represent a tear.[73]

Several other ankle ligaments can also demonstrate heterogeneous or striated areas of relatively increased signal intensity in normal subjects. These include the posterior talofibular, posterior tibiofibular, deep deltoid, and talocalcaneal ligaments.[23,54] An irregularity involving the superior margin of the posterior talofibular ligament has been noted that can simulate the presence of a tear.[73] The ankle ligaments can undergo ossification, which results in heterogeneous signal intensity on both T1-weighted and T2-weighted images.

Although MR is capable of depicting most ankle injuries, their severity as depicted on MR images may not correlate with the degree of instability documented by physical examination or stress radiography.[12,79] This is probably because stress is not applied to the ankle joint during MR imaging. In one series, 12 of 23 patients who showed ligamentous abnormalities on MR had normal stress radiographs.[12] In such situations, MR findings probably reflect relatively low-grade ligamentous injuries that do not result in functional instability.

Because of their low signal intensity, ankle ligaments that are viewed in cross-section can simulate nonossified loose bodies.[23,54] For example, the posterior talofibular and posterior tibiofibular ligaments can simulate loose bodies within the posterior ankle joint on sagittal images.

Tendons

Imaging technique

Poor visualization of ankle tendons and ligaments may result from excessive slice thickness or interslice gap, or may be related to the oblique course of these structures relative to the plane of image acquisition.[42] In some individuals, undocumented remote trauma may have resulted in disruption of these structures, precluding visualization with MR images.

In most situations, the ankle tendons are evaluated using standard orthogonal images. The transaxial plane is particularly useful for evaluating abnormal signal intensity within these tendons or involving their surrounding sheaths. The Achilles, anterior tibial, and flexor hallucis longus tendons are consistently visualized on images acquired in all orthogonal planes.[42] However, the remaining ankle tendons are not; complete evaluation of all ankle tendons usually requires image acquisition in all three orthogonal planes.[42] Oblique images can also be useful for evaluation of the medial ankle tendons, including the flexor hallucis longus, flexor digitorum longus, and posterior tibial tendons.[24] Oblique axial images can also assist in evaluation of the peroneal tunnel; these images demonstrate considerable variability in the thickness of the peroneal retinaculum among normal subjects.[110] Three-dimensional Fourier transform gradient echo images can also improve depiction of the ankle tendons, because they can be reformatted along the anatomic course of these structures.[44]

Tendon injury

The diagnosis of a tendon tear is made when a fluid-filled gap is visualized separating retracted ends of a torn tendon or when severe focal morphologic and signal intensity abnormalities are observed (Fig. 13-38). These findings may not be evident in all tears. For example, signal intensity may be only minimally altered in some torn tendons because of scarring.[88] Therefore, secondary signs should be sought in making this diagnosis. In the evaluation of the posterior tibial tendon, for example, useful secondary signs of a tear include a hypertrophied medial tubercle, an accessory navicular bone, and a talonavicular abnormality.[86]

On the other hand, some signs that are frequently used to diagnose tendon injury, such as alteration in tendon size and signal intensity, may be observed in normal sub-

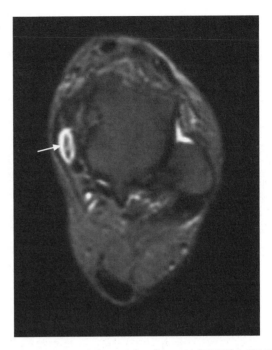

Fig. 13-38. Transaxial T2-weighted image (TR 3600, TE 80, 1 Nex) demonstrates marked thinning and heterogeneous signal intensity involving the posterior tibial tendon (*arrow*) and fluid distending its tendon sheath. These findings indicate a partial thickness tear of this structure.

jects. The normal Achilles tendon is concave on transaxial images, except near its insertion, where it can be rounded.[88] The posterior tibial tendon has a bulbous appearance near its insertion into the navicular, potentially simulating a tear.[44,86] Similarly, many normal subjects exhibit foci of relatively increased signal intensity within the posterior tibial tendon on both T1-weighted and T2-weighted images. Small foci of relatively increased signal intensity may be observed within the Achilles tendons, presumably because of interposed fibrofatty tissue (Fig. 13-39).

Other ankle tendons, such as the flexor hallucis longus and flexor digitorum longus tendons, also demonstrate relative increased signal intensity near their attachments, presumably because of the "magic angle" phenomenon.[44] This refers to the observation of relatively increased signal intensity within collagenous structures oriented at approximately 55 degrees relative to the main magnetic field.[22,54] These findings can simulate tendinous degeneration, inflammation, or a tear. Increased signal intensity is unrelated to the plane of imaging, but is affected by the angle formed between the tendinous structure and the magnetic field. These effects are most prominent when a short echo time is used on either spin echo or gradient echo images.

Distinction of this cause of artifactually increased

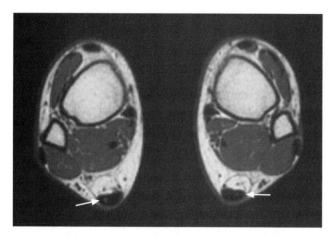

Fig. 13-39. A small focus of relatively increased signal intensity *(arrows)* representing fibrofatty tissue is noted within the central aspect of both Achilles tendons on this transaxial T1-weighted image (TR 450, TE 12, 2 Nex).

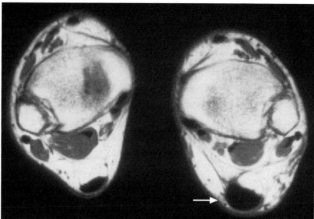

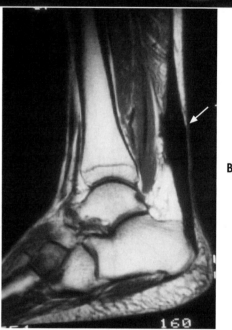

Fig. 13-40. Transaxial **(A)** and sagittal **(B)** T1-weighted images demonstrate fusiform enlargement of the left Achilles tendon *(arrow)* in a patient who underwent tendon repair.

signal intensity from actual pathology is based on the following observations. First, the "magic angle" phenomenon does not result in apparent morphologic abnormalities within the involved tendon. When evidence of tendon thinning, enlargement, or disruption is seen, the possibility of actual injury should be strongly considered. Second, the "magic angle" phenomenon does not result in fluid-like increased signal intensity on T2-weighted images. Thus, visualization of fluid collections involving the tendon sheath or, particularly, filling a gap within a tendon also raises the possibility of tendinous injury. Third, when "magic angle" phenomenon is suspected as the cause of increased tendinous signal intensity, the orientation of that tendon in relation to the magnetic field should be evaluated. In problematic cases, repeat imaging with the involved tendon placed in a different orientation should be performed.

Another cause of apparent increased tendinous signal intensity is partial volume averaging with adjacent fat. This can result in apparent increased signal intensity within the distal aspect of the posterior tibial and other tendons.[15] Relatively increased signal intensity may be observed within the Achilles tendon near its insertion.[88] Longitudinal foci of relatively increased signal intensity can be observed as a result of fibrofatty tissue interposed between divisions of the posterior tibial tendon, possibly mimicking a longitudinal tear.[44] Relatively increased signal intensity due to fatty marrow within a sesamoid bone can simulate tendon injury.[54] Inflammatory changes (i.e., tendinitis) can result in relatively increased signal intensity within ankle tendons that may be indistinguishable from partial thickness tendon tears.[15] Inflammatory and degenerative changes of the flexor hallucis longus and Achilles tendons may be observed in asymptomatic long-distance runners.[100] Tendinous enlargement and

signal heterogeneity can also result from previous surgical repair.[53] For example, a focal increase in tendon caliber with associated relatively increased signal intensity can be observed at the site of a repaired Achilles tendon (Figs. 13-40, *A* and *B*).[45]

It may be difficult to distinguish tendons from adjacent low signal intensity bone cortex or osseous abnormalities.[15] Similarly, blending of distal tendon with adjacent low signal intensity bone cortex can simulate tendon expansion.[45]

Fluid collections

The observation of fluid within tendon sheaths is often regarded as ancillary evidence of tenosynovitis or

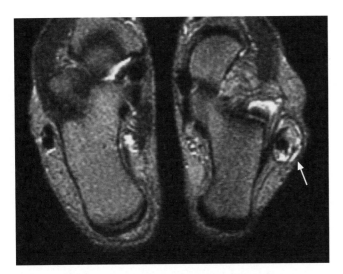

Fig. 13-41. Transaxial T2-weighted image (TR 3400, TE 80, 1 Nex) demonstrates distention of the peroneal tendon sheath of the left ankle *(arrow)* as a result of tenosynovitis. A small amount of physiologic fluid is seen within the contralateral tendon sheath.

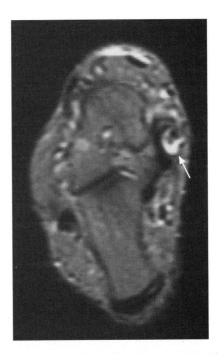

Fig. 13-42. Fluid is seen distending the posterior tibial tendon sheath *(arrow)* on this transaxial T2-weighted image (TR 2400, TE 80, 1 Nex) in a patient who underwent tenography and steroid injection for tenosynovitis.

tendon injury. However, fluid can be seen on MR images within many ankle tendon sheaths in normal subjects (Fig. 13-41).[54,87] A relatively large volume of fluid can be seen within the flexor hallucis longus tendon sheath in asymptomatic subjects. The peroneal tendon sheaths are another common site where fluid can be observed in normal subjects.[88] Fluid within the common peroneal tendon sheaths can simulate a longitudinal tendon tear.[73] Fluid is usually not associated with the anterior (i.e., extensor) ankle tendons and the distal posterior tibial tendon in normal subjects.[88] Distention of a tendon sheath with fluid may also be related to previous tenography with steroid injection for the treatment of tendinitis (Fig. 13-42).

WRIST
Osseous Structures

The radius or the ulna may be partially or completely absent.[6] The carpal bones can vary considerably in number, and the metacarpals and phalanges may be of variable length and thickness.[6] A variety of sesamoid bones and ossicles may be present about the wrist and hand. Small, rounded foci of relatively decreased signal intensity are commonly observed within the carpal bones, usually representing small bone islands or subchondral cysts (Fig. 13-43). These are of no clinical significance. Variability in the distribution of hyaline cartilage overlying the carpal bones can be observed among normal subjects.[94]

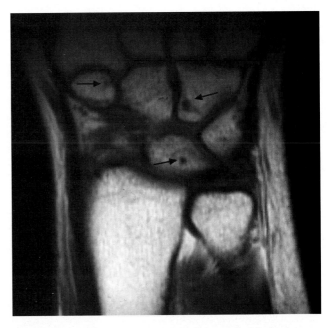

Fig. 13-43. There are scattered, small, rounded foci of relatively decreased signal intensity *(arrows)* throughout several carpal bones on this coronal T1-weighted image (TR 430, TE 15, 2 Nex).

Soft Tissues

The palmaris longus muscle is absent in 11% of individuals.[6] Anomalous muscles have been observed on MR images in the region of the ulnar tunnel (Guyon's canal).[109] These anomalous muscles may occur bilaterally.

Increased soft tissue signal intensity can be observed on MR images obtained immediately following wrist and forearm exercise. Significant variation in recruitment of individual muscles has been observed among normal subjects following the performance of a standardized protocol involving wrist flexion.[25]

Ganglions are cystic structures that contain mucinous material and are commonly present about the wrist (Figs. 13-44, 13-45). They are most frequently observed along the dorsal wrist, flexor tendon sheath, and palmar radial wrist, in descending frequency.[111] The appearance of many benign and malignant soft tissue masses about the wrist is often nonspecific on MR images.[7]

Triangular Fibrocartilage

The normal triangular fibrocartilage complex has sometimes been characterized as uniformly hypointense on all pulse sequences. However, foci of relatively increased signal intensity can be observed within this structure in the absence of injury (Figs. 13-46, 13-47). Foci of increased intensity are particularly frequent within the triangular fibrocartilage near its radial and ulnar attachments.[41,111]

In one study, relatively increased signal intensity was observed in 70% of normal subjects.[59] These signal alterations may be the result of degenerative changes within the triangular fibrocartilage and are most frequently observed in older subjects. However, they can occur in all age groups, including young, asymptomatic subjects.[59]

Degenerative changes of the triangular fibrocartilage can simulate a posttraumatic tear of this structure, but degenerative changes tend to have a more central location than posttraumatic tears.[89] Another distinction is that tears often demonstrate high signal intensity on T2-weighted images, whereas degenerative changes do not.[41,111] Linear signal abnormalities, particularly those extending to an articular surface, have been considered to be indicative of a tear rather than of globular degenerative changes. However, in their study of 70 asymptomatic wrists, Sugimoto et al. found that 50% had linear signal abnormalities extending to an articular surface.[97] Many of these subjects were in their teens or twenties, raising the question of whether all of the observed findings reflected degenerative changes. The morphology of the triangular fibrocartilage was also abnormal in some subjects, consisting of a band shape or an amorphous shape rather than the usual triangular configuration and/or demonstrating irregular rather than smooth edges. The high prevalence of such findings in asymptomatic subjects indicates that when signal intensity and/or morphologic alterations are present within the triangular fibrocartilage, close correlation with clinical examination must be performed to assign significance to these observations.

It is difficult to identify a site of superimposed tearing in patients with underlying degenerative changes in-

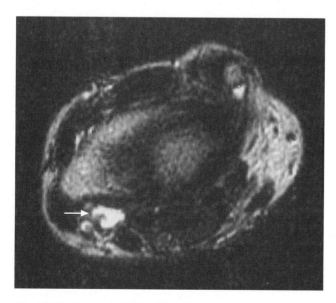

Fig. 13-44. Transaxial T2-weighted image (TR 2400, TE 80, 1 Nex) demonstrates a small ganglion cyst *(arrow)* along the volar aspect of the wrist near the radial styloid on this transaxial T2-weighted image.

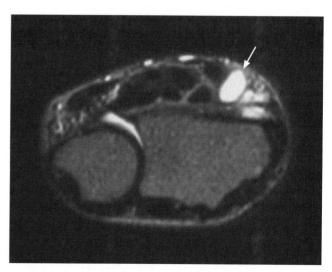

Fig. 13-45. A ganglion cyst *(arrow)* is demonstrated with uniform hyperintensity along the dorsum of the wrist on this transaxial T2-weighted image (TR 2000, TE 80, 2 Nex).

volving the triangular fibrocartilage.[75] It may not be possible to distinguish between degenerative and traumatic tears.[59] Fluid in the distal radioulnar joint is frequently seen as an ancillary finding in patients with triangular fibrocartilage tears.[85]

Coronal images may demonstrate an apparent defect of the triangular fibrocartilage, representing the boundary between the dorsal edge of this structure and the joint capsule.[97]

Ligaments
Imaging technique

Optimization of the imaging technique is important for visualizing the wrist ligaments on MR images. Adequate spatial resolution requires the use of a small field-of-view, a high-resolution matrix, and thin sections with a minimal intersection gap. A local coil is essential for an adequate signal-to-noise ratio. Imaging is ideally performed with the wrist at the patient's side using an off-center field of view, since this position is most comfortable and hence reduces motion artifact.[111]

The selection of imaging planes is also very important for evaluating the wrist ligaments. In general, coronal and sagittal images provide the best depiction of these ligaments. Sagittal images have been particularly useful for visualizing the radioscaphocapitate and radiolunate ligaments, whereas coronal images are used to depict the radioscapholunate and interosseous ligaments

of the scaphoid, lunate, and triquetrum.[5] Transaxial images provide optimal depiction of the flexor and extensor retinacula.

Anatomic variations

The carpal ligaments are subject to considerable anatomic variation. In one study, the radiotriquetral ligament appeared to have a single origin in 84% and a dual origin in 16% of normal subjects.[93] The dorsal intercarpal ligament was even more variable, having a single band-like structure, a branched appearance, and a separation into distinct fascicles in 14%, 44%, and 38% of subjects, respectively.

Ligament visualization

Even when optimized imaging techniques are used, all wrist ligaments may not be consistently visualized on MR images. This can be problematic, since it may not be clear whether the apparent absence of the ligament is the result of a tear, an anatomic variation, or factors related to the imaging technique. Absence of some carpal ligaments, such as the scapholunate ligament, usually indicates a tear. However, other ligaments, such as the lunotriquetral ligament, may not be visualized even when they are intact.[32,85] The radioscaphocapitate, radiolunotriquetral, radiolunate, ulnolunate, ulnotriquetral, and triquetroscaphoid ligaments are visible in most normal subjects on three-dimensional Fourier transform gradient echo images.[95] However, the radioscaphoid and radioscapholunate ligaments are often somewhat more difficult to identify.

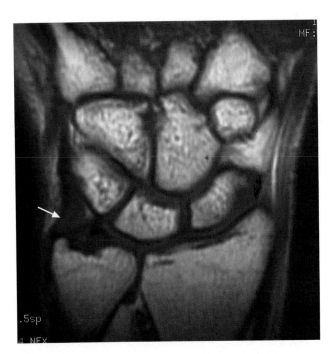

Fig. 13-46. Coronal T1-weighted image (TR 400, TE 14, 4 Nex) demonstrates moderately increased signal intensity *(arrow)* within the triangular fibrocartilage complex near its ulnar attachment.

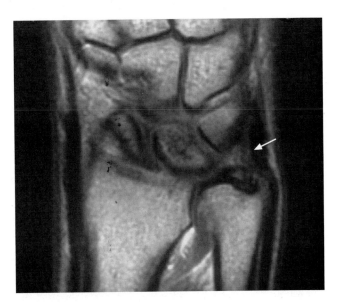

Fig. 13-47. A globular focus of relatively increased signal intensity is noted within the midsubstance of the triangular fibrocartilage complex *(arrow)* on coronal proton density–weighted image (TR 2000, TE 30, 1 Nex).

Images of the contralateral wrist may be useful for patients with an apparently absent ligament, although ligamentous wrist anatomy is not bilaterally symmetric in all individuals.[95] In one study, the dorsal intercarpal ligaments had a bilaterally symmetric appearance in only 16 of 25 normal subjects.[93]

Alterations in signal intensity and morphology

The scapholunate and lunotriquetral ligaments exhibit somewhat variable morphology and signal intensity. In most patients, a deltalike configuration is present, but a linear configuration can also be seen.[92,94] Although these ligaments are of uniformly low signal intensity in most patients, in many patients, foci of intermediate signal intensity are observed on gradient-echo images. In some normal subjects, the volar ligaments demonstrate a striated appearance.[101] Apparent discontinuity of the lunotriquetral ligament can also be observed along its volar portion, simulating a tear.[111] Intermediate signal intensity is observed within wrist tendons and ligaments oriented at approximately 55 degrees relative to the magnetic field. This so-called "magic angle" phenomenon can simulate inflammatory, degenerative, or posttraumatic changes involving these structures.[22]

Injuries

In studies of ligament tears using cadaveric wrists, significant numbers of false-negative and false-positive MR findings have also been observed.[101] Success of detecting wrist ligament tears varies with the size and orientation of each ligament. In one study, only 50% of scapholunate ligament tears and 40% of lunotriquetral tears that were proven with arthroscopy could be identified with MR.[80] Other studies also indicate that tears of the scapholunate ligament are somewhat more reliably seen than those involving the lunotriquetral ligament.[85] Kinematic MR studies, in which images are acquired at various increments of motion, may better demonstrate ligamentous abnormalities that result in wrist instability. Defects involving the wrist ligaments identified with MR images may result from chronic use or degeneration rather than from acute traumatic tears.[28]

Carpal Tunnel Syndrome

MR findings in patients with carpal tunnel syndrome can include abnormally increased signal intensity of the median nerve on T2-weighted images, alteration in size of the median nerve, convexity of the flexor retinaculum, and fluid within the flexor tendon sheaths.[57]

Anatomic variations can simulate some of these findings. For example, the normal median nerve may appear slightly flattened at the level of the pisiform bone, and mild convexity of the flexor retinaculum may also be observed (Figs. 13-48, A and B).[58] Some anatomic variations

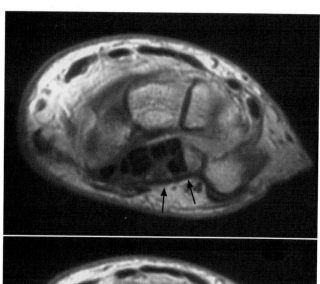

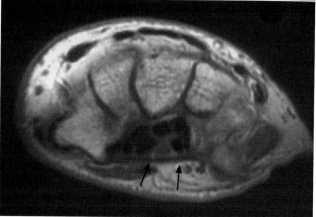

A

B

Fig. 13-48. Transaxial T1-weighted image **(A)** (TR 500, TE 15, 2 Nex) demonstrates mild convexity of the flexor retinaculum *(arrows)* in a normal subject. The adjacent image **(B)** demonstrates that the retinaculum has a straight course.

contribute to median nerve compression. These include the presence of abundant fat within the carpal tunnel, a large adductor pollicis muscle, or a persistent median artery.[57] Fibrolipomatous infiltration of the median nerve can also result in carpal tunnel syndrome (Fig. 13-49).[106]

Whereas increased signal intensity of the median nerve on T2-weighted images is usually associated with carpal tunnel syndrome, paradoxically decreased intensity of this structure can result from fibrosis.[111]

Usually, the morphology of the carpal tunnel is assessed with the wrist in a neutral position. Significant alterations in the configuration of the carpal tunnel may be observed due to wrist positioning. In the extended wrist, the carpal tunnel decreases in cross-sectional area at the level of the pisiform bone, which may contribute to median nerve impingement.[107] The cross-sectional area of the carpal tunnel is decreased during wrist flexion at the pisiform and hamate hook levels.[91,107] Furthermore, the flexor tendons undergo rearrangement during

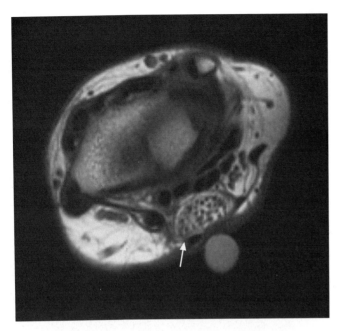

Fig. 13-49. Fibrolipomatous infiltration of the median nerve *(arrow)* is demonstrated on this transaxial T1-weighted image (TR 450, TE 15, 2 Nex) in a patient who underwent previous retinacular release for carpal tunnel syndrome.

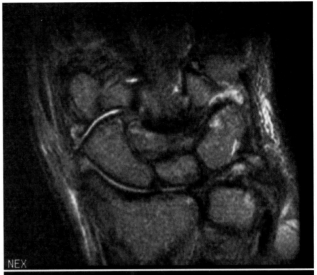

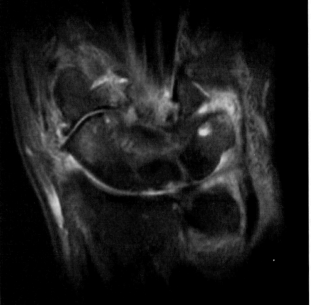

Fig. 13-50. The presence of synovial inflammation (i.e., pannus) is poorly depicted on coronal T2-weighted image **(A)** (TR 2000, TE 80, 1 Nex). However, the corresponding fat-suppressed T1-weighted image **(B)** (TR 500, TE 15, 2 Nex) obtained following intravenous administration of gadolinium chelate demonstrates extensive abnormal contrast material enhancement in this patient with rheumatoid arthritis.

wrist flexion, which may also contribute to compression of the median nerve.[91] With the wrist in the neutral position, the median nerve is located anterior to the superficial flexor tendon of the index finger. However, with wrist flexion, the nerve may become interposed among the flexor tendons. When the median nerve remains anteriorly positioned during wrist flexion, it often appears flattened along its anteroposterior dimension, whereas more posteriorly positioned nerves can appear round or flattened along their mediolateral dimension.

Volar migration of the carpal tunnel contents can be observed following surgical release of the flexor retinaculum.[111] Residually increased signal intensity within the median nerve may be observed following successful surgical treatment.[111]

Synovial Arthritis

Standard T1-weighted and T2-weighted images have not proven to be very beneficial in the evaluation of patients with inflammatory arthritis. However, contrast-enhanced images demonstrate prominent enhancement of inflamed synovium (Figs. 13-50, *A* and *B*, 13-51, *A* and *B*). In patients with rheumatoid arthritis, contrast-enhanced T1-weighted images demonstrate a wide range of findings, even among patients with a similar clinical presentation.[39] These findings range from mild inhomogeneous synovial enhancement, to discrete curvilinear or nodular enhancing foci, to diffuse synovial enhancement.

Findings of synovitis observed on MR images in patients with rheumatoid arthritis correlate poorly with the clinical assessment of disease activity.[40,71,83] MR often demonstrates pannus and tendon sheath effusions, even in patients with clinically mild disease; these findings do not differentiate more active disease. Osseous cysts in patients with rheumatoid arthritis do not undergo signifi-

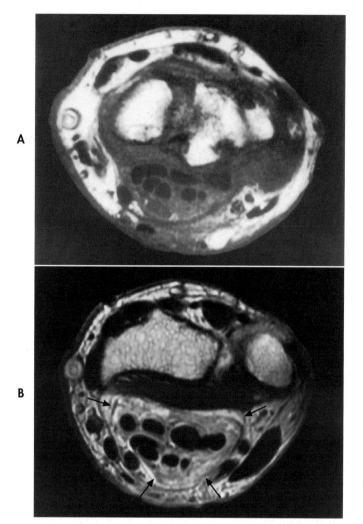

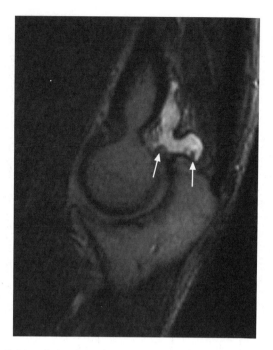

Fig. 13-52. Distention of the joint space by fluid allows for observation of multiple small, osteochondral bodies *(arrows)* within the posterior elbow joint space on this sagittal T2-weighted image (TR 2600, TE 80, 1 Nex).

Fig. 13-51. Transaxial T1-weighted images (TR 500, TE 15, 2 Nex) obtained before **(A)** and after **(B)** intravenous administration of gadolinium chelate. There is marked thickening of the flexor tendon sheaths with associated abnormal contrast material enhancement *(arrows)* and osseous erosion in a patient with rheumatoid arthritis.

cant contrast enhancement and may be indistinguishable from degenerative or other osseous cysts.[31]

ELBOW
Osseous and Soft Tissue Structures

Evaluation of the elbow requires particular attention to imaging technique, including the use of a small-surface coil for a high signal-to-noise ratio. A single-loop coil, designed for shoulder imaging, also accommodates the elbow and provides a relatively uniform signal intensity profile across the elbow. Volume coils, into which the arm is inserted, or Helmholtz or phased-array coil arrangements are also used successfully. Thin sections (i.e., 3 to 4 mm thick) with small intersection gaps should be used to maximize spatial resolution, since many important structures about the elbow are quite small. The elbow must be immobilized within the coil to prevent motion artifacts.

Standard spin-echo sequences continue to be used for elbow imaging. However, subtle osseous abnormalities about the elbow may be poorly depicted on such images. Three-dimensional Fourier transform gradient-echo imaging may be advantageous for the depiction of elbow lesions such as osteochondral bodies, small osteophytes, and fragmentation of the olecranon.[69]

In the presence of joint effusion, osteochondral bodies are easily visualized as defects within the joint space on T2-weighted images (Fig. 13-52). However, such bodies may not be visible in patients without joint fluid because of isointensity between such fragments and adjacent soft tissues.[35] Fragments containing marrow fat can be missed because of isointensity with adjacent fat planes (Fig. 13-53).

An osteochondral fracture of the distal humerus can be simulated on coronal and transaxial MR images; this "pseudodefect" is attributable to a groove situated at the junction of the capitellum and lateral humeral epicondyle.[81] An apparent defect involving the distal humerus

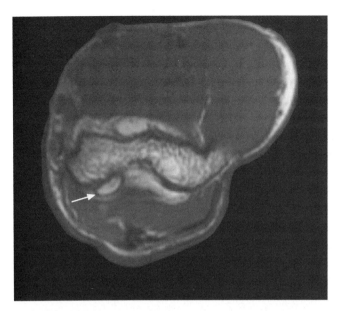

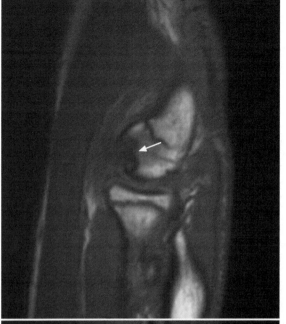

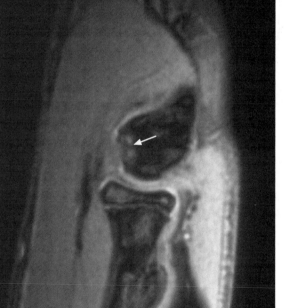

Fig. 13-53. The presence of a low signal intensity cortical rim allows the identification of an osteochondral body *(arrow)*, which is otherwise isointense with the adjacent posterior fat pad, on this transaxial T1-weighted image (TR 400, TE 15, 2 Nex).

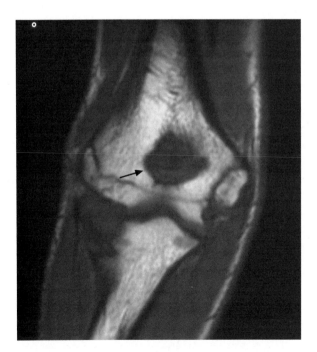

Fig. 13-54. Coronal T1-weighted image (TR 400, TE 15, 2 Nex) demonstrates apparent low-intensity marrow abnormality within the distal humerus *(arrow)*, which is due to normal osseous thinning at the olecranon fossa.

Fig. 13-55. Sagittal T1-weighted image **(A)** (TR 530, TE 15, 2 Nex) demonstrates focus of osteonecrosis *(arrow)* involving the capitellum. Corresponding gradient echo image **(B)** (TR 450, TE 7, 2 Nex, 90-degree flip angle) demonstrates interruption of high signal intensity hyaline cartilage overlying this defect.

may also be created by the normal osseous thinning that occurs in the region of the olecranon fossa (Fig. 13-54).

Direct evidence of epicondylitis may be poorly displayed on MR images in some patients. However, a secondary sign that may be seen in patients with lateral humeral epicondylitis (i.e., tennis elbow) is abnormally increased signal intensity on T2-weighted images within the anconeous muscle.[16] This finding is presumed to reflect muscular inflammation and/or edema, which may contribute to symptoms. Chondromalacia is another entity that is difficult to appreciate on MR images.[69] Gradient-echo images may help to determine the status of hyaline cartilage in the region of the elbow (Figs. 13-55, *A* and *B).*

Ligaments

The ulnar collateral ligament may be injured in throwing athletes, resulting in medial joint pain and valgus instability. The ulnar collateral ligament is usually best visualized on coronal images, although these should be supplemented by transaxial images. However, because of its oblique anterior-posterior course, the ligament may not be visualized in continuity on a single coronal image. Retrospective reformation of two-dimensional coronal images on a computer workstation can be useful for aligning the plane of image display along that of the collateral ligament.[1] In patients with ulnar collateral ligament injury, the ligament appears lax, poorly defined, and of relatively increased signal intensity on all pulse sequences (Fig. 13-56).[62]

Whereas the above abnormalities indicate injury involving the collateral ligament, the precise definition of such injury may be difficult to determine in some pa-

tients. For example, distinction between partial thickness and small, full thickness tears can be difficult unless there is retraction of torn ligament fibers in the latter situation. Another limitation of MR is its relative insensitivity to demonstrating partial thickness tears involving the undersurface of the medial collateral ligament; these tears can be visualized using CT arthrography.[99]

Moderate signal intensity may be observed within the proximal aspect of the ulnar collateral ligament on coronal images in patients without injury to this structure.[70] The radial collateral ligament—a much less functionally important structure—is poorly depicted on coronal images[69] and appears as a complete signal void. The components of the radial (i.e., lateral) collateral ligament are also highly variable among individuals.

REFERENCES

1. Apicella P, Mirowitz SA: Interactive multiplanar interpolation of two-dimensional MR images, Clin Imaging 19:287-290, 1995.
2. Asnis SE, Gould ES, Bansal M et al: Magnetic resonance imaging of the hip after displaced femoral neck fractures, Clin Orthop 298:191-198, 1994.
3. Beltran J, Chandnani V, McGhee RA Jr et al: Gadopentetate dimeglumine–enhanced MR imaging of the musculoskeletal system AJR 156:457-466, 1991.
4. Beltran J, Noto AM, Herman LJ et al: Joint effusions: MR imaging, Radiology 158:133-137, 1986.
5. Berger RA, Linscheid RL, Berquist TH: Magnetic resonance imaging of the anterior radiocarpal ligaments, J Hand Surg [Am] 19:295-303, 1994.
6. Bergman NA, Thompson SA, Afifi AK et al: Compendium of human anatomic variation: text, atlas, and world literature, Baltimore, 1988, Urban & Schwarzenberg.
7. Binkovitz LA, Berquist TH, McLeod RA: Masses of the hand and wrist: detection and characterization with MR imaging, AJR 154:323-326, 1990.
8. Blandino A, Salvi L, Chirico G et al: Synovial osteochondromatosis of the ankle: MR findings, Clin Imaging 16:34-36, 1992.
9. Bloem JL: Transient osteoporosis of the hip: MR imaging, Radiology 167:753-755, 1988.
10. Bongartz G, Bock E, Horbach T et al: Degenerative cartilage lesions of the hip—magnetic resonance evaluation, Magn Reson Imaging 7:179-186, 1989.
11. Canoso JJ, Liu N, Traill MR et al: Physiology of the retrocalcaneal bursa, Ann Rheum Dis 47:910-912, 1988.
12. Cardone BW, Erickson SJ, Den Hartog BD et al: MRI of injury to the lateral collateral ligamentous complex of the ankle, J Comput Assist Tomogr 17:102-107, 1993.
13. Chan TW, Dalinka MK, Steinberg ME et al: MRI appearance of femoral head osteonecrosis following core decompression and bone grafting, Skeletal Radiol 20:103-107, 1991.
14. Chandnani VP, Harper MT, Ficke JR et al: Chronic ankle instability: evaluation with MR arthrography, MR imaging, and stress radiography, Radiology 192:189-194, 1994.

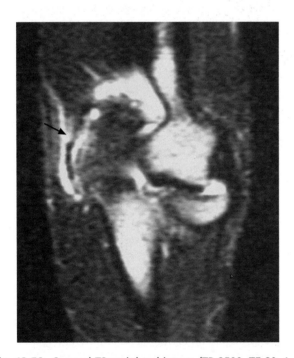

Fig. 13-56. Coronal T2-weighted image (TR 2500, TE 80, 1 Nex) demonstrates moderately increased signal intensity within the proximal aspect of a partially torn ulnar collateral ligament *(arrow),* with fluid surrounding this structure.

15. Cheung Y, Rosenberg ZS, Magee T et al: Normal anatomy and pathologic conditions of ankle tendons: current imaging techniques, Radiographics 12:429-444, 1992.

16. Coel M, Yamada CY, Ko J: MR imaging of patients with lateral epicondylitis of the elbow (tennis elbow): importance of increased signal of the anconenus muscle, AJR 161:1019-1021, 1993.

17. Crabbe JP, Martel W, Matthews LS: Rapid growth of femoral herniation pit, AJR 159:1038-1040, 1992.

18. Dawson KL, Moore SG, Rowland JM: Age-related marrow changes in the pelvis: MR and anatomic findings, Radiology 183:47-51, 1992.

19. De Smet AA, Fisher DR, Burnstein MI et al: Value of MR imaging in staging osteochondral lesions of the talus (osteochondritis dissecans): results in 14 patients, AJR 154:555-558, 1990.

20. Ebraheim NA, Savolaine ER, Zeiss J et al: Titanium hip implants for improved magnetic resonance and computed tomography examinations, Clin Orthop 275:194-198, 1992.

21. Ekstrom JE, Shuman WP, Mack LA: MR imaging of accessory soleus muscle, J Comput Assist Tomogr 14:239-242, 1990.

22. Erickson SJ, Cox IH, Hyde JS et al: Effect of tendon orientation on MR imaging signal intensity: a manifestation of the "magic angle" phenomenon, Radiology 181:389-392, 1991.

23. Erickson SJ, Smith JW, Ruiz ME et al: MR imaging of the lateral collateral ligament of the ankle, AJR 156:131-136, 1991.

24. Ferkel RD, Flannigan BD, Elkins BS: Magnetic resonance imaging of the foot and ankle: correlation of normal anatomy with pathologic conditions, Foot Ankle 11:289-305, 1991.

25. Fleckenstein JL, Watumull D, Bertocci LA et al: Muscle recruitment variations during wrist flexion exercise: MR evaluation, J Comput Assist Tomogr 18:449-453, 1994.

26. Genenz BM, Wilson MR, Houk RW et al: Early osteonecrosis of the femoral head: detection in high-risk patients with MR imaging, Radiology 168:521-524, 1988.

27. Genez BM: MR diagnosis of a prosthesis pseudobursa, [letter] AJR 151:837, 1988.

28. Gilula LA, Palmer AK: Is it possible to diagnose a tear at arthrography or MR imaging? [letter] Radiology 187:582, 1993.

29. Glickstein MF, Burk DL, Schiebler ML et al: Avascular necrosis versus other diseases of the hip: sensitivity of MR imaging, Radiology 169:213-215, 1988.

30. Grimm J, Higer HP, Benning R et al: MRI of transient osteoporosis of the hip, [review] Arch Orthop Trauma Surg 110:98-102, 1991.

31. Gubler FM, Algra PR, Maas M et al: Gadolinium-DTPA enhanced magnetic resonance imaging of bone cysts in patients with rheumatoid arthritis, Ann Rheum Dis 52:716-719, 1993.

32. Gundry CR, Kursunoglu-Brahme S, Schwaighofer B et al: Is MR better than arthrography for evaluating the ligaments of the wrist? In vitro study, AJR 154:337-341, 1990.

33. Hauzeur JP, Hanquinet S, Gevenois PA et al: Study of magnetic resonance imaging in transient osteoporosis of the hip, J Rheumatol 18:1211-1217, 1991.

34. Hayes CW, Conway WF, Daniel WW: MR imaging of bone marrow edema pattern: transient osteoporosis, transient bone marrow edema syndrome, or osteonecrosis, Radiographics 13:1001-1012, 1993.

35. Ho VW, Peterfy C, Helms CA: Tarsal tunnel syndrome caused by strain of an anomalous muscle: an MRI-specific diagnosis, J Comput Assist Tomogr 17:822-823, 1993.

36. Hodler J, Resnick D: Chondromalacia patellae, AJR 158:106-107, 1992.

37. Hoffinger SA, Henderson RC, Renner JB et al: Magnetic resonance evaluation of "metaphyseal" changes in Legg-Calve-Perthes disease, J Pediatr Orthop 13:602-606, 1993.

38. Hofman S, Engel A, Neuhold A et al: Bone-marrow oedema syndrome and transient osteoporosis of the hip. An MRI-controlled study of treatment by core decompression, J Bone Joint Surg Br 75:210-216, 1993.

39. Jevtic V, Watt I, Rozman B et al: Precontrast and postcontrast (Gd-DTPA) magnetic resonance imaging of hand joints in patients with rheumatoid arthritis, Clin Radiol 48:176-181, 1993.

40. Jorgensen C, Cyteval C, Anaya JM et al: Sensitivity of magnetic resonance imaging of the wrist in very early rheumatoid arthritis, Clin Exp Rheumatol 11:163-168, 1993.

41. Kang HS, Kindynis P, Brahme SK et al: Triangular fibrocartilage and intercarpal ligaments of the wrist: MR imaging. Cadaveric study with gross pathologic and histologic correlation, Radiology 181:401-404, 1991.

42. Kier R, Dietz MJ, McCarthy SM et al: MR imaging of the normal ligaments and tendons of the ankle, J Comput Assist Tomogr 15:477-482, 1991.

43. Klein MA: MR imaging of the ankle: normal and abnormal findings in the medial collateral ligament, AJR 162:377-383, 1994.

44. Klein MA: Reformatted three-dimensional Fourier transform gradient-recalled echo MR imaging of the ankle: spectrum of normal and abnormal findings, AJR 161:831-836, 1993.

45. Kneeland JB, Dalinka MK: Magnetic resonance imaging of the foot and ankle, Magn Reson Q 8:97-115, 1992.

46. Kokubo T, Takatori Y, Ninomiya S et al: Fat intensity within the hypointense zone on MR imaging of avascular necrosis of the femoral head, J Comput Assist Tomogr 15:470-473, 1991.

47. Kopecky KK, Braunstein EM, Branmdt KD et al: Apparent avascular necrosis of the hip: appearance and spontaneous resolution of MR findings in renal allograft recipients, Radiology 179:523-527, 1991.

48. Laakman RW, Kaufman B, Han JS et al: MR imaging in patients with metallic implants, Radiology 157:711-714, 1985.

49. Lafforgue P, Dahan E, Chagnaud C et al: Early-stage avascular necrosis of the femoral head: MR imaging for prognosis in 31 cases with at least 2 years of follow-up, Radiology 187:199-204, 1993.

50. Lang P, Genant HK, Jergesen HE et al: Imaging of the hip joint. Computed tomography versus magnetic resonance imaging, Clin Orthop 274:135-153, 1992.

51. Lang P, Jergesen HE, Moseley ME et al: Avascular necrosis of the femoral head: high–field-strength MR imaging with histologic correlation, Radiology 169:517-524, 1988.

52. Li KC, Hiette P: Contrast-enhanced fat saturation magnetic resonance imaging for studying the pathophysiology of osteonecrosis of the hips, Skeletal Radiol 21:375-379, 1992.

53. Liem MD, Zegel HG, Balduini FC et al: Repair of Achilles tendon ruptures with a polylactic acid implant: assessment with MR imaging, AJR 156:769-773, 1991.

54. Link SC, Erickson SJ, Timins ME: MR imaging of the ankle and foot: normal structures and anatomic variants that may simulate disease, AJR 161:607-612, 1993.

55. Lupetin AR, Daffner RH: Rheumatoid iliopsoas bursitis: MR findings, J Comput Assist Tomogr 14:1035-1036, 1990.

56. Mayer DP, Jay RM, Schoenhaus H et al: Magnetic resonance arthrography of the ankle, J Foot Surg 31:584-587, 1992.

57. Mesgarzadeh M, Schneck CD, Bonakdarpour A et al: Carpal tunnel: MR imaging. Part II. Carpal tunnel syndrome, Radiology 171:749-754, 1989.

58. Mesgarzadeh M, Schneck CD, Bonakdarpour A: Carpal tunnel: MR imaging. Part I. Normal anatomy, Radiology 171:743-748, 1989.

59. Metz VM, Schratter M, Dock WI et al: Age-associated changes of the triangular fibrocartilage of the wrist: evaluation of the diagnostic performance of MR imaging, Radiology 184:217-220, 1992.

60. Mirowitz SA, Apicella P, Reinus WR et al: MR imaging of bone marrow lesions: relative conspicuousness of lesions on T_1-weighted, fat suppressed T_2-weighted, and STIR images, AJR 162:215-221, 1994.

61. Mirowitz SA: Hematopoietic bone marrow within the proximal humeral epiphysis in normal adults: investigation with MR imaging, Radiology 188:689-693, 1993.

62. Mirowitz SA, London SL: Ulnar collateral ligament injury in baseball pitchers: MR imaging evaluation, Radiology 185:573-576, 1992.

63. Mitchell DG, Kressel HY, Arger PH et al: Avascular necrosis of the femoral head: morphologic assessment by MR imaging, with CT correlation, Radiology 161:739-742, 1986.

64. Mitchell DG, Rao V, Dalinka M et al: MRI of joint fluid in the normal and ischemic hip, AJR 146:1215-1218, 1986.

65. Mitchell DG, Rao VJ, Dalinka M et al: Hematopoietic and fatty bone marrow distribution in the normal and ischemic hip: new observations with 1.5-T MR imaging, Radiology 161:199-202, 1986.

66. Mitchell DG, Rao VM, Dalinka MK et al: Femoral head avascular necrosis: correlation of MR imaging, radiographic staging, radionuclide imaging, and clinical findings, Radiology 162:709-715, 1987.

67. Modl JM, Sether LA, Haughton VM et al: Articular cartilage: correlation of histologic zones with signal intensity at MR imaging, Radiology 181:853-855, 1991.

68. Moore SG, Bisset GS III, Siegel MJ et al: Pediatric musculoskeletal MR imaging, Radiology 179:345-360, 1991.

69. Murphy BJ: MR imaging of the elbow, Radiology 184:525-529, 1992.

70. Nadel SN, Debatin JF, Richardson WJ et al: Detection of acute avascular necrosis of the femoral head in dogs: dynamic contrast-enhanced MR imaging vs spin-echo and STIR sequences, AJR 159:1255-1261, 1992.

71. Nagele M, Kunze V, Koch W et al: Rheumatoid arthritis of the wrist. Dynamic Gd-DTPA enhanced MRT, ROFO 158:141-146, 1993.

72. Nokes SR, Vogler JB, Spritzer CE et al: Herniation pits of the femoral neck: appearance at MR imaging, Radiology 172:231-234, 1989.

73. Noto AM, Cheung Y, Rosenberg ZS et al: MR imaging of the ankle: normal variants, Radiology 170:121-124, 1989.

74. Pay NT, Singer WS, Bartal E: Hip pain in three children accompanied by transient abnormal findings on MR images, Radiology 171:147-149, 1989.

75. Pederzini L, Luchetti R, Soragni O et al: Evaluation of the triangular fibrocartilage complex tears by arthroscopy, arthrography, and magnetic resonance imaging, Arthroscopy 8:191-197, 1992.

76. Peterson DA, Stinson W, Carter J: Bilateral accessory soleus: a report on four patients with partial fasciectomy, (review) Foot Ankle 14:284-288, 1993.

77. Potter H, Moran M, Schneider R et al: Magnetic resonance imaging in diagnosis of transient osteoporosis of the hip, Clin Orthop 280:223-229, 1992.

78. Pritchard RS, Shah HR, Nelson CL et al: MR and CT appearance of iliopsoas bursal distention secondary to diseased hips, J Comput Assist Tomogr 14:797-800, 1990.

79. Rijke AM, Goitz HT, McCue FC 3d et al: Magnetic resonance imaging of injury to the lateral ankle ligaments, Am J Sports Med 21:528-534, 1993.

80. Rominger MB, Bernreuter WK, Kenney PJ et al: MR imaging of anatomy and tears of wrist ligaments, Radiographics 13:1233-1246, 1993.

81. Rosenberg ZS, Beltran J, Cheung YY: Pseudodefect of the capitellum: potential MR imaging pitfall, Radiology 191:821-823, 1994.

82. Rosenberg ZS, Cheung Y, Jahss MH et al: Rupture of posterior tibial tendon: CT and MR imaging with surgical correlation, Radiology 169:229-235, 1988.

83. Rubens DJ, Blebea JS, Totterman SM et al: Rheumatoid arthritis: evaluation of wrist extensor tendons with clinical examination versus MR imaging—a preliminary report, Radiology 187:831-838, 1993.

84. Schenk CD, Mesgarzadeh M, Bonakdarpour A et al: MR imaging of the most commonly injured ankle ligaments. Part I. Normal anatomy, Radiology 184:499-506, 1992.

85. Schweitzer ME, Brahme SK, Hodler J et al: Chronic wrist pain: spin-echo and short tau inversion recovery MR imaging and conventional and MR arthrography, Radiology 182:205-211, 1992.

86. Schweitzer ME, Caccese R, Karasick D et al: Posterior tibial tendon tears: utility of secondary signs for MR imaging diagnosis, Radiology 188:655-659, 1993.

87. Schweitzer ME, van Leersum M, Ehrlich SS et al: Fluid in normal and abnormal ankle joints: amount and distribution as seen on MR images, AJR 162:111-114, 1994.

88. Schweitzer ME: Magnetic resonance imaging of the foot and ankle, (review) Magn Reson Q 9:214-234, 1993.

89. Shahabpour M, Lacotte B, David P et al: MRI of the wrist joint, Ann Radiol 35:341-348, 1992.

90. Shuman WP, Castagno AA, Baron RL et al: MR imaging of avascular necrosis of the femoral head: value of small-field-of-view sagittal surface-coil images, AJR 150:1073-1078, 1988.

91. Skie M, Zeiss J, Ebraheim NA et al: Carpal tunnel changes and median nerve compression during wrist flexion and extension seen by magnetic resonance imaging, J Hand Surg [Am] 15:934-939, 1990.

92. Smith DK, Snearly WN: Lunotriquetral interosseous ligament of the wrist: MR appearances in asymptomatic volunteers and arthrographically normal wrists, Radiology 191:199-202, 1994.

93. Smith DK: Dorsal carpal ligaments of the wrist: normal appearance on multiplanar reconstructions of three-dimensional Fourier transform MR imaging, AJR 161:119-125, 1993.

94. Smith DK: Scapholunate interosseous ligament of the wrist: MR appearances in asymptomatic volunteers and arthrographically normal wrists, Radiology 192:217-221, 1994.

95. Smith DK: Volar carpal ligaments of the wrist: normal appearance on multiplanar reconstructions of three-dimensional Fourier transform MR imaging, AJR 161:353-357, 1993.

96. Sugimoto H, Okubo RS, Ohsawa: Chemical shift and the double-line signal in MRI of early femoral avascular necrosis, J Comput Assist Tomogr 16:727-730, 1992.

97. Sugimoto H, Shinozaki T, Ohsawa T: Triangular fibrocartilage in asymptomatic subjects: investigation of abnormal MR signal intensity, Radiology 191:193-197, 1994.

98. Takatori Y, Kokubo T, Ninomiya S et al: Transient osteoporosis of the hip. Magnetic resonance imaging, Clin Orthop 271:190-194, 1991.

99. Timmerman LA, Schwartz ML, Andrews JR: Preoperative evaluation of the ulnar collateral ligament by magnetic resonance imaging and computed tomography arthrography. Evaluation in 25 baseball players with surgical confirmation, Am J Sports Med 22:26-31, 1994.

100. Tosch U, Sander B, Schubeus P et al: Magnetic resonance tomographic and sonographic imaging of the ankle in marathon runners, ROFO 154:150-154, 1991.

101. Totterman SM, Miller R, Wasserman B et al: Intrinsic and extrinsic carpal ligaments: evaluation by three-dimensional Fourier transform MR imaging, AJR 160:117-123, 1993.

102. Turner DA, Templeton AC, Selzer PM et al: Femoral capital osteonecrosis: MR finding of diffuse marrow abnormalities without focal lesions, Radiology 171:135-140, 1989.

103. Vande Berg BE, Malghem JJ, Labaisse MA et al: MR imaging of avascular necrosis and transient marrow edema of the femoral head, Radiographics 13:501-520, 1993.

104. Varma DGK, Richli WR, Charnsangavej C et al: MR appearance of the distended iliopsoas bursa, AJR 156:1025-1028, 1991.

105. Vogler JB III, Murphy WA: Bone marrow imaging, Radiology 168:679-693, 1988.

106. Walker CW, Adams BD, Barnes CL et al: Case report 667. (Fibrolipomatous hamartoma of the median nerve), Skeletal Radiol 20:237-239, 1991.

107. Yoshioka S, Okuda Y, Tamai K et al: Changes in carpal tunnel shape during wrist joint motion. MRI evaluation of normal volunteers, J Hand Surg [Br] 18:620-623, 1993.

108. Zeiss J, Ebraheim N, Rusin J et al: Magnetic resonance imaging of the calcaneus: normal anatomy and application in calcaneal fractures, Foot Ankle 11:264-273, 1991.

109. Zeiss J, Jakab E, Khimji T et al: The ulnar tunnel at the wrist (Guyon's canal): normal MR anatomy and variants, AJR 158:1081-1085, 1992.

110. Zeiss J, Skie M, Ebraheim N et al: Anatomic relations between the median nerve and flexor tendons in the carpal tunnel: MR evaluation in normal volunteers, AJR 153:533-536, 1989.

111. Zlatkin MB, Greenan T: Magnetic resonance imaging of the wrist, Magn Reson Q 8:65-96, 1992.

14

Bone Marrow

Magnetic resonance (MR) imaging is highly sensitive for detecting bone marrow lesions and is often the imaging method of choice for bone marrow evaluation in a limited anatomic region. Marrow lesions are generally depicted as foci of relative reduced signal intensity on T1-weighted images, as contrasted against the high signal intensity of normal marrow fat. Marrow lesions can have variable signal characteristics on T2-weighted images, appearing hypointense, isointense, or hyperintense relative to surrounding normal marrow.

MARROW DISTRIBUTION PATTERNS

Regional signal intensity variations are observed throughout the marrow space of normal individuals. These variations reflect the relative proportion of fatty (i.e., yellow) and hematopoietic (i.e., cellular or red) marrow present. Familiarity with patterns of hematopoietic and fatty marrow distribution is important, so that normal marrow elements are not misdiagnosed as pathology (Figs. 14-1 and 14-2, A and B).

Diffusely prominent hematopoietic marrow is routinely observed in infants and children.* This results in relative hypointensity on T1-weighted images throughout the axial and appendicular skeleton. With development of skeletal maturity, there is conversion of hematopoietic to fatty marrow, which initially occurs peripherally within the skeleton and then progresses centrally.[74] Fatty marrow is first observed within the distal extremities and only later within the proximal extremities.

In adults, the appendicular skeleton is comprised primarily of fatty marrow, resulting in increased signal intensity on T1-weighted images and intermediate signal intensity on T2-weighted images. Hematopoietic marrow elements are largely confined to the axial skeleton (i.e., skull, spinal column, and pelvis) in the normal adult. Hematopoietic marrow appears relatively hypointense on both T1- and T2-weighted images. Within the axial skeleton, a heterogeneous signal intensity pattern can be caused by scattered islands of hematopoietic and fatty marrow elements.

In addition to the axial skeleton, hematopoietic marrow is also commonly present in the proximal metaphyses of the humerus and femur in normal adults.[74] Long bone epiphyses appear hypointense during infancy, because of their cartilaginous composition and residual hematopoietic marrow.[35,47] The epiphyses and apophyses are generally comprised of strictly fatty marrow in normal adults.[74] However, reserves of hematopoietic marrow can be present within the proximal humeral ephiphysis, and possibly other epiphyses, in normal adults[45] (Figs. 14-3 and 14-4, A and B).

The expected high signal intensity of fatty marrow is often not observed on gradient echo images, even when T1-weighted imaging parameters are used,[65,74] because of susceptibility effects resulting in artifactual signal loss. These artifacts arise at interfaces of marrow fat,

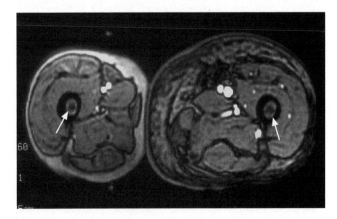

Fig. 14-1. Transaxial spoiled gradient echo image (TR 50, TE 12, 2 Nex, 60-degree flip angle) demonstrates apparent hypointense abnormality *(arrows)* within the marrow space of the femurs. These findings are due to hematopoietic marrow elements.

*References 15, 17, 19, 35, 38, 47, 57.

375

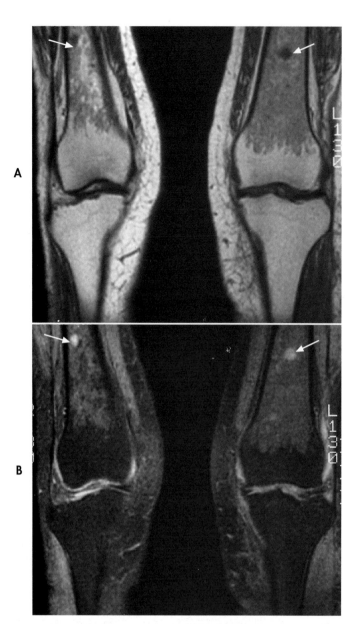

Fig. 14-2. Coronal T1-weighted **(A)** (TR 400, TE 19, 2 Nex) and fat suppressed proton-density weighted **(B)** (TR 2250, TE 20, 1 Nex) images demonstrate diffuse hypointensity and mild hyperintensity respectively, throughout the distal femoral metadiaphyses. These findings are due to hyperplastic hematopoietic marrow in response to anemia. In addition, two small foci of more profound signal alteration are noted *(arrows)*, representing metastatic foci from lung cancer.

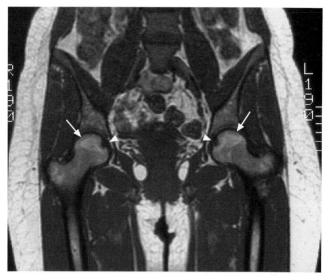

Fig. 14-3. Coronal T1-weighted image (TR 466, TE 12, 2 Nex) in anemic patient demonstrates hypointensity within the peripheral femoral capital epiphyses *(arrows)*, extending into the femoral neck. These findings are due to hyperplastic hematopoietic marrow. The normal fovea capitis can also be visualized bilaterally *(arrowheads).*

marrow and because lesions can be obscured by susceptibility artifacts.

Reconversion of fatty to hematopoietic marrow can occur in patients with anemia or marrow replacement (Figs. 14-5, *A* and *B*). Reconversion can also occur in patients receiving chemotherapy.[46] Reconversion occurs in a proximal to distal progression, first involving the axial skeleton and only subsequently the appendicular skeleton. Therefore decreased signal intensity corresponding to hematopoietic marrow is usually first observed in the spine and pelvis and later progresses to involve the proximal and then distal long bones. In most patients, the epiphyses and apophyses do not undergo reconversion to hematopoietic marrow.[74] However, epiphyseal reconversion can occur in response to severe anemia or marrow replacement.[45]

Women of reproductive age often demonstrate prominent hematopoietic marrow on MR images. This finding is due to physiologic anemia related to menstrual blood loss and the effects of previous pregnancies. In such patients, prominent hematopoietic marrow is often observed within the long bones and can simulate neoplastic lesions. Prominence of hematopoietic marrow within the appendicular skeleton is also more frequent in obese patients, cigarette smokers, and endurance athletes such as marathon runners.[17]

Diffuse skeletal involvement by hyperplastic hematopoietic marrow can lead to diagnostic difficulties on MR images because the signal intensity alterations of hema-

cellular elements, and bone trabeculae as a result of the differences in magnetization among these tissues. The marrow space is thus depicted as hypointense on gradient echo images. Marrow lesions are generally not well depicted on gradient echo images because such images provide suboptimal contrast between lesions and normal

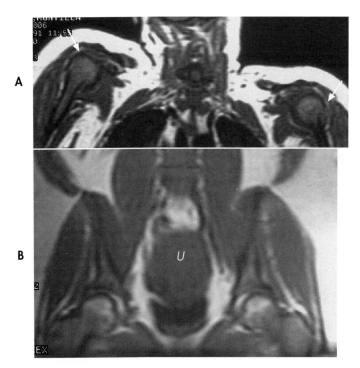

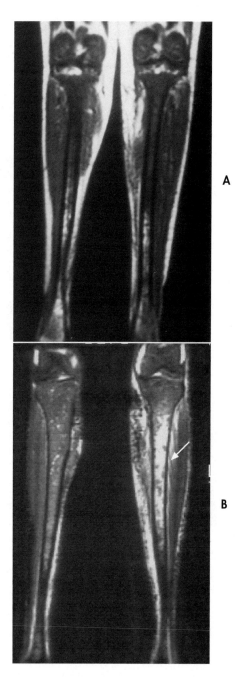

Fig. 14-4. A, Coronal T1-weighted images (TR 500, TE 11, 4 Nex) demonstrate apparent diffuse replacement of marrow fat, including portions of the humeral and femoral epiphyses *(arrows)*. These findings are due to hyperplastic hematopoietic bone marrow attributable to menorrhagia caused by large uterine leiomyomata, which are partially seen in **B** *(U)*.

Fig. 14-5. A, Coronal T1-weighted image (TR 500, TE 11, 2 Nex) in patient with sickle cell anemia. There is reduced signal intensity throughout the marrow space of both tibias, caused by hyperplastic hematopoietic marrow. This limits the sensitivity for detection of marrow lesions on this image. **B,** The corresponding fast spin echo STIR image (TR 4000, effective TE 48, 4 Nex, inversion time 150) demonstrates extensive abnormal signal intensity within the proximal left tibia *(arrow)*, resulting from osteomyelitis.

topoietic marrow can simulate marrow infiltration by tumor[17] (Figs. 14-5, *A* and *B* and 14-6, *A* and *B*). Conversely, actual diffuse marrow involvement by tumor can be misinterpreted as representing prominent hematopoietic marrow.[13,61] Furthermore, signal alterations caused by hematopoietic marrow can cause marrow lesions to be less conspicuous. This latter point applies primarily to T1-weighted images, which are most frequently used for marrow lesion detection. Because of difficulty in distinguishing hematopoietic marrow from marrow lesions on T1-weighted images, T2-weighted or STIR images are more efficacious for detecting marrow lesions in regions dominated by hematopoietic marrow (Figs. 14-5, *A* and *B*).

Schweitzer et al[64] have observed that hematopoietic marrow often demonstrates a focus of high signal intensity within a larger zone of low signal intensity on T1-weighted images. This focus of increased signal inten-

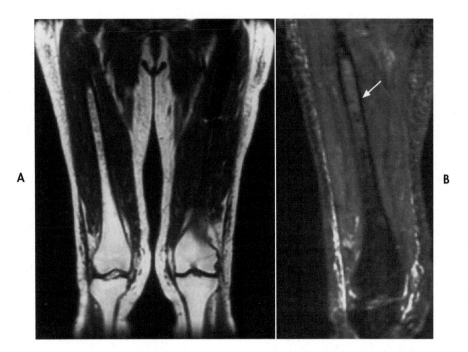

Fig. 14-6. Coronal T1-weighted **(A)** (TR 450, TE 10, 2 Nex) and fast spin echo STIR **(B)** (TR 4000, effective TE 51, 2 Nex, inversion time 150) images demonstrate soft tissue edema within the subcutaneous tissues of the legs. There is relative decreased and increased signal intensity on T1-weighted and STIR images, respectively, within the marrow space of the proximal right femur *(arrow)*. This is due to hematopoietic marrow and should not be interpreted as evidence of marrow edema or infiltration.

sity represents yellow marrow and gives rise to a "bull's-eye" appearance. This contrasts with the "halo" appearance of bony metastases, which is manifested as diffuse or peripheral hyperintensity of a lesion on T2-weighted images. While the halo sign is very specific for malignancy, it is not observed in all such cases.

Distinction between residual or reconverted hematopoietic marrow and neoplastic marrow involvement is based on several criteria. First, residual or reconverted hematopoietic marrow should correspond to the distribution patterns described previously. Second, hematopoietic marrow tends to be relatively symmetric bilaterally. However, the extremities do not necessarily depict mirror image marrow patterns; some asymmetry does exist. Third, hematopoietic marrow appears relatively hypointense on T2-weighted images. Although marrow neoplasms have variable signal intensity characteristics on T2-weighted images, most are of relatively higher signal intensity than hematopoietic marrow. However, some marrow neoplasms, such as sclerotic or blastic lesions (e.g., osteosarcoma, metastatic prostate carcinoma), can appear markedly hypointense on T2-weighted images. (Hematopoietic marrow is also unassociated with soft tissue abnormalities, and demonstrates relatively subtle en-

hancement following intravenous contrast material administration.)

Quantitative techniques have been investigated for improving detection of marrow replacement as compared with strict visual assessment. For example, quantitative reduction in percentage marrow fat on phase contrast chemical shift images has enabled marrow replacement to be determined with higher sensitivity than visual inspection.[29]

Unfused ossification centers can simulate fractures, by appearing to represent avulsed bone fragments (Fig. 14-7). Small defects can be observed within the marrow space; these represent normal marrow vessels (Figs. 14-8 and 14-9). A ringlike pattern of high signal intensity can also be observed within the marrow space of long bones on transaxial T1-weighted images in normal individuals.

RADIATION CHANGES

Radiation therapy depletes cellular marrow elements and results in increases in marrow fat; this produces uniform increased marrow signal intensity on T1-weighted images. Signal alterations resulting from radiation therapy can be observed as early as 9 days following a 1

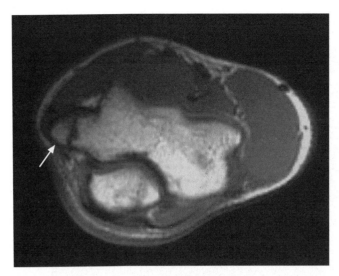

Fig. 14-7. Transaxial T1-weighted image (TR 500, TE 12, 2 Nex) in 15-year-old male with medial elbow pain. Unfused ossification center of the medial humeral epicondyle is noted *(arrow),* which bears resemblance to a fracture involving the medial humerus.

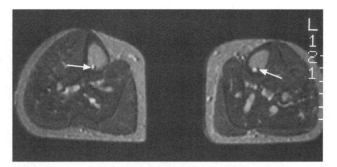

Fig. 14-9. Symmetrical foci of increased signal intensity are noted within the posterior aspect of the marrow space of the femoral shafts *(arrows)* on transaxial T2-weighted image (TR 3000, TE 80, 1 Nex). These findings represent marrow vessels and can simulate the appearance of lesions involving the marrow space. Note chemical shift misregistration artifact related to these vessels along the frequency encode direction of the image, at the position of a fat-fluid interface. Multiple rounded structures of increased signal intensity throughout the soft tissues of the posterior thighs represent soft tissue vessels on this flow-compensated image.

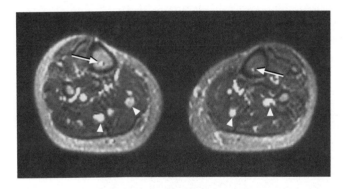

Fig. 14-8. Transaxial fat suppressed fast spin echo T2-weighted image (TR 4300, effective TE 102, 4 Nex, 16 echo train) of the lower legs. There is marked asymmetric signal intensity of tibial marrow, with relative increased intensity on the right. This is due to inhomogeneous fat saturation using a relatively large field-of-view (30 cm). Also note nodular high signal intensity foci in the soft tissues bilaterally *(arrowheads),* reflecting prominent vessels. A circular high signal intensity structure within the marrow space of both tibiae *(arrows)* also represents a vessel.

month treatment course of 3000 rad.[56] However, some reports indicate that such findings are not evident for approximately 3 weeks following treatment completion.[25a] A sharp interface between normal and irradiated marrow is typically observed, corresponding to the margins of the radiation port. While postradiation marrow alterations do not resemble tumor involvement, normal marrow located adjacent to marrow that has been irradiated appears unusually hypointense on T1-weighted images and thus can be misdiagnosed as pathologic. Relative increased marrow signal intensity on T1-weighted images can also occur following successful medical treatment for osteomyelitis.[72]

IRON OVERLOAD

Iron deposition within the marrow space can produce marrow hypointensity on T2-weighted, and in some cases, T1-weighted images. This most often occurs in patients with severe iron overload caused by previous transfusions (i.e., hemosiderosis), and it can simulate diffuse marrow involvement with metastatic tumor. The presence of iron leads to extreme signal intensity loss on gradient echo images.

FAT SUPPRESSION

Fat suppression techniques can also improve sensitivity for marrow lesion detection[27,30,37,76] (Figs. 14-10, *A* and *B*). These methods are particularly valuable when evaluating regions populated by hematopoietic marrow. In such locations, marrow lesions may be obscured on T1-weighted images, as discussed previously. While T2-weighted images may depict marrow lesions that are surrounded by hematopoietic marrow, the conspicuousness of such lesions can be increased when fat suppressed T2-weighted sequences are used. The use of fat suppression

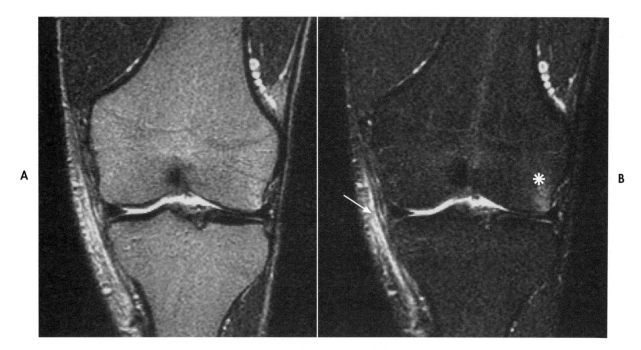

Fig. 14-10. Coronal conventional **(A)** and fat suppressed **(B)** T2-weighted images (TR 2250, TE 75, 1 Nex) in patient who underwent recent knee trauma. There is improved conspicuousness of bone marrow edema *(asterisk)* from traumautic trabecular bone injury on fat-suppressed image, despite use of shorter echo time, as well as improved depiction of soft tissue edema related to medial collateral ligament injury *(arrow)*.

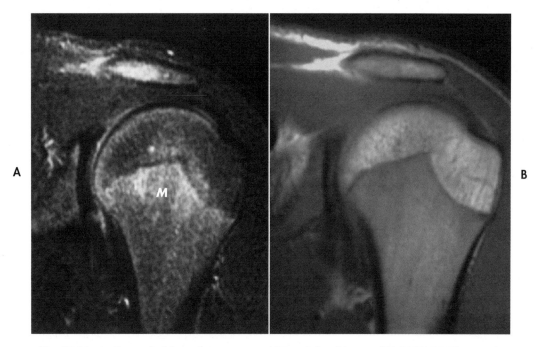

Fig. 14-11. A, Coronal oblique fat suppressed T2-weighted image (TR 2200, TE 70, 1 Nex) demonstrates hyperintensity in the marrow space of the proximal humeral metaphysis *(M)* as a result of normal residual hematopoietic marrow, which is also demonstrated on corresponding T1-weighted image **(B)** (TR 400, TE 18, 2 Nex).

also allows adequate tissue contrast to be achieved using a shorter repetition time (TR) and echo time (TE), thus reducing imaging time. Furthermore, narrow receiver bandwidth can be implemented on fat suppressed sequences for improved signal-to-noise ratio, because chemical shift misregistration artifacts are essentially eliminated.[30]

Fat suppression can be accomplished using several different techniques. Among these are short tau inversion recovery (STIR), phase contrast (i.e., Dixon) methods, and radiofrequency presaturation of the lipid peak (i.e., fat saturation). While these techniques are useful in improving the conspicuousness of marrow lesions, several pitfalls may be encountered. Hematopoietic marrow can appear relatively hyperintense on fat suppressed T2-weighted images, potentially simulating neoplastic or other marrow lesions (Figs. 14-6, *A* and *B*, 14-11, *A* and *B* and 14-12). Hematopoietic marrow can also appear hyperintense when some gradient echo sequences are used. A highly uniform magnetic field is necessary to achieve uniform fat saturation throughout the field-of-view. Nonuniform fat suppression can occur because of inhomogeneity of the main magnetic field, in regions adjacent to a local coil, or in the vicinity of ferromagnetic materials[40] (Figs. 14-13, *A-C*). Susceptibility artifacts related to metal, air, and other causes are accentuated when fat

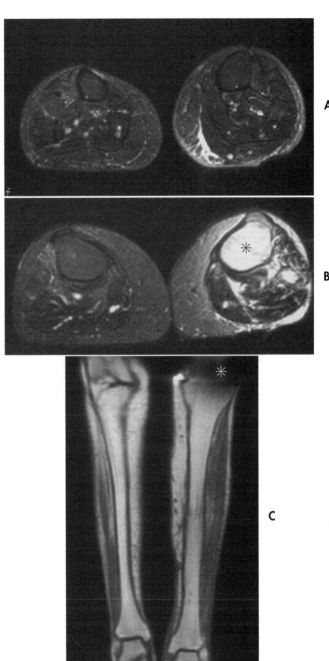

Fig. 14-13. A and **B,** Transaxial fat suppressed fast spin echo T2-weighted images (TR 4200, effective TE 102, 2 Nex, 8 echo train) in patient with suspected osteomyelitis. The image at the lower tibial level **(A)** is unremarkable, whereas a higher image **(B)** demonstrates relative increased signal intensity throughout the left tibial *(asterisk)* and fibular marrow space. These findings reflect inadequate fat suppression caused by proximity of metallic knee prosthesis. **C,** Corresponding T1-weighted coronal image (TR 500, TE 10, 2 Nex) verifies normal marrow signal intensity throughout the lower leg and shows susceptibility artifact (asterisk) related to knee prosthesis.

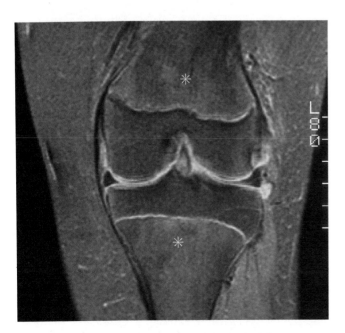

Fig. 14-12. Coronal fat suppressed T2-weighted (TR 2250, TE 75, 1 Nex) image demonstrates relative hyperintensity of residual hematopoietic marrow in distal femur and proximal tibia *(asterisks)* in 14-year-old female. Also note linear hyperintensity along the physeal plates.

ENTITIES THAT CAN SIMULATE BONE MARROW LESIONS

- Residual hematopoietic marrow
- Reconverted hematopoietic marrow
- Susceptibility artifact
- Adjacent radiation changes
- Iron overload
- Nonuniform fat suppression
- Local decreased signal-to-noise ratio
- Chemical shift misregistration artifact
- Motion artifact

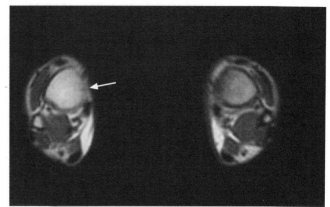

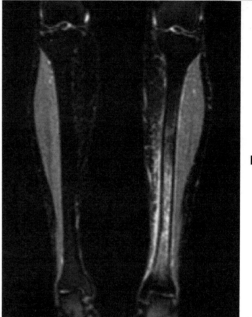

A

B

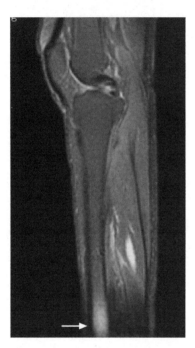

Fig. 14-14. Sagittal proton density–weighted image (TR 2500, TE 30, 1 Nex) using fat saturation demonstrates heterogeneous suppression of marrow fat throughout the field-of-view. Fat along the inferior aspect of the tibial shaft *(arrow)* demonstrates increased signal intensity, and there is inadvertent suppression of water signal in this location, as manifest by the reduced signal intensity of the adjacent musculature.

Fig. 14-15. **A,** There is apparent thinning and increased signal intensity related to the medial tibial cortex of the right leg *(arrow)* on transaxial T1-weighted image (TR 500, TE 15, 2 Nex). These findings are due to partial volume averaging of the cortex with underlying subcutaneous fat, as well as to chemical shift misregistration artifact. The opposite leg demonstrates marrow replacement caused by metastatic disease, as well as actual cortical involvement. **B,** The corresponding coronal STIR image (TR 2500, TE 20, 1 Nex, inversion time 160) demonstrates increased signal intensity within the left tibia and adjacent soft tissues.

saturation is used.[40,54] Heterogeneous fat suppression can result in foci of variable size and configuration that appear relatively intense compared with adjacent fat suppressed marrow; these findings can simulate marrow neoplasms or osteomyelitis (Figs. 14-8 and 14-13, *A-C*). In extreme cases, inadvertent suppression of water signals can occur on fat saturation images, potentially obscuring marrow lesions (Fig. 14-14).

STIR images are less vulnerable—though not resistant—to magnetic field inhomogeneities (Figs. 14-15, *A* and *B*). Adequate fat suppression using STIR is highly dependent on proper choice of inversion time (TI). The appropriate TI is usually calculated based on the field strength at which imaging is performed. Fat suppression can be further improved when the TI value is determined on the basis of spectral information acquired as the patient is being imaged.[67]

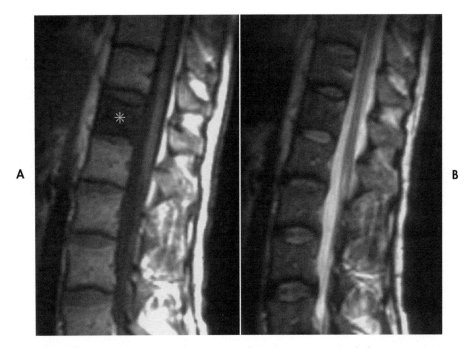

Fig. 14-16. A, Midsagittal T1-weighted image (TR 500, TE 12, 2 Nex) demonstrates marrow replacement throughout the T12 vertebral body *(asterisk)* caused by lymphoma. The presence of this marrow abnormality is inconspicuous on the corresponding T2-weighted fast spin echo image **(B)** (TR 4000, effective TE 96, 4 Nex, 16 echo train).

Fat suppressed images provide reduced signal-to-noise ratio, because the fat contribution to signal intensity is eliminated. This results in image graininess and accentuation of motion artifacts, which can limit evaluation of small lesions.

FAST SPIN ECHO SEQUENCES

Fast spin echo (i.e., rapid acquisition relaxation enhanced, RARE) sequences are used with increasing frequency for musculoskeletal imaging because they provide high-quality images in markedly reduced acquisition times. While T2-weighted fast spin echo images resemble conventional T2-weighted images in most respects, one important difference is the markedly increased intensity of fat on fast spin echo images.[31] This applies not only to subcutaneous fat but also to marrow fat, and it has important implications for detecting marrow lesions. Because of the increased signal intensity of marrow fat on T2-weighted fast spin echo images, lesions that would usually be visualized on the basis of their long T2 relaxation may be obscured (Figs. 14-16, *A* and *B*). Thus fat suppression (e.g., fat saturation or STIR) should be used in conjunction with fast spin echo T2-weighted sequences when evaluating for marrow abnormalities.

MAGNETIC FIELD INHOMOGENEITIES

Local magnetic field inhomogeneities can result in heterogeneous marrow signal intensity on conventional spin echo images. Shading artifacts, manifested as artifactually decreased marrow signal intensity, can occur when the patient is in direct contact with the body coil. When a local coil is used, signal intensity decreases dramatically with increasing distance from the coil.[50] Normal marrow can appear of decreased signal intensity in these situations, which can simulate or obscure marrow lesions (Fig. 14-17).

CHEMICAL SHIFT MISREGISTRATION ARTIFACTS

Chemical shift misregistration artifacts result in artifactual displacement of signal intensity from a fat-water interface along the frequency encoding direction of the image. This occurs because of the different precessional frequency of fat and water protons. Chemical shift misregistration artifacts occur at the interface between bone marrow and surrounding soft tissues and can simulate thinning or destruction of normal bone cortex[18] (Fig. 14-13). Chemical shift effects can also arise at the interface between tumor and surrounding normal marrow, potentially creating aberrant signal characteristics.[55] Measure-

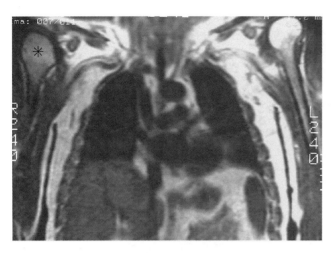

Fig. 14-17. Decreased signal intensity is noted throughout the right humeral head *(asterisk)* as compared with the left on coronal T1-weighted image (TR 500, TE 12, 2 Nex). While this finding is suggestive of marrow replacement, it results from shading artifact on this large field-of-view body coil image.

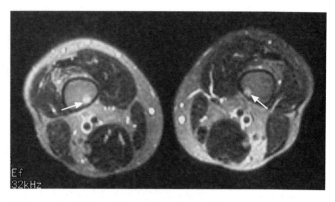

Fig. 14-18. High signal intensity foci are noted within the marrow space of both femoral shafts *(arrows)* on T2-weighted fast spin echo image (TR 4300, effective TE 104, 2 Nex, 16 echo train). While these findings may simulate lesions, they are due to phase encode artifacts caused by pulsation of the femoral artery and can be visualized coursing across the image.

ment of chemical shift misregistration artifacts can be used to estimate marrow cellularity.[34] Chemical shift misregistration frequently occurs at the unfused physis on T2-weighted images; the resultant band of hyperintensity can simulate (marrow edema resulting from) a Salter fracture.

MOTION ARTIFACTS

Phase encoding errors caused by pulsation of large vessels appear as rounded foci of alternating increased and decreased signal intensity. When these ghosting artifacts traverse the marrow space, they can simulate marrow lesions (Fig. 14-18). Pulsation artifacts can be reduced with use of spatial presaturation and gradient moment nulling. These artifacts can also be shifted with reorientation of the phase and frequency encoding gradients, which allows their artifactual nature to be verified and permits more accurate evaluation of underlying marrow.

ANATOMIC DISTORTION

Gradient echo images can result in artifactual distortion of bone contours, because of susceptibility differences occurring at bone and soft tissue interfaces.[14] Such artifacts are frequently observed in the vicinity of metallic prosthesis, fixation devices, or other orthopedic hardware. These artifacts are minimized when short echo times and small voxel sizes are used. Gradient nonlinearity is another cause for distortion of bone and soft tissues contours.[3]

CHARACTERIZATION OF MARROW LESIONS

Despite the pitfalls that have been discussed, MR is usually exceptionally sensitive for detecting bone marrow lesions. Once a lesion has been identified, however, it is often difficult to specify its nature on the basis of its MR signal intensity characteristics. While certain lesions have characteristic signal intensity patterns that allow for reasonable specificity, most marrow lesions do not. Consequently, it is usually not possible to confidently determine whether a given marrow lesion is malignant or benign or whether it is of neoplastic, inflammatory, or other etiology.

Most marrow lesions display similar nondescript signal intensity characteristics, consisting of hypointensity on T1-weighted images and variable hyperintensity on T2-weighted images relative to surrounding uninvolved marrow.[70] When the signal intensity characteristics of a marrow lesion vary from this pattern, signal intensity data may be used to improve lesion characterization. For example, cortical bone and fibrous tissue have relatively short T2 relaxation. Thus lesions comprised of these tissues usually have decreased rather than increased signal intensity on T2-weighted images. Yet some fibrous marrow lesions (e.g., fibrous dysplasia) can have paradoxically increased signal intensity on T2-weighted images[51,73] (Fig. 14-19). In one study of 13 patients with fibrous dysplasia, nearly half of the lesions showed areas of increased signal intensity on T2-weighted images.[51] This emphasizes that even when signal intensity patterns suggest a limited differential diagnosis, MR does not substitute for the histospecific information provided by biopsy.

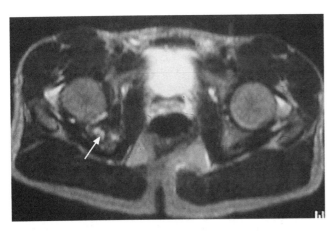

Fig. 14-19. Transaxial T2-weighted image (TR 3000, TE 90) in patient with fibrous dysplasia involving the right acetabular region *(arrow)*. The lesion demonstrates heterogeneous areas of relative increased and decreased signal intensity.

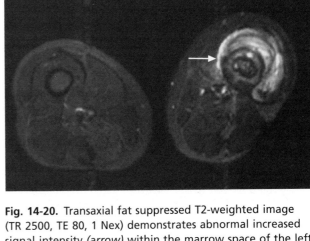

Fig. 14-20. Transaxial fat suppressed T2-weighted image (TR 2500, TE 80, 1 Nex) demonstrates abnormal increased signal intensity *(arrow)* within the marrow space of the left femur. There is also an adjacent soft tissue mass involving the anterior compartment. Although these findings resemble those of neoplasm, they represent osteomyelitis with associated cellulitis in this patient.

Whereas the signal intensity characteristics of marrow lesions are usually nonspecific, analysis of lesion morphology can be useful in distinguishing benign from malignant lesions. This involves evaluation of lesion definition, regularity of margins, internal homogeneity, adjacent marrow edema, and associated soft tissue abnormalities. Benign lesions typically appear well defined, with smooth and regular margins, are internally homogeneous, and are not associated with adjacent marrow edema or soft tissue masses. Malignant lesions are typified by the converse of these findings. These criteria do not, however, allow for definitive lesion characterization. Many benign lesions display features associated with malignant lesions[41,46,59,70] (Fig. 14-20). Such lesions may include eosinophilic granuloma, osteoid osteoma,[75] chondroblastoma, cortical and/or trabecular fracture,[8] Paget disease, skeletal tuberculosis,[1] and bone infarct, among others. In the appropriate clinical setting, these entities could also simulate osteomyelitis.[20] In patients with osteoid osteoma, reactive marrow edema can be prominent and simulate entities such as sarcoma, osteonecrosis, stress fracture, and inflammatory arthritis.[26] The nidus of such osteoid osteomas may not be evident on MR images, further contributing to confusion. Abnormal marrow signal intensity suggestive of osteomyelitis can result from reactive marrow edema in the juxtaarticular regions surrounding a septic joint.[20]

Observation of fluid-fluid levels within a bone lesion is primarily associated with an aneurysmal bone cyst.

However, fluid-fluid levels can be observed with a variety of benign as well as malignant lesions.[5,49,71]

Bursal fluid collections can arise adjacent to benign osteochondromas. The resultant high signal intensity soft tissue mass can simulate sarcomatous degeneration of the osteochondroma.[28] Concern regarding malignant transformation is heightened by a reported history of recent enlargement of the mass and associated pain.

Fibrous cortical defects, which typically involve the distal metaphysis of the femur, are often observed in adolescent patients as incidental findings. These benign lesions can demonstrate heterogeneous areas of relative increased and decreased signal intensity on T2-weighted images, simulating an aggressive lesion.[58,68]

The signal intensity characteristics of fatty marrow are largely preserved in patients with Paget disease, in the absence of complicating factors such as fracture or sarcomatous degeneration.[39] However, small regions of relative decreased marrow signal intensity on T1-weighted images can be observed in patients with uncomplicated Paget disease and do not necessarily indicate neoplastic involvement.

CONTRAST ENHANCEMENT PATTERNS

The role of contrast agents such as gadopentetate dimeglumine for evaluating marrow lesions has not yet been clearly defined. Contrast agents do not significantly improve detection of marrow lesions and often have counterproductive results. In one study in which gadopentetate dimeglumine was administered to a series of patients with various musculoskeletal masses, unenhanced T2-weighted images consistently provided equal or greater diagnostic information than contrast enhanced T1-weighted images.[60] Enhancement of marrow lesions frequently causes them to become isointense with surrounding normal marrow fat on conventional T1-weighted images.[4,10,21,60,66] This requires that T1-weighted images be acquired prior to contrast material administration in all patients. Depiction of contrast enhancing marrow lesions is markedly improved when fat suppressed T1-weighted images are acquired.[48]

Contrast material has also been used in an attempt to better characterize marrow lesions. Serial rapid image acquisition during and following bolus contrast material administration (i.e., dynamic contrast enhanced imaging) can provide useful information regarding lesion aggressiveness and activity. Such information may not, however, be available by visual inspection of these images; quantitative time-enhancement analysis must be performed.[21] Visual analysis of lesion enhancement patterns on dynamic contrast enhanced rapid images demonstrates considerable overlap between the enhancement patterns of various lesions.[22,23a,44] Furthermore, the enhancement pattern of specific lesion types also varies considerably. Therefore, it does not appear that contrast material is generally beneficial for detecting or characterizing marrow lesions in most clinical settings.

POSTTHERAPY CHANGES

MR is frequently used to monitor the response of marrow lesions to therapy. In general, a positive response is marked by a decrease in lesion size and signal intensity on T2-weighted images, as well as decreased intensity of lesion contrast enhancement as compared with pretreatment studies. However, lesions can undergo a variety of alterations on MR images in response to chemotherapy, radiation therapy, and/or surgical intervention.

Observation of decreased lesion signal intensity on T2-weighted images may not signify tumor eradication. In one study of patients who underwent chemotherapy for Ewing sarcoma, active tumor cells were present in areas of low signal intensity on T2-weighted images in 71% of patients.[42] Conversely, areas of high signal intensity on T2-weighted images do not necessarily indicate a residual or recurrent tumor. These findings may also represent necrotic tumor, hemorrhage, or granulation tissue.[42] Osteosarcomas can demonstrate homogeneous, speckled, cystic, target-like, and other signal intensity patterns following preoperative chemotherapy.[16,32,33,53] Neither T2-weighted images nor contrast enhanced T1-weighted images have allowed for reliable distinction between residual viable tumor, inflammatory changes, and areas of necrosis or hemorrhage.[16]

Marrow lesions may not undergo decreases in size, despite their responsiveness to an administered chemo-

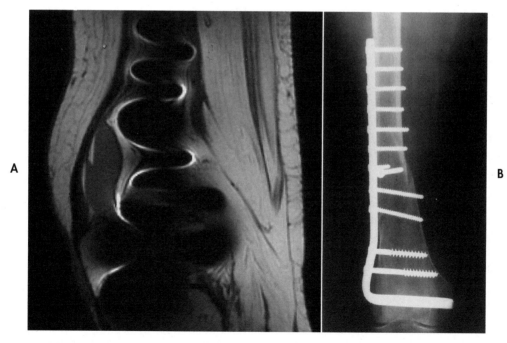

Fig. 14-21. A, Sagittal T1-weighted image (TR 400, TE 15, 2 Nex) of the knee demonstrates a series of high and low signal intensity artifacts that obscure visualization of the marrow space of the femur. These are related to a ferromagnetic metallic fixation device, as demonstrated on plain film **(B).**

therapeutic regimen.[32,33,62] This differs from soft tissue tumors, in which tumor response is usually associated with reduction in tumor volume. Rates of tumor regression following radiotherapy are also variable.[43] Irradiated marrow can demonstrate abnormal contrast material enhancement, which simulates a residual or recurrent marrow tumor.[43]

Bone infarcts can occur in patients treated with intraarterial chemotherapy for osteosarcoma and can simulate an extension of tumor.[52] Abnormal marrow and soft tissue signal intensity can be caused by edema and hemorrhage following bone biopsy. These findings can obscure underlying lesions or lead to overestimation of their size and extent.[70]

A bone chip allograft placed within a cystic marrow lesion following currettage can simulate a neoplasm.[36] Orthopedic devices including fixation pins, rods, and screws produce signal void artifacts that interfere with assessment of nearby marrow lesions (Figs. 14-21, *A* and *B* and 14-22). Marked decreased marrow signal intensity on T1-weighted images can be observed in patients who have undergone bone marrow transplantation.[9,69] This may reflect hyperplastic hematopoietic marrow or iron overload resulting from transfusions.[6,9] For all of the above reasons, MR imaging of marrow lesions should be performed prior to any intervention whenever possible. This will not only provide the most accurate representation of the sig-

nal characteristics and extent of the lesion but will also serve as a baseline examination for comparison with subsequent examinations performed following therapy.

STAGING OF MARROW LESIONS

MR provides valuable information regarding the extent of marrow lesions. These data are used to define surgical options and plans, as well as for prognostic purposes. Signal alterations on MR images tend to result in slight overestimation of lesion extent. This is often due to abnormal signal intensity caused by reactive marrow edema adjacent to the tumor margin. Peritumoral edema can occur in conjunction with benign lesions such as osteoblastoma and chondroblastoma,[11,12] as well as with primary malignant bone tumors.[70] In some patients with malignant lesions, the zone of peritumoral edema can harbor tumor cells. Therefore, the entire zone of abnormal marrow signal intensity should be conservatively regarded as representing the tumor margins, though this can lead to mild overestimation. Chemical shift selective imaging sequences such as fat saturation or STIR cause marrow lesions as well as surrounding edema to be more conspicuous; this can result in further overestimation of lesion extent.[27,30,37,63] Extensive reactive marrow edema can also surround nonneoplastic lesions such as osteonecrosis. The resultant signal intensity alterations can obscure the underlying lesion or cause its extent to be overestimated (Fig. 14-23).

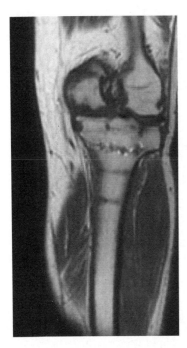

Fig. 14-22. Coronal T1-weighted image (TR 450, TE 10, 2 Nex) demonstrates signal intensity alterations within the marrow space of the proximal tibia at site of previous osteotomy and placement of surgical fixation pins. Metallic artifact at the osteotomy site is also noted.

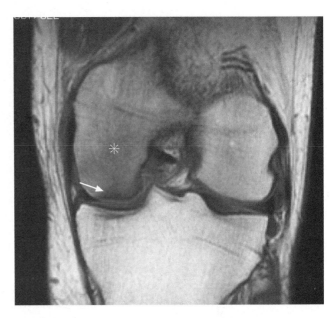

Fig. 14-23. There is reduced signal intensity throughout the medial femoral condyle *(asterisk)* on coronal T1-weighted image (TR 550, TE 19, 2 Nex). This is due to extensive reactive marrow edema, which nearly obscures visualization of a small osteonecrotic nidus along the weight-bearing surface of the condyle *(arrow)*.

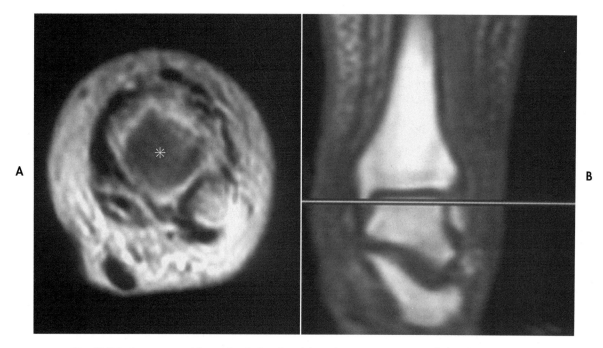

Fig. 14-24. An apparent irregular lesion involving the marrow space of the distal tibia *(asterisk)* is demonstrated on transaxial proton density–weighted image **(A)** (TR 2200, TE 30, 1 Nex). This is due to partial volume averaging of marrow with hyaline cartilage of the tibiotalar joint, as confirmed on coronal T1-weighted image **(B)** (TR 500, TE 11, 2 Nex), in which position of **A** is denoted.

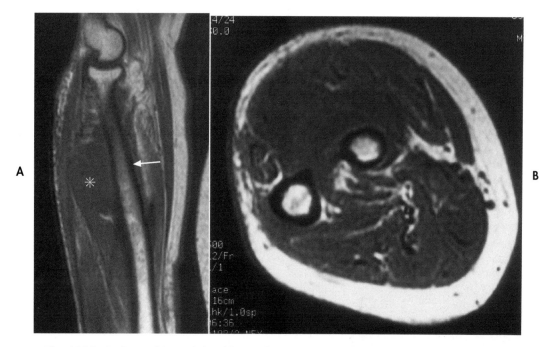

Fig. 14-25. A, Coronal T1-weighted image (TR 500, TE 12, 2 Nex) of the forearm demonstrates soft tissue mass *(asterisk)* caused by metastatic lung cancer. There is low signal intensity within the marrow space of the radius *(arrows),* suggestive of tumor involvement. However, this latter finding is due to partial volume averaging of marrow fat with low signal intensity bone cortex, as verified on transaxial T1-weighted **(B)** (TR 500, TE 12, 2 Nex) and other images.

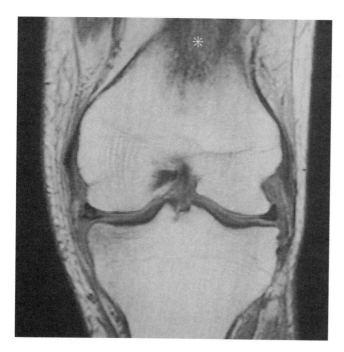

Fig. 14-26. Coronal T1-weighted image (TR 550, TE 19, 2 Nex) demonstrates apparent marrow lesion involving the distal femur *(asterisk)*. This is due to partial volume averaging of marrow fat with adjacent bone cortex. Also note torn medial collateral ligament and medial meniscus, as well as marrow contusion involving medial tibial plateau.

Large amounts of hemosiderin may be present in some tumors, such as giant cell tumors of bone. This can result in decreased signal intensity on all pulse sequences and interfere with evaluation of the adjacent bone cortex.[2]

MR has limited ability to depict calcium; this can make abnormalities of the bone cortex and periosteum difficult to detect. For example, subtle cortical destruction may be obscure on MR images; computed tomography (CT) should be considered when such information is specifically sought. Periosteal new bone formation is also suboptimally demonstrated on MR images in some patients.[46] Among the entities that can simulate periosteal reaction are (1) partial volume averaging of bone cortex with adjacent soft tissues or juxtacortical soft tissue masses and (2) normal cortical irregularity found in sites such as the posterior femur.[46] Partial volume averaging of marrow fat with adjacent bone cortex or with overlying hyaline cartilage can simulate marrow lesions (Figs. 14-24, *A* and *B,* 14-25, *A* and *B,* and 14-26).

REFERENCES

1. Abdelwahab IF, Kenan S, Hermann G et al: Atypical skeletal tuberculosis mimicking neoplasm, Br J Radiol 64:551-555, 1991.

2. Aoki J, Moriya K, Yamashita K et al: Giant cell tumors of bone containing large amounts of hemosiderin: MR-pathologic correlation, J Comput Assist Tomogr 15:1024-1027, 1991.

3. Bakker CJ, Moerland MA, Bhagwandien R et al: Analysis of machine-dependent and object-induced geometric distortion in 2DFT MR imaging, Magn Reson Imaging 10:597-608, 1992.

4. Beltran J, Chandnani V, McGhee RA Jr et al: Gadopentetate dimeglumine-enhanced MR imaging of the musculoskeletal system, Am J Roentgenol 156:457-466, 1991.

5. Beltran J, Simon DC, Levy M et al: Aneurysmal bone cysts: MR imaging at 1.5 T, Radiology 158:689-690, 1986.

6. Berdon WE: Letter to the editor, Pediatr Radiol 21:605-607, 1991.

7. Bergman RA, Thompson SA, Afifi AK et al: Compendium of human anatomic variation: text, atlas, and world literature, Baltimore, 1988, Urban & Schwarzenberg.

8. Blomlie V, Lien HH, Iversen T et al: Radiation-induced insufficiency fractures of the sacrum: evaluation with MR imaging, Radiology 188:241-244, 1993.

9. Boothroyd AE, Sebag G, Brunelle F: MR appearances of bone marrow in children following bone marrow transplantation, Pediatr Radiol 21:291-292, 1991.

10. Breger RK, Williams AL, Daniels DL et al: Contrast enhancement in spinal MR imaging, Am J Roentgenol 153:387-391, 1989.

11. Brower AC, Moser RP, Kransdorf MJ: The frequency and diagnostic significance of periostitis in chondroblastoma, Am J Roentgenol 154:309-314, 1990.

12. Crim JR, Mirra JM, Eckardt JJ et al: Widespread inflammatory response of osteoblastoma: the flare phenomenon, Radiology 177:835-836, 1990.

13. Czarnecki DJ, Goell WS: Metastatic carcinoma of the proximal femur closely resembling hematopoietic hyperplasia on MR (letter), Am J Roentgenol 154:902-903, 1990.

14. Czervionke LF, Daniels DL, Wehrli FW et al: Magnetic susceptibility artifacts in gradient-recalled echo MR imaging, Am J Neuroradiol 9:1149-1155, 1988.

15. Dawson KL, Moore SG, Rowland JM: Age-related marrow changes in the pelvis: MR and anatomic findings, Radiology 183:47-51, 1992.

16. de Baere T, Vanel D, Shapeero LG et al: Osteosarcoma after chemotherapy: evaluation with contrast material-enahanced subtraction MR imaging, Radiology 185:587-592, 1992.

17. Deutsch AL, Mink JH, Rosenfelt FP et al: Incidental detection of hematopoietic hyperplasia on routine knee MR imaging, Am J Roentgenol 152:333-336, 1989.

18. Dick BW, Mitchell DG, Burk DL et al: The effect of chemical shift misrepresentation on cortical bone thickness on MR imaging, Am J Roentgenol 151:537-538, 1988.

19. Dooms GC, Fisher MR, Hricak H et al: Bone marrow imaging: magnetic resonance studies related to age and sex, Radiology 155:429-432, 1985.

20. Erdman WA, Tamburro F, Jayson HT et al: Osteomyelitis: characteristics and pitfalls of diagnosis with MR imaging, Radiology 180:533-539, 1991.

21. Erlemann R, Reiser MF, Peters PE et al: Musculoskeletal neoplasms: static and dynamic Gd-DTPA-enhanced MR imaging, Radiology 171:767-773, 1989.

22. Erlemann R, Vassallo P, Bongartz G et al: Musculoskeletal neoplasms: fast low-angle shot MR imaging with and without Gd-DTPA, Radiology 176:489-495, 1990.

23. Erlemann R: Dynamic gadolinium-enhanced MR imaging to monitor tumor response to chemotherapy (letter), Radiology 186:904, 1993.

23a. Fletcher BD, Hanna SL: Musculoskeletal neoplasms: dynamic Gd-DTPA-enhanced MR imaging (letter), Radiology 177:287-288, 1990

24. Fletcher BD, Hanna SL, Fairclough DL et al: Pediatric musculoskeletal tumors: use of dynamic, contrast-enhanced MR imaging to monitor response to chemotherapy, Radiology 184:243-248, 1992.

25. Fletcher BD, Hanna SL, Fairclough DL et al. Reply to Erlemann R: dynamic gadolinium-enhanced MR imaging to monitor tumor response to chemotherapy (letter), Radiology 186:905, 1993.

25a. Fletcher BD, Hanna SL, Kun LE: Changes in MR signal intensity and contrast enhancement of therapeutically irradiated soft tissue, Magn Reson Imaging 8:771-777, 1990.

26. Goldman AB, Schneider R, Pavlov H: Osteoid osteomas of the femoral neck: report of four cases evaluated with isotopic bone scanning, CT, and MR imaging, Radiology 186:227-232, 1993.

27. Golfieri R, Baddeley H, Pringle JS et al: The role of the STIR sequence in magnetic resonance imaging examination of bone tumours, Br J Radiol 63:251-256, 1990.

28. Griffiths HJ, Thompson RC Jr, Galloway HR et al: Bursitis in association with solitary osteochondromas presenting as mass lesions, Skeletal Radiol 20:513-516, 1991.

29. Guckel F, Brix G, Semmler W et al: Systemic bone marrow disorders: characterization with proton chemical shift imaging, J Comput Assist Tomogr 14:633-642, 1990.

30. Harned EM, Mitchell DG, Burk DL Jr et al: Bone marrow findings on magnetic resonance images of the knee: accentuation by fat suppression, Magn Reson Imaging 8:27-31, 1990.

31. Henkelman RM, Hardy PA, Bishop JE et al: Why fat is bright in RARE and fast spin-echo imaging, J Magn Reson Imaging 2:533-540, 1992.

32. Holscher HC, Bloem JL, Nooy MA et al: The value of MR imaging in monitoring the effect of chemotherapy on bone sarcomas, Am J Roentgenol 154:763-769, 1990.

33. Holscher HC, Bloem JL, Vanel D et al: Osteosarcoma: chemotherapy-induced changes at MR imaging, Radiology 182:839-844, 1992.

34. Ishizaka H, Tomiyoshi K, Matsumoto M: MR quantification of bone marrow cellularity: use of chemical-shift misregistration artifact, Am J Roentgenol 160:572-574, 1993.

35. Jaramillo D, Laor T, Hoffer FA et al: Epiphyseal marrow in infancy: MR imaging, Radiology 180:809-812, 1991.

36. Jelinek JS, Kransdorf MJ, Moser RP et al: MR imaging findings in patients with bone-chip allografts, Am J Roentgenol 155:1257-1260, 1990.

37. Jones KM, Unger EC, Granstrom P et al: Bone marrow imaging using STIR at 0.5 and 1.5 T, Magn Reson Imaging 10:169-176, 1992.

38. Kangarloo H, Dietrich RB, Taira RT et al: MR imaging of bone marrow in children, J Comput Assist Tomogr 10:205-209, 1986.

39. Kaufmann GA, Sundaram M, McDonald DJ: Magnetic resonance imaging in symptomatic Paget's disease, Skeletal Radiol 20:413-418, 1991.

40. Keller PJ, Hunter WW Jr, Schmalbrock P: Multisection fat-water imaging with chemical shift selective presaturation, Radiology 164:539-541, 1987.

41. Lee JK, Yao L: Stress fractures: MR imaging, Radiology 169:217-220, 1988.

42. MacVicar D, Olliff JFC, Pringle J et al: Ewing sarcoma: MR imaging of chemotherapy-induced changes with histologic correlation, Radiology 184:859-864, 1992.

43. Mayr NA, Tali ET, Yuh WTC et al: The application of MRI in the management of patients undergoing radiation therapy for gynecological malignancies, SMRM Book of Abstracts, 1992, p 3202.

44. Mirowitz SA, Totty WG, Lee JKT: Characterization of musculoskeletal masses using dynamic Gd-DTPA enhanced spin-echo MRI, J Comput Assist Tomogr 16:120-125, 1992.

45. Mirowitz SA: Hematopoietic bone marrow within the proximal humeral epiphysis in normal adults: investigation with MR imaging, Radiology 188:689-693, 1993.

46. Moore SG, Bisset GS III, Siegel MJ et al: Pediatric musculoskeletal MR imaging, Radiology 179:345-360, 1991.

47. Moore SG, Dawson KL: Red and yellow marrow in the femur: age-related changes in appearance at MR imaging, Radiology 175:219-223, 1990.

48. Morrison WB, Schweitzer ME, Bock GW et al: Diagnosis of osteomyelitis: utility of fat-suppressed contrast-enhanced MR imaging, Radiology 189:251-257, 1993.

49. Munk PL, Helms CA, Holt RG et al: MR imaging of aneurysmal bone cysts, Am J Roentgenol 153:99-101, 1989.

50. Narayana PA, Brey WW, Kulkarni MV et al: Compensation for surface coil sensitivity variation in magnetic resonance imaging, Magn Reson Imaging 6:271-274, 1988.

51. Norris MA, Kaplan PA, Pathria M et al: Fibrous dysplasia: magnetic resonance imaging appearance at 1.5 tesla, Clin Imaging 14:211-215, 1990.

52. Ollivier L, Leclere J, Vanel D et al: Femoral infarction following intraarterial chemotherapy for osteosarcoma of the leg: a possible pitfall in magnetic resonance imaging, Skeletal Radiol 20:329-332, 1991.

53. Pan G, Raymond AK, Carrasco CH et al: Osteosarcoma: MR imaging after preoperative chemotherapy, Radiology 174:517-526, 1990.

54. Pope JM, Walker RR, Kron T: Artifacts in chemical shift selective imaging, Magn Reson Imaging 10:695-698, 1992.

55. Redmond OM, Stack JP, Dervan PA et al: Osteosarcoma: use of MR imaging and MR spectroscopy in clinical decision making, Radiology 172:811-815, 1989.

56. Remedios PA, Colletti PM, Raval JK et al: Magnetic resonance imaging of bone after radiation, Magn Reson Imaging 6:301-304, 1988.

57. Ricci C, Cova M, Kang YS et al: Normal age-related patterns of cellular and fatty bone marrow distribution in the axial skeleton: MR imaging study, Radiology 177:83-88, 1990.

58. Ritschl P, Hajek PC, Pechmann U: Fibrous metaphyseal defects: magnetic resonance imaging appearances, Skeletal Radiol 18:253-259, 1989.

59. Roberts MC, Kressel HY, Fallon MD et al: Paget disease: MR imaging findings, Radiology 173:341-345, 1989.

60. Rosenthal RE, Wozney P: Diagnostic value of gadopentetate dimeglumine for 1.5-T MR imaging of musculoskeletal masses: comparison with unenhanced T1- and T2-weighted imaging, J Magn Resonan Imaging 1:547-551, 1991.

61. Ruzal-Shapiro C, Berdon WE, Cohen MD et al: MR imaging of diffuse bone marrow replacement in pediatric patients with cancer, Radiology 181:587-589, 1991.

62. Sanchez RB, Quinn SF, Walling A et al: Musculoskeletal neoplasms after intraarterial chemotherapy: correlation of MR images with pathologic specimens, Radiology 174:237-240, 1990.

63. Schick F, Bongers H, Aicher K et al: Subtle bone marrow edema assessed by frequency selective chemical shift MRI, J Comput Assist Tomogr 16:454-460, 1992.

64. Schweitzer ME, Levine C, Mitchell DG et al: Bull's-eyes and halos: useful MR discriminators of osseous metastases, Radiology 188:249-252, 1993.

65. Sebag GH, Moore SG: Effect of trabecular bone on the appearance of marrow in gradient-echo imaging of the appendicular skeleton, Radiology 174:855-859, 1990.

66. Seeger LL, Widoff BE, Bassett LW et al: Preoperative evaluation of osteosarcoma: value of gadopentetate dimeglumine-enhanced MR imaging, Am J Roentgenol 157:347-351, 1991.

67. Shuman WP, Lambert DT, Patten RM et al: Improved fat suppression in STIR MR imaging: selecting inversion time through spectral display, Radiology 178:885-887, 1991.

68. Sklar DH, Phillips JJ, Lachman RS: Case report 683, Skeletal Radiol 20:394-396, 1991.

69. Stevens SK, Moore SG, Amylon MD: Repopulation of marrow after transplantation: MR imaging with pathologic correlation, Radiology 175:213-218, 1990.

70. Sundaram M, McLeod RA: MR imaging of tumor and tumor-like lesions of bone and soft tissue, Am J Roentgenol 155:817-824, 1990.

71. Tsai JC, Dalinka MK, Fallon MD et al: Fluid-fluid level: a nonspecific finding in tumors of bone and soft tissue, Radiology 175:779-782, 1990.

72. Unger E, Moldofsky P, Gatenby R et al: Diagnosis of osteomyelitis by MR imaging, Am J Roentgenol 150:605-610, 1988.

73. Utz JA, Kransdorf MJ, Jelinek JS et al: MR appearance of fibrous dysplasia, J Comput Assist Tomogr 13:845-851, 1989.

74. Vogler JB III, Murphy WA: Bone marrow imaging, Radiology 168:679-693, 1988.

75. Woods ER, Martel W, Mandell SH et al: Reactive soft-tissue mass associated with osteoid osteoma: correlation of MR imaging features with pathologic findings, Radiology 186:221-225, 1993.

76. Yuh WTC, Corson JD, Baraniewski HM et al: Osteomyelitis of the foot in diabetic patients: evaluation with plain film, 99mTc-MDP bone scintigraphy, and MR imaging, Am J Roentgenol 152:795-800, 1989.

77. Zawin JK, Jaramillo D: Conversion of bone marrow in the humerus, sternum, and clavicle: changes with age on MR images, Radiology 188:159-164, 1993.

15

Soft Tissues

PULSE SEQUENCES

The ability of magnetic resonance (MR) to depict soft tissue abnormalities is unrivaled among all imaging modalities. Soft tissue lesions surrounded by muscle are usually most evident on T2-weighted images. T1- and proton density–weighted images are not reliable for demonstrating such lesions, particularly when they are small or do not result in significant mass effect or other morphologic alterations. In order to provide an adequate degree of T2 weighting for lesion visualization, a sufficiently long repetition time (TR) and echo time (TE) must be chosen. Mildly T2-weighted images also display fat and some soft tissues with signal intensity similar to fluid, which can complicate lesion characterization. In regard to lesions arising in muscle, soft tissue lesions surrounded by fat are better depicted on T1- rather than T2-weighted images. Because many soft tissue lesions have components that border both fat and muscle, a combination of T1- and T2-weighted sequences is generally required.

FAT SUPPRESSION

While standard T1- and T2-weighted spin echo images allow for detection of most soft tissue masses, some lesions may be isointense with surrounding soft tissues and are therefore rendered inconspicuous. One approach for improving the conspicuousness of soft tissue lesions is the use of fat suppression techniques. Fat suppression can be useful for several reasons. Suppression of the relatively high signal intensity of fat leads to more efficient use of the dynamic range for display of tissue contrast on MR images.[63] Thus differences among tissues in terms of either T1 or T2 relaxation are often heightened as compared with comparable sequences in which fat suppression is not used. This effect is most prominent on T2-weighted sequences, where fat suppression can markedly increase the conspicuousness of fluid and improve sensitivity for detection of many lesions. Similarly, the conspicuousness of abnormal enhancement after injection of paramagnetic contrast material is increased on T1-weighted images by using fat suppression.[84] This does not, however, eliminate the need to obtain unenhanced fat suppressed images; these are necessary for accurate interpretation. Fat suppressed T2-weighted sequences can also reduce imaging time, since TR and TE can be reduced while maintaining acceptable tissue contrast.

In addition to improved sensitivity for lesion detection, characterization of some soft tissue lesions is better when fat suppression is used. For example, high signal intensity on T1-weighted images can indicate hemorrhagic, proteinaceous, or lipid components within a lesion. Reduction of a lesion's signal intensity on fat suppressed images, however, can specifically indicate the presence of fatty tissue.

Fat suppression can also be helpful for improving image quality. The conspicuousness of phase-encoding errors caused by motion is proportional to the signal intensity of the moving structure. Because fat is a major contributor to motion artifacts, fat suppression is effective in reducing their prominence. Chemical shift misregistration artifacts arise at fat-water interfaces along the frequency-encoding direction; these artifacts can be eliminated with the use of fat suppression. This allows for use of narrow receiver bandwidth sampling to improve the signal-to-noise ratio.[63]

With the phase contrast technique, originally described by Dixon,[20] the echo time is altered so that sampling occurs when fat and water protons are out of phase with one another. The appropriate echo time depends on the field strength at which imaging is performed. Signal cancellation occurs in voxels containing both fat and water protons on opposed phase images. These chemical shift phase cancellation artifacts outline muscle groups

A portion of this chapter is reproduced with permission from Mirowitz SA: Fast scanning and fat-suppression MR imaging of musculoskeletal disorders, *Am J Roentgenol*, Dec 1993.

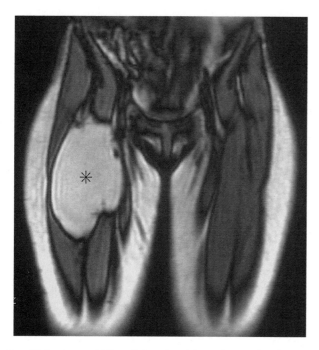

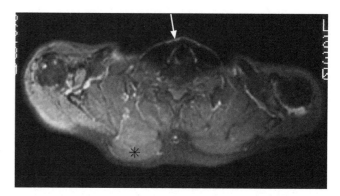

Fig. 15-2. Soft tissue mass located along the right back (*asterisk*) is isointense with surrounding muscle on fat suppressed proton density–weighted image (TR 2250, TE 30, 1 Nex) as well as all other pulse sequences. Note heterogeneous fat suppression on this large field-of-view image, with inadvertent suppression of water-containing tissues along the anterior neck (*arrow*).

Fig. 15-1. Coronal T1-weighted rapid gradient echo image (TR 113, TE 2.6, 1 Nex, 90-degree flip angle) demonstrates signal loss at fat-water interfaces caused by use of an opposed phase echo time. However, there is preservation of signal intensity within a right anterior thigh lipoma (*asterisk*).

along fascial planes. This artifactual decreased signal intensity line should not be interpreted as representing the actual margin of a soft tissue lesion. In-phase images, on which fat signals and water signals are additive, are also acquired, and these data sets are then postprocessed to render fat-only or water-only images. This method can be used in conjunction with spin echo or gradient echo sequences. Disadvantages include the need to perform two sequences and to use postprocessing.[85] Misregistration can result from motion between acquisition of the in-phase and out-of-phase sequences. Chopper is a phase-sensitive variant of the Dixon method that does not require postprocessing and eliminates misregistration.[92] Phase contrast images will display signal loss only where fat and water protons occupy the same voxels; purely lipomatous lesions will not be suppressed (Fig. 15-1).

The short tau inversion recovery (STIR) technique uses an initial 180-degree inverting radiofrequency pulse followed by a standard 90 to 180-degree spin echo sequence.[85] The time allowed to elapse between the inversion pulse and the subsequent 90-degree pulse is chosen to approximate the null point of fat, resulting in suppression of fat signal. Most often, the inversion time is determined by using field strength–dependent reference values. However, improved fat suppression can be achieved by performing a spectral analysis, allowing the inversion time that is optimal for suppressing the fat of

a given patient to be determined.[83] Inversion recovery images can be displayed in phase sensitive or magnitude modes. The latter format, which is used most often, displays positive signal intensity for tissues with magnetization either above or below the baseline.

Because they display additive T1 and T2 contrast, STIR images sensitively depict alterations in tissue signal intensity.[97] However, their specificity for characterizing abnormal signal intensity is somewhat reduced compared with conventional T1- and T2-weighted images, since observed signal alterations may occur on the basis of either T1 or T2 relaxation effects. Other limitations of STIR include relatively long imaging times for acquisition of a limited number of imaging slices, vulnerability to motion artifacts, and poor signal-to-noise ratio.[85] In addition, although suppression of signal intensity on STIR images usually implies that fat is present, it is important to be aware that fat suppression on STIR images is based strictly on relaxation phenomena. Therefore any nonlipid tissue will also be suppressed if it has a short T1 value similar to that of fat. Inadvertent suppression of short T1 tissues on STIR images is referred to as "bounce point artifact."[37] When paramagnetic contrast agents are used, inadvertent suppression of contrast enhancing tissue can occur on STIR images. Although fat suppression on STIR images is not directly affected by minor inhomogeneities in the magnetic field, it may be indirectly affected because fat within different locations in the magnetic field can have slightly different relaxation behavior. This can result in uneven fat suppression throughout the field-of-view.

Fat saturation involves use of a chemical shift selective radiofrequency presaturation pulse applied at the resonant frequency of lipid protons.[50] This is followed

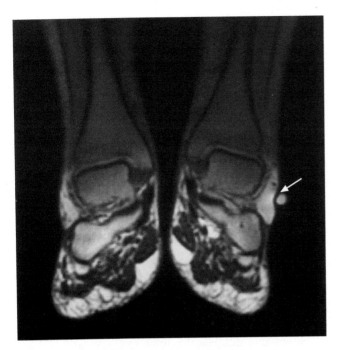

Fig. 15-3. Coronal T1-weighted image (TR 500, TE 11, 2 Nex) using fat suppression demonstrates lack of suppression of fat throughout the distal ankle and foot. This results in unexpected lack of signal decrease within the lateral portion of a lipoma *(arrow)*. Also note distortion of soft tissues caused by an oil bead taped to the skin surface to serve as a marker.

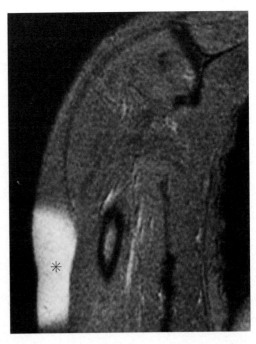

Fig. 15-4. Coronal proton density–weighted fat suppressed image (TR 2900, TE 30, 1 Nex) of the upper arm. There is a region of relative increased signal intensity along the lateral inferior arm *(asterisk)* in which the signal intensity of fat has not been effectively suppressed.

by a gradient pulse that spoils any residual signal intensity of fat. Fat saturation can be used in conjunction with T1- or T2-weighted spin echo sequences or with gradient echo sequences. This technique is most effectively implemented on high field strength systems, because the separation between fat and water peaks increases proportional to magnetic field strength.

Fat saturation can be used to achieve fat suppression without loss of familiar T1- or T2-weighted tissue contrast. This feature is advantageous for performing lesion characterization. Suppression of signal intensity with fat saturation is specific for fat, since other tissues with short T1 relaxation are not affected. However, to be effective, fat saturation requires a highly uniform magnetic field. Any intrinsic or extrinsic nonuniformities can result in incomplete fat suppression or even inadvertent suppression of water signal. In the latter situation, soft tissue lesions that contain high water content can be obscured (Fig. 15-2). Furthermore, the signal intensity of lipomatous lesions may not be suppressed when fat saturation is performed in the presence of a nonuniform magnetic field (Fig. 15-3). Such nonuniformities can result from imperfections in the magnet, improper shimming, or the presence of air or ferromagnetic objects, which distort local magnetic field gradients. Artifacts associated with

failure of fat suppression can simulate or obscure soft tissue lesions[3] (Fig. 15-4). Because of its sensitivity to nonuniformities in the magnetic field, fat saturation is less effective on images acquired using a large field-of-view.

Susceptibility artifacts related to ferromagnetic items are accentuated on fat saturation images. These artifacts appear as a signal void with surrounding hyperintensity and can obscure or simulate soft tissue abnormalities. Another limitation of fat saturation is that it reduces the number of imaging slices that can be acquired during a given TR by approximately 15% to 25%. Finally, as with all fat suppression methods, images obtained using fat saturation have reduced signal-to-noise ratio as compared with comparable conventional images. This can result in a grainy image appearance and limit detection of small or subtle abnormalities.

The fat suppression techniques described here are not mutually exclusive. In fact, combinations of these methods can result in improved effectiveness and uniformity of fat suppression. For example, the phase contrast method and its variants can be effectively used in conjunction with fat saturation.[14]

FAST SPIN ECHO IMAGING

Fat appears considerably more intense on T2-weighted fast spin echo (i.e., rapid acquisition relaxation

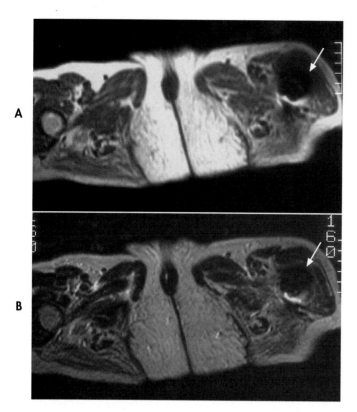

Fig. 15-5. Transaxial T1-weighted spin echo **(A)** (TR 500, TE 11, 4 Nex) and T2-weighted fast spin echo **(B)** (TR 4000, effective TE 119, 4 Nex, 16 echo train) images at corresponding levels. The signal void artifact related to the left femoral head prosthesis *(arrow)* is reduced on the fast spin echo image, despite the use of a considerably longer echo time.

enhancement) images as compared with conventional spin echo images using comparable parameters. This effect is due to decoupling of J-modulation effects[16,39] and possibly other mechanisms, and it can cause high signal intensity soft tissue lesions surrounded by fat to be obscured on T2-weighted fast spin echo images. Skeletal muscle and lesions composed of muscle, such as leiomyomas, may appear lower in signal intensity on fast spin echoes compared with conventional spin echo images.[16] Fast spin echo images are predisposed to blurring, particularly when short echo times and/or relatively long echo trains are used.[16] Susceptibility artifacts, such as those related to air or metal, are generally less conspicuous on fast spin echo images (Figs. 15-5, *A* and *B*) because of the rephasing effects of multiple 180-degree refocusing pulses.

PERILESIONAL SIGNAL INTENSITY ALTERATIONS

Increased signal intensity frequently surrounds soft tissue lesions on T2-weighted images. These findings usually reflect reactive edema incited by the lesion. When peritumoral signal alterations are present, the size and extent of the lesion may be overestimated on MR images.[7] Distinction between soft tissue lesions and surrounding edema is particularly difficult on STIR images, where overestimation of lesion size and extent are more likely to occur.[73,82] Peritumoral edema can lead to difficulty in precisely determining lesion margins for treatment planning.[82] Reactive edema can also simulate soft tissue infection.[21]

Observation of perilesional edema does not indicate that the underlying lesion is malignant or even neoplastic.[7] In one study of 46 patients, Hanna et al observed perilesional signal alterations with equal frequency in benign and malignant lesions.[35] Perilesional edema can be associated with various benign soft tissue lesions including hematoma, myositis, eosinophilic granuloma, hemangioma, myositis ossificans, and others.[35] Extensive signal alterations can sometimes involve entire muscles or compartments. This "massive edema pattern" can also be observed with benign or malignant lesions.

CONTRAST ENHANCEMENT PATTERNS

Intravenous contrast agents have been used in an effort to improve definition of lesion margins and to distinguish soft tissue lesions from surrounding edema. When paramagnetic agents are given and standard imaging sequences performed, contrast material enhancement occurs not only within the lesion but also in the zone of peritumoral signal changes. This is attributed to widening of intercellular spaces in the perilesional zone, among other factors.[35] However, when images are rapidly acquired during the bolus injection of contrast material, differences between lesions and surrounding tissues are improved. On dynamic contrast enhanced images, the perilesional zone enhances less rapidly than does the lesion itself.[35]

POSTTREATMENT ALTERATIONS

The diagnosis and staging of soft tissue lesions can be complicated by a number of iatrogenic factors. For example, percutaneous or open surgical biopsy of a soft tissue lesion results in hemorrhage and edema. This can obscure visualization of the underlying lesion, limit its characterization on the basis of signal characteristics, and interfere with determination of its extent.[19] Similar limitations are encountered for lesions that have undergone spontaneous or posttraumatic intratumoral hemorrhage. In such cases, the signal alterations exhibited by hemorrhagic breakdown products can obscure the underlying lesion.

Substantial soft tissue edema is often present in patients who have undergone radiation therapy. Abnormal enhancement following gadopentetate dimeglumine ad-

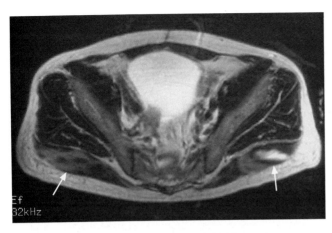

Fig. 15-6. Foci of relative increased signal intensity are noted within the gluteal soft tissues bilaterally *(arrows)* on fast spin echo T2-weighted image (TR 3500, effective TE 117, 4 Nex, 16 echo train), with central fluid-like signal intensity on the left. These findings were caused by recent intramuscular injections.

ministration can also be observed. The onset of these findings is variable but has been observed as early as 6 weeks after treatment completion and can persist for more than 1 year.[32] Radiation induced signal alterations may be accompanied by muscular atrophy.[32] Another finding suggestive of radiation induced soft tissue alterations is its geometric pattern, with sharply defined margins corresponding to the treatment port.

Edema, hemorrhage, and necrosis resulting from previous surgery or radiation therapy can also interfere with MR assessment for response of the lesion to treatment.* When contrast material is given, necrotic or nonviable tumor usually does not enhance. However, such enhancement can occur, simulating residual viable tumor.[30] Distinction between these entities is improved with use of dynamic contrast enhanced imaging, which allows the rate of tissue enhancement to be determined.[30]

In patients who have undergone treatment (chemotherapy or radiation therapy) for soft tissue masses, decreasing signal intensity on T2-weighted images usually indicates a positive response, reflecting conversion of viable tumor to fibrotic tissue.[42] A fibrous pseudocapsule can develop around the periphery of the lesion following chemotherapy treatment.[15] When the lesion becomes uniformly isointense with muscle on T2-weighted images, a residual tumor is unlikely. In the follow-up evaluation of patients with posttherapeutic fibrosis, observation of a focus of high signal intensity on T2-weighted images usually suggests tumor recurrence. However, high signal intensity may not be observed on T2-weighted images with some malignant lesions, particularly those with a prominent fibrous component.

*References 30, 40, 47, 54, 89, 90, 98.

Conversely, postoperative fluid collections, vascular structures, bowel loops, and other sources of hyperintensity can simulate tumor recurrence.[77] These entities can often be recognized through careful evaluation of their morphologic characteristics.

Another iatrogenic cause for soft tissue signal alterations is intramuscular injection (Fig. 15-6). Signal alterations are visualized immediately following injection, become progressively more conspicuous over the course of the next day, and can remain evident for up to 36 days.[43]

SIMULATION OF SOFT TISSUE LESIONS

Altered signal intensity can be observed within specific muscle groups following recent exercise.[4,18,26-28,80,81] This is manifested as relative increased signal intensity on T2-weighted or STIR images (Figs. 15-7, *A* and *B*). Accentuated tissue perfusion is a factor in increasing relaxation parameters in exercised muscle.[4] There is also a more delayed increase in muscle signal intensity, which can be seen 2 to 3 days following exercise, which is reflective of ultrastructural injury.[66]

Denervation is another entity that can result in abnormal soft tissue signal intensity. Increased signal intensity can be observed within denervated muscle groups on T2-weighted and STIR images in the subacute stage. This appearance can simulate inflammatory myositis, exertional muscle injury, or soft tissue neoplasia.[29,96] In the chronic stage, fatty infiltration predominates, resulting in increased signal intensity on T1-weighted images.

A number of other entities can simulate soft tissue neoplasms. Bursae can appear to represent a hemorrhagic or necrotic soft tissue neoplasm, since they contain fluid and possibly cellular debris or hemorrhagic products (Fig. 15-8). Their proximity to joints or bony prominences is characteristic. A synovial cyst can simulate a necrotic soft tissue neoplasm, particularly when it is in an unusual location, remote from a joint; when it has dissected through the soft tissues; or when its communication with the joint space cannot be visualized (Figs. 15-9, *A* and *B*). Conversely, when cystic or necrotic soft tissue neoplasms happen to be located near a joint, they may

A

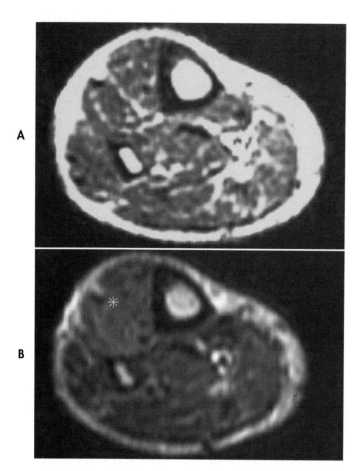

B

Fig. 15-7. Transaxial T2-weighted images (TR 2500, TE 80, 1 Nex) obtained before **(A)** and after **(B)** repeated dorsiflexion of the foot. There is relative increased signal intensity within the anterior compartment of the lower leg on postexercise image *(asterisk)*.

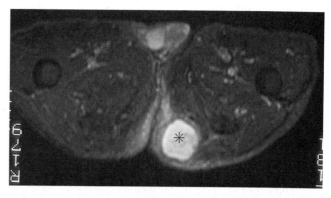

Fig. 15-8. A rounded mass of increased signal intensity *(asterisk)* is observed on transaxial fat suppressed T2-weighted image (TR 3200, TE 80, 2 Nex). While this appearance resembles that of neoplasm (e.g., sarcoma), the mass was found to represent bursitis at surgery.

be mistaken for synovial cysts (Figs. 15-10, *A* and *B*). In problematic cases, reimaging following intraarticular injection of air or contrast material may be necessary to distinguish these entities.

Deformation of the soft tissues resulting from extrinsic objects can simulate a lesion. For example, when external markers are taped to the skin surface, subtle distortion of the underlying soft tissues can occur[100] (Figs. 15-3, 15-11, and 15-12). Prominent vessels, such as venous varicosities, can simulate angiodysplastic or cystic soft tissue lesions (Fig. 15-13). High flow vascular malformations such as arteriovenous malformations typically demonstrate flow void, whereas slower flow venous structures are hyperintense on T2-weighted images. In the latter situation, the vascular nature of the lesion may not be evident (Fig. 15-14), and flow sensitive gradient echo images may be useful. When veins contain phleboliths, calcification can result in signal void that spuriously indicates rapid flow.[75]

SOFT TISSUE HEMORRHAGE

Posttraumatic hematomas can simulate soft tissue neoplasms. The signal intensity of blood breakdown products evolves through a relatively predictable pattern. Immediately after the onset of hemorrhage, oxyhemoglobin appears similar to simple fluid—that is, hypointense on T1-weighted images and markedly hyperintense on T2-weighted images. Within hours, deoxygenation of hemoglobin results in preferential T2-shortening, leading to marked decreased signal intensity on T2-weighted images. This is followed over the next several days by formation of methemoglobin, which is hyperintense on T1-weighted images. As long as methemoglobin is contained within red blood cells, it appears hypointense on T2-weighted images, whereas hyperintensity occurs following cellular lysis. This appearance of subacute hematoma can persist for up to 1 year. It is followed by a chronic stage, in which the center of the hematoma again assumes signal characteristics compatible with fluid and is surrounded by peripheral hypointensity on T2-weighted images caused by hemosiderin accumulation.

When the signal intensity of a soft tissue lesion follows the above progression, the diagnosis of hematoma is indicated in the proper clinical setting. However, the possibility of hemorrhage into an underlying neoplasm should always be considered, particularly if any deviation from this pattern is observed.[25] Observation of marginal irregularity or internal heterogeneity resulting from

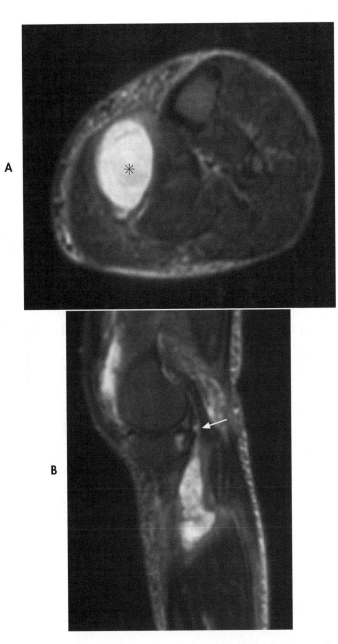

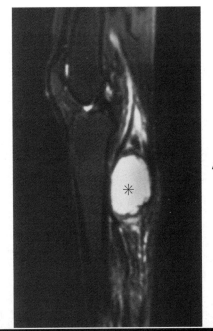

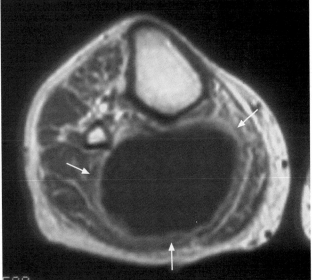

Fig. 15-9. A, Cystic mass is noted within the soft tissues of the medial lower leg *(asterisk)* on transaxial T2-weighted image (TR 2500, TE 80, 1 Nex). This represents an atypical synovial cyst that has dissected inferiorly from the knee joint in a patient with rheumatoid arthritis as demonstrated in **B** *(arrow)* (fast spin echo TR 4000, effective TE 104, 4 Nex, 8 echo train).

Fig. 15-10. A, Sagittal fast spin echo T2-weighted image (TR 4000, effective TE 104, 4 Nex, 8 echo train) demonstrates cystic mass *(asterisk)* in posterior calf. There is some *(arrows)* peripheral enhancement on transaxial gadopentetate enhanced T1-weighted image **(B)** (TR 500, TE 11, 2 Nex). While the location and configuration of this lesion are suggestive of synovial cyst, this pathologically represented a necrotic squamous cell metastasis from lung carcinoma.

soft tissue components should raise suspicion for an underlying lesion.[90] However, these latter features are not specific for malignancy. Simple hematomas and some benign lesions such as hemophilic pseudotumor can appear very heterogeneous and disorganized.[40,101] Hemorrhagic breakdown products can also be observed within

the soft tissues at sites of previous intramuscular injection.[43,76] Hemorrhage into a soft tissue lesion can simulate rapid tumor growth and increased aggressiveness.[67]

T1 shortening caused by subacute hemorrhage can be isointense with surrounding fatty tissue. This can obscure its presence or cause hematoma to simulate a lipomatous

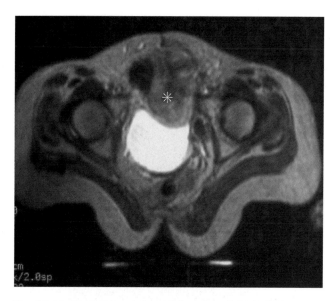

Fig. 15-11. There is apparent deformity of the soft tissues of the buttocks demonstrated on this transaxial T2-weighted image (TR 2200, TE 90, 2 Nex) caused by placement of a bedpan beneath the patient. Also noted is a large bladder carcinoma *(asterisk)* that has extended anteriorly to involve the pubic bones.

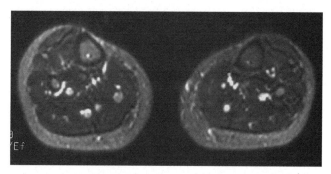

Fig. 15-13. Transaxial fat suppressed T2-weighted fast spin echo image (TR 4300, effective TE 102, 4 Nex, 16 echo train) of the lower legs in patient with suspected soft tissue mass. There is marked asymmetric signal intensity of tibial marrow, with relative increased signal intensity on the right. This is due to inhomogeneous fat saturation using a relatively large field-of-view (30 cm). Also note nodular high signal intensity in soft tissues resulting from prominent vessels, which could potentially simulate soft tissue lesions. A circular high signal intensity structure within the marrow space of both tibias also represents a vascular structure.

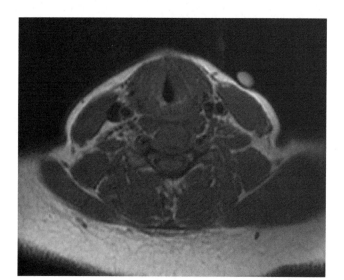

Fig. 15-12. A vitamin E capsule serving as a skin marker has been taped along the anterolateral left neck to mark the site of patient's discomfort. The pressure of the marker and tape results in subtle distortion of underlying soft tissues, with apparent soft tissue prominence in this location on T1-weighted image (TR 450, TE 11, 2 Nex). There are no corresponding alterations in signal intensity noted within this region.

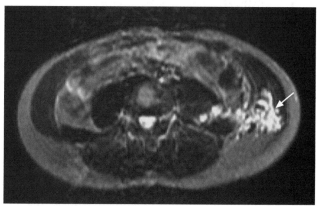

Fig. 15-14. Transaxial T2-weighted image (TR 3000, TE 90, 1 Nex) demonstrates a multilobular soft tissue mass *(arrow)* with markedly increased signal intensity within the left flank. This represents an angiodysplasia with hyperintensity caused by slow blood flow.

lesion. Fat saturated T1-weighted images can be very helpful in distinguishing these entities (Figs. 15-15, *A* and *B*). Marked reduction of lesion signal intensity on fat saturation images is specific for lipoma. However, as noted previously, some hematomas can undergo suppression on STIR images when their T1 relaxation value is similar to that of fat.

FATTY LESIONS

Lipomatous lesions are among the most common soft tissue masses. The distinction between a benign lipoma and liposarcoma is based on observation of soft tissue nodularity and/or stranding or signal characteristics that vary from those of fat in malignant lesions. However, these criteria are not entirely reliable, since soft tissue components can be observed in histologically benign lesions. Conversely, malignant lesions can appear deceptively homogeneous and devoid of soft tissue components.

Atypical lipomas are a distinct entity that straddle the characteristics of benign and malignant lesions histologically as well as on MR images (Fig. 15-16). Such lesions consist largely of mature fat cells but also have some soft tissue components. These soft tissue components are generally hypointense relative to fat on T1-weighted images and hyperintense relative to fat on T2-weighted images. Histologically, they contain collagen bundles, multinucleated cells, and fat cells with hyperchromic nuclei.[13,59] The fat contained within atypical lipomas may be indistinguishable from normal subcutaneous fat.[59] While atypical lipomas do not result in widespread metastases, they can be locally recurrent. When soft tissue components are observed within lipomatous lesions, liposarcoma cannot be excluded, and biopsy is necessary.[13]

Some lipomatous lesions display signal intensity characteristics that are not typical for fat.[87] Myxoid liposarcomas—the most frequent variety of liposarcoma—can appear generically hypointense on T1-weighted images and hyperintense on T2-weighted images (Figs. 15-17, *A*

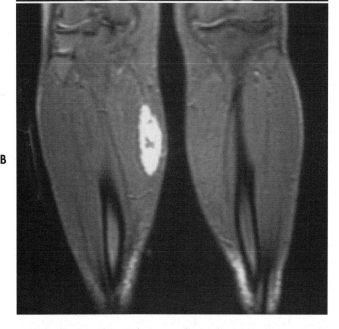

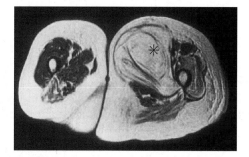

Fig. 15-15. A, A lenticular mass *(arrow)* with signal characteristics similar to those of subcutaneous fat is noted within the medial calf on coronal T1-weighted image (TR 400, TE 10, 1 Nex). **B,** Fat suppressed T1-weighted image (TR 450, TE 10, 2 Nex) demonstrates absence of suppression within this lesion, indicating that it represents hemorrhage rather than a lipoma.

Fig. 15-16. Transaxial proton density–weighted image demonstrates a large lipomatous lesion *(asterisk)* with multiple soft tissue septations coursing through it. This represented an atypical lipoma pathologically.

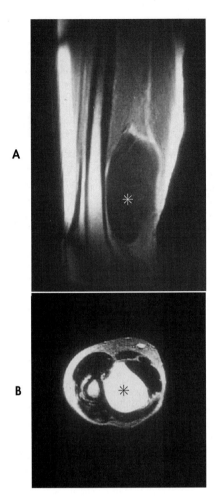

Fig. 15-17. Sagittal T1-weighted **(A)** and transaxial T2-weighted **(B)** images of the lower thigh reveal a large soft tissue mass with water-like signal intensity characteristics. Despite the absence of any apparent fatlike components, this was proven to represent a myxoid liposarcoma pathologically.

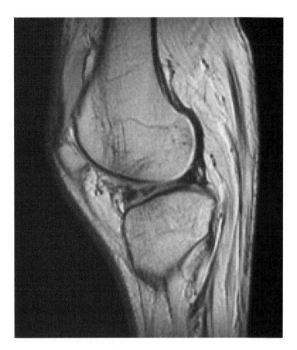

Fig. 15-18. Sagittal proton density–weighted image (TR 2250, TE 20, 1 Nex) demonstrates extensive fatty replacement of the musculature about the knee in a patient with previous poliomyelitis. A tear involving the anterior horn of the lateral meniscus and a joint effusion are also noted.

and *B*). Amorphous or linear foci of increased signal intensity on T1-weighted images are often observed, representing fatty components, though the majority of the lesion is often comprised of nonfatty tissue.[59,87] These lesions frequently display morphologic features that are usually associated with benign entities. For example, they typically have well-defined margins and no evidence of infiltration of surrounding tissues. Septations are, however, frequently observed. For all of these reasons, it is recommended that when a small amount of apparent fat is observed within an otherwise benign-appearing soft tissue mass, the diagnosis of myxoid liposarcoma should be considered.[87] The uniform high signal intensity of some myxoid liposarcomas on T2-weighted or STIR images can suggest the diagnosis of a benign cyst.[45,95] Dedifferentiated liposarcomas can also display predominant nondescript soft tissue signal

intensity characteristics that do not suggest the presence of fat,[45,55] though some fatty components are usually apparent.

Atypical increased—rather than decreased—signal intensity has also been observed on STIR images in some patients with lipid-containing tumors, including myxoid liposarcoma and tendon sheath lipoma.[65]

CHARACTERIZATION OF SOFT TISSUE LESIONS

Soft tissue hemangiomas can have variable signal characteristics on MR images. Although these lesions are usually hyperintense on T2-weighted images, their signal intensity on T1-weighted images varies from hypointense to markedly hyperintense.[90] In the latter situation, T1 shortening can be due to fatty components within the hemangioma; these findings can simulate a primary lipomatous lesion.[11] Foci of hyperintensity on T1-weighted images can also be observed in patients with myositis ossificans, representing marrow fat. Myositis ossificans can have markedly heterogeneous signal intensity that simulates malignancy.[56] Atrophic muscle groups may also appear hyperintense on T1-weighted images because of fatty infiltration. These findings are particularly prominent in patients with paralysis or polio-

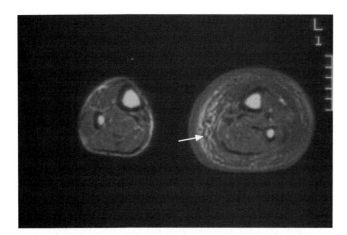

Fig. 15-19. There is marked soft tissue swelling of the left thigh with associated hyperintensity *(arrow)* demonstrated on transaxial T1-weighted image (TR 500, TE 15, 2 Nex). This is due to lymphedema in a patient who underwent previous left pelvic lymph node dissection. This appearance may simulate that of soft tissue hemorrhage.

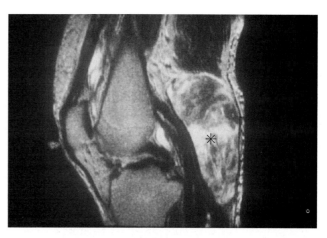

Fig. 15-20. Sagittal T2-weighted image demonstrates large heterogeneous mass *(asterisk)* in the popliteal region. This represents a popliteal cyst containing hemorrhagic debris. This appearance can simulate a sarcoma or other soft tissue lesion.

myelitis (Fig. 15-18). Lymphedema and lymphocele are additional causes for soft tissue hyperintensity on T1-weighted images.[88] The proteinaceous and lipid components of lymph fluid contribute to T1 shortening, which can simulate soft tissue hemorrhage or lipomatous infiltration (Fig. 15-19). Some nerve sheath tumors can also display high signal intensity on T1-weighted images.[79,86]

Intramuscular myxoma appears as a sharply marginated lesion confined within muscle, with low signal intensity on T1-weighted images and marked increased signal intensity on T2-weighted images.[1] This appearance can simulate fluid containing soft tissue lesions, including ganglia and other cystic entities, and vice versa.[95] While most myxoid soft tissue lesions are benign, myxoid material can be found within malignant lesions as well, and it can be difficult to distinguish between benign and malignant myxoid lesions.[68] Heterogeneous enhancement can be observed following intravenous contrast material administration in malignant myxoid tumors, although atypical patterns have also been observed in association with their benign counterparts.[58]

Ganglia are benign cystic lesions that are usually found near joints, though they can occur in any location. They can appear unilocular or multilocular, with frequent septations, and are markedly intense on T2-weighted images because of their gelatinous contents.[24] High signal intensity can occasionally be seen on T1-weighted images. These common lesions can be mistaken for malignant soft tissue neoplasm.

As indicated by these examples, the most significant limitation of MR in the evaluation of soft tissue lesions is that there is often significant overlap in the appearance of various lesions. As a result, it can be difficult to use signal intensity or morphologic characteristics to characterize a lesion as to etiology (e.g., inflammatory versus neoplastic) or even more generally to determine whether the lesion is malignant or benign[9,36,46,54,70,88,90,94] (Fig. 15-20).

Crim et al analyzed traditional criteria for determining benign versus malignant etiology in a series comprising 83 soft tissue masses.[17] These criteria included lesion size, homogeneity, signal intensity characteristics, margination, surrounding edema, and involvement of bone or neurovascular structures. Using these criteria, 53% of benign lesions were predicted to be malignant by one or more blinded reviewers. Among these lesions were hemangioma, hematoma, desmoid, neural tumor, myositis ossificans, lipoma, bursitis, and others. Conversely, 12% of sarcomas were called benign by one or more reviewers. In another study of patients with synovial sarcoma, most of the lesions demonstrated a benign appearance.[48] There can be considerable overlap in nearly all of the criteria listed between benign and malignant lesions (Fig. 15-21). The observation of fluid-fluid levels or internal septations within a soft tissue mass have both proven to be nonspecific findings.[12,49,64]

Lesions having signal characteristics different from the usual pattern can sometimes be characterized more completely on MR images. High signal intensity on T1-weighted images may indicate that a lesion contains fat,

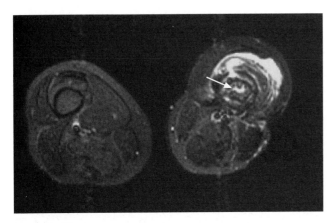

Fig. 15-21. Transaxial fat suppressed T2-weighted image (TR 2500, TE 80, 1 Nex) of the thighs demonstrates abnormal increased signal intensity within the marrow space of the left femur *(arrow)*, with adjacent soft tissue mass in the anterior compartment. While these findings are suggestive of neoplasm, in this patient they represented chronic osteomyelitis with associated cellulitis.

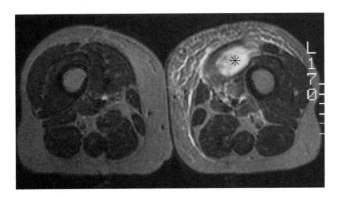

Fig. 15-22. Transaxial T2-weighted image (TR 2500, TE 90, 1 Nex) depicts hyperintense soft tissue mass *(asterisk)* involving left vastus medialis muscle, with surrounding high signal intensity. Excisional biopsy revealed nodular fasciitis. Calcifications within the lesion as depicted on CT are not visualized on corresponding MR image.

blood products, melanin, or proteinaceous fluid, as discussed previously. Lesions that are hypointense on T2-weighted images may contain hemorrhagic products, fibrous tissue, hemosiderin, calcification, or gas. Soft tissue masses that can contain hemosiderin include pigmented villonodular synovitis and giant cell tumor of tendon sheath.[40,47,52,54,89,90]

MR is relatively insensitive for depiction of small amounts of calcium or soft tissue gas[10,69,88,94] (Fig. 15-22). Gradient echo images are most likely to reveal foci of hypointensity when these entities are present. However, complementary use of CT should be considered when identification of calcium or gas is essential. Both calcification and iron can result in marked decreased sig-

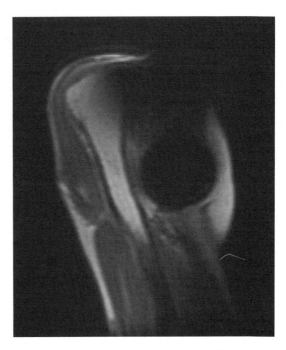

Fig. 15-23. Sagittal T1-weighted image (TR 500, TE 11, 2 Nex) of the shoulder demonstrates a large area of signal void which was caused by a small metal disk within a pillow located beneath the patient.

nal intensity on all pulse sequences, making them difficult to distinguish from one another. Phase reconstructions of gradient echo acquisitions have been used to improve depiction of calcification and help distinguish calcification from ferrous material.[34]

Fibromatous lesions can appear uniformly hypointense on T2-weighted images, though variable signal characteristics including hyperintensity may be observed.[74] Atypical signal intensity characteristics have also been observed for some fibrous lesions on gradient echo images. In one report, relatively proton density–weighted gradient echo images depicted a fibrosarcoma with unusually high signal intensity for unclear reasons.[91] Some fibromatous lesions, such as soft tissue desmoid and nodular fasciitis, are notorious for simulating sarcomatous lesions.[36,60] These lesions can have very heterogeneous signal intensity, which contributes to their malignant appearance.[53] Foci of linear or curvilinear relative decreased signal intensity are often observed within the lesion.[24] Although these lesions are initially well marginated, recurrent lesions often have infiltrative margins. Furthermore, a recurrent tumor can have signal characteristics similar to those of postoperative edema, granulation tissue, and fibrosis.[24] Nodular fasciitis is a related entity that also has highly variable signal characteristics because of mucoid or fibrous components; it can also closely simulate sarcoma[60] (Fig. 15-23). Focal myositis, pyomyositis, and myonecrosis are other entities that can simulate soft tissue sarcoma.[44,103]

Decreased signal intensity within the soft tissues can indicate the presence of metal. For example, these findings are observed in patients with bullets or pellets[93] or with implanted drug pumps.[99] Susceptibility artifacts associated with these entities can simulate or obscure soft tissue lesions (Fig. 15-23).

Intravenous contrast material has been used as an adjunct to unenhanced images for soft tissue lesion characterization. However, there is considerable overlap in contrast enhancement patterns among different lesion types and among malignant and benign lesion categories.[22,33,61] There is continued controversy regarding the accuracy of time-intensity data in characterization of soft tissue lesions and in predicting responsiveness of malignant lesions to chemotherapy.[23,31] Nonneoplastic conditions such as soft tissue infection can undergo prominent enhancement, and similar findings can be seen following radiation therapy[6] or surgical excision[51] of a soft tissue mass. Furthermore, the interface between tumor and adjacent fat can be obscured when contrast material is given, creating difficulty in defining lesion extent.[41] In one study of 26 patients with suspected masses, in no case did contrast enhanced images provide information superior to that available on unenhanced T1- and T2-weighted images.[78] Enhanced T1-weighted images were considerably less useful than unenhanced images in several patients, primarily because the interface between lesion and adjacent fat was often obscured following contrast material administration.

REFERENCES

1. Abdelwahab AF, Kenan S, Hermann G et al: Intramuscular myxoma: magnetic resonance features, Br J Radiol 65:485-490, 1992.
2. Abdelwahab IF, Kenan S, Hermann G et al: Periosteal ganglia: CT and MR imaging features, Radiology 188:245-248, 1993.
3. Anzai Y, Lufkin RB, Jabour BA et al: Fat-suppression failure artifacts simulating pathology on frequency-selective fat-suppression MR images of the head and neck, Am J Neuroradiol 13:879-884, 1992.
4. Archer BT, Fleckenstein JL, Bertocci LA et al: Effect of perfusion on exercised muscle: MR imaging evaluation, Magn Reson Imaging 2:407-413, 1992.
5. Baran GA, Sundaram M, Janney C: Paradoxical signals (short T2, long T2) in a patient with a soft-tissue tumor (letter), Am J Roentgenol 157:648-649, 1991.
6. Beltran J, Chandnani V, McGhee RA Jr et al: Gadopentetate dimeglumine-enhanced MR imaging of the musculoskeletal system, Am J Roentgenol 156:457-466, 1991.
7. Beltran J, Simon DC, Katz W et al: Increased MR signal intensity in skeletal muscle adjacent to malignant tumors: pathologic correlation and clinical relevance, Radiology 162:251-255, 1987.
8. Bergman RA, Thompson SA, Afifi AK et al. Compendium

of human anatomic variation: text, atlas, and world literature, Baltimore, 1988, Urban & Schwarzenberg.
9. Berquist TH, Ehman RL, King BF et al: Value of MR imaging in differentiating benign from malignant soft-tissue masses: study of 95 lesions, Am J Roentgenol 155:1251-1255, 1991.
10. Boyko OB, Cory DA, Cohen MD et al: MR imaging of osteogenic and Ewing's sarcoma, Am J Roentgenol 148:317-322, 1987.
11. Buetow PC, Kransdorf MJ, Moser RP Jr et al: Radiologic appearance of intramuscular hemangioma with emphasis on MR imaging, Am J Roentgenol 154:563-567, 1990.
12. Burk DL Jr, Dalinka MK, Kanal E et al: Meniscal and ganglion cysts of the knee: MR evaluation, Am J Roentgenol 150:331-336, 1988.
13. Bush CH, Spanier SS, Gillespy T III: Imaging of atypical lipomas of the extremities: report of three cases, Skeletal Radiol 17:472-475, 1988.
14. Chan TW, Listerud J, Kressel HY: Combined chemical-shift and phase-selective imaging for fat suppression: theory and initial clinical experience, Radiology 181:41-47, 1991.
15. Chandnani VP, Beltran J, Morris CS et al: Acute experimental osteomyelitis and abscesses: detection with MR imaging versus CT, Radiology 174:233-236, 1990.
16. Constable RT, Anderson AW, Zhong J et al: Factors influencing contrast in fast spin-echo MR imaging, Magn Reson Imaging 10:497-511, 1992.
17. Crim JR, Seeger LL, Yao L et al: Diagnosis of soft-tissue masses with MR imaging: can benign masses be differentiated from malignant ones? Radiology 185:581-586, 1992.
18. de Kerviler E, Leroy-Willig A, Jehenson P et al: Exercise-induced muscle modifications: study of healthy subjects and patients with metabolic myopathies with MR imaging and P-31 spectroscopy, Radiology 181:259-264, 1991.
19. Demas BE, Heelan RT, Lane J et al: Soft-tissue sarcomas of the extremities: comparison of MR and CT in determining the extent of disease, Am J Roentgenol 150:615-620, 1988.
20. Dixon WT: Simple proton spectroscopic imaging, Radiology 153:189-194, 1984.
21. Erdman WA, Tamburro F, Jayson HT et al: Osteomyelitis: characteristics and pitfalls of diagnosis with MR imaging, Radiology 180:533-539, 1991.
22. Erlemann R, Vassallo P, Bongartz G et al: Musculoskeletal neoplasms: fast low-angle shot MR imaging with and without Gd-DTPA, Radiology 176:489-495, 1990.
23. Erlemann R: Dynamic gadolinium-enhanced MR imaging to monitor tumor response to chemotherapy (letter), Radiology 186:904, 1993.
24. Feld R, Burk DL Jr, McCue P et al: MRI of aggressive fibromatosis: frequent appearance of high signal intensity on T2-weighted images, Magn Reson Imaging 8:583-588, 1990.
25. Fleckenstein FL, Weatherall PT, Parkey RW et al: Sports-related muscle injuries: evaluation with MR imaging, Radiology 172:793-798, 1989.
26. Fleckenstein JL, Bertocci LA, Nunnally RL et al: Exercise-enhanced MR imaging of variations in forearm muscle anatomy and use: importance in MR spectroscopy, Am J Roentgenol 153:693-698, 1989.
27. Fleckenstein JL, Canby RC, Parkey RW et al: Acute effects of exercise on MR imaging of skeletal muscle in normal volunteers, Am J Roentgenol 151:231-237, 1988.

28. Fleckenstein JL, Haller RG, Bertocci LA et al: Glycogenolysis, not perfusion, is the critical mediator of exercise-induced muscle modifications on MR images, Radiology 183:25-26, 1992.

29. Fleckenstein JL, Watumull D, Conner KE et al: Denervated human skeletal muscle: MR imaging evaluation, Radiology 187:213-218, 1993.

30. Fletcher BD, Hanna SL, Fairclough DL et al: Pediatric musculoskeletal tumors: use of dynamic, contrast-enhanced MR imaging to monitor response to chemotherapy, Radiology 184:243-248, 1992.

31. Fletcher BD, Hanna SL, Fairclough DL et al: Reply to Erlemann R: dynamic gadolinium-enhanced MR imaging to monitor tumor response to chemotherapy (letter), Radiology 186:905, 1993.

32. Fletcher BD, Hanna SL, Kun LE: Changes in MR signal intensity and contrast enhancement of therapeutically irradiated soft tissue, Magn Reson Imaging 8:771-777, 1990.

33. Fletcher BD, Hanna SL: Musculoskeletal neoplasms: dynamic Gd-DTPA-enhanced MR imaging (letter), Radiology 177:287-288, 1990.

34. Gronemeyer SA, Langston JW, Hanna SL et al: MR imaging detection of calcified intracranial lesions and differentiation from iron-laden lesions, Magn Reson Imaging 2:271-276, 1992.

35. Hanna SL, Fletcher BD, Parham DM et al: Muscle edema in musculoskeletal tumors: MR imaging characteristics and clinical significance, Magn Reson Imaging 1:441-449, 1991.

36. Hartman TE, Berquist TH, Fetsch JF: MR imaging of extra-abdominal desmoids: differentiation from other neoplasms, Am J Roentgenol 158:581-585, 1992.

37. Hearshen DO, Ellis JH, Carson PL et al: Boundary effects from opposed magnetization artifact in IR images, Radiology 160:543-547, 1986.

38. Henck ME, Simpson EL: Superiority of cod liver oil as a marker for lesions in MR images of the extremities (letter), Am J Roentgenol 161:904-905, 1993.

39. Henkelman RM, Hardy PA, Bishop JE et al: Why fat is bright in RARE and fast spin-echo imaging, Magn Reson Imaging 2:533-540, 1992.

40. Hermann G, Gilbert MS, Abdelwahab IF: Hemophilia: evaluation of musculoskeletal involvement with CT, sonography, and MR imaging, Am J Roentgenol 158:119-123, 1992.

41. Herrlin K, Ling LB, Pettersson H et al: Gadolinium-DTPA enhancement of soft tissue tumors in magnetic resonance imaging, Acta Radiol 31:233-236, 1990.

42. Holscher HC, Bloem JL, Nooy MA et al: The value of MR imaging in monitoring the effect of chemotherapy on bone sarcomas, Am J Roentgenol 154:763-769, 1990.

43. Huber DJ, Sumers E, Klein M: Soft tissue pseudotumor following intramuscular injection of "DPT": a pitfall in magnetic resonance imaging, Skeletal Radiol 16:469-473, 1987.

44. Janzen DL, Connell DG, Vaisler BJ: Calcific myonecrosis of the calf manifesting as an enlarging soft-tissue mass: imaging features, Am J Roentgenol 160:1072-1074, 1993.

45. Jelinek JS, Kransdorf MJ, Shmookler BM et al: Liposarcoma of the extremities: MR and CT findings in the histologic subtypes, Radiology 186:455-459, 1993.

46. Jelinek JS, Kransdorf MJ: MR imaging of soft-tissue masses (letter), Am J Roentgenol 155:423-424, 1990.

47. Jelinek JS, Kransdorf MJ, Utz JA et al: Imaging of pigmented villonodular synovitis with emphasis on MR imaging, Am J Roentgenol 152:337-342, 1989.

48. Jones BC, Sundaram M, Kransdorf MJ: Synovial sarcoma: MR imaging findings in 34 patients, Am J Roentgenol 161:827-830, 1993.

49. Kaplan PA, Williams SM: Mucocutaneous and peripheral soft-tissue hemangiomas: MR imaging, Radiology 163:163-166, 1987.

50. Keller PJ, Hunter WW Jr, Schmalbrock P: Multisection fat-water imaging with chemical shift selective presaturation, Radiology 164:539-541, 1987.

51. Kim EE, Alekhteyar KM: Follow-up MRI findings of soft tissue sarcomas after treatment with surgery, radiotherapy, chemotherapy or their combination, SMRM Book of Abstracts, 1992, p 2621.

52. Kottal RA, Vogler JB III, Matamoros A et al: Pigmented villonodular synovitis: a report of MR imaging in two cases, Radiology 163:551-553, 1987.

53. Kransdorf MJ, Jelinek JS, Moser RP Jr et al: Magnetic resonance appearance of fibromatosis: a report of 14 cases and review of the literature, Skeletal Radiol 19:495-499, 1990.

54. Kransdorf MJ, Jelinek JS, Moser RP Jr et al: Soft-tissue masses: diagnosis using MR imaging, Am J Roentgenol 153:541-547, 1989.

55. Kransdorf MJ, Meis JM, Jelinek JS: Dedifferentiated liposarcoma of the extremities: imaging findings in four patients, Am J Roentgenol 161:127-130, 1993.

56. Kransdorf MJ, Meis JM, Jelinek JS: Myositis ossificans: MR appearance with radiologic-pathologic correlation, Am J Roentgenol 157:1243-1248, 1991.

57. Kransdorf MJ, Meis JM, Montgomery E: Elastofibroma: MR and CT appearance with radiologic-pathologic correlation, Am J Roentgenol 159:575-579, 1992.

58. Kransdorf MJ, Moser RP Jr, Jelinek JS et al: Intramuscular myxoma: MR features, J Comput Assist Tomogr 13:836-839, 1989.

59. London J, Kim EE, Wallace S et al: MR imaging of liposarcomas: correlation of MR features and histology, J Comput Assist Tomogr 13:832-835, 1989.

60. Meyer CA, Kransdorf MJ, Jelinek JS, Moser RP Jr: MR and CT appearance of nodular fasciitis, J Comput Assist Tomogr 15:276-279, 1991.

61. Mirowitz SA, Totty WG, Lee JKT: Characterization of musculoskeletal masses using dynamic Gd-DTPA enhanced spin-echo MRI, J Comput Assist Tomogr 16:120-125, 1992.

62. Mirowitz SA, London SL: Ulnar collateral ligament injury in baseball pitchers: MR imaging evaluation, Radiology 185:573-576, 1992.

63. Mitchell DG, Vinitski S, Rifkin MD, Burk DL Jr: Sampling bandwidth and fat suppression: effects on long TR/TE MR imaging of the abdomen and pelvis at 1.5 T, Am J Roentgenol 153:419-425, 1989.

64. Morton MJ, Berquist TH, McLeod RA et al: MR imaging of synovial sarcoma, Am J Roentgenol 156:337-340, 1991.

65. Murphy WD, Hurst GC, Duerk JL et al: Atypical appearance of lipomatous tumors on MR images: high signal intensity with fat-suppression STIR sequences, Magn Reson Imaging 1:477-480, 1991.

66. Nurenberg P, Giddings CJ, Stray-Gundersen J et al: MR imaging-guided muscle biopsy for correlation of increased

signal intensity with ultrastructural change and delayed-onset muscle soreness after exercise, Radiology 184:865-869, 1992.

67. Panicek DM, Casper ES, Brennan MF et al: Hemorrhage simulating tumor growth in malignant fibrous histiocytoma at MR imaging, Radiology 181:398-400, 1991.

68. Peterson KK, Renfrew DL, Feddersen RM et al: Magnetic resonance imaging of myxoid containing tumors, Skeletal Radiol 20:245-250, 1991.

69. Pettersson H, Gillespy T III, Hamlin DJ et al: Primary musculoskeletal tumors: examination with MR imaging compared with conventional modalities, Radiology 164:237-241, 1987.

70. Pettersson H, Slone RM, Spanier S et al: Musculoskeletal tumors: T1 and T2 relaxation times, Radiology 167:783-785, 1988.

71. Plante E, Turkstra L: Sources of error in the quantitative analysis of MRI scans, Magn Reson Imaging 9:589-595, 1992.

72. Podo F: Tissue characterization by MRI: a multidisciplinary and multi-centre challenge today, Magn Reson Imaging 6:173-174, 1988.

73. Porter BA: High-field-strength STIR imaging: limitations (letter), Am J Roentgenol 153:1104, 1989.

74. Quinn SF, Erickson SJ, Dee PM et al: MR imaging in fibromatosis: results in 26 patients with pathologic correlation, Am J Roentgenol 156:539-542, 1991.

75. Rak KM, Yakes WF, Ray RL et al: MR imaging of symptomatic peripheral vascular malformations, Am J Roentgenol 159:107-112, 1992.

76. Resendes M, Helms CA, Fritz RC et al: MR appearance of intramuscular injections, Am J Roentgenol 158:1293-1294, 1992.

77. Reuther G, Mutschler W: Detection of local recurrent disease in musculoskeletal tumors: magnetic resonance imaging versus computed tomography, Skeletal Radiol 19:85-90, 1990.

78. Rosenthal RE, Wozney P: Diagnostic value of gadopentetate dimeglumine for 1.5- T MR imaging of musculoskeletal masses: comparison with unenhanced T1- and T2-weighted imaging, Magn Reson Imaging 1:547-551, 1991.

79. Sakai F, Sone S, Kiyono K et al: Intrathoracic neurogenic tumors: MR-pathologic correlation, Am J Roentgenol 159:279-283, 1992.

80. Shellock FG, Fukunaga T, Mink JH, Edgerton VR: Acute effects of exercise on MR imaging of skeletal muscle: concentric vs eccentric actions, Am J Roentgenol 156:765-768, 1991.

81. Shellock FG, Fukunaga T, Mink JH, Edgerton VR: Exertional muscle injury: evaluation of concentric versus eccentric actions with serial MR imaging, Radiology 179:659-664, 1991.

82. Shuman WP, Baron RL, Peters MJ, Tazioli PK: Comparison of STIR and spin-echo MR imaging at 1.5 T in 90 lesions of chest, liver, and pelvis, Am J Roentgenol 152:853-859, 1989.

83. Shuman WP, Lambert DT, Patten RM et al: Improved fat suppression in STIR MR imaging: selecting inversion time through spectral display, Radiology 178:885-887, 1991.

84. Simon JH, Szumowski J: Chemical shift imaging with paramagnetic contrast material enhancement for improved lesion depiction, Radiology 171:539-543, 1989.

85. Simon JH, Szumowski J: Proton (fat/water) chemical shift imaging in medical magnetic resonance imaging: current status, Invest Radiol 27:865-874, 1992.

86. Suh J-S, Abenoza P, Galloway HR et al: Peripheral (extracranial) nerve tumors: correlation of MR imaging and histologic findings, Radiology 183:341-346, 1992.

87. Sundaram M, Baran G, Merenda G, McDonald DJ: Myxoid liposarcoma: magnetic resonance imaging appearances with clinical and histological correlation, Skeletal Radiol 19:359-362, 1990.

88. Sundaram M, McGuire MH, Herbold DR: Magnetic resonance imaging of soft tissue masses: an evaluation of fifty-three histologically proven tumors, Magn Reson Imaging 6:237-248, 1988.

89. Sundaram M, McGuire MH, Schajowicz F: Soft-tissue masses: histologic basis for decreased signal (short T2) on T2-weighted MR images, Am J Roentgenol 148:1247-1250, 1987.

90. Sundaram M, McLeod RA: MR imaging of tumor and tumorlike lesions of bone and soft tissue, Am J Roentgenol 155:817-824, 1990.

91. Sundaram M, Perman W: Paradoxical signals on spin- and gradient-echo MR pulse sequences in a soft-tissue sarcoma (letter), Am J Roentgenol 161:904, 1993.

92. Szumowski J, Plewes DB: Separation of lipid and water MR imaging signals by chopper averaging in the time domain, Radiology 165:247-250, 1987.

93. Teitelbaum GP, Yee CA, Van Horn DD et al: Metallic ballistic fragments: MR imaging safety and artifacts, Radiology 175:855-859, 1990.

94. Totty WG, Murphy WA, Lee JKT: Soft-tissue tumors: MR imaging, Radiology 160:135-141, 1986.

95. Turner DA: Musculoskeletal tumors mimicking cysts (letter), Radiology 188:584, 1993.

96. Uetani M, Hayashi K, Matsunaga N et al: Denervated skeletal muscle: MR imaging: work in progress, Radiology 189:511-515, 1993.

97. Unger EC, Summers TB: Bone marrow, Top Magn Reson Imaging 1:31-52, 1989.

98. Vanel D, Lacombe M-J, Couanet D et al: Musculoskeletal tumors: follow-up with MR imaging after treatment with surgery and radiation therapy, Radiology 164:243-245, 1987.

99. von Roemeling R, Lanning RM, Eames FA: MR imaging of patients with implanted drug infusion pumps, Magn Reson Imaging 1:77-81, 1991.

100. Widder DJ: Simple localization device for MR imaging (letter), Am J Roentgenol 151:616, 1988.

101. Wilson DA, Prince JR: MR imaging of hemophilic pseudotumors, Am J Roentgenol 150:349-350, 1988.

102. Woods ER, Martel W, Mandell SH, Crabbe JP: Reactive soft-tissue mass associated with osteoid osteoma: correlation of MR imaging features with pathologic findings, Radiology 186:221-225, 1993.

103. Yuh WT, Schreiber AE, Montgomery WJ, Ehara S: Magnetic resonance imaging of pyomyositis, Skeletal Radiol 17:190-193, 1988.

Section Five

SPINE

16

Spinal Column and Paravertebral Soft Tissues

VERTEBRAL BODIES
Anatomic Variations

The vertebral bodies are subject to considerable variation in size and configuration. Variation is particularly evident at the cranial and caudal aspects of the spinal column. For example, the cervical spinous processes are often bifid and may demonstrate lateral tubercles at lower cervical levels[7]. Similar tubercles may also be present along the laminae in the lower cervical spine.[7] The foramen transversarium of C7 can be of variable size and may be absent, whereas accessory foramina transversaria can also exist.[7] The atlas and axis can have a variety of configurations. The dens may not be united with the body of C2 (i.e., os odontoideum), simulating the appearance of a fracture (Fig. 16-1). Other variations at this level include absence of the dens or origination of the dens from the anterior arch of the atlas.[7] The second cervical vertebra can be fused with the atlas or with the third cervical vertebra, and the atlas may be partially or completely fused with the occipital bone.[7] Incomplete ossification of the anterior and posterior arch of the atlas can occur.[7] There is marked variability in the prominence of the transverse and costal processes of the cervical vertebrae, and cervical ribs can arise from the lower cervical vertebrae.

Hemivertebrae can be present throughout the vertebral column and may be fused with adjacent vertebrae. Congenital variations in vertebral configuration must be distinguished from acquired abnormalities, such as may occur in patients with sickle cell anemia and other conditions.

The sacrococcygeal elements are of variable number and size. Schmorl's nodes represent herniation of intervertebral disk material into the endplate of an adjacent vertebral body. Although these are relatively common and of no clinical significance, they must be distinguished from vertebral lesions.

Determination of Vertebral Level

The number of vertebral bodies may appear decreased as a result of congenital fusion of one or more elements. The lumbar vertebrae can appear either increased or decreased in number because of lumbarization of the first sacral element or sacralization of the fifth lumbar element, respectively. The presence of transitional vertebrae can result in errors in designating the location of spinal

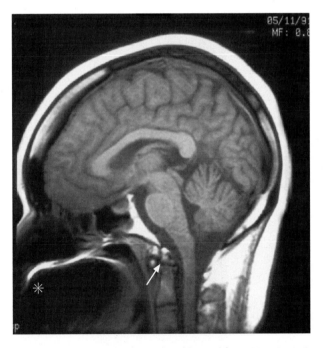

Fig. 16-1. Midsagittal T1-weighted image (TR 433, TE 11, 2 Nex) demonstrates lack of fusion of a corticated odontoid process *(arrow)* with the base of the C2 vertebral body (os odontoideum) in 27-year-old female. Also note artifactual signal void related to metallic dental device *(asterisk).*

abnormalities, including those involving the vertebral column or intervertebral disks.[24] The correct level can usually be determined if a large field-of-view image encompassing the odontoid process is available. The position of each vertebral body can then be determined by noting its position relative to anatomic structures that can be visualized (e.g., the main pulmonary artery). However, when an anterior presaturation band is used to decrease aortic pulsation artifacts, such structures may be obscured. Using a large field-of-view body coil image that shows the odontoid process, one can also localize vertebral bodies on subsequent surface coil images by using an electronic cursor to determine craniocaudal position or by placing an external marker over a particular vertebral body.[66] Another method is to identify the position of the right renal artery where it is interposed between the inferior vena cava and diaphragmatic crus on parasagittal images. This method has indicated the L1-2 intervertebral disk level in 86% of patients,[48] but it has not achieved universal acceptance, because some physicians believe that it is not sufficiently reliable[23] (Fig. 16-2). Nevertheless, the right renal artery is considerably more consistent in position than the insertion of the right diaphragmatic crus, which varies from the L1-2 to L3-4 levels.[48] Despite use of the methods just described, incorrect localization of spinal abnormalities can occur when the patient moves between acquisition of the initial body coil image and subsequent surface coil images (Fig. 16-3, A-C).

The number of vertebral elements varies between 32 and 35.[7] It has been stated that the "standard" complement of seven cervical, twelve thoracic, five lumbar, five sacral, and four coccygeal vertebrae is actually present in only approximately 20% of persons.[7]

POSTERIOR ELEMENTS

The posterior spinal elements are also of variable morphology. Spina bifida occulta is frequently observed in the lumbar spine, appearing as incomplete fusion of the spinous process. The transverse process of the fifth lumbar vertebra may form a pseudarthrosis with the sacrum. Variations in the morphology of the central spinal canal are frequent. The pedicles may be congenitally short, predisposing to stenosis of the spinal canal (Fig. 16-4).

Congenital defects in the pars interarticularis (i.e., spondylolysis defects) can appear similar to normal facet joints on axial images (Figs. 16-5 to 16-7, B) and may therefore go unrecognized.[22] Conversely, sclerosis involving the pars interarticularis can simulate spondylolysis defects.[29,30] Another cause for apparent spondylolysis defects is partial volume averaging with degenerative osteophytes projecting from the facet joints.[29] Spondylolysis defects may be more easily recognized in the sagittal than in the transaxial plane.[29]

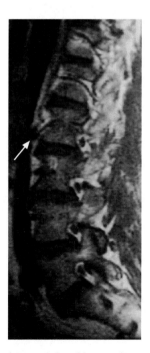

Fig. 16-2. Sagittal T1-weighted image (TR 500, TE 12, 2 Nex) demonstrates the right renal artery *(arrow)* to be located at the level of the lower margin of the L2 vertebral body.

CAUSES OF REDUCED VERTEBRAL MARROW SIGNAL INTENSITY SIMULATING A TUMOR

- Hematopoietic marrow
- Fibrous tissue (e.g., odontoid process)
- Partial volume averaging with intervertebral disk
- Chronic illness (e.g., acquired immune deficiency syndrome [AIDS])
- Chronic disuse
- Iron overload
- Normal marrow adjacent to site of increased marrow fat
- Motion artifacts
- Unintended radiofrequency presaturation
- Extension beyond sensitive range of surface coil
- Chemical shift misregistration artifact
- Susceptibility (ferromagnetic) artifact
- Marrow edema (i.e., trauma)
- Fibrosis, sclerosis, or eburnation
- Inflammatory endplate changes
- Postoperative changes

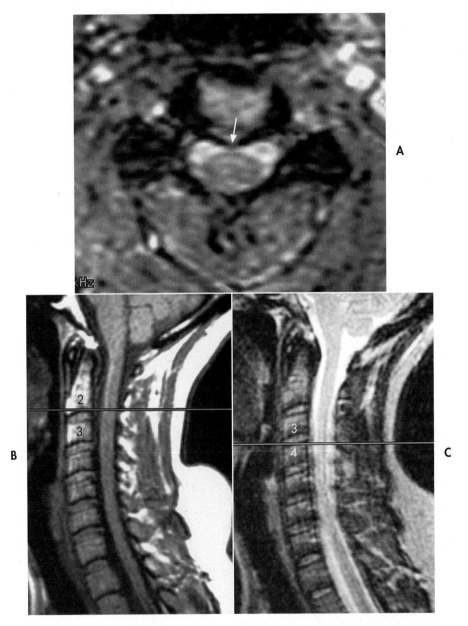

Fig. 16-3. A, Transaxial three-dimensional spoiled gradient echo image (TR 35, TE 15, 5-degree flip angle, 2 Nex) depicts small midline disk herniation *(arrow).* **B,** Based on the original localizer image (TR 566, TE 19, 2 Nex), the herniation appears to be located at the C2-3 interspace *(line).* However, the patient moved cranially in the magnet bore between acquisition of the localizer image and subsequent images. When **A** is referenced to **C,** the T2-weighted image (TR 2200, TE 80, 1 Nex), which was also acquired after the patient moved, it can be seen that the herniation is actually located at the C3-4 interspace *(line).*

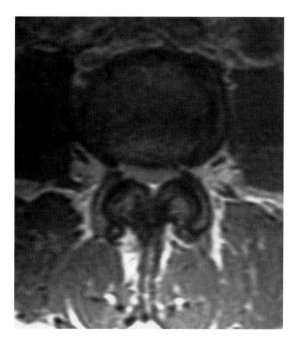

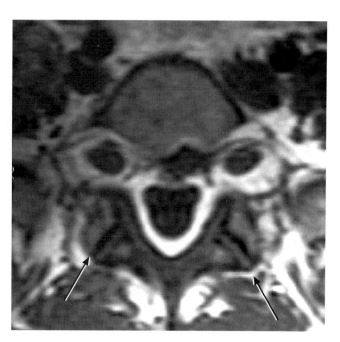

Fig. 16-4. Moderate to severe stenosis of the central spinal canal is noted on this transaxial proton density–weighted image (TR 2500, TE 35, 2 Nex) through the lumbar spine. Stenosis is primarily related to congenitally short pedicles, with superimposed narrowing attributed to hypertrophic degenerative changes involving the facet joints and ligamenta flava.

Fig. 16-5. Bilateral defects of the pars interarticularis (i.e., spondylolysis defects) *(arrows)* are noted on this transaxial T1-weighted image (TR 500, TE 15, 2 Nex) in a 36-year-old female. These defects can simulate the appearance of the normal facet joint.

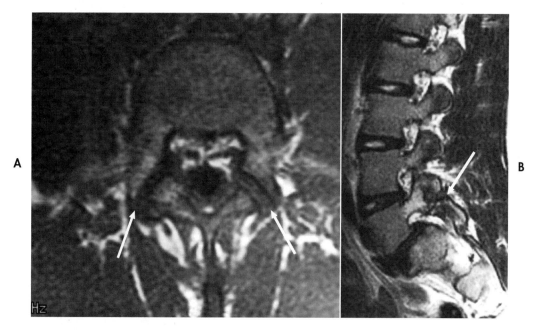

Fig. 16-6. A, Transaxial T1-weighted image (TR 400, TE 13, 4 Nex) demonstrates bilateral defects of the pars interarticularis *(arrows)* that simulate the appearance of normal facet joints. The spondylolysis defect *(arrow),* as well as the associated spondylolisthesis, is depicted on **B,** parasagittal T2-weighted fast spin echo image (TR 4000, effective TE 91, 4 Nex, 8 echo train length).

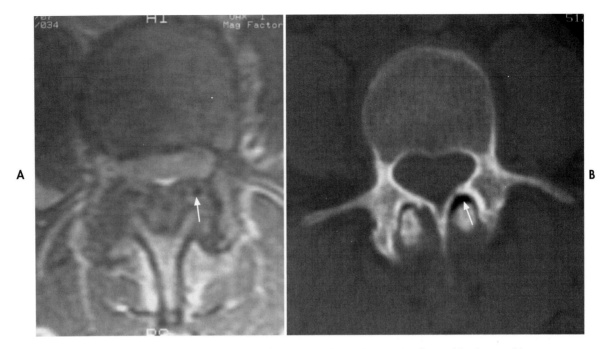

Fig. 16-7. A, A small focus of markedly decreased signal intensity *(arrow)* is observed in the region of the left facet joint on this transaxial proton density–weighted image (TR 2500, TE 35, 2 Nex). This represents air within the degenerative facet joint (i.e., vacuum phenomenon), as confirmed on the corresponding CT image *(arrow),* **B.**

MARROW SPACE

Anatomic Variations and Imaging Artifacts

Hematopoietic marrow

Heterogeneous signal intensity is frequently observed throughout the marrow space of the spinal column, with foci of relative increased or decreased signal intensity of variable size and configuration (Fig. 16-8). Hematopoietic (i.e., cellular) marrow appears as hypointense foci on both T1- and T2-weighted images, whereas fatty marrow appears hyperintense on T1-weighted images and moderately hypointense on T2-weighted images. Heterogeneous signal intensity resulting from normal cellular marrow elements can simulate metastatic involvement, multiple myeloma, Waldenstrom's macroglobulinemia, or other infiltrative marrow conditions affecting the spine[42] (Figs. 16-9 to 16-11).

Marrow heterogeneity is usually more conspicuous on images acquired using high field strength systems, because the hypointensity of iron-containing hematopoietic elements increases with magnetic field strength. Heterogeneous vertebral signal intensity is also generally more prominent in older adults.[50] Heterogeneous marrow patterns not only can simulate malignancy but may also obscure visualization of multiple myeloma or subtle meta-

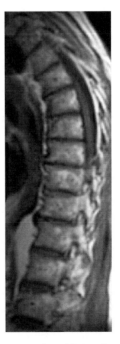

Fig. 16-8. Heterogeneous signal intensity pattern is observed throughout the marrow space of the vertebral column on midsagittal T1-weighted image (TR 500, TE 12, 2 Nex) in normal 74-year-old female.

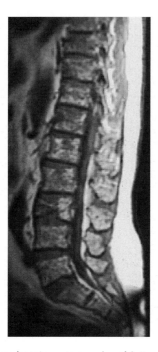

Fig. 16-9. Diffuse heterogeneous signal intensity is present throughout the marrow space of the vertebral column on this sagittal T1-weighted image (TR 600, TE 11, 2 Nex) in 69-year-old male with multiple myeloma.

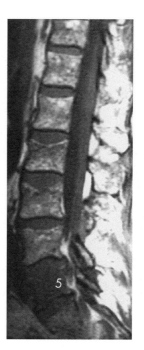

Fig. 16-10. Midsagittal T1-weighted image (TR 500, TE 12, 2 Nex) in 74-year-old male with multiple myeloma. Confluent abnormal marrow signal intensity is present in the L5 vertebral body. The remainder of the lumbar spine demonstrates heterogeneous marrow signal intensity.

DISTINCTION OF HEMATOPOIETIC MARROW FROM A TUMOR

- Relative hypointensity on T2-weighted images
- Absence of marked hyperintensity on fat-suppressed images
- Hyperintense versus intervertebral disks on T1-weighted images
- Absence of significant contrast material enhancement
- Absence of bone expansion
- Absence of cortical destruction
- Absence of abnormal morphology
- Absence of associated soft tissue mass

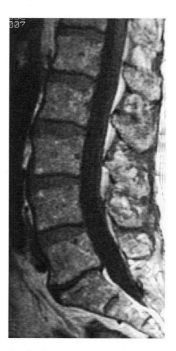

Fig. 16-11. Markedly heterogeneous signal intensity throughout the marrow space of the lumbar spine is observed on sagittal T1-weighted image (TR 500, TE 12, 2 Nex) in 73-year-old male with multiple myeloma. Narrowing of the L5-S1 intervertebral disk space is also present.

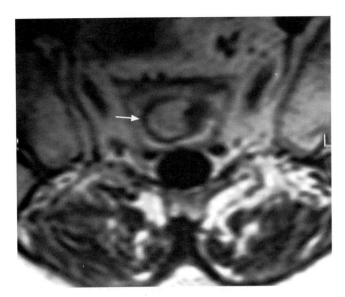

Fig. 16-12. Transaxial T1-weighted image (TR 400, TE 14, 4 Nex) obtained through the upper sacrum in 75-year-old female. There is a suggestion of a ringlike marrow lesion *(arrows),* although this area of low signal intensity represents the normal S1-2 intervertebral disk.

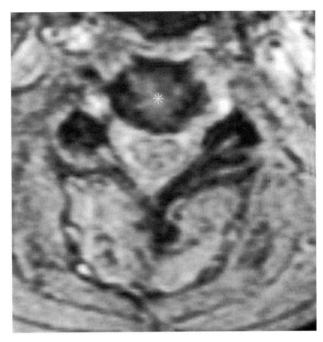

Fig. 16-13. Transaxial three-dimensional spoiled gradient echo image (TR 35, TE 15, 5-degree flip angle, 1 Nex) demonstrates rounded hyperintense focus *(asterisk)* that is suggestive of normal intervertebral disk material. However, this hyperintense focus actually represented a vertebral metastasis.

static involvement.[36,43] In one study, myelomatous involvement was not detectable in 31% of patients.[43]

The odontoid process typically demonstrates reduced signal intensity relative to other vertebral elements. This is present on all pulse sequences but usually is most noticeable on T1-weighted images. This is due to the presence of fibrous tissue components and can simulate marrow edema or replacement.[18]

Transaxial T1-weighted images can demonstrate partial volume averaging of the vertebral body and adjacent intervertebral disk, which simulates vertebral marrow replacement (Fig. 16-12). Conversely, focal increased or decreased signal intensity within the vertebral body caused by neoplasm may be overlooked when it is assumed to represent the normal intervertebral disk (Fig. 16-13).

Hematopoietic marrow elements are prominent in infants and children. During the first month of life, the vertebral bodies appear hypointense on T1-weighted images, except for linear hyperintensity along the course of the basivertebral vein, and they are also hypointense on T2-weighted images.[63] Hyaline cartilage, which surrounds the ossification centers, appears hyperintense on both T1- and T2-weighted images. Between 1 and 6 months of age, there is an increase in vertebral body signal intensity, which progresses from the endplates centrally, with relative isointensity of vertebral bodies and cartilage achieved at approximately 7 months.[63] When contrast material is administered, enhancement of nor-

mal marrow elements as well as vertebral hyaline cartilage can be observed in children.[65]

Very prominent hematopoietic marrow stores are also present in adults with anemia or infiltrative marrow disorders (Figs. 16-14, A to 16-16). Under these conditions, fatty marrow undergoes reconversion to hematopoietic marrow in an attempt to increase red blood cell production. Females of reproductive age frequently demonstrate prominent hematopoietic marrow caused by physiologic anemia.

Diffuse homogeneous hypointense spinal marrow on T1-weighted images is frequently observed in patients with chronic debilitating illnesses, such as AIDS (Figs. 16-17, A and B).[20] This finding reflects abundant marrow iron stores related to anemia of chronic disease and can be difficult to distinguish from diffuse tumor involvement. Conversely, diffuse marrow hypointensity caused by tumor replacement can also be misinterpreted as related to anemia (Figs. 16-18, A and B). As noted previously, T2-weighted images depict hematopoietic marrow as hypointense, whereas tumor frequently displays moderate hyperintensity. However, the signal characteristics of marrow neoplasm vary; necrotic lesions can be markedly hyperintense, whereas sclerotic lesions will be markedly hypointense on T2-weighted images. Fat sup-

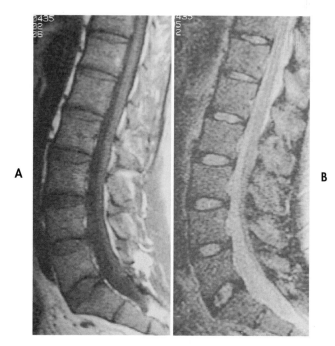

Fig. 16-14. A, Midsagittal T1-weighted image (TR 500, TE 12, 2 Nex) demonstrates diffusely reduced signal intensity throughout the marrow space of the lumbar spine caused by prominent hematopoietic bone marrow. B, There is no evidence of corresponding hyperintensity within the marrow space on T2-weighted image (TR 2000, TE 75, 1 Nex).

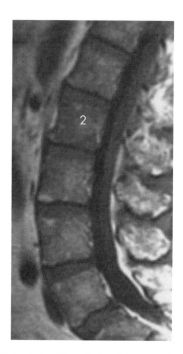

Fig. 16-15. Midsagittal T1-weighted image (TR 500, TE 12, 2 Nex) in 67-year-old female with lung carcinoma. Relative decreased marrow signal intensity within the L2 vertebral body (2) was initially interpreted as possible evidence of metastatic involvement. However, subsequent vertebral biopsy revealed only prominent hematopoietic marrow.

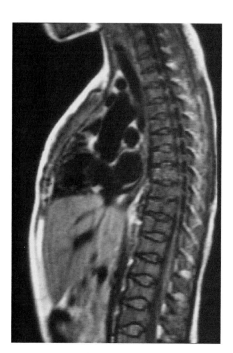

Fig. 16-16. Sagittal T1-weighted image of the spine in patient with sickle cell anemia. Characteristic morphologic alterations of the vertebral bodies are noted. In addition, there is diffusely reduced signal intensity throughout the marrow space.

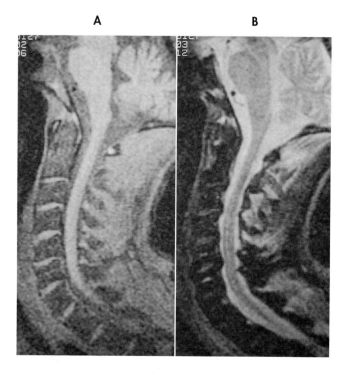

Fig. 16-17. A, Sagittal T1-weighted image (TR 567, TE 19, 2 Nex) and, B, T2-weighted image (TR 2200, TE 80, 1 Nex) in 50-year-old male with AIDS. There is prominent diffuse hypointensity throughout the marrow space of the spinal column. This results in relative hyperintensity of the intervertebral disks as compared with adjacent vertebral bodies on the T1-weighted image.

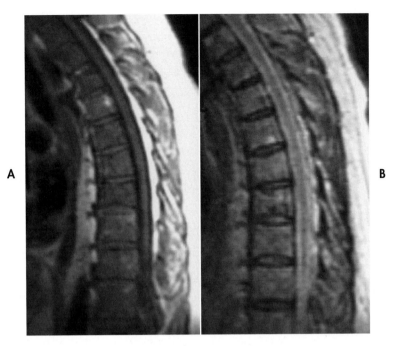

Fig. 16-18. A, Sagittal T1-weighted image (TR 500, TE 10, 2 Nex) and **B,** T2-weighted image (TR 2000, TE 80, 1 Nex) in 59-year-old female with breast carcinoma. Metastatic involvement of the spinal column is present, although it is somewhat difficult to recognize because of its diffuse nature and could potentially be interpreted as prominent hematopoietic marrow.

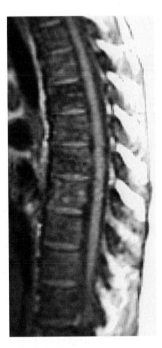

Fig. 16-19. Diffusely decreased marrow signal intensity is present on sagittal T1-weighted image (TR 500, TE 11, 2 Nex) in 60-year-old female with metastatic breast carcinoma. Observation of marrow hypointensity relative to intervertebral disks assists in distinction of marrow replacement by tumor from prominent hematopoietic marrow.

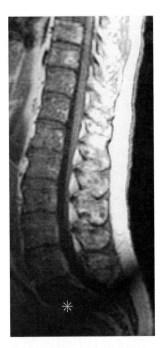

Fig. 16-20. Metastatic involvement of the spinal column by prostate cancer in 67-year-old male is manifested as diffuse marked reduction in marrow signal intensity on T1-weighted sagittal image (TR 500, TE 11, 2 Nex). Artifactual reduced signal intensity is noted along the bottom of the image *(asterisk),* where the effective field-of-view of the surface coil has been exceeded.

pressed T2-weighted or STIR images will depict hematopoietic marrow elements as moderately hyperintense, which can cause further confusion for tumor involvement.

In patients with prominent hematopoietic marrow, the vertebral bodies usually maintain a somewhat higher signal intensity than intervertebral disks on T1-weighted images; with diffuse tumor involvement, this relationship is reversed (Figs. 16-19 and 16-20). This has been termed the *hyperintense disk sign* of diffuse vertebral column tumor involvement,[12] and it can be useful in equivocal cases (Fig. 16-21). However, hyperintensity of disk material relative to adjacent marrow can be very subtle in some patients, and the conspicuousness of this finding can be affected by photographic image display (i.e., window width and level) settings.[12] Further, the intervertebral disks can appear hyperintense relative to the vertebral bodies in some severely anemic patients with hyperplastic hematopoietic marrow or in patients with iron overload affecting the marrow space (Figs. 16-22 and 16-23). Thus, when this sign is observed, correlation with clinical history and laboratory data remains important to establish whether the patient has known anemia or malignancy. In patients with equivocal findings or those in whom the vertebral bodies are relatively isointense with the intervertebral disks on T1-weighted im-

ages, further data can be obtained using intravenous contrast material. The disks will often become noticeably hypointense relative to the enhancing vertebral bodies in patients with diffuse tumor replacement on contrast enhanced T1-weighted images.[43] Use of fat suppressed T1-weighted images will render these findings more conspicuous. In addition, bone scintigraphy can be very useful in characterizing these signal abnormalities in equivocal cases.

Chronic disuse also results in generalized decreased signal intensity throughout the vertebral column on T2-weighted images.[32] Decreased height of the intervertebral disks can also be observed in patients with chronic disuse.

High signal intensity foci

Discrete foci of relative increased signal intensity are frequently observed in the spinal column on T1-weighted images. These findings usually represent either lipid rests or vertebral hemangiomas[25,45] (Fig. 16-24). The hyperintense appearance of hemangiomas on T1-weighted images is related to fat interspersed among their trabeculae.[54] Fatty marrow changes can potentially simulate hemorrhagic lesions or cystic lesions containing proteinaceous material, although both of these entities are

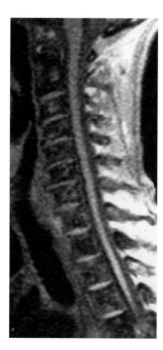

Fig. 16-21. Midsagittal T1-weighted image (TR 550, TE 10, 2 Nex) in patient with prostate cancer. Note diffuse hypointensity of the marrow space caused by metastatic involvement and relative hyperintensity of the intervertebral disks as compared with adjacent bone marrow.

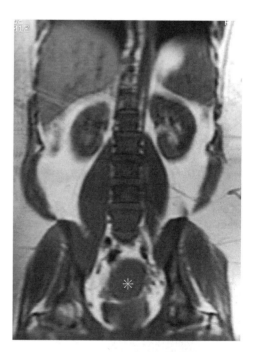

Fig. 16-22. Coronal T1-weighted image (TR 500, TE 11, 2 Nex) in 34-year-old female with menorrhagia caused by a myomatous uterus *(asterisk)* and secondary severe anemia. There is diffuse marked reduction of marrow signal intensity, with hypointensity of the vertebral bodies relative to adjacent intervertebral disks. These findings are the result of hyperplastic hematopoietic marrow and not tumor replacement.

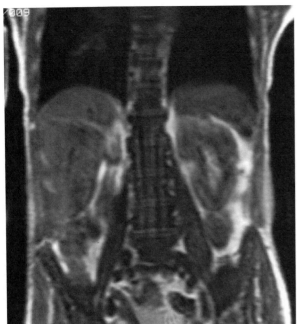

Fig. 16-23. Coronal T1-weighted image (TR 300, TE 12, 4 Nex) in 78-year-old male with iron overload. There is markedly decreased marrow signal intensity throughout the vertebral column, resulting in hypointensity of the vertebrae relative to intervertebral disks. These findings are due to increased iron stores within the marrow space and simulate the appearance of diffuse metastatic involvement.

distinctly unusual in the spinal column. However, in equivocal cases, fat suppressed T1-weighted or STIR images will allow differentiation between these entities.

Linear regions of increased signal intensity can be observed in normal individuals on T1-weighted images within the midportion of the vertebral body. This also represents focal fatty changes within the marrow space, which have a predilection to occur along the course of the basivertebral vein (Figs. 16-25 and 16-26). This can cause the vertebral column to have a horizontally striated appearance, with alternating laminae of relative increased and decreased signal intensity.

The basivertebral venous complex itself demonstrates linear low signal intensity on T1-weighted images and increased signal intensity on T2-weighted images (Fig. 16-27). The latter findings are due to slow blood flow within these veins and are accentuated on the second echo of dual echo sequences and when gradient moment nulling is used for artifact reduction. Absence of the high signal intensity of the basivertebral vein on such images may be a subtle indication of marrow replacement.[3] The vertebral endplate veins can be shown on MR images, particularly when contrast material is given.[56] Chemical shift misregistration artifacts can simulate or obscure these endplate veins.

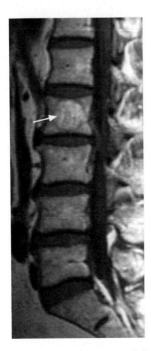

Fig. 16-24. A rounded focus of increased signal intensity *(arrow)* is observed within the L2 vertebral body on sagittal T1-weighted image (TR 500, TE 12, 2 Nex) in 69-year-old female, representing a lipid rest.

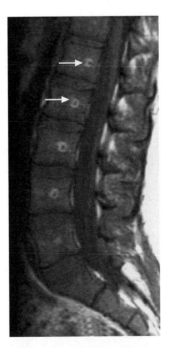

Fig. 16-25. Midsagittal T1-weighted image (TR 500, TE 12, 2 Nex) in 18-year-old male demonstrates linear high signal intensity within the midportion of each visualized vertebral body *(arrows).* These findings reflect focal increased proportion of marrow fat that occurs along the course of basivertebral veins.

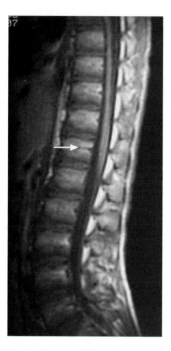

Fig. 16-26. Midsagittal T1-weighted image (TR 600, TE 12, 2 Nex) of 11-year-old male. Decreased signal intensity within the thoracolumbar vertebral bodies is demonstrated in the region of the basivertebral veins *(arrow)*. Note relative hyperintensity surrounding the basivertebral vein caused by focal fatty changes.

HYPERINTENSE FOCI VERTEBRAL BODIES

- Fatty marrow along basivertebral vein
- Hyperintensity of basivertebral vein
- Lipid rests
- Hemangiomas
- Chemical shift misregistration artifact
- Postradiation changes
- Motion (respiratory, cardiac) artifacts
- Fat suppression failure artifacts
- Aliasing artifacts
- Susceptibility (ferromagnetic) artifact
- Inflammatory endplate changes
- Postoperative changes

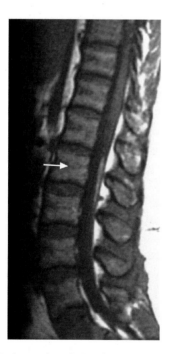

Fig. 16-27. Relative reduced signal intensity is observed within the vertebral bodies along the course of the basivertebral veins *(arrow)* on midsagittal T1-weighted image (TR 500, TE 12, 2 Nex).

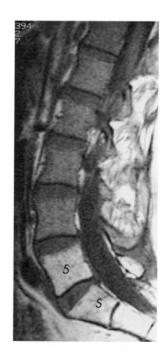

Fig. 16-28. A 49-year-old male with history of lymphoma. There is markedly increased marrow signal intensity within the L5 vertebral body *(5)* and upper sacrum *(S)* on this sagittal T1-weighted image (TR 500, TE 12, 2 Nex), corresponding to the port that was used for administration of radiation therapy. A sharp demarcation in marrow signal intensity is observed along the margins of the radiation port.

Radiation changes

Depletion of cellular marrow elements occurs in patients who have undergone prior radiation therapy to the spine. Consequently, irradiated marrow demonstrates signal intensity characteristics compatible with those of fat on all pulse sequences.[49,51,69] This is most noticeable as markedly increased marrow signal intensity on T1-weighted images (Fig. 16-28). A sharp interface between normal-appearing and hyperintense marrow is observed, corresponding to the margins of the radiation port. The onset of visible signal alterations in the vertebral column following radiation therapy is variable; it appears to depend on elapsed time as well as administered dose.[49] In patients who have received spinal radiation, relative decreased signal intensity of nonirradiated normal marrow can simulate metastatic involvement (Fig. 16-29). Increased vertebral marrow signal on T1-weighted images also occurs following bone marrow transplantation.[60]

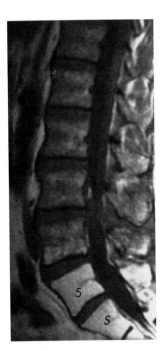

Fig. 16-29. There is relative decreased marrow signal intensity involving the T12 through L4 vertebral bodies on this midsagittal T1-weighted image (TR 500, TE 12, 2 Nex), which suggests the presence of metastatic involvement. However, these levels are normal, with their apparent hypointensity related to increased signal intensity within the L5 vertebral body (5) and sacrum (S) as a result of previous radiation therapy. Several observations help to distinguish these normal vertebrae from tumor involvement, including lack of vertebral expansion, small foci of preserved marrow fat, and preservation of the basivertebral veins. Absence of vertebral metastases was confirmed on subsequent CT scan and radionuclide bone scan.

Role of pulse sequence

The conspicuousness of vertebral lesions depends on the degree to which such lesions and surrounding normal marrow are of different signal intensity. Contrast between these tissues can be affected by many of the variations in marrow composition already discussed, as well as by pulse sequence parameters. When fatty marrow predominates, vertebral lesions are generally more conspicuous on T1- rather than T2-weighted images (Figs. 16-30, A-C). In patients who have received spinal radiation, the increased proportion of fatty marrow can therefore improve the conspicuousness of marrow lesions on T1-weighted images (Fig. 16-31, A and B). Conversely, when hematopoietic elements predominate, T2-weighted images are generally more sensitive (Fig. 16-32, A and B). Because neither T1- nor T2-weighted sequences are consistently superior for detection of vertebral lesions, both should be employed when such lesions are suspected.

Fat suppression sequences

Fat suppression may be used in conjunction with T2-weighted spin echo or inversion recovery (i.e., STIR) sequences to further improve the conspicuousness of vertebral lesions as compared with standard T2-weighted images. However, fat suppression will decrease the conspicuousness of marrow lesions when used on T1-weighted sequences, although water suppression can be helpful for improving lesion contrast (Fig. 16-33, A and B).

Fast spin echo sequences

Fast spin echo, or RARE (rapid acquisition relaxation enhanced), T2-weighted images can be acquired considerably faster than conventional T2-weighted spin echo images. Tissue contrast on fast spin echo images generally parallels that displayed on conventional images, although one important difference is that fat is of considerably higher signal intensity. As a result, contrast between vertebral lesions and surrounding marrow can

---

CAUSES FOR REDUCED DEPICTION OF VERTEBRAL LESIONS

- Surrounding hematopoietic marrow (T1-weighted images)
- Surrounding fatty marrow (T2-weighted images)
- Fat-suppressed T1-weighted images
- Fast spin echo T2-weighted images
- Contrast material–enhanced T1-weighted images
- Gradient echo images
- Motion artifacts
- Located beyond sensitive range of surface coil
- Aliasing artifacts

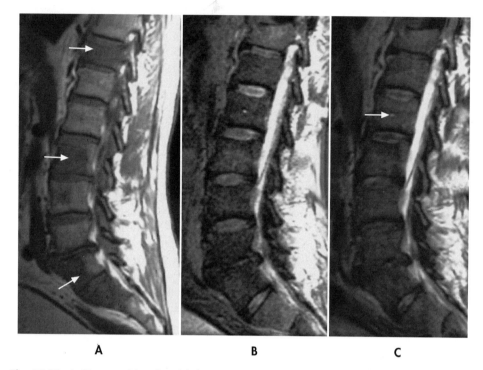

A   B   C

Fig. 16-30. A 65-year-old male with lung carcinoma. **A,** Sagittal T1-weighted image (TR 500, TE 12, 2 Nex) demonstrates extensive metastatic involvement of the thoracolumbar spine *(arrows)*. The conspicuousness and apparent extent of involvement are considerably greater than on **B,** the corresponding T2-weighted image (TR 2000, TE 75, 1 Nex). **C,** Further reduction in lesion conspicuousness occurs on fast spin echo T2-weighted image (TR 4000, effective TE 102, 4 Nex, 16 echo train length) because of isointensity between lesions and hyperintense marrow fat. Incidental note is made of a focus of relative increased signal intensity within the L1 vertebral body *(arrow)* caused by slow flow within the basivertebral vein.

be considerably decreased on fast spin echo T2-weighted images (Figs. 16-30, A-C and 16-34, A and B). The use of fat saturation will render marrow lesions more conspicuous for T2-weighted fast spin echo imaging. Fast spin echo images are also predisposed to blurring, particularly when short echo times or long echo train lengths are used (Fig. 16-35, A and B).

Contrast enhanced imaging

Spinal column lesions are also generally less conspicuous on T1-weighted images acquired after contrast material administration. In such circumstances, marrow lesions may become completely obscured as the high signal intensity of enhancing lesions approaches that of surrounding fatty marrow (Figs. 16-36, A to 16-38, B). Thus if contrast material is to be used, unenhanced T1-weighted images should always be acquired first. Fat suppressed T1-weighted images can be used to markedly improve the conspicuousness of enhancing marrow lesions as compared with conventional enhanced T1-weighted images.[46]

In patients who have received chemotherapy or radiotherapy, it has been observed that reduction in the intensity of vertebral lesion enhancement indicates a favorable treatment response, whereas persistent strong enhancement implies lack of response.[62] However, post-treatment contrast enhancement patterns are highly variable, even among patients with the same tumor type.[47]

Gradient echo imaging

The conspicuousness of vertebral lesions varies on gradient echo images and depends on the particular TR, TE, and flip angle, as well as the type of gradient echo sequence used. In general, gradient echo images are somewhat less sensitive for depicting vertebral lesions than are spin echo images. This is due in part to susceptibility effects generated by different components of the marrow space, including bony trabeculae, fat, and cellular elements. Differences in magnetization among these components leads to accentuation of artifactual signal intensity loss on gradient echo images, which can obscure underlying lesions.

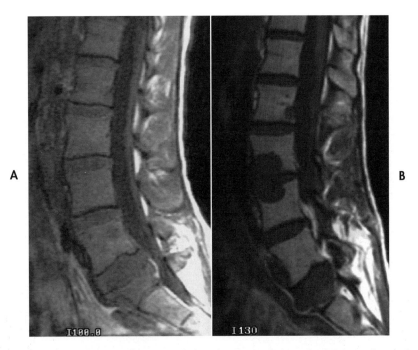

Fig. 16-31. A, The presence of metastatic involvement of the spinal column is relatively inconspicuous on initial T1-weighted sagittal image (TR 500, TE 12, 2 Nex) in 31-year-old female with breast cancer. However, repeat image, **B,** acquired 1 month later, following initiation of radiation therapy, shows markedly increased signal intensity caused by fatty elements throughout the marrow space. This renders the metastatic lesions easier to detect.

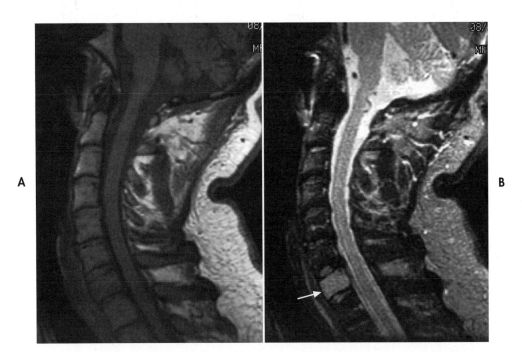

Fig. 16-32. A, Sagittal T1-weighted image (TR 566, TE 19, 2 Nex) in 52-year-old male with renal carcinoma is essentially unremarkable. However, **B,** corresponding T2-weighted image (TR 2200, TE 80, 1 Nex), reveals large focus of abnormal signal intensity within the C6 vertebral body *(arrow)*, representing a focus of metastatic involvement. Although the reason for lack of visualization of this lesion on T1-weighted image is unclear, it is possible that hemorrhagic breakdown products within the lesion rendered it isointense with surrounding marrow fat.

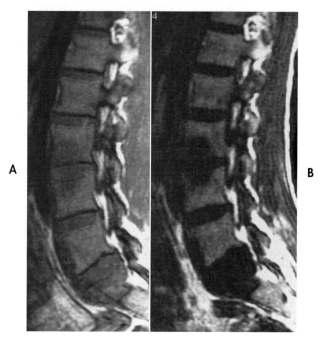

Fig. 16-33. A, Conventional T1-weighted image (TR 500, TE 12, 2 Nex) and **B,** T1-weighted image acquired using identical parameters with water suppression. Metastatic lesions as a result of breast carcinoma are considerably more conspicuous on the water suppressed image. This is due to heightened differentiation in signal intensity between the suppressed lesion and surrounding preserved marrow fat.

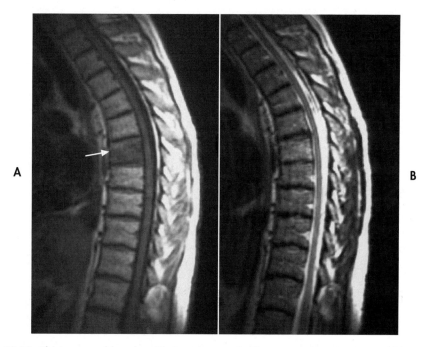

Fig. 16-34. Thirty-year-old male with lymphoma. **A,** Marrow replacement caused by tumor involvement of the T6 vertebral body *(arrow)* is evident on sagittal T1-weighted image (TR 500, TE 10, 2 Nex). However, tumor involvement is inconspicuous on **B,** corresponding fast spin echo T2-weighted image (TR 4000, effective TE 96, 4 Nex, 16 echo train length), because of isointensity between tumor and surrounding marrow fat.

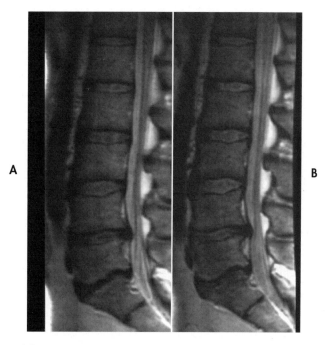

Fig. 16-35. Sagittal fast spin echo proton density–weighted images of the lumbar spine (TR 4000, TE 17, 4 Nex) obtained using an echo train length of, **A,** 16 and, **B,** 8. Accentuated image blurring, observable at the diskovertebral junctions, is present on the longer echo train image.

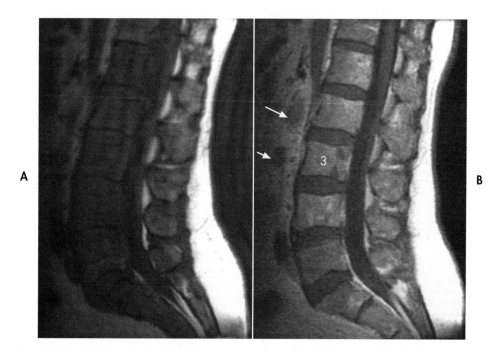

Fig. 16-36. A 59-year-old male with prostate cancer. **A,** Diffuse metastatic involvement of the lumbar spinal column is evident on midsagittal T1-weighted image (TR 500, TE 12, 2 Nex). **B,** Tumor involvement is largely obscured on T1-weighted image acquired following gadolinium chelate administration using identical imaging parameters. Two small foci of abnormality continue to be evident within the posterior L3 vertebra (3), although the extent of disease would be greatly underestimated on the basis of the contrast enhanced image alone. Enlarged retroperitoneal lymph nodes *(arrows)* are also noted.

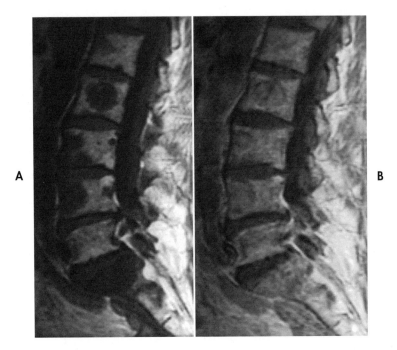

Fig. 16-37. A, Multiple foci of abnormal signal intensity, representing foci of metastatic tumor involvement, are evident on sagittal T1-weighted image (TR 600, TE 12, 2 Nex). **B,** Following gadolinium chelate administration, T1-weighted image acquired using identical parameters shows markedly decreased lesion conspicuousness compared to the precontrast image.

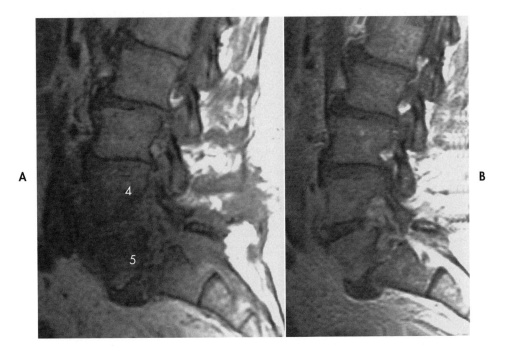

Fig. 16-38. A, Abnormal marrow signal intensity involving the L4 (4) and L5 (5) vertebral bodies because of osteomyelitis is evident on sagittal T1-weighted image (TR 600, TE 12, 2 Nex). Extensive inflammatory soft tissue component is also present and extends into the spinal canal and neural foramina. Alterations within the posterior paraspinal soft tissues are related to previous spinal surgery. **B,** Following gadolinium chelate administration, the marrow abnormality is essentially obscured, although the soft tissue abnormalities remain evident.

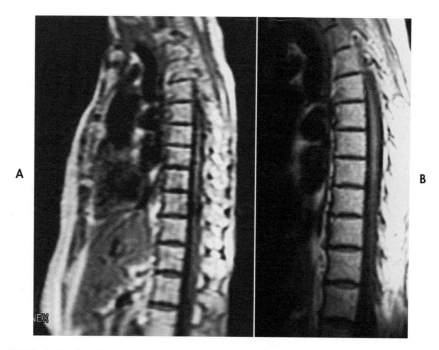

Fig. 16-39. A, Sagittal T1-weighted body coil image (TR 500, TE 10, 2 Nex) in 72-year-old female with breast cancer. Heterogeneous low signal intensity foci are evident involving several mid-lower thoracic vertebral bodies, raising suspicion for metastatic tumor involvement. These findings, however, are due to phase-encoding errors related to cardiac pulsation. **B,** The use of a posteriorly positioned surface coil and presaturation band placed over the heart (TR 500, TE 10, 2 Nex) allows the vertebrae to be better visualized and demonstrate a normal appearance.

Motion artifacts

Artifactual increased or decreased signal intensity involving the vertebral column and paravertebral soft tissues can arise from motion. When motion occurs during image acquisition, there can be blurring of anatomic structures and/or structured "ghosting" artifacts. These artifacts can obscure or simulate vertebral lesions (Figs. 16-39, A and B and 16-40). In the cervical spine, motion artifacts are most often due to swallowing, whereas in the thoracolumbar region respiratory motion and vascular pulsation artifacts emanating from the heart and aorta are prevalent (Fig. 16-41). These structured motion artifacts are consistently expressed along the phase-encoding axis of the image; this is usually the antero-posterior direction when spinal imaging is performed (Fig. 16-42).

Several options exist for reducing the severity of motion artifacts for spinal imaging. Sagittal images can be acquired with the phase-encoding gradient aligned along the craniocaudal direction, so that motion artifacts do not directly traverse the spinal canal.[27] This presents several disadvantages, including aliasing or wraparound of tissue extending beyond the field-of-view into the image. Phase-encoding steps can be reordered with reference

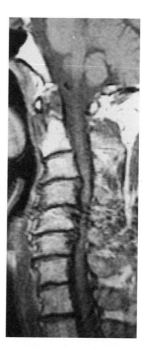

Fig. 16-40. A band of artifactual signal intensity related to swallowing traverses the midcervical spine along the phase-encoding direction on this midsagittal T1-weighted image (TR 600, TE 19, 2 Nex). This artifact obscures detail in a region affected by spondylosis and central spinal stenosis.

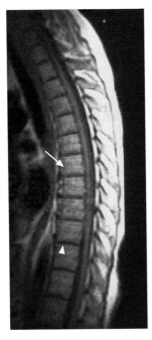

Fig. 16-41. Artifactual signal reduction is evident within the marrow space of the lower thoracic vertebrae on this midsagittal T1-weighted image (TR 500, TE 10, 2 Nex) because of reduced signal-to-noise ratio beyond the sensitive range of the surface coil. Also noted is artifactual signal intensity overlying the vertebral column and spinal cord because of cardiac pulsations *(arrow)*. A dark line is evident along the inferior endplate of each vertebral body *(arrowhead),* which is not observed along the superior endplate. This latter finding is caused by a chemical shift misregistration artifact, which occurs at the diskovertebral junction.

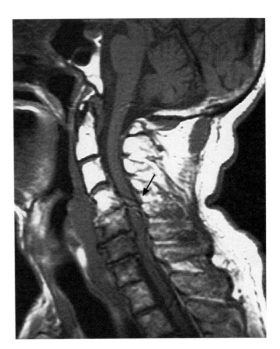

Fig. 16-42. Midsagittal T1-weighted image (TR 500, TE 11, 2 Nex) in patient with marked cervical spondylosis and central canal stenosis. There is a band of relative increased signal intensity *(arrow)* extending along the phase-encoding direction of the image, caused by swallowing artifact. Artifacts overlie the spinal cord, simulating pathologically increased signal intensity.

REDUCTION OF MOTION ARTIFACTS FOR SPINAL IMAGING

- Gradient reorientation
- Respiratory-ordered phase encoding
- Electrocardiogram (ECG) gating
- Radiofrequency presaturation bands
- Surface coils
- Gradient moment nulling
- Patient reassurance, communication
- Two-dimensional (versus three-dimensional) Fourier transform

---

to the cardiac cycle to decrease pulsation artifacts related to motion of cerebrospinal fluid (CSF).[13] Radiofrequency presaturation bands can be positioned over moving structures (e.g., aorta, heart, esophagus) to reduce the signal intensity of motion artifacts arising from these structures (Fig. 16-41). When doing so, one must be cautious to avoid positioning the presaturation band too close to the spine. Artifactual decreased vertebral signal intensity can occur because of the proximity of presaturation bands, simulating marrow replacement (Fig. 16-43A and B).

Surface coils

Surface coils are important for spinal imaging so that an adequate signal-to-noise ratio can be achieved in combination with relatively small voxel sizes.[27] Surface coils are also useful in that reception of signal intensity is limited to the immediate vicinity of the coil. Consequently, there is little signal generated from fat in the anterior thoracic or abdominal wall, and artifacts caused by motion of such tissues are therefore limited. Surface coils receive signal over a limited distance, with the sensitive volume of the coil approximately equal to its radius. Rapid decline in signal intensity occurs beyond this sensitive volume; this can cause normal marrow to appear hypoin-

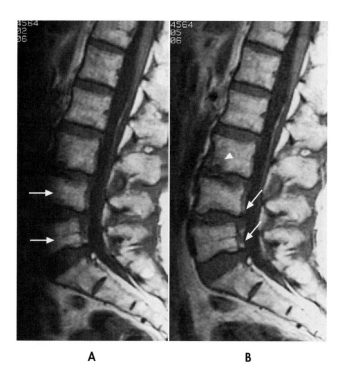

A   **B**

Fig. 16-43. A, Reduced signal intensity is observed within the anterior aspect of the lower lumbar vertebral bodies *(arrows)* on this sagittal T1-weighted image (TR 500, TE 12, 2 Nex). An anterior spatially selective presaturation band was used on this image to reduce vascular pulsation artifacts arising from the aorta. **B,** When the presaturation band was moved further anterior, the signal intensity of the vertebral bodies is seen to be normal. Note relative increased signal intensity immediately posterior to the vertebral bodies *(arrows),* caused by slow flow within the anterior epidural venous plexus. In addition, a focus of decreased marrow signal intensity is present within the anteroinferior aspect of L3 *(arrowhead),* representing a Schmorl's node.

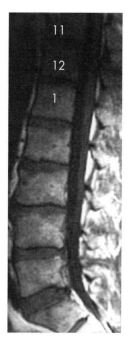

Fig. 16-44. Reduced signal intensity is present within the T11 (11), T12 (12), and L1 (1) vertebral bodies on this midsagittal T1-weighted image (TR 500, TE 12, 2 Nex). Whereas this signal reduction may suggest marrow replacement, it relates to decreased signal-to-noise ratio within tissue that extends beyond the sensitive range of the surface coil.

tense, thus simulating marrow replacement[4] (Figs. 16-20, 16-41, and 16-44). Further, vertebral lesions located beyond the sensitive range of the coil may be obscured as a result of the low signal-to-noise ratio. Software algorithms that compensate for signal drop-off encountered with surface coils are available; the result is a more uniform signal profile across the image.[44]

On fat suppressed sequences, failure to suppress fat signal intensity may occur in the vicinity of the surface coil because of local variations in the magnetic field (see Fig. 18-26). These fat suppression failure artifacts can simulate or obscure either marrow or soft tissue lesions in this location.

Phase-encoding steps can be reordered according to the respiratory cycle to allow for a reduction in respiratory motion artifacts; this technique is known as respiratory-ordered phase encoding, or respiratory compensation. Gradient moment nulling (i.e., flow compensation) techniques cause moving spins to be rephased at the time of echo collection. The additional gradient lobes introduced with this method require relatively long echo times, and they are therefore usually implemented on T2-weighted sequences. Gradient moment nulling is helpful for reducing vascular pulsation as well as respiratory motion artifacts.

Patient reassurance and communication are helpful in decreasing gross patient motion, although sedation may be necessary in patients who are particularly anxious or uncomfortable. As mentioned previously, in patients who are moving, one must be cautious that errors in numbering of vertebrae and intervertebral disks do not occur. For example, numbering errors can arise when transaxial images are numbered by referencing them to previously acquired sagittal images. Motion of the patient between acquisition of the sagittal and transaxial sequences will cause potentially serious errors in identification of vertebral levels and associated pathologic conditions.

Motion artifacts are accentuated on three-dimensional Fourier transform sequences, which are frequently used to evaluate the cervical spine,[68,71] because phase encoding is performed along the conventional phase-encoding

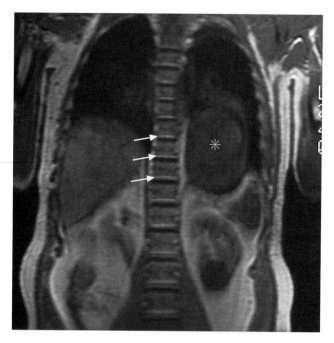

Fig. 16-45. There is relative hyperintensity along the inferior endplate region *(arrows)* and corresponding hypointensity along the superior endplates of all thoracic vertebral bodies on coronal T1-weighted image (TR 833, TE 12, 4 Nex). This is due to chemical shift misregistration artifact, occurring along the frequency-encoding direction of the image. Also noted is a large left thoracic mass representing a left ventricular pseudoaneurysm *(asterisk).*

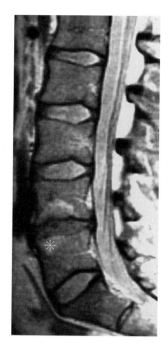

Fig. 16-46. Midsagittal fast spin echo proton density–weighted image (TR 4000, effective TE 13, 4 Nex, 8 echo train length). There is focal absence of low signal intensity along the superior endplate of the L5 vertebral body. This is due to chemical shift misregistration artifact related to focal fatty changes within the vertebral body *(asterisk).*

axis as well as along the slice selection axis. Three-dimensional sequences also display aliasing (i.e., wraparound) artifacts along the slice selection as well as the conventional phase-encoding direction.[68,71] Images of structures situated along the upper spine can thus be represented on images acquired through the lower spine. These aliasing artifacts can simulate or obscure lesions involving the spinal column or paravertebral soft tissues or those found within the spinal canal.

Chemical shift misregistration artifacts

Chemical shift misregistration artifacts are due to differences in the precessional frequency of fat and water protons. This results in artifactual shift of signal intensity at fat-water interfaces along the frequency-encoding direction of the image, which is usually superior-inferior for sagittal spine imaging. Because the diskovertebral junction represents a fat-water interface, chemical shift misregistration can result in artifactual shift of signal intensity from one vertebral endplate to the opposite endplate on sagittal spine images[17] (Figs. 16-41, 16-45, and 16-46). This effect can be observed on both T1- and T2-weighted images and is more prominent with use of high field strength magnets and large voxel sizes and when a

narrow receiver bandwidth is used to increase the signal-to-noise ratio (Fig. 16-47).

Metallic artifacts

Ferromagnetic objects distort local magnetic field gradients in their vicinity, resulting in artifactual signal void, which can be associated with peripheral hyperintensity. These "susceptibility" artifacts can simulate or obscure vertebral lesions (Fig. 16-2). They are of increased prominence on images acquired using high field strength magnets, long echo times, large voxel sizes, and gradient echo rather than spin echo sequences[15,70] (Fig. 16-48A-D). In the spine these artifacts can be related to spinal fixation rods, bullet fragments or other metallic foreign bodies, or surgical clips in the posterior mediastinum or retroperitoneum. They may also be due to metal filings or hardware associated with previous spinal surgery[10,33,45] (Fig. 16-49). Stainless steel fixation wires produce severe susceptibility artifacts; titanium wire is far less damaging to image quality.[40] Severe artifacts can also result from many cervical spine braces, halos, and orthoses, although nonferrous orthoses made of aluminum, graphite-composite, and plastic components are available.[14] Some nonferrous stabilization devices can

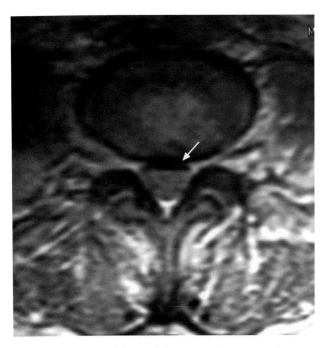

Fig. 16-47. Transaxial proton density–weighted image (TR 2500, TE 35, 2 Nex) demonstrates artifactual loss of signal intensity along the anterior margin of the thecal sac *(arrow)* caused by chemical shift misregistration artifact. When there is bulging of the intervertebral disk, this artifact can result in overestimation of the extent of disk protrusion. The phase-encoding direction is assigned along the right-left direction to direct aortic pulsation artifacts away from the spinal canal.

also cause artifacts because of generation of eddy currents and other effects.[38]

In addition to obscuring anatomy, susceptibility effects generated at bone-tissue-CSF interfaces can create artifactual distortion of the spinal canal and cause overestimation of spinal stenosis[15] (Fig. 16-50). Inhomogeneity of the main magnetic field or nonlinearity of the gradient magnetic fields can also result in distortion of anatomic features.[6] Fast spin echo sequences are generally less vulnerable than standard spin echo sequences to susceptibility artifacts because of the refocusing effect of the multiple 180-degree pulses applied.

Vertebral Disorders
Vertebral endplate signal alterations

Vertebral signal intensity alterations can occur within the endplates bordering degenerated intervertebral disks. These changes generally progress through three phases.[16,41] Initially, there is decreased marrow signal intensity on T1-weighted images and increased intensity on T2-weighted images. These type I changes are due to edema and/or granulation tissue and can demonstrate abnormal enhancement when intravenous contrast material

is given.[28,55,57] The above findings can simulate vertebral infection, tumor, or other lesions. Fatty metamorphosis characterizes type II endplate changes, which appear as markedly hyperintense on T1-weighted images and mildly hyperintense on T2-weighted images (Fig. 16-51). Sclerosis ultimately develops, appearing markedly hypointense on all sequences (type III changes).

Distinction of these signal changes from other pathologic conditions is based on their characteristic involvement of the vertebral endplate and visualization of associated disk degeneration. Degeneration presents as decreased signal intensity of the affected disk on T2-weighted images, often with associated loss of height and disk protrusion. When the adjacent intervertebral disk has a normal appearance, other etiologies for the vertebral signal alterations should be considered.

Other forms of vertebral pathologic conditions also demonstrate considerable overlap in their MR appearance. For example, signal intensity and morphologic alterations resulting from vertebral neoplasm, infection, avascular necrosis, Paget's disease, and fracture may be difficult to distinguish in some patients[59] (Figs. 16-52, A and B). Involvement of two contiguous vertebral bodies and the intervertebral disk between them often characterizes spinal infection rather than neoplasia. There are, however, exceptions to this rule. Infectious processes, including tuberculosis, can involve a single vertebral body, sparing the adjacent disk.[1] This appearance simulates neoplasia, particularly when there is an associated soft tissue mass. Bone destruction usually indicates an aggressive process, such as tumor or infection. However, large disk fragments can occasionally result in bone erosion.

Vertebral compression fractures

MR imaging has been used to differentiate osteoporotic (i.e., insufficiency) vertebral fractures from pathologic (i.e., neoplastic) vertebral fractures. Such distinction is based on observation of preserved marrow signal intensity in association with insufficiency fractures. On the other hand, pathologic fractures are typified by marrow replacement as well as decreased vertebral height. Although these criteria are useful in many patients, several pitfalls have been recognized. In patients who have sustained acute simple vertebral compression fracture, marrow edema and hemorrhage can appear to represent underlying tumor or infection[5,19,72] (Figs. 16-53 and 16-54). Less frequently, signal alterations caused by fibrosis or sclerosis can be present in patients with chronic insufficiency fractures, which can also result in misdiagnosis for tumor involvement.[5] Sacral insufficiency fractures can closely simulate neoplastic involvement (Fig. 16-55).

In an effort to improve distinction between simple and pathologic vertebral compression fractures, a quantitative

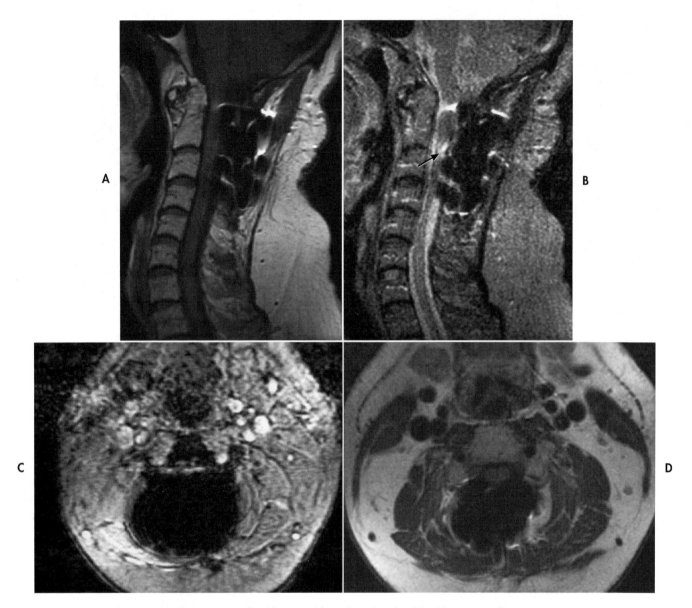

Fig. 16-48. A large zone of artifact manifested as signal void with surrounding hyperintensity is present on **A,** sagittal T1-weighted image (TR 550, TE 19, 2 Nex) and, **B,** T2-weighted (TR 2200, TE 80, 1 Nex) image in patient who underwent previous posterior cervical fusion. These susceptibility artifacts are more extensive on T2-weighted rather than T1-weighted images, and hyperintensity simulates intramedullary lesion *(arrow)* on the former. **C,** Also note blooming of artifact on transaxial three-dimensional spoiled gradient echo image (TR 35, TE 15, 5-degree flip angle, 1 Nex), where the spinal cord is completely obscured, as compared with **D,** corresponding T1-weighted image (TR 400, TE 20, 4 Nex).

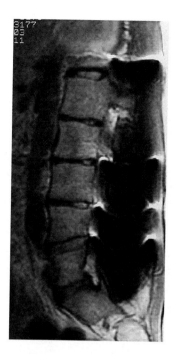

Fig. 16-49. Susceptibility artifacts manifested as areas of signal void with intervening foci of increased signal intensity, obscure visualization of the spinal canal on this sagittal proton density–weighted image (TR 2000, TE 30, 1 Nex) in a 27-year-old female with Harrington rods.

index of signal intensity has been used. When the signal intensity of the collapsed vertebral body is divided by the mean signal intensity of three adjacent vertebrae, a ratio of 0.8 or greater indicates that tumor involvement is unlikely.[35] Although contrast material can be considered as another tool for differentiating these entities, abnormal enhancement can occur in association with benign as well as malignant compression fractures.[43]

Vertebral avascular necrosis

In patients with vertebral compression, visualization of an intravertebral vacuum cleft on plain radiographs indicates avascular necrosis. This cleft may be difficult to visualize on MR images because of their relative insensitivity to depiction of small air collections. Malghem et al. have shown that paradoxical signal alterations can be observed in patients with vertebral avascular necrosis.[37] Initial images may demonstrate a signal void, compatible with air, whereas a region of increased signal intensity on T2-weighted images can be observed in the same location 20 to 40 minutes later. The latter finding indicates accumulation of fluid within the vacuum cleft, which occurs with supine positioning and can simulate malignancy or infection.

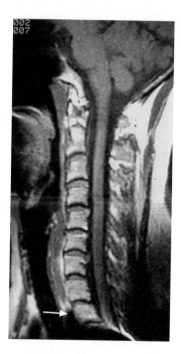

Fig. 16-50. Susceptibility artifacts related to metallic bra snaps obscure portions of the upper thoracic spine on this midsagittal T1-weighted (TR 567, TE 19, 2 Nex) image. Also note that portions of the spine *(arrow)* demonstrate anatomic distortion as a result of alteration in local magnetic field gradients.

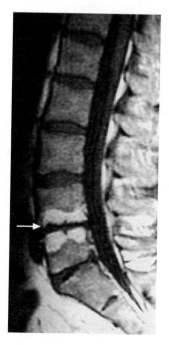

Fig. 16-51. Fatty changes result in markedly increased signal intensity involving the endplates bordering the L4-5 intervertebral disk *(arrow)* on this sagittal T1-weighted image (TR 500, TE 12, 2 Nex). These findings are secondary to degenerative disk disease, which has also resulted in narrowing and irregularity of the affected disk space.

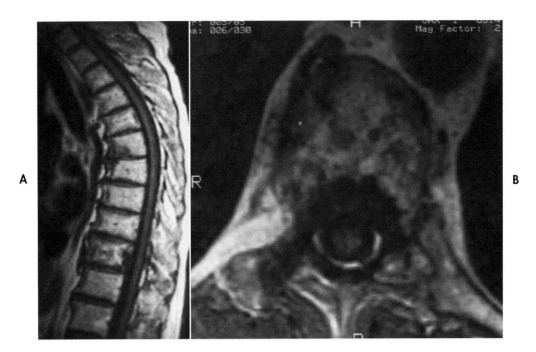

Fig. 16-52. Sagittal **(A)** and transaxial **(B)** T1-weighted images (TR 500, TE 17, 2 Nex) demonstrate marked heterogeneous signal intensity throughout the marrow space of the thoracic vertebral column. These findings, which are due to Paget's disease, closely simulate the appearance of metastatic involvement.

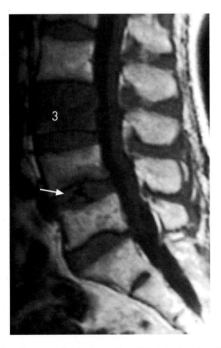

Fig. 16-53. Abnormal marrow signal intensity simulating tumor replacement involves the compressed L3 (3) vertebral body on this sagittal T1-weighted image (TR 500, TE 12, 2 Nex). These signal intensity alterations were due to marrow edema and hemorrhage in a patient who had sustained a recent simple compression fracture. Also note foci of relative decreased signal intensity within the L4-5 intervertebral disk *(arrow)* as a result of the vacuum phenomenon.

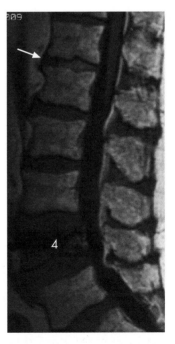

Fig. 16-54. Markedly reduced signal intensity is present throughout the compressed L4(4) vertebral body on this sagittal T1-weighted image (TR 350, TE 12, 2 Nex). Although this appearance suggests a pathologic compression fracture, this represents a posttraumatic compression fracture with secondary marrow edema. Increased signal intensity within the T12-L1 intervertebral disk *(arrow)* is due to calcification.

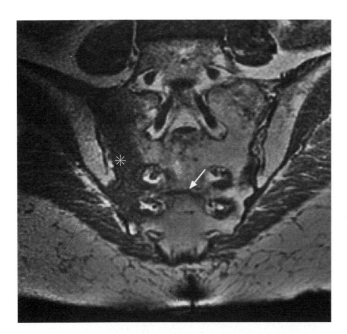

Fig. 16-55. Coronal oblique T1-weighted image (TR 350, TE 13, 2 Nex) in 68-year-old female with history of rectal carcinoma and back pain. Extensive decreased signal intensity is observed within the right sacral ala *(asterisk),* suggestive of possible tumor involvement. However, linear focus extending transversely across the midsacrum *(arrow)* indicates sacral insufficiency fracture with marrow edema, caused by previous radiation therapy in this patient.

Contrast enhanced imaging

Vertebral lesions demonstrate variable intensity and pattern of enhancement following contrast material administration (Fig. 16-56). As noted previously, vertebral metastases and other lesions may become less conspicuous on T1-weighted images acquired following contrast material administration as compared with unenhanced images,[9,43,61] because enhancement of lesions causes their signal intensity to become similar to that of surrounding normal marrow (Figs. 16-39 and 16-40). Use of fat suppressed T1-weighted images allows for a marked increase in conspicuousness of enhancing vertebral lesions. Limitations of fat suppressed imaging, however, include increased vulnerability to motion and magnetic susceptibility artifacts.[67]

Enhancement of vertebral lesions is not specific for malignancy; some benign vertebral lesions (e.g., hemangioma, osteomyelitis) also prominently enhance following contrast material administration[67] (Fig. 16-40).

POSTOPERATIVE SPINE

Many alterations in morphology and signal intensity are encountered in patients who have undergone previous spinal surgery. Bone fusion grafts have variable signal intensity, and their appearance varies according to whether autograft or allograft material has been used[52] (Figs. 16-57 and 16-58). In the lumbar spine the verte-

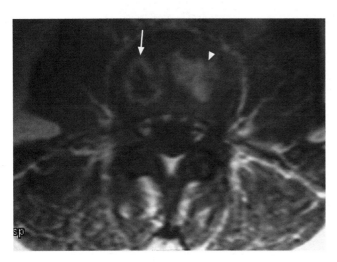

Fig. 16-56. Transaxial gadopentetate enhanced T1-weighted image (TR 500, TE 15, 2 Nex) in 54-year-old man with prostate cancer illustrates variable contrast enhancement patterns caused by metastatic involvement. Regions of ring enhancement *(arrow),* as well as separate foci of diffuse or nodular enhancement *(arrowhead),* are present at this single level, with additional variability noted on other images.

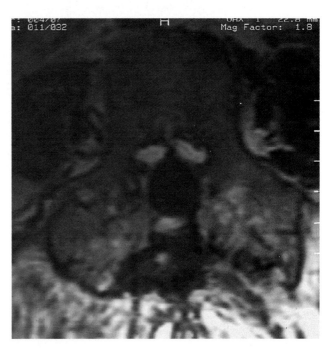

Fig. 16-57. T1-weighted transaxial image (TR 550, TE 15, 4 Nex) demonstrates absence of the spinous process as a result of previous posterior decompression and considerable hypertrophic bone related to lateral fusion masses.

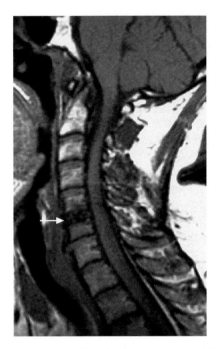

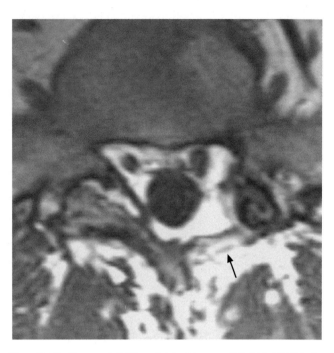

Fig. 16-58. Midsagittal T1-weighted image (TR 560, TE 20, 2 Nex) demonstrates relative decreased signal intensity at the C5-6 interspace *(arrow)* in patient who underwent previous fusion at this level.

Fig. 16-59. Transaxial T1-weighted image (TR 500, TE 15, 4 Nex) indicates large left laminectomy defect (arrow).

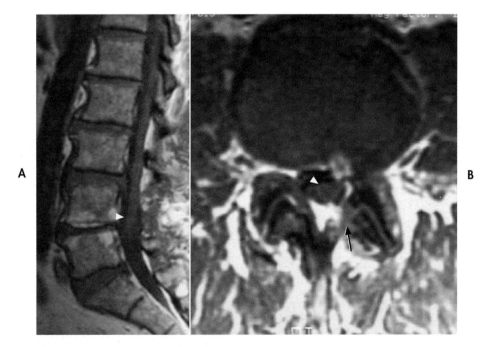

Fig. 16-60. Patient who had undergone previous laminectomy and diskectomy. **A,** Sagittal T1-weighted image (TR 500, TE 12, 2 Nex) before gadopentetate administration. **B,** Transaxial T1-weighted image (TR 500, TE 15, 4 Nex) after gadopentetate administration. The left laminectomy defect can be seen *(arrow),* with associated contrast enhancement caused by the presence of granulation tissue. Also noted is clumping of cava equina nerve roots *(arrowhead)* due to postoperative arachnoiditis.

bral endplates demonstrate signal intensity alterations in patients who have received chymopapain injections involving the adjacent intervertebral disk.[39] Laminectomy defects present a familiar appearance, although small laminotomy defects may be difficult to visualize on MR images[11] (Fig. 16-59). When gadopentetate dimeglumine is administered, contrast enhancement is often observed within the laminectomy site because of postoperative granulation tissue (Figs. 16-60A and B). Contrast enhancement of the facet joints has also been noted in postoperative patients,[8] and distortion as well as abnormal enhancement of the posterior paraspinal musculature can also occur.[53]

PARASPINAL SOFT TISSUES

Soft tissue inflammatory processes such as tuberculous spondylitis can simulate the appearance of neoplasm.[59] A hiatal hernia can appear to represent a cystic or necrotic mass anterior to the thoracic spinal column. Hernias of the inferior lumbar space can also simulate paravertebral mass lesions.[58] Soft tissue pseudotumors of the cervical spine can result from pannus material in patients with rheumatoid arthritis[2,10,31] (Fig. 16-61). Similar pseudotumors can also occur because of the reactive inflammatory tissue in patients with chronic vertebral subluxation.[64]

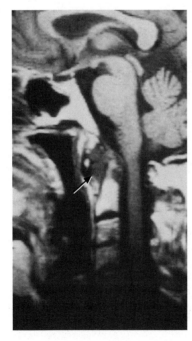

Fig. 16-61. Sagittal T1-weighted image (TR 500, TE 21) in patient with rheumatoid arthritis. There is a soft tissue mass noted in the atlantoaxial region *(arrow),* representing pannus formation. Atlantoaxial subluxation is also demonstrated.

Anatomic Variations

Normal anatomic structures can also appear to represent paravertebral soft tissue masses. Prominent ascending lumbar veins may display intermediate intraluminal signal intensity, similar to that of soft tissue, as a result of slow flow. These veins are recognized by their tubular course over multiple adjacent images. In equivocal cases, gradient echo sequences can be used to confirm the presence of blood flow. Prominent azygos or hemiazygos veins can simulate lymph nodes or other prevertebral masses in the thoracic region. In the cervical spine the pterygoid and posterior digastric muscles can appear rounded and masslike, particularly on coronal images. The collapsed esophagus and prevertebral fat stripe demonstrate relative increased signal intensity on T2-weighted images and can simulate a cervical prevertebral mass.[34] Fibrofatty tissue surrounding the superior aspect of the odontoid process is another cause for an apparent paravertebral soft tissue lesion.[18]

Fatty changes

Focal or diffuse regions of relative increased signal intensity on T1-weighted images can result from fatty replacement of the paraspinal muscles in paraplegic patients and others with chronic disuse (Fig. 16-62). Discrete, masslike fat collections may represent paraspinal lipomatosis in patients receiving corticosteroid therapy or those with adrenocortical tumors or hyperplasia.[21] Fat appears relatively hyperintense on T2-weighted fast spin echo (RARE) images[26]; this can potentially cause fat-containing soft tissue lesions to simulate other high signal intensity soft tissue lesions. Paraspinal fat, as well as other tissues, can also appear artifactually hyperintense because of its proximity to a posteriorly positioned sur-

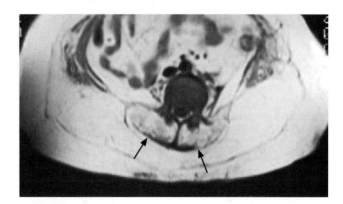

Fig. 16-62. Severe atrophy and fatty replacement of the paravertebral musculature (arrows) and psoas muscles bilaterally are evident on this transaxial T1-weighted image (TR 450, TE 11, 4 Nex) in 30-year-old paraplegic male. Relative decreased marrow signal intensity is also noted within the spinal column, caused by hyperplastic hematopoietic marrow secondary to anemia.

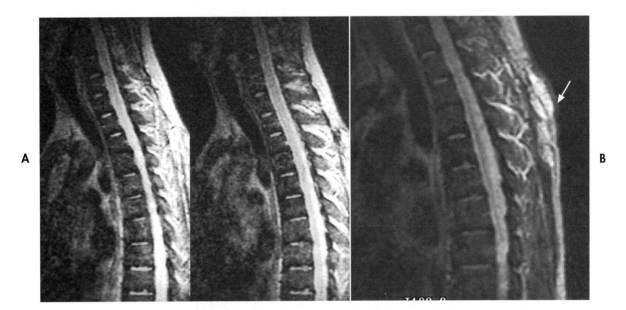

Fig. 16-63. A, Two-on-one filming protocol for sagittal T2-weighted images (TR 2000, TE 75, 1 Nex) results in partial exclusion of posterior subcutaneous soft tissue mass from image display. **B,** When the entire field-of-view is photographed, the mass *(arrow)* can be visualized.

face coil. This may also contribute to difficulty in distinguishing fat from fluid or other high signal intensity tissues on T2-weighted images.

Imaging Artifacts
Image display

Use of consistent image display settings (i.e., window width and level) is important for accurate representation of signal intensity characteristics of tissues in and around the spine. Inappropriate window and level settings (e.g., excessively narrow window width) can hinder visualization of some lesions and make characterization of some lesions difficult. Proper photographic practices must also be followed, since they can affect lesion detection. For example, sagittal spine images are frequently photographed using a two-on-one format. However, without proper attention, superficial lesions located within the posterior paraspinal soft tissues can be excluded from the image and will go undetected (Figs. 16-63, A and B).

Phase cancellation artifact

Curvilinear artifactual decreased signal intensity is often observed along the fascial planes of the paravertebral soft tissues on gradient echo images (Fig. 16-64). These represent chemical shift phase cancellation artifacts, which arise in voxels containing both fat and water protons when the magnetization of these tissues is of opposed phase at the time of echo collection. Use of a

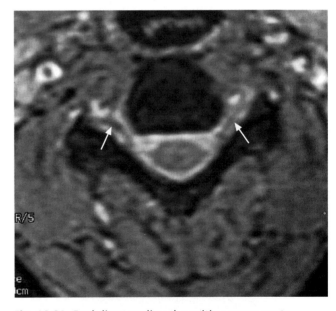

Fig. 16-64. Dark lines outline the exiting nerve roots *(arrows)* and fascial planes on this transaxial three-dimensional spoiled gradient echo image (TR 35, TE 15, 5-degree flip angle, 1 Nex). These findings represent chemical shift phase cancellation artifact, caused by use of an opposed phase echo time.

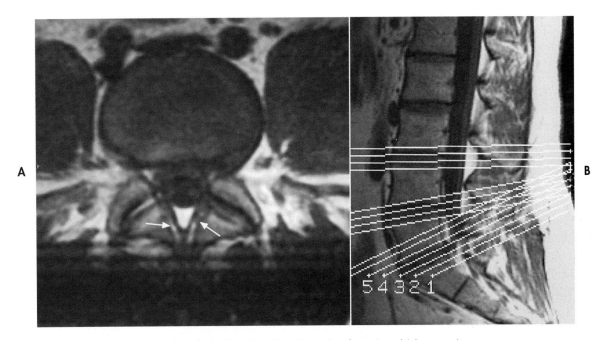

Fig. 16-65. A, A series of parallel signal void bands of varying thicknesses is present within the posterior paraspinal region, obscuring visualization of underlying soft tissue and bony structures on this axial oblique T1-weighted image (TR 500, TE 15, 4 Nex). This is due to overlap of imaging sections, which were acquired parallel to the intervertebral disks. This is depicted on T1-weighted sagittal reference image (TR 500, TE 12, 2 Nex), **B.** Relative hyperintensity of the ligamentum flavum *(arrows)* is also noted on the transaxial image **(A).**

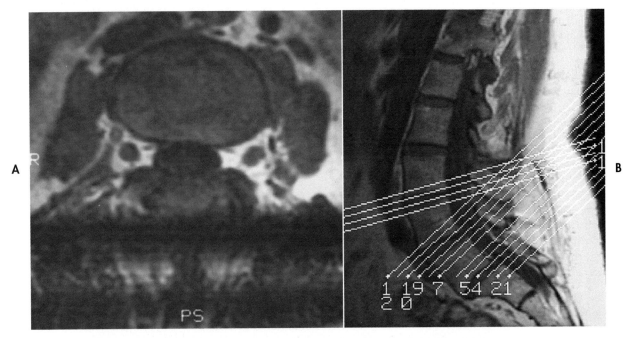

Fig. 16-66. A, Two broad linear foci of relative decreased signal intensity obscure portions of the posterior paraspinal musculature and bony structures on oblique axial T1-weighted image (TR 550, TE 15, 4 Nex). These represent areas of saturation where adjacent imaging sections overlap one another. The relationship between these overlapping sections is demonstrated in **B** (TR 500, TE 12, 2 Nex).

field strength–dependent in-phase echo time eliminates this artifact. This artifact is usually not present on spin echo images because of the refocusing effects of the 180-degree radiofrequency pulse.

Saturation artifact

Because the lumbar intervertebral disks are oblique with reference to the transaxial plane of the magnet, angled oblique images are frequently acquired. The amount of angulation required depends on the degree of lumbar lordosis. In patients with accentuated lumbar lordosis, oblique imaging slices often overlap posteriorly. This results in saturation effects, which are manifested as a series of linear foci of artifactually decreased signal intensity within the posterior paraspinal soft tissues (Figs. 16-65, A and B and 16-65, A and B). These artifacts can obscure lesions located within the posterior paraspinal soft tissues and possibly intraspinal lesions. When the initial sagittal series indicates that overlap of oblique axial images is likely to occur, a less acutely oblique angle can be prescribed or direct transaxial images may be substituted.

REFERENCES

1. Ahmadi J, Bajaj A, Destian S et al: Spinal tuberculosis: atypical observations at MR imaging, Radiology 189:489-493, 1993.
2. Aisen AM, Martel W, Ellis JH et al: Cervical spine involvement in rheumatoid arthritis: MR imaging, Radiology 165:159-163, 1987.
3. Algra PR, Bloem JL, Valk J: Disappearance of the basivertebral vein: a new MR imaging sign of bone marrow disease (letter), Am J Roentgenol 157:1129-1130, 1991.
4. Axel L, Costantini J, Listerud J: Intensity correction in surface-coil MR imaging, Am J Roentgenol 148:418-420, 1987.
5. Baker LL, Goodman SB, Perkash I et al: Benign versus pathologic compression fractures of vertebral bodies: assessment with conventional spin-echo, chemical-shift, and STIR MR imaging, Radiology 174:495-502, 1990.
6. Bakker CJ, Moerland MA, Bhagwandien R et al: Analysis of machine-dependent and object-induced geometric distortion in 2DFT MR imaging, Magn Reson Imaging 10:597-608, 1992.
7. Bergman RA, Thompson SA, Afifi AK et al: Compendium of human anatomic variation: text, atlas, and world literature, Baltimore, 1988, Urban & Schwarzenberg.
8. Boden SD, Davis DO, Dina TS et al: Contrast-enhanced MR imaging performed after successful lumbar disk surgery: prospective study, Radiology 182:59-64, 1992.
9. Breger RK, Williams AL, Daniels DL et al: Contrast enhancement in spinal MR imaging, Am J Neuroradiol 10:633-637, 1989.
10. Bundschuh CV, Modic MT, Kearney F et al: Rheumatoid arthritis of the cervical spine: surface-coil MR imaging, Am J Roentgenol 151:181-187, 1988.
11. Bundschuh CV, Modic MT, Ross JS et al: Epidural fibrosis and recurrent disk herniation in the lumbar spine: MR imaging assessment, Am J Roentgenol 150:923-932, 1988.
12. Castillo M, Malko JA, Hoffman JC Jr: The bright intervertebral disk: an indirect sign of abnormal spinal bone marrow on T1-weighted MR images, Am J Neuroradiol 11:23-26, 1990.
13. Cho MH, Kim WS, Cho ZH: CSF flow artifact reduction using cardiac cycle ordered phase-encoding method, Magn Reson Imaging 8:395-405, 1990.
14. Clayman DA, Murakami ME, Vines FS: Compatibility of cervical spine braces with MR imaging: a study of nine nonferrous devices, Am J Neuroradiol 11:385-390, 1990.
15. Czervionke LF, Daniels DL, Wehrli FW et al: Magnetic susceptibility artifacts in gradient-recalled echo MR imaging, Am J Neuroradiol 9:1149-1155, 1988.
16. de Roos A, Kressel H, Spritzer C et al: MR imaging of marrow changes adjacent to end plates in degenerative lumbar disk disease, Am J Roentgenol 149:531-534, 1987.
17. Dwyer AJ, Knop RH, Hoult DI: Frequency shift artifacts in MR imaging, J Comput Assist Tomogr 9:16-18, 1985.
18. Ellis JH, Martel W, Lillie JH et al: Magnetic resonance imaging of the normal craniovertebral junction, Spine 16:105-111, 1991.
19. Frager D, Elkin C, Swerdlow M et al: Subacute osteoporotic compression fracture: misleading magnetic resonance appearance, Skeletal Radiol 17:123-126, 1988.
20. Geremia GK, McCluney KW, Adler SS et al: The magnetic resonance hypointense spine of AIDS, J Comput Assist Tomogr 14:785-789, 1990.
21. Glickstein MF, Miller WT, Dalinka MK et al: Paraspinal lipomatosis: a benign mass, Radiology 163:79-80, 1987.
22. Grenier N, Greselle J-F, Vital J-M et al: Normal and disrupted lumbar longitudinal ligaments: correlative MR and anatomic study, Radiology 171:197-205, 1989.
23. Hahn PY, Strobel JJ, Hahn FJ: Verification of lumbar vertebral bodies: response to letter to editor, Radiology 185:616, 1992.
24. Hahn PY, Strobel JJ, Hahn FJ: Verification of lumbosacral segments on MR images: identification of transitional vertebrae, Radiology 182:580-581, 1992.
25. Hajek PC, Baker LL, Goobar JE et al: Focal fat deposition in axial bone marrow: MR characteristics, Radiology 162:245-249, 1987.
26. Henkelman RM, Hardy PA, Bishop JE et al: Why fat is bright in RARE and fast spin-echo imaging, J Magn Reson Imaging 2:533-540, 1992.
27. Holtas SL, Plewes DB, Simon JH et al: Technical aspects on magnetic resonance imaging of the spine at 1.5 tesla, Acta Radiol 28:375-381, 1987.
28. Hueftle MG, Modic MT, Ross JS et al: Lumbar spine: postoperative MR imaging with Gd-DTPA, Radiology 167:817-824, 1988.
29. Jinkins JR, Matthes JC, Sener RN et al: Spondylolysis, spondylolisthesis, and associated nerve root entrapment in the lumbosacral spine: MR evaluation, Am J Roentgenol 159:799-803, 1992.
30. Johnson DW, Farnum GN, Latchaw RE et al: MR imaging of the pars interarticularis, Am J Roentgenol 152:327-332, 1989.

31. Larsson EM, Holtas S, Zygmunt S: Pre- and postoperative MR imaging of the craniocervical junction in rheumatoid arthritis, Am J Roentgenol 152:561-566, 1989.

32. LeBlanc AD, Schonfeld E, Schneider VS et al: The spine: changes in T2 relaxation times from disuse, Radiology 169:105-107, 1988.

33. Levitt M, Benjamin V, Kricheff II: Potential misinterpretation of cervical spondylosis with cord compression caused by metallic artifacts in magnetic resonance imaging of the postoperative spine, Neurosurgery 27:126-130, 1990.

34. Lewis CA, Castillo M, Hudgins PA: Cervical prevertebral fat stripe: a normal variant simulating prevertebral hemorrhage, Am J Roentgenol 155:559-560, 1990.

35. Li KC, Poon PY: Sensitivity and specificity of MRI in detecting malignant spinal cord compression and in distinguishing malignant from benign compression fractures of vertebrae, Magn Reson Imaging 6:547-556, 1988.

36. Libshitz HI, Malthouse SR, Cunningham D et al: Multiple myeloma: appearance at MR imaging, Radiology 182:833-837, 1992.

37. Malghem J, Maldague B, Labaisse M-A et al: Intravertebral vacuum cleft: changes in content after supine positioning, Radiology 187:483-487, 1993.

38. Malko JA, Hoffman JC, Jarrett PJ: Eddy-current-induced artifacts caused by an "MR-compatible" halo device, Radiology 173:563-564, 1989.

39. Masaryk TJ, Boumphrey F, Modic MT, et al: Effects of chemonucleolysis demonstrated by MR imaging, J Comput Assist Tomogr 10:917-923, 1986.

40. Mirvis SE, Geisler F, Joslyn JN et al: Use of titanium wire in cervical spine fixation as a means to reduce MR artifacts, Am J Neuroradiol 9:1229-1231, 1988.

41. Modic MT, Steinberg PM, Ross JS et al: Degenerative disk disease: assessment of changes in vertebral body marrow with MR imaging, Radiology 166:193-199, 1988.

42. Moulopoulos LA, Dimopoulos MA, Varma DGK et al: Waldenstrom macroglobulinemia: MR imaging of the spine and CT of the abdomen and pelvis, Radiology 188:669-673, 1993.

43. Moulopoulos LA, Varma DGK, Dimopoulos MA et al: Multiple myeloma: spinal MR imaging in patients with untreated newly diagnosed disease, Radiology 185:833-840, 1992.

44. Narayana PA, Brey WW, Kulkarni MV et al: Compensation for surface coil sensitivity variation in magnetic resonance imaging, Magn Reson Imaging 6:271-274, 1988.

45. Peterman SB, Hoffman JC Jr, Malko JA: Magnetic resonance artifact in the postoperative cervical spine: a potential pitfall, Spine 16:721-725, 1991.

46. Rahmouni A, Divine M, Mathieu D et al: Detection of multiple myeloma involving the spine: efficacy of fat-suppression and contrast-enhanced MR imaging, Am J Roentgenol 160:1049-1052, 1993.

47. Rahmouni A, Divine M, Mathieu D et al: MR appearance of multiple myeloma of the spine before and after treatment, Am J Roentgenol 160:1053-1057, 1993.

48. Ralston MD, Dykes TA, Applebaum BI: Verification of lumbar vertebral bodies (letter), Radiology 185:615-616, 1992.

49. Remedios PA, Colletti PM, Raval JK et al: Magnetic resonance imaging of bone after radiation, Magn Reson Imaging 6:301-304, 1988.

50. Ricci C, Cova M, Kang YS et al: Normal age-related patterns of cellular and fatty bone marrow distribution in the axial skeleton: MR imaging study, Radiology 177:83-88, 1990.

51. Rosenthal DI, Hayes CW, Rosen B et al: Fatty replacement of spinal bone marrow due to radiation: demonstration by dual energy quantitative CT and MR imaging, J Comput Assist Tomogr 13:463-465, 1989.

52. Ross JS, Masaryk TJ, Modic MT: Postoperative cervical spine: MR assessment, J Comput Assist Tomogr 11:955-962, 1987.

53. Ross JS, Masaryk TJ, Modic MT et al: Lumbar spine: postoperative assessment with surface-coil MR imaging, Radiology 164:851-860, 1987.

54. Ross JS, Masaryk TJ, Modic MT et al: Vertebral hemangiomas: MR imaging, Radiology 165:165-169, 1987.

55. Ross JS, Modic MT, Masaryk TJ et al: Assessment of extradural degenerative disease with Gd-DTPA-enhanced MR imaging: correlation with surgical and pathologic findings, Am J Neuroradiol 10:1243-1249, 1989.

56. Saywell WR, Crock HV, England JPS et al: Demonstration of vertebral body end plate veins by magnetic resonance imaging, Br J Radiol 62:290-292, 1989.

57. Sether LA, Yu S, Haughton VM et al: Intervertebral disk: normal age-related changes in MR signal intensity, Radiology 177:385-388, 1990.

58. Siffring PA, Forrest TS, Frick MP: Hernias of the inferior lumbar space: diagnosis with US, Radiology 170:190, 1989.

59. Smith AS, Weinstein MA, Mizushima A et al: MR imaging characteristics of tuberculous spondylitis vs vertebral osteomyelitis, Am J Roentgenol 153:399-405, 1989.

60. Stevens SK, Moore SG, Amylon MD: Repopulation of marrow after transplantation: MR imaging with pathologic correlation, Radiology 175:213-218, 1990.

61. Stimac GK, Porter BA, Olson DO et al: Gadolinium-DTPA-enhanced MR imaging of spinal neoplasms: preliminary investigation and comparison with unenhanced spin-echo and STIR sequences, Am J Neuroradiol 9:839-846, 1988.

62. Sugimura K, Kajitani A, Okizuka H et al: Assessing response to therapy of spinal metastases with gadolinium-enhanced MR imaging, J Magn Reson Imaging 1:481-484, 1991.

63. Sze G, Baierl P, Bravo S: Evolution of the infant spinal column: evaluation with MR imaging, Radiology 181:819-827, 1991.

64. Sze G, Brant-Zawadzki MN, Wilson CR et al: Pseudotumor of the craniovertebral junction associated with chronic subluxation: MR imaging studies, Radiology 161:391-394, 1986.

65. Sze G, Bravo S, Baierl P et al: Developing spinal column: gadolinium-enhanced MR imaging, Radiology 180:497-502, 1991.

66. Tien R, Newton TH, Dillon WP et al: A simple method for spinal localization in MR imaging, Am J Neuroradiol 10:1232, 1989.

67. Tien RD, Olson EM, Zee CS: Diseases of the lumbar spine: findings on fat-suppression MR imaging, Am J Roentgenol 159:95-99, 1992.

68. Tsuruda JS, Norman D, Dillon W et al: Three-dimensional gradient-recalled MR imaging as a screening tool for the diagnosis of cervical radiculopathy, Am J Roentgenol 154:375-383, 1990.

69. Yankelevitz DF, Henschke CI, Knapp PH et al: Effect of radiation therapy on thoracic and lumbar bone marrow: evaluation with MR imaging, Am J Roentgenol 157:87-92, 1991.

70. Young IR, Cox IJ, Bryant DJ et al: The benefits of increasing spatial resolution as a means of reducing artifacts due to field inhomogeneities, Magn Reson Imaging 6:585-590, 1988.

71. Yousem DM, Atlas SW, Goldberg HI et al: Degenerative narrowing of the cervical spine neural foramina: evaluation with high-resolution 3DFT gradient-echo MR imaging, Am J Roentgenol 156:1229-1236, 1991.

72. Yuh WTC, Zachar CK, Barloon TJ et al: Vertebral compression fractures: distinction between benign and malignant causes with MR imaging, Radiology 172:215-218, 1989.

17

Intervertebral Disk, Extradural Space, and Neural Foramen

INTERVERTEBRAL DISK

The most frequent indication for performing spinal MR imaging is to evaluate for potential abnormalities related to the intervertebral disks. A number of variations and pitfalls related to the intervertebral disk can simulate or obscure the appearance of disk herniation.

Anatomic Variations

Disk degeneration

The intervertebral disk is relatively prominent during infancy,[91] and undergoes progressive loss in volume during aging. The normal adult disk is depicted as hypointense on T1-weighted images and hyperintense on T2-weighted images. Decreased signal intensity of the intervertebral disk on T2-weighted images can be caused by disk degeneration (Fig. 17-1). These signal intensity changes reflect decreased disk hydration as well as alterations in the connective tissue components of the disk. Hypointensity associated with disk degeneration is accentuated on images acquired using long echo times and on those acquired using some relatively T2-weighted gradient echo and fast spin echo (i.e., RARE) pulse sequences (Figs. 17-2A and B). Quantitative measurements of disk signal intensity indicate significant diurnal variation in diskal T1 and T2 relaxation behavior.[10]

Although disk degeneration is most frequently observed in older patients, these findings can be observed in patients of all ages, including children.[81] The observation of disk degeneration does not necessarily correlate with patient symptoms,[33] and such findings are often observed in asymptomatic individuals. Conversely, altered disk signal intensity may not be evident on MR images in some patients with significant disk degeneration.[6] Partial volume averaging of a normal disk with adjacent vertebral cortex, osteophyte, or paravertebral muscle can lead to artifactual decreased signal intensity on sagittal T2-weighted images, simulating disk degeneration.

Disk calcification can also result in decreased signal intensity on both T1- and T2-weighted images. The resultant signal alterations are usually more focal than those caused by disk degeneration. In some patients, calcification can lead to atypical hyperintensity of the affected intervertebral disk on T1-weighted images[46] (Figs. 17-3 and 17-4).

The vacuum phenomenon—accumulation of nitrogen within a degenerated disk—is another cause for markedly decreased signal intensity of the disk on all se-

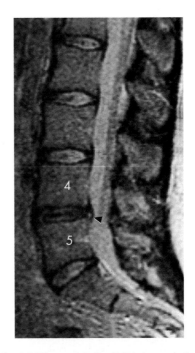

Fig. 17-1. The L4-5 intervertebral disk has relative decreased signal intensity on this sagittal T2-weighted image (TR 2000, TE 75, 1 Nex) because of degenerative changes. There is mild bulging of the posterior disk margin, and a small focus of increased signal intensity (*arrowhead*) is present posteriorly, representing an annular tear.

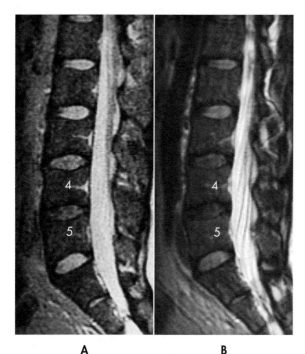

A B

Fig. 17-2. A, Sagittal T2-weighted spin echo image (TR 2000, TE 75, 1 Nex) depicts relative reduced signal intensity of the L4-5 intervertebral disk, indicating degenerative disk disease. **B,** Disk hypointensity is accentuated on corresponding fast spin echo T2-weighted image (TR 4000, effective TE 102, 4 Nex, 16 echo train length) and appears to involve additional disk levels.

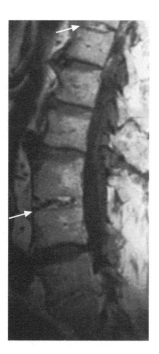

Fig. 17-3. Hyperintensity within the L3-4 and T11-12 intervertebral disks (*arrows*) is depicted on sagittal T1-weighted image (TR 500, TE 12, 2 Nex), corresponding to the presence of diskal calcification on plain radiographs.

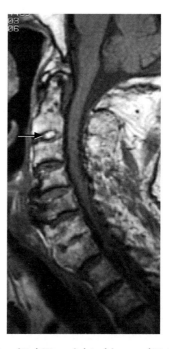

Fig. 17-4. Midsagittal T1-weighted image (TR 600, TE 19, 2 Nex) in 84-year-old male with diffuse idiopathic skeletal hyperostosis. Flowing hyperostosis is observed along the anterior margins of the cervical vertebral bodies, as well as posterior osteophytes and disk protrusions that result in significant stenosis of the central spinal canal. Increased signal intensity is also present within the C2-3 intervertebral disk (*arrow*), corresponding to a site of diskal calcification on plain radiographs.

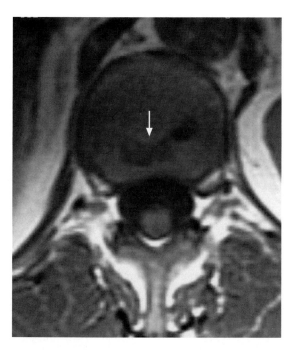

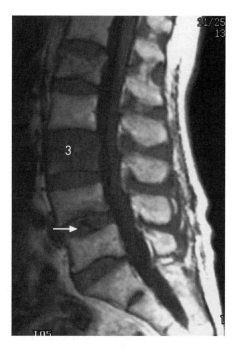

Fig. 17-5. Transaxial T1-weighted image (TR 550, TE 15, 4 Nex) demonstrates a crescentic region of decreased signal intensity within the intervertebral disk (*arrow*), representing gas related to the vacuum phenomenon.

Fig. 17-6. Foci of relative decreased signal intensity within the L4-5 intervertebral disk (*arrow*) reflect the presence of gas (i.e., vacuum phenomenon) on this sagittal T1-weighted image (TR 500, TE 12, 2 Nex). Decreased height and abnormal signal intensity of the L3 vertebral body (3) are also present, related to an acute posttraumatic compression fracture.

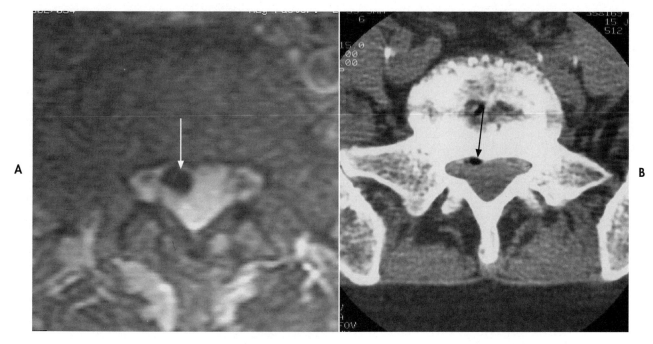

Fig. 17-7. A, A large focus of signal void (*arrow*) is present within the right anterior epidural space on this transaxial T2-weighted image (TR 2500, TE 75, 2 Nex). This represents a susceptibility artifact caused by air within a herniated disk fragment (*arrow*), as confirmed on CT, **B**.

quences[29,52] (Figs. 17-5 and 17-6). When signal void is related to calcium, air, or metal, peripheral hyperintensity can also be observed. Air within a herniated disk fragment can simulate an epidural abscess (Figs. 17-7A and B). Signal void resulting from calcium or air within the disk is more prominent on gradient echo as compared with spin echo images.[5,55] These signal voids are also more prominent when a relatively long echo time is used.[5]

Differentiation of disk from bone

The markedly decreased signal intensity of calcified or degenerated disk material can be difficult to distinguish from osteophytes.[31,37,52,67] The markedly hypointense appearance of bone on gradient echo images can assist in distinguishing bone from normal disk material. However, degenerated disk material, with its associated hypointensity, can be difficult to distinguish from bone.[42] Thus, gradient echo images have been considered to have reduced ability to distinguish between "hard" and "soft" disk herniation.[71] However, nondegenerated disk material can be isointense with osteophytes on spin echo images. In such cases, gradient echo images are often bet-

ter able to distinguish disk from bone, with the latter having significantly lower signal intensity (Figs. 17-8A-C).

Other causes for decreased disk signal intensity

Decreased signal intensity on T2-weighted images as well as decreased height of the intervertebral disks can result from disuse, as in paraplegic patients.[43] Patients who have undergone chymopapain injections for chemonucleolysis demonstrate markedly decreased signal intensity of the treated disk on T2-weighted images,[47] with an associated decrease in disk height.[39] Decreased signal intensity can be observed 2 weeks following treatment, with subsequent return to baseline appearance approximately 2 years later, as degenerated disk material becomes transformed into scar tissue.[39] Hypointensity is also routinely observed in patients who have undergone previous diskectomy at the operated level.

A central linear focus of relatively decreased signal intensity is observed within the nucleus pulposus in normal individuals (Figs. 17-9A and B). This "intranuclear disk cleft" represents a fibrous remnant of the noto-

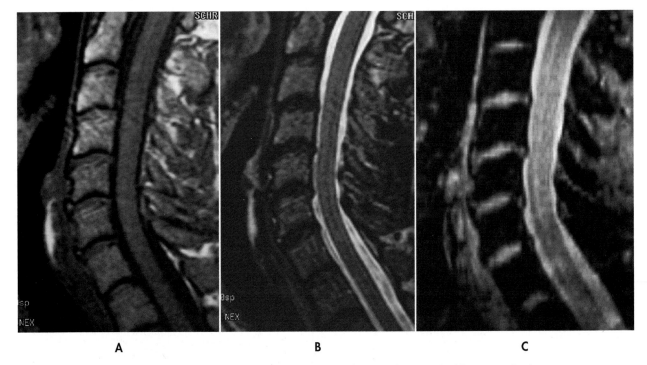

A   B   C

Fig. 17-8. Isointensity of posterior osteophytes and protruding cervical intervertebral disks is present on **A,** midsagittal T1-weighted image (TR 566, TE 19, 2 Nex) and, **B,** fast spin echo T2-weighted image (TR 4000, effective TE 102, 4 Nex, 16 echo train) resulting in poor distinction between these tissues. **C,** Distinction between disk material and bone is improved on sagittal reformation from three-dimensional Fourier transform spoiled gradient echo series (TR 35, TE 15, 5-degree flip angle, 1 Nex).

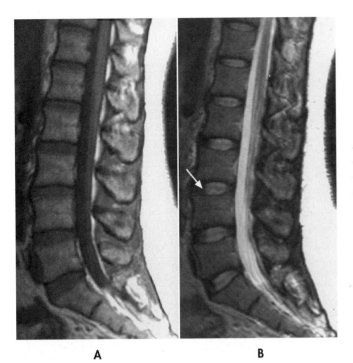

A   **B**

Fig. 17-9. The precise level of termination of the conus medullaris is difficult to determine on **A,** sagittal T1-weighted image (TR 500, TE 12, 2 Nex) and, **B,** T-fast spin echo T2-weighted image (TR 4000, effective TE 102, 4 Nex, 16 echo train) because of blending of the conus medullaris with the proximal cauda equina nerve roots. The T2-weighted image demonstrates the appearance of a normal intranuclear cleft of the intravertebral disk at all levels (*arrow*).

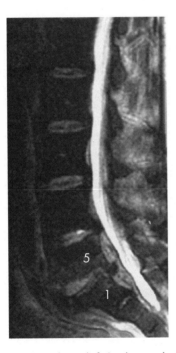

Fig. 17-10. The intranuclear cleft is obscured at the L5-S1 intervertebral disk level on sagittal fast spin echo T2-weighted image (TR 4000, effective TE 104, 4 Nex, 16 echo train) in a patient with diskitis at this level. Some reactive marrow edema can also be seen within the vertebral endplates bordering the affected disk space. The intranuclear cleft can be visualized at all remaining intervertebral levels.

chord.[61] Absence of this cleft is a secondary sign of disk space infection (Fig. 17-10).

Imaging Artifacts
Motion artifacts

Motion occurring during image acquisition can cause phase-encoding errors (i.e., ghosting artifacts) that project artifactual increased signal intensity over the intervertebral disk. These motion artifacts can be due to respiratory motion, vascular pulsation, or gross patient motion. Because they propagate along the phase-encoding axis of the image, gradient reorientation can be used to realign these artifacts (Figs. 17-11A and B). Other methods that can be used to reduce the severity of motion artifacts include respiratory-ordered phase encoding, spatial presaturation, multiexcitation pulse sequences, and other techniques discussed elsewhere in this book. Motion artifacts are considerably more severe on three-dimensional Fourier transform images than on standard two-dimensional acquisitions.[90]

Chemical shift misregistration artifact

Fat within the vertebral marrow space and water within the intervertebral disk present a fat-water interface where chemical shift misregistration artifacts can arise. Because frequency encoding is usually performed along the superior-inferior direction, this creates artifactual increased signal intensity in the region of the intervertebral disk–vertebral endplate junction, which can obscure visualization of the endplate (Figs. 17-11A and

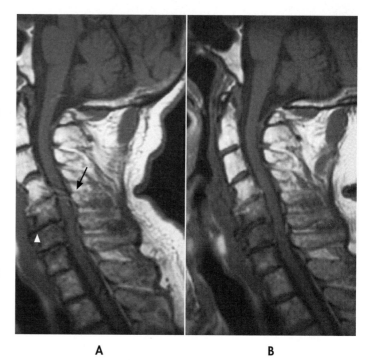

Fig. 17-11. A, T1-weighted sagittal image (TR 500, TE 11, 2 Nex) obtained with phase-encoding direction oriented along the anteroposterior axis of the body demonstrates ghosting artifacts related to swallowing motion (*arrow*) projected across the spinal canal. **B,** On reorientation of the phase- and frequency-encoding gradients, motion artifacts are aligned along the superior-inferior axis of the body. Chemical shift misregistration at the diskovertebral junction results in artifactual linear decreased signal intensity (*arrowhead*) on image in **A.** In **B** the low signal intensity component of chemical shift misregistration at the vertebral body–CSF interface causes overestimation of the severity of spinal stenosis. Diffuse spondylotic changes are noted, as well as marrow replacement involving the C5 and C6 vertebral bodies.

A   **B**

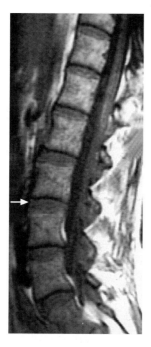

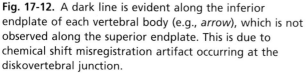

Fig. 17-12. A dark line is evident along the inferior endplate of each vertebral body (e.g., *arrow*), which is not observed along the superior endplate. This is due to chemical shift misregistration artifact occurring at the diskovertebral junction.

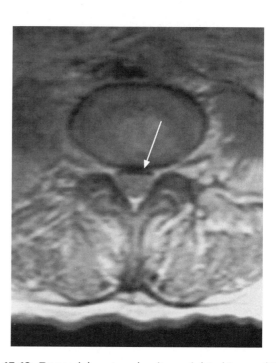

Fig. 17-13. Transaxial proton density–weighted image (TR 2500, TE 35, 2 Nex) demonstrates artifactual loss of signal intensity along the anterior margin of the thecal sac (*arrow*), caused by chemical shift misregistration artifact.

B and 17-12). It simultaneously results in artifactual decreased signal intensity along the opposite diskovertebral junction; this can increase the apparent size of a bulging or herniated intervertebral disk (Fig. 17-13). When frequency encoding is assigned along the anteroposterior direction, artifactual decreased signal intensity related to chemical shift misregistration can obscure visualization of herniated disk material[19,21] and also result in apparent narrowing of the subarachnoid space[19,20] (Fig. 17-11). Reduced receiver bandwidth techniques—used to improve the signal-to-noise ratio—accentuate chemical shift misregistration artifacts.[40] Such artifacts are also more prominent on images acquired using high field strength systems and with large voxel sizes. T2-weighted images generally display more prominent chemical shift misregistration than do corresponding T1-weighted images.

Truncation artifact

Truncation artifacts appear as linear foci of alternating high and low signal intensity that usually propagate along the phase-encoding direction of the image. These artifacts arise at high tissue-contrast interfaces, such as at the diskovertebral junction.[13,52] They can be reduced in prominence when a moderate to high resolution matrix is used (e.g., 192 to 256 × 256) or with the use of various filtration mechanisms.

Postoperative changes

Diffuse decreased signal intensity of the disk is usually observed following diskectomy. The cervical disks can display signal alterations following performance of anterior cervical fusion.[65,71] A focus of markedly increased signal intensity is often observed on T2-weighted images within the posterior disk margin in patients who have undergone previous diskectomy. In the immediate postoperative period this represents fluid within the site of disk curettage, which is subsequently replaced by granulation tissue.[66] Following intravenous contrast material administration, granulation tissue within the posterior margin of the disk undergoes enhancement; this does not indicate disk space infection (Figs. 17-14 and 17-15). However, when abnormally increased disk signal intensity on T2-weighted images and abnormal contrast enhancement are also observed within the adjacent vertebral endplates, postoperative diskitis should be considered.[8] It is important to verify that these

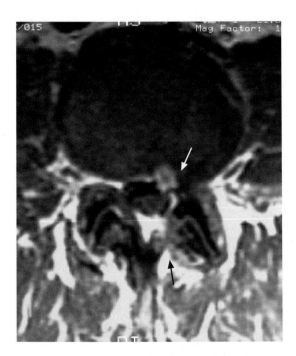

Fig. 17-14. Transaxial T1-weighted image following gadolinium chelate administration (TR 500, TE 15, 4 Nex) in patient who underwent previous laminectomy and diskectomy. The laminectomy defect can be seen on the left (*black arrow*), with associated contrast enhancement because of granulation tissue. Contrast enhancement within the intervertebral disk is also noted (*white arrow*), at the site of curettage, because of granulation tissue ingrowth. Clumping of the cauda equina nerve roots is due to arachnoiditis.

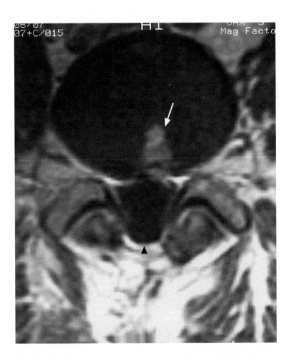

Fig. 17-15. Gadopentetate enhanced T1-weighted image (TR 500, TE 15, 4 Nex) in patient who underwent previous diskectomy demonstrates contrast enhancement within the intervertebral disk curettage site (*arrow*). There is also postoperative expansion of the posterior aspect of the thecal sac (*arrowhead*).

endplate abnormalities were not present preoperatively, since similar findings can be caused by degenerative disk disease (type I changes).

Annular disk tears

Annular disk tears are frequently present in bulging and degenerative disks and may play a role in the etiology of back pain.[1] Annular tears can have variable signal intensity characteristics; in some cases focal high signal intensity is present on T2-weighted images, whereas in other cases the tear cannot be visualized because of the absence of signal alterations.[1,68,74,92] The presence of focal increased intensity within annular tears on T2-weighted images is due to fluid or mucoid material within the tear site[92] (Fig. 5-1). Generalized hypointensity of the disk on T2-weighted images, as occurs with disk degeneration, can also occur in the presence of a radial disk tear.[51,73,74,92] T1-weighted images acquired following paramagnetic contrast material injection frequently show abnormal contrast enhancement at sites of annular disk tears.[68] The presence of granulation tissue within the tear site is responsible for such enhancement, which appears to be a more sensitive indicator of annu-

lar tear than signal alterations on T2-weighted images.[68] However, the sensitivity of MR for detection of annular disk tears appears to be lower than that of diskography.[92]

Disk expansion

Marked enlargement and increased signal intensity on T2-weighted images can be observed in intervertebral disks located adjacent to a site of vertebral collapse (Figs. 17-16 to 17-18). These findings are apparently due to increased hydration of the disk in an effort to occupy the volume lost by the compressed vertebra. This phenomenon can be observed in conjunction with acute as well as chronic vertebral compressions, which may occur due to insufficiency or pathologic vertebral involvement. These findings should be distinguished from disk space infection. Although diskitis also results in increased diskal signal intensity on T2-weighted images, the affected disk is usually not enlarged.

Disk Herniation

Disk bulging appears as a generalized convexity of the disk margins without a focal component. This contrasts with the appearance of disk herniation, in which a focal disk fragment can be seen extending beyond the confines of the remainder of the disk, possibly with associated mass effect on the thecal sac or nerve roots. Difficulty

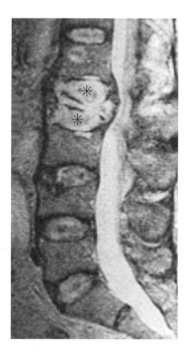

Fig. 17-16. Marked collapse of the L2 vertebral body because of osteomyelitis is present on this sagittal T2-weighted image (TR 2000, TE 75, 1 Nex). The involved vertebra demonstrates increased signal intensity, caused by marrow edema and infection, and protrudes into the spinal canal, resulting in stenosis. There is significant enlargement of the adjoining intervertebral disks (*asterisks*), which also appear hyperintense because of increased water content.

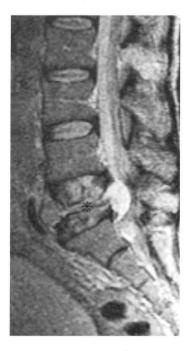

Fig. 17-17. Metastatic involvement from colon carcinoma has resulted in collapse and posterior extrusion of the L5 vertebral body (*asterisk*). On this T2-weighted image (TR 2000, TE 75, 1 Nex), marked expansion and relative increased signal intensity of the intervertebral disks bordering the collapsed vertebral body are also observed.

in classification may be encountered in patients who demonstrate evidence of generalized disk bulging, although with a slight focal component. In some centers such entities are referred to as disk protrusions or focal bulges rather than herniations. Although this terminology may be useful if the referring physicians are familiar with its implications, it should be recognized that small disk herniations may be present in many such cases.

Clinical correlation of MR observations

The full functional impact of disk-related morphologic alterations may not be evident on MR images because imaging is performed with the patient supine and without application of any external stressors. It is likely that alterations in the morphology of many disk herniations, and their impact on critical surrounding structures, may be altered or accentuated when the patient assumes an upright position[57] and when axial loading forces resulting from weight bearing are applied to the intervertebral disks. Additional alterations may occur when flexion and extension maneuvers are performed. These limitations may explain some of the discrepancies between MR images and clinical symptomatology. However, it is likely

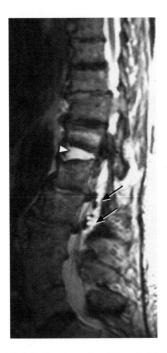

Fig. 17-18. Sagittal fast spin echo T2-weighted image (TR 4000, effective TE 96, 4 Nex, 16 echo train) demonstrates multiple punctate foci of decreased signal intensity in the anterior epidural space (*arrows*). These represent air bubbles in a patient who underwent recent administration of epidural anesthesia. Enlargement and hyperintensity of the T12-L1 intervertebral disk (*arrowhead*) can also be observed related to compression fracture of the T12 vertebral body.

that a number of important factors in the pathogenesis of low back pain and sciatica are not amenable to visualization on MR images.

For these and other reasons, correlation between morphologic abnormalities depicted on MR images and patient symptomatology is frequently discrepant.[53] MR images often depict morphologic abnormalities that do not account for patient symptoms or neurologic signs, and conversely, a morphologic correlate is frequently not found on MR images to correlate with such symptoms and signs.[88] This discrepancy is particularly evident in the thoracic spine, where disk herniations are observed on MR with high frequency in asymptomatic patients. Williams et al. observed such findings in 14.5% of oncology patients using a limited survey protocol.[87] Teresi et al. have made similar observations in the cervical spine.[80] In some asymptomatic patients, large disk herniations are observed with evidence of mass effect on the spinal cord or nerve roots.[80,86]

Time-dependent changes in disk herniations

MR images can depict significant differences in the appearance of disk herniations over time. Bozzao et al.[11] found that 63% of conservatively treated disk herniations displayed greater than 30% reduction in size on follow-up MR examination. These changes may be due to dehydration of herniated disk material, disk fragmentation, or resorption of surrounding granulation tissue.[11] Thus, the appearance of the intervertebral disk and any related pathologic condition should be correlated with the time course of patient symptoms.

Simulation of disk herniation

In patients with spondylolisthesis, the appearance of disk protrusion or herniation can be simulated (Figs. 17-19A and B). In this situation the posterior margins of the disk should be compared with the posterior cortex of the vertebral body located below the affected disk. Comparison with the slipped cephalad vertebral body will lead

---

SIMULATION OF DISK HERNIATION

- Spondylolisthesis
- Partial volume averaging with soft tissue or bone
- Lumbosacral junction
- Dilated epidural veins
- Basivertebral vein
- Conjoined nerve roots
- Epidural soft tissue masses (neoplasm, inflammation, hemorrhage)
- Postoperative epidural granulation tissue or fibrosis
- Postoperative edema or hemorrhage

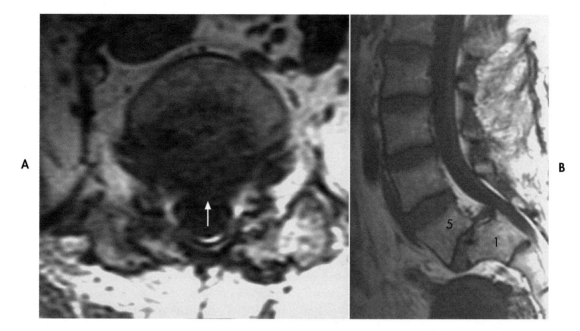

Fig. 17-19. A, Apparent central herniation of disk material (*arrow*) at the L5-S1 level is present on this transaxial T1-weighted image (TR 500, TE 14, 2 Nex). **B,** Corresponding midsagittal T1-weighted image (TR 500, TE 12, 2 Nex), however, indicates that the posterior margin of the L5-S1 disk does not extend beyond the posterior margin of the upper sacrum and that the appearance on the axial image is due to grade II spondylolisthesis at this level.

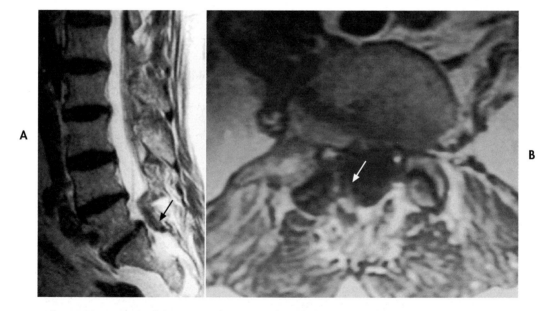

Fig. 17-20. A, Sagittal fast spin echo T2-weighted image (TR 4000, effective TE 104, 4 Nex, 16 echo train) in 72-year-old male patient receiving anticoagulant therapy was obtained for clinically suspected epidural hematoma. An apparent extradural mass at the L5 level (*arrow*) represents partial volume averaging with hypertrophic facet joint and ligamentum flavum in this scoliotic patient, as verified on corresponding transaxial T1-weighted image (TR 500, TE 14, 2 Nex) (*arrow*), **B.**

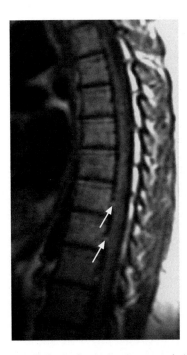

Fig. 17-21. Multiple foci of relative increased signal intensity within the anterior epidural space (*arrows*) are visualized on this sagittal T1-weighted image (TR 500, TE 17, 2 Nex), representing slow flow within the epidural venous plexus.

to a false impression of disk protrusion or herniation. Disk protrusion can also be simulated by partial volume averaging of the disk with adjacent soft tissue and bony structures. This is most likely to occur in patients with scoliosis. In these patients, partial volume averaging of the facet joint and ligamentum flavum with epidural fat can simulate an epidural mass, and partial volume effects can also lead to a false appearance of lateral disk herniation along the apex of the curvature (Figs. 17-20A and B). At the lumbosacral junction, the normal L5-S1 intervertebral disk often has a convex posterior margin, which should not be interpreted as abnormal. Transaxial images acquired through the sacral body can also simulate disk protrusion.

In patients with low back pain or sciatica, MR images are often acquired along the plane of the intervertebral disks. This results in images oriented transaxial with reference to the disk rather than to the magnetic field. The degree of image angulation can affect the apparent prominence of protruding disk material.

Epidural venous plexus. The anterior epidural venous plexus can be unusually prominent in some patients. Relative increased signal intensity can be observed within these veins on T1- and T2-weighted images as a result of slow flow and second-echo rephasing, respectively (Fig. 17-21). These findings can simulate herni-

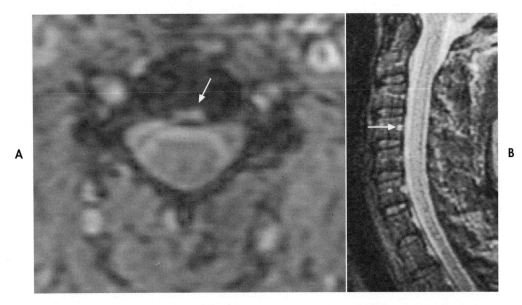

Fig. 17-22. A, Transaxial spoiled gradient echo image (TR 35, TE 15, 5-degree flip angle, 1 Nex) of the cervical spine demonstrates hyperintense focus (*arrow*) along the posterior vertebral margin. This represents flow-related enhancement within a prominent basivertebral vein, as confirmed on sagittal T2-weighted image (TR 2200, TE 80, 1 Nex) (*arrow*), **B.**

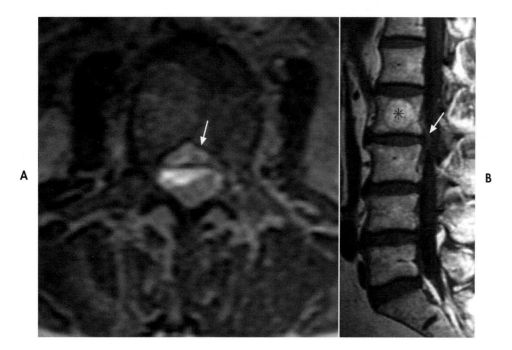

Fig. 17-23. A, A hyperintense structure (*arrow*) is located ventral to the thecal sac on this transaxial T2-weighted image (TR 2800, TE 75, 2 Nex), representing a dilated anterior epidural vein with high signal intensity caused by slow blood flow and use of flow compensation for motion artifact suppression. **B,** Venous dilatation is secondary to disk herniation at adjacent level (*arrow*), as depicted on sagittal T1-weighted image (TR 500, TE 12, 2 Nex). Rounded focus of increased signal intensity within the L2 vertebral body (*asterisk*) represents a lipid rest.

ated disk material[15,23,60] or other anterior epidural soft tissue lesions. Focal prominence of the basivertebral vein can simulate a small disk herniation on sagittal or transaxial images (Figs. 17-22A and B). Confusion with a neoplastic or vascular mass may be further heightened when intravenous contrast material is given, since prominent contrast enhancement can be observed with each of these entities.[24] Enhancement within the epidural venous plexus is variably prominent among individuals.[14] Recognition of epidural veins is based on their tubular nature, characteristic fusiform shape with a midline septum, flow-related enhancement on gradient echo images, and enhancement following contrast material administration. Dilatation of the epidural veins often occurs proximal to a site of impingement as a result of disk herniation or spinal stenosis (Figs. 17-23A and B and 17-24).

Conjoined nerve roots. Conjoined nerve roots can also simulate the appearance of disk herniation (Figs. 17-25A and B). Conjoined roots can be seen to divide as they are observed over the course of several consecutive images. Epidural soft tissue masses, including neoplasm, inflammation, or hemorrhage, can also simulate a herniated disk fragment.

Failure to detect migrated disk fragments

Oblique axial images are often prescribed in clusters that are targeted to the intervertebral disk spaces. Images may not be acquired through the mid–vertebral body level in order to conserve imaging slices and time. However, one must be aware that herniated disk fragments can undergo considerable migration in some patients and that such fragments may not be detected when the previously described imaging protocol is used[72] (Figs. 17-26A-C). Sagittal images should be carefully inspected in all patients; when a migrated disk fragment is suspected, complete transaxial coverage of the relevant portion of the spine should be carried out.

Impact of pulse sequence on detection of disk herniation

The size of a herniated disk fragment may be underestimated on T1-weighted images, since the relatively low signal intensity of disk (particularly the anulus) may be imperceptible when applied against the similarly hypointense anterior dural margin and cerebrospinal fluid (CSF).[63] Another limitation of T1-weighted images is that osteophytes and ligaments appear isointense with

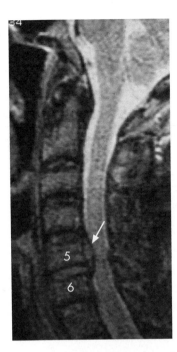

Fig. 17-24. Sagittal T2-weighted image (TR 2200, TE 80, 1 Nex) in patient with C5-6 disk herniation. There is focal dilatation of the anterior epidural venous plexus (*arrow*) above the level of disk herniation. The dilated epidural vein is isointense with disk material because of slow flow and use of flow compensating gradient pulses. This can lead to difficulty in establishing actual cephalad extent of herniated disk material.

CSF. Therefore spin echo or gradient echo images depicting CSF as hyperintense (i.e., T2- or T2*-weighted sequences) are often preferable for defining extradural abnormalities. When gradient echo imaging is used, careful attention to TR, TE, and flip angle is necessary to optimize the signal intensity difference between disk material and CSF.[56,85]

Postoperative Changes
Immediate postoperative changes

Immediately following diskectomy, MR images can demonstrate apparent residual herniated disk material at the operated interspace. The configuration of this interspace may, in fact, be identical to its preoperative appearance[8,9,66] (Figs. 17-27A and B). The appearance of residual herniated disk material is caused by hemorrhage and edema related to the recent surgical procedure. These findings generally remit over the ensuing months. The usefulness of MR for detecting residual or recurrent disk herniation in the perioperative period is therefore quite limited.

Delayed postoperative changes

Signal intensity characteristics. MR is often very useful for evaluating patients with back or leg pain fol-

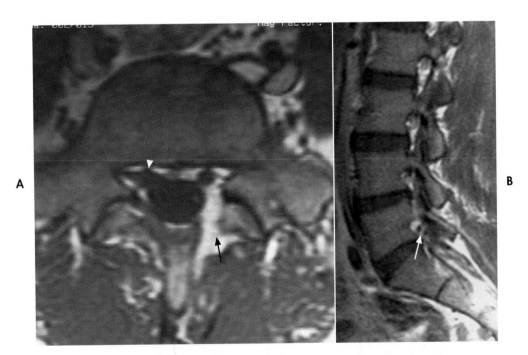

Fig. 17-25. A, Transaxial T1-weighted image (TR 500, TE 15, 4 Nex) in patient who underwent previous left L5 hemilaminectomy. The laminectomy defect (*arrow*) is filled with fat packing. There is asymmetry of the nerve roots, with apparent enlargement on the right (*arrowhead*) caused by conjoined L5 and S1 nerve roots. This is confirmed on sagittal T1-weighted image (TR 500, TE 12, 2 Nex), **B,** where the two individual components of the conjoined complex (*arrow*) can be distinguished.

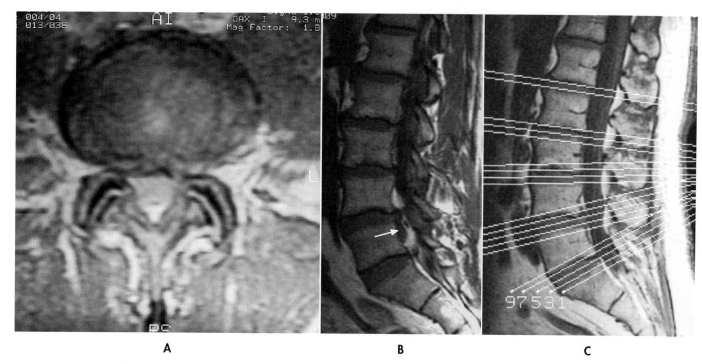

Fig. 17-26. A, Transaxial proton density–weighted image (TR 2000, TE 35, 2 Nex) acquired at the L4-5 interspace fails to depict large herniated disk fragment that has extended inferiorly from the L4-5 interspace and lies behind the upper L5 vertebral body (TR 600, TE 12, 2 Nex) (*arrow*), **B.** This is because the transaxial images were targeted to the disk spaces, and the intervening tissue was not imaged, as demonstrated in **C** (TR 600, TE 12, 2 Nex).

lowing previous lumbar diskectomy beyond the immediate postoperative period. In such patients, anterior epidural soft tissue masses are frequently observed, which can represent herniated disk material or postoperative granulation tissue or fibrosis. The signal intensity characteristics of the mass on T2-weighted images can help distinguish among these entities. Epidural granulation tissue or fibrosis generally has a signal intensity greater than that of herniated disk material. However, extruded disk fragments that have become detached from the parent disk (i.e., sequestered fragments) can appear hyperintense on T2-weighted images, simulating inflammatory tissue[15] (Fig. 17-28). Conversely, mature fibrosis can appear hypointense on T2-weighted images, which also presents an opportunity for diagnostic error. Following the initial months after surgery, the proportion of extracellular space within sites of epidural fibrosis declines, resulting in decreasing signal intensity on T2-weighted images.[16] The signal intensity of epidural fibrosis also varies according to its location. Hyperintensity is observed in the anterior epidural space, lateral recess, lateral epidural space, and posterior epidural space, in decreasing order of frequency.[16]

Morphologic characteristics. Morphologic evaluation of the epidural lesion is also helpful in its charac-

terization but is similarly subject to pitfalls. Contiguity of the mass with the adjacent intervertebral disk on sagittal images is suggestive—although not diagnostic—of disk herniation. Herniated disk material is often associated with mass effect on the adjacent thecal sac or nerve roots, whereas epidural fibrosis is not. In fact, epidural fibrosis can lead to retraction of these structures in some patients (i.e., "negative mass effect"). However, mass effect can be observed in some patients as a result of epidural granulation tissue or fibrosis,[32,50,67] and all disk herniations do not, of course, produce observable mass effect.

Contrast enhancement characteristics. The use of intravenous contrast agents such as gadopentetate dimeglumine has become an important part of the MR evaluation of patients with failed back surgery syndrome and has improved the ability to distinguish disk herniation from postoperative inflammatory tissue. Because disk material is avascular, it does not undergo significant contrast enhancement, whereas the numerous vessels and leaky intercellular junctions contained within inflammatory tissue usually result in prominent enhancement. It is important to note that enhancement of herniated disk material can be observed on images acquired 20 minutes or more following contrast material administration.[32,69]

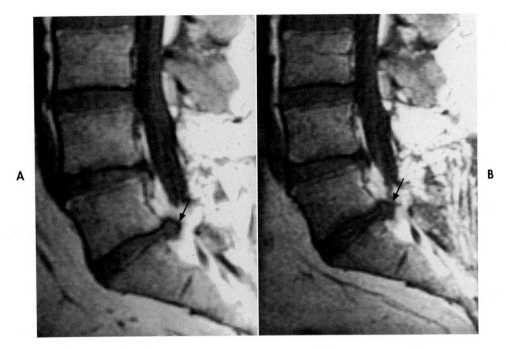

Fig. 17-27. Sagittal T2-weighted fast spin echo images (TR 500, TE 16, 2 Nex) obtained, **A,** before and, **B,** 5 days following surgical removal of herniated L5-S1 disk fragment (*arrow,* **A**). The immediate postoperative examination demonstrates apparent residual disk herniation at the L5-S1 level (*arrow,* **B**), with little apparent change as compared to the preoperative examination. However, subsequent examination revealed progressive resolution of changes at this level.

PITFALLS IN DISTINGUISHING DISK HERNIATION FROM EPIDURAL FIBROSIS

- Hyperintensity of extruded disk fragment on T2-weighted image
- Hypointensity of mature fibrosis on T2-weighted image
- Relative decreased signal intensity fibrosis in lateral and posterior epidural space
- Mass effect caused by epidural fibrosis
- Absence of mass effect because of disk herniation
- Delayed enhancement of disk fragment
- Reduced intensity enhancement of mature epidural fibrosis
- Reduced enhancement of posterior epidural fibrosis
- Heterogeneous enhancement of epidural fibrosis
- Epidural fibrosis surrounding nerve root
- Partial volume averaging of small fragments with enhancing fibrosis or epidural veins
- Invasion of herniated disk fragment by fibrosis
- Partial volume averaging of fibrosis with nonenhancing bone, soft tissue, disk material

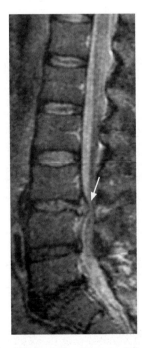

Fig. 17-28. Sagittal T2-weighted image (TR 2000, TE 75, 1 Nex) in 35-year-old male who underwent previous diskectomy. Recurrent disk herniation (*arrow*) demonstrates hyperintensity caused by extrusion of the herniation fragment, which simulates signal intensity characteristics of epidural fibrosis. The posterior longitudinal ligament is uplifted by the disk fragment.

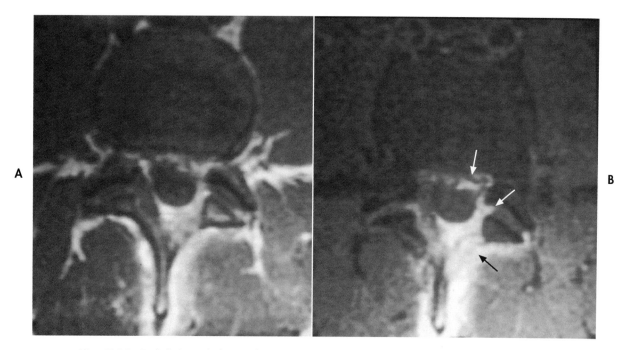

Fig. 17-29. Gadolinium chelate enhanced transaxial T1-weighted images obtained, **A,** without and, **B,** with fat saturation in patient who has undergone previous left laminectomy. The extent of enhancing epidural fibrosis is difficult to determine on conventional image because of isointensity with adjacent epidural fat. Visualization of complete extent of enhancing tissue (*arrows*) is improved with use of fat suppression.

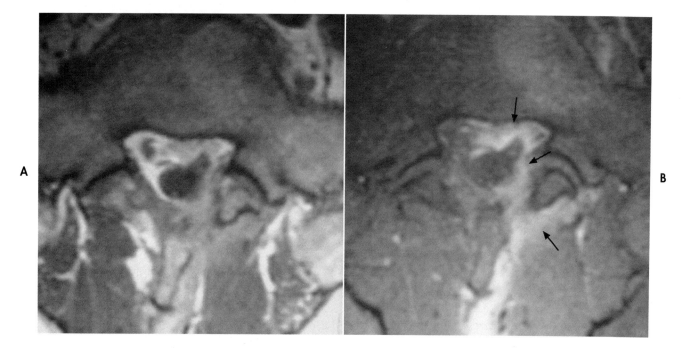

Fig. 17-30. Gadolinium chelate enhanced transaxial T1-weighted images obtained, **A,** without and, **B,** with fat saturation in patient who underwent left laminectomy and diskectomy. Enhancement of epidural fibrosis (*arrows*) is more conspicuous on the fat suppressed image, allowing for improved identification and definition of its extent.

This can cause disk herniation to simulate epidural fibrosis and mandates that images be acquired immediately following contrast material administration in postoperative patients.

Sites of epidural fibrosis have been observed to undergo enhancement for up to 20 years following surgery.[70] The intensity of enhancement, however, varies over time. Enhancement is most intense during the initial 9 months following surgery and progressively diminishes thereafter.[26] This may ultimately result in relatively subtle or even absent contrast enhancement, causing potential confusion with recurrent disk herniation. The conspicuousness of contrast material enhancement is accentuated when contrast enhanced T1-weighted images are acquired using fat suppression[7,50] (Figs. 17-29A and B and 17-30A and B). In equivocal cases, region-of-interest measurements can be used to ascertain the level of contrast material enhancement. However, for such measurements to be meaningful, precontrast and postcontrast enhanced images should be obtained without alteration of receiver gain settings, or measurements of the epidural tissue should be normalized to uninvolved muscle or fat, which undergo insignificant enhancement.

The time course for contrast enhancement of anterior epidural scar differs from that of posterior epidural scar. Maximal enhancement of posterior epidural scar occurs 1 month following laminectomy, with a subsequent decrease in intensity.[64] By the fourth postoperative month, the scar has matured by conversion to collagen fibers, which do not enhance significantly.

Distinction between enhancing epidural fibrosis and surrounding epidural fat can be difficult on contrast enhanced T1-weighted images, because these tissues have similar signal intensity. They can generally be differentiated through close comparison of precontrast and postcontrast enhanced T1-weighted images. The use of fat suppressed T1-weighted images can also greatly facilitate this distinction.[50]

Epidural fibrosis usually undergoes relatively uniform enhancement, although in some patients enhancement can be quite heterogeneous. In such cases, small hypointense foci are observed within the fibrotic mass, which do not significantly enhance or enhance less intensely than the tissue that surrounds them.[50] In this situation it may be difficult to exclude a small disk fragment that is surrounded by inflammatory tissue.[4,8,32] This occurs fre-

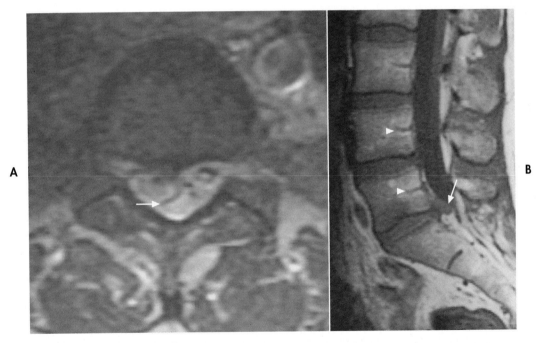

Fig. 17-31. A, A large extruded disk fragment located anterolateral to the thecal sac on the right is difficult to visualize on transaxial T2-weighted image (TR 2500, TE 75, 2 Nex) because of isointensity with CSF in adjacent thecal sac. A dark line (*arrow*), representing chemical shift misregistration, highlights the boundary between the two structures. **B,** The herniated fragment (*arrow*), which has ruptured through the posterior longitudinal ligament, is more easily identified on the sagittal T1-weighted image (TR 500, TE 12, 2 Nex). Also note high signal intensity within the vertebral bodies along the course of the basivertebral veins (*arrowheads*), caused by fatty changes in the marrow space.

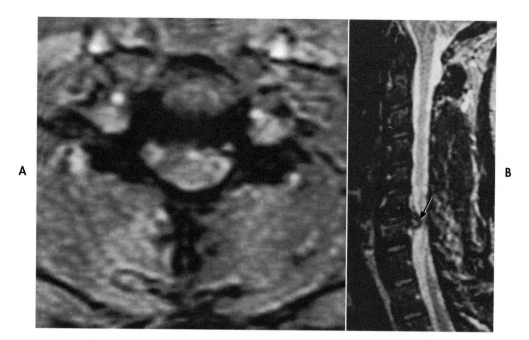

Fig. 17-32. A, The presence of a large extruded disk fragment in the C5-6 right lateral recess is difficult to appreciate on this transaxial three-dimensional spoiled gradient echo image (TR 35, TE 15, 5-degree flip angle, 1 Nex) because of isointensity between the fragment and adjacent CSF. **B,** The fragment (*arrow*) is easily visualized, however, on corresponding parasagittal T2-weighted image (TR 2200, TE 80, 1 Nex).

quently, because disk herniations in the postoperative as well as nonoperated spine are often surrounded by reactive inflammatory tissue. When contrast material is given in such patients, a target appearance is observed, consisting of a central nonenhancing disk fragment with peripherally enhancing fibrosis.[32,50,51,69] This target appearance can be simulated when enhancing epidural fibrosis surrounds a nerve root within the lateral recess or neural foramen. In this situation the nerve root can appear to represent a herniated disk fragment. Careful analysis of both contrast enhanced contiguous transaxial as well as sagittal images will demonstrate the typical course of the nerve root.

Because herniated disk fragments are often surrounded by inflammatory tissue, their size can be overestimated on unenhanced images.[69] Surrounding inflammatory tissue can also result in partial volume effects between central nonenhancing disk fragments and adjacent enhancing inflammatory tissue on contrast enhanced images.[2,32,67] In this situation the central focus of herniated disk material can become inconspicuous or may appear to undergo enhancement. Partial volume averaging of small disk fragments with adjacent enhancing anterior epidural veins can lead to similar diagnostic difficulties.[2] Frank invasion of a herniated disk fragment by surrounding epidural fibrosis can also occur, resulting in nonvisualization of the fragment.[70] Conversely, there is a poten-

tial for confusion of posterior vertebral or facet joint osteophytes with nonenhancing disk material.[67] Contrast enhancement of the extradural segment of lumbar nerve roots has also been noted in postoperative patients.[8]

Sequestered Disk Fragments

When a herniated disk fragment becomes detached from its parent disk, it often appears hyperintense on T2-weighted images because of increased hydration[25] (Figs. 17-31A and B). In this situation the sequestered fragment can become isointense with epidural fat or CSF. Its identification may therefore be difficult on T2-weighted images unless it results in obvious mass effect on the thecal sac or nerve roots[48] (Figs. 17-32A and B and 17-33A and B). Extruded disk fragments can appear similar to anterior epidural hematomas; such hematomas can result from rupture of epidural veins as a result of small disk herniations.[30]

EPIDURAL SOFT TISSUES

Anatomic Variations and Imaging Artifacts

Ligamentum flavum

The ligamentum flavum has a higher signal intensity than most other ligaments on T1-weighted images (Fig. 17-34). This is due to its higher concentration of elastin.

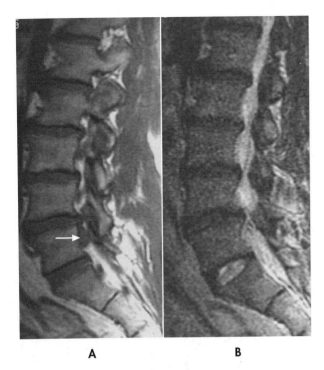

A   **B**

Fig. 17-33. A, Sagittal T1-weighted image (TR 600, TE 12, 2 Nex) demonstrates large extruded disk fragment (*arrow*), which has extended inferiorly from the L4-5 interspace and is lodged behind the upper L5 vertebral body. **B,** The herniated fragment is not identified on the corresponding T2-weighted sagittal image (TR 2000, TE 75, 1 Nex) because of isointensity between the fragment and adjacent epidural fat as well as CSF.

Accentuated increased intensity on T1-weighted images within the ligamentum flavum can indicate ossification, with T1 shortening as a result of marrow fat.[29] However, ligamentous ossification may also be associated with hypointensity on all pulse sequences,[77] which can also occur because of ligamentous calcification. Focal globular calcifications of the ligamentum can appear masslike, simulating a synovial cyst.[29] The ligamentum flavum can appear bulging when axial loading forces are applied to the spine.[57] In patients who have undergone previous laminectomy, the ligamentum flavum is often absent[66] (Fig. 17-35).

Posterior longitudinal ligament

The posterior longitudinal ligament can be obscured because of chemical shift misregistration artifact, which can be suggestive of rupture of this structure.[28] Ossification of the posterior longitudinal ligament may be difficult to distinguish from ligamentous hypertrophy, unless high signal intensity because of marrow elements can be visualized.[59,89] When the posterior longitudinal ligament is prominent or redundant, the appearance of posterior vertebral osteophytes can be simulated.[71] This

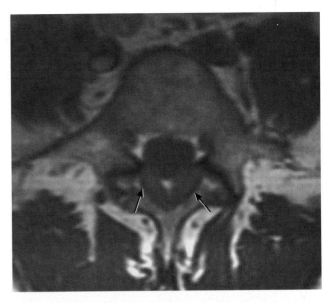

Fig. 17-34. Transaxial T1-weighted image (TR 500, TE 14, 4 Nex) demonstrates relative hyperintensity of the hypertrophied ligamentum flavum (*arrows*).

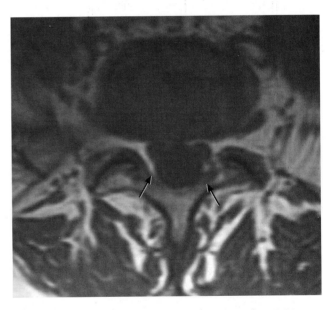

Fig. 17-35. The ligamenta flava are absent at the L5-S1 level (*arrows*) in this patient who underwent previous laminectomy (TR 500, TE 14, 4 Nex).

is most likely to occur on gradient echo images, particularly when the ligament is calcified. Fat suppression is useful for improving the conspicuousness of vertebral lesions and myelographic effect on T2-weighted images of the spine. However, the posterior longitudinal ligament can be difficult to visualize on fat-suppressed T2-weighted images (Figs. 17-36A and B and 17-37A and B).

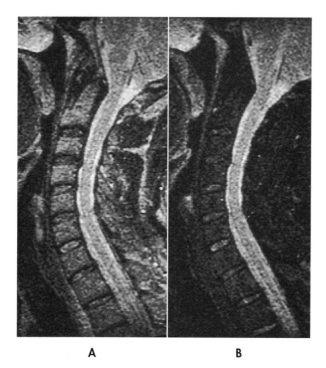

Fig. 17-36. Midsagittal T2-weighted images (TR 2500, TE 80, 1 Nex) obtained, **A,** without fat saturation and, **B,** with fat saturation. The fat saturation image demonstrates somewhat better myelographic effect. However, there is decreased visualization of the posterior longitudinal ligament on the fat saturation image.

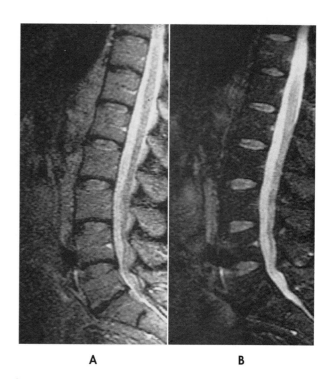

Fig. 17-37. Midsagittal T2-weighted images (TR 2200, TE 80, 1 Nex) obtained, **A,** without fat saturation and, **B,** with fat saturation. Whereas there is improved myelographic effect on the fat saturation image, there is decreased ability to visualize the posterior longitudinal ligament. (From Mirowitz SA, Reinus WR, Hammerman AM: Evaluation of fat saturation technique for T2-weighted imaging of the spine, Magn Reson Imag 12:599-604, 1994.)

Facet joints

Another entity that can simulate an epidural mass is hypertrophy of the posterior spinal elements.[29] Synovial cysts of the facet joints projecting into the spinal canal can also be mistaken for an epidural neoplasm[34] (Fig. 17-38). The facet joint capsule can extend into or behind the ligamentum flavum in some patients, creating an atypical appearance. Hypointensity can be observed within the facet joints as a result of the vacuum phenomenon. Synovial cysts exhibit variable signal intensity characteristics on T2-weighted images, ranging from hypointensity to marked hyperintensity.[45] When they are hyperintense, synovial cysts can be difficult to detect, because they may be isointense with adjacent CSF.[44] A low signal intensity rim may surround some synovial cysts.[3] When contrast material is administered, peripheral enhancement can be observed around the cyst.[17,75]

Characterization of Epidural Soft Tissue Lesions

Epidural soft tissue masses often have a nondescript appearance, which can lead to difficulty in their characterization. For example, distinction between epidural ab-

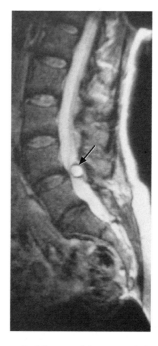

Fig. 17-38. A rounded focus of increased signal intensity (*arrow*) is demonstrated within the posterior epidural space on this sagittal T2-weighted image (TR 2000, TE 90) representing a synovial cyst.

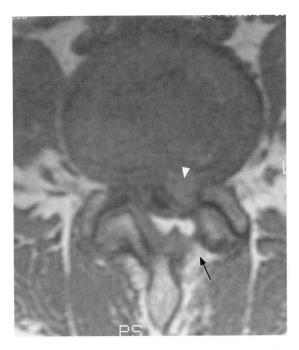

Fig. 17-39. Fat graft is observed filling laminectomy site (*arrow*) on this T1-weighted transaxial image (TR 500, TE 15, 4 Nex). A large soft tissue mass (*arrowhead*) can also be seen anterior to the thecal sac on the left, representing a recurrent disk herniation.

scess and neoplasm can be difficult,[48] particularly given the limited ability of MR to depict small air collections. Because of fat packing of the operative site, collections of fat can be observed within the posterior epidural space in patients who have undergone previous laminectomy,[66] (Figs. 17-21, 17-39, and 17-40). Such fat can potentially simulate the T1 shortening effects of methemoglobin within an epidural hematoma. The postoperative site can demonstrate extensive alterations in morphology and signal intensity, particularly early after surgery.[66] Heterogeneous signal intensity at the laminectomy site can also be seen because of Gelfoam or methylmethacrylate[66]; these materials can simulate an abscess. In patients who have undergone recent epidural anesthesia, small collections of air, manifested as foci of signal void, can be observed in the epidural space (see Fig. 17-18).

Epidural fat is variably prominent; when abundant it can result in neurologic symptoms (lipomatosis)[62] (Figs. 17-41A to 17-43). Epidural lipomas are most frequent in the thoracic spine and are associated with obesity and treatment with corticosteroids.[54] Epidural lipoma can be indistinguishable from CSF on T2-weighted images, particularly those that are acquired using fast spin echo or

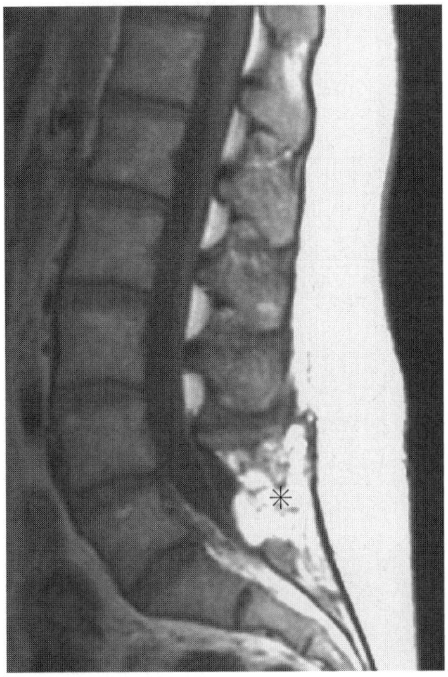

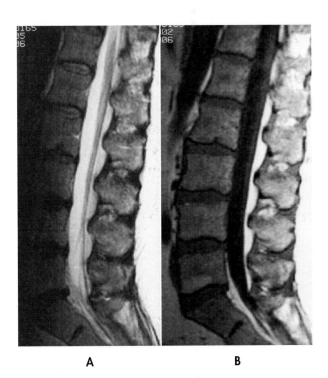

A   B

Fig. 17-41. A, Midsagittal fast spin echo T2-weighted image (TR 4000, effective TE 102, 2 Nex, 8 echo train) and, **B,** corresponding T1-weighted image (TR 500, TE 12, 2 Nex) are shown. There is relative isointensity of CSF and prominent posterior epidural fat on the fast spin echo image. However, these tissues can be easily distinguished on the T1-weighted image.

Fig. 17-40. Sagittal T1-weighted image in 47-year-old female after L5 laminectomy demonstrates fat packing (*asterisk*) filling bony defects (TR 500, TE 12, 2 Nex).

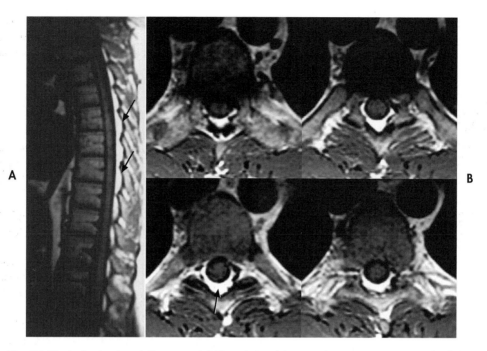

Fig. 17-42. A, Sagittal and, **B,** transaxial T1-weighted images (TR 500, TE 11, 2 Nex) of the thoracic spine demonstrate prominent collections of fat (*arrows*) within the posterior epidural space.

related sequences[22] (see Fig. 17-42). Determination of abnormal contrast material enhancement of epidural lesions can be difficult because of isointensity of enhancing tissue with surrounding epidural fat.[78,79] Close comparison with precontrast images and use of T1-weighted, fat suppressed, contrast-enhanced sequences can be helpful. Epidural lipomas can appear similar to subacute hematomas; fat suppressed T1-weighted images will allow for distinction.

Screening Examination of the Entire Spine

MR is frequently used to check for epidural tumor masses that compress the thecal sac and spinal cord. In such cases it is often important to survey the entire spine, since multiple sites of cord compression can be present.[76] The need for complete spine screening is heightened by difficulty in precisely determining the location of cord compression by clinical examination. One method for imaging the entire spine in a reasonable time period is the use of large field-of-view body coil sagittal images. Although this method is efficient, subtle extradural tumor involvement may not be appreciated on such images.[38] Thus, a detailed examination using a surface coil and small field-of-view, with image acquisition in two planes, should be considered in areas with a high likelihood of involvement based on clinical information or preliminary MR images.

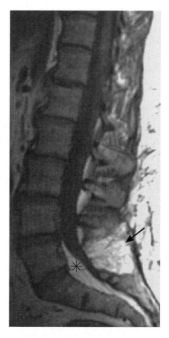

Fig. 17-43. Midsagittal T1-weighted image (TR 500, TE 12, 2 Nex) demonstrates prominent collection of fat (*asterisk*) within the anterior epidural space of the lower lumbar and upper sacral regions. Signal alterations related to previous lumbar laminectomy (*arrow*) are also noted posteriorly.

Lateral disk herniations

Lateral (i.e., foraminal and extraforaminal) disk herniations are often difficult to visualize on MR images. In one study 15 of 50 lateral herniations were not detected.[58] This is because distal to the neural foramen low signal intensity disk material is not contrasted against the high signal intensity of fat on T1-weighted images or fluid on T2-weighted images. Lateral disk herniations may be somewhat easier to visualize when they are calcified, because of accentuation of low signal intensity (Fig. 17-44). Coronal images can be helpful in demonstrating lateral disk bulging or herniation. Nonstandard coronal and sagittal oblique images can also be useful in the detection of lateral disk herniations.[27,41] These images are useful as problem-solving tools, particularly for evaluation of small herniations located within the neural foramina.

Anterior disk herniations

Anterior disk herniations are frequently observed on spine MR images[36] (Figs. 17-45 and 17-46). The clinical significance of such herniations is often obscure, because direct nerve root compression does not usually result in this location.

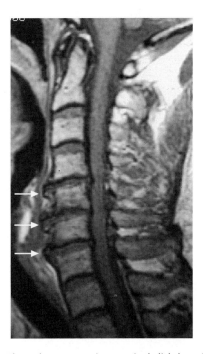

Fig. 17-45. Three large anterior cervical disk herniations (*arrows*) are present at adjacent levels on this midsagittal T1-weighted image (TR 600, TE 19, 2 Nex). Posterior protrusion of disk material is also present at the affected levels, with mild impression on the anterior surface of the cervical spinal cord.

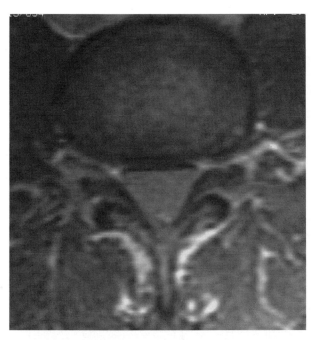

Fig. 17-44. The presence of a left lateral calcified disk herniation is difficult to visualize on this transaxial proton density–weighted image (TR 2500, TE 35, 2 Nex). The corresponding T1- and T2-weighted images were similarly unrevealing, although the herniation was present on postmyelography CT and CT diskography and was verified surgically.

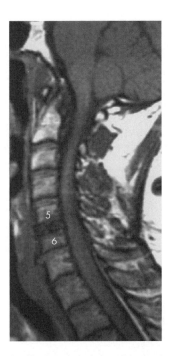

Fig. 17-46. Markedly decreased signal intensity as well as mild enlargement of the C5-6 intervertebral disk is present on this sagittal T1-weighted image (TR 566, TE 19, 2 Nex). These findings are related to previous anterior disk fusion. Anterior protrusion of the C6-7 disk is also present.

NEURAL FORAMEN

The dorsal root ganglion routinely undergoes enhancement following intravenous contrast material administration[14,18,69] (Figs. 17-47A and B). Such enhancement is particularly prominent when fat suppressed T1-weighted images are acquired[50]. The foraminal venous plexus of the cervical spine also enhances prominently,[69] which can assist in the definition of small foraminal disk herniations.

To adequately evaluate the neural foramina, the use of relatively small slice thickness and interslice gaps is required.[21,63,70] This has led to frequent use of three-dimensional Fourier transform gradient echo sequences for axial imaging of the cervical spine. Three-dimensional imaging provides thin contiguous slices with adequate signal-to-noise ratio, minimizing partial volume averaging.[83] Further, three-dimensional images can be retrospectively reformatted into any plane. This feature is useful in the cervical spine, where the neural foramina are better profiled on oblique image reformations rather than standard sagittal images.

Limitations of three-dimensional imaging include its increased vulnerability to motion artifacts and potential for aliasing and truncation artifacts to occur along the slice select in addition to the conventional phase-encoding direction.[83] Further, the observed contrast among CSF, cord, and disk can vary on different imaging slices with some three-dimensional gradient echo sequences.[21] Higher contrast between CSF and soft tissue may be observed on images acquired near the beginning of the imaging volume, because of inflow of unsaturated CSF spins.[21] However, inflow phenomenon is generally not as prominent on three-dimensional as on two-dimensional gradient echo images. This results in relative reduced intensity of CSF on the former images. In addition, the distribution of flip angles throughout the imaging volume may not be uniform, which can lead to variable tissue contrast on individual partition images.[70]

The neural foramina can appear artifactually reduced in size on images acquired using either two- or three-dimensional Fourier transform gradient echo technique (Figs. 17-48A and B). This is due to the difference in magnetization of bone and soft tissue, which results in susceptibility artifacts at their interface. These artifacts lead to a "blooming" of low signal intensity that can simulate hypertrophic bone. Susceptibility artifacts are increased in prominence in proportion to the echo time used.[82,84] Tsuruda and Remley found that an 11-msec echo time resulted in overestimation of foraminal stenosis by 8%, whereas an echo time of 22 msec led to 27% overestimation.[84] Image display settings can also affect the apparent severity of foraminal narrowing on MR im-

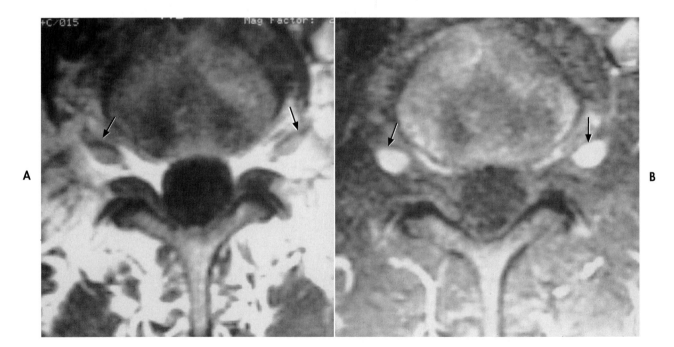

Fig. 17-47. Transaxial gadolinium chelate enhanced T1-weighted images obtained, **A,** without fat saturation and, **B,** with fat saturation demonstrate contrast enhancement of normal dorsal root ganglia (*arrows*). The conspicuousness of enhancement of these structures is markedly increased on the fat suppressed image.

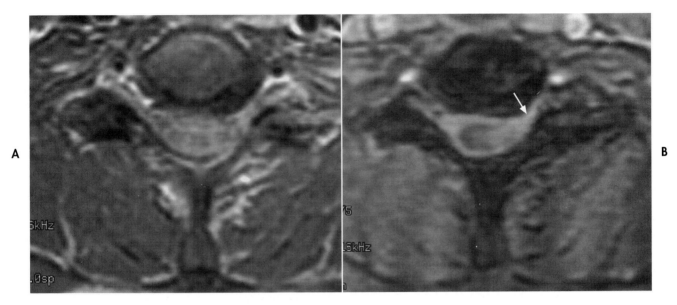

Fig. 17-48. Corresponding, **A,** transaxial proton density–weighted image (TR 2700, TE 30, 1 Nex) and, **B,** three-dimensional spoiled gradient echo image (TR 35, TE 15, 5-degree flip angle, 2 Nex) of the cervical spine. There is artifactual accentuation of narrowing of the left neural foramen (*arrow*) on the gradient echo image as compared with the spin echo image because of susceptibility artifacts arising at the bone–soft tissue interface.

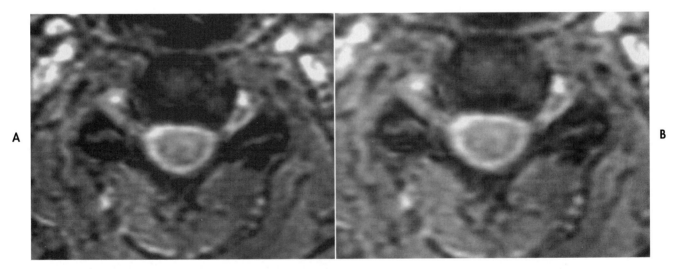

Fig. 17-49A and **B.** Transaxial image from three-dimensional spoiled gradient echo (TR 35, TE 15, 5-degree flip angle, 2 Nex) series is shown with two different photographic settings. **A** indicates artifactual decreased diameter of the neural foramina because of narrower window width setting.

ages, with narrow window settings causing potential overestimation of such narrowing (Figs. 17-49A and B).

Motion artifacts are another contributor to apparent foraminal narrowing and also increase in prominence with increasing echo time.[84] Application of axial loading forces can cause the neural foramen to appear narrowed.[57] The neural foramen may appear to be patent on axial images that are acquired through its inferior recess.[35] However, images acquired at a slightly higher level may depict significant foraminal root encroachment.

Artifactual linear areas of hypointensity can be observed along the course of the exiting nerve roots on gradient echo images. This is due to chemical shift phase cancellation that occurs at the interface between the perineurium and surrounding foraminal fat.

Synovial cysts can occasionally extend into the neural foramen, where they may simulate a foraminal disk herniation.[49] Tortuous and looping vertebral arteries can erode into the neural foramen, simulating neural tumors or other masses.

REFERENCES

1. Aprill C, Bogduk N: High-intensity zone: a diagnostic sign of painful lumbar disc on magnetic resonance imaging, Br J Radiol 65:361-369, 1992.
2. Araki Y, Ootani M, Furukawa T et al: Pseudoenhancement of intervertebral disc herniation, Neuroradiology 34:271-272, 1992.
3. Awwad EE, Martin DS, Smith KR Jr et al: MR imaging of lumbar juxtaarticular cysts, J Comput Assist Tomogr 14:415-417, 1990.
4. Beltran J, Chandnani V, McGhee RA Jr et al: Gadopentetate dimeglumine-enhanced MR imaging of the musculoskeletal system, Am J Roentgenol 156:457-466, 1991.
5. Berns DH, Ross JS, Kormos D et al: The spinal vacuum phenomenon: evaluation by gradient echo MR imaging, J Comput Assist Tomogr 15:233-236, 1991.
6. Blumberg ML, Ostrum BJ, Ostrum DM: Changes in MR signal intensity of the intervertebral disk, Radiology 179:584-585, 1991.
7. Bobman SA, Atlas SW, Listerud J et al: Postoperative lumbar spine: contrast-enhanced chemical shift MR imaging, Radiology 179:557-562, 1991.
8. Boden SD, Davis DO, Dina TS et al: Contrast-enhanced MR imaging performed after successful lumbar disk surgery: prospective study, Radiology 182:59-64, 1992.
9. Boden SD, Davis DO, Dina TS et al: Postoperative diskitis: distinguishing early MR imaging findings from normal postoperative disk space changes, Radiology 184:765-771, 1992.
10. Boos N, Wallin A, Gbedegbegnon T et al: Quantitative MR imaging of lumbar intervertebral disks and vertebral bodies: influence of diurnal water content variations, Radiology 188:351-354, 1993.
11. Bozzao A, Gallucci M, Masciocchi C et al: Lumbar disk herniation: MR imaging assessment of natural history in patients treated without surgery, Radiology 185:135-141, 1992.
12. Brant-Zawadzki M: Pitfalls of contrast-enhanced imaging in the nervous system, Magn Reson Med 22:243-248, 1991.
13. Breger RK, Czervionke LF, Kass EG et al: Truncation artifact in MR images of the intervertebral disk, Am J Neuroradiol 9:825-828, 1988.
14. Breger RK, Williams AL, Daniels DL et al: Contrast enhancement in spinal MR imaging, Am J Neuroradiol 10:633-637, 1989.
15. Bundschuh CV, Modic MT, Ross JS et al: Epidural fibrosis and recurrent disk herniation in the lumbar spine: MR imaging assessment, Am J Roentgenol 150:923-932, 1988.
16. Bundschuh CV, Stein L, Slusser JH et al: Distinguishing between scar and recurrent herniated disk in postoperative patients: value of contrast-enhanced CT and MR imaging, Am J Neuroradiol 11:949-958, 1990.
17. Chiang KS, Lee Y-Y, Mawad ME: MR of intraspinal synovial cyst: rim enhancement with gadopentetate dimeglumine, Am J Roentgenol 157:416, 1991.
18. Czervionke LF, Daniels DL, Ho PSP et al: Cervical neural foramina: correlative anatomic and MR imaging study, Radiology 169:753-759, 1988.
19. Dwyer AJ, Knop RH, Hoult DI: Frequency shift artifacts in MR imaging, J Comput Assist Tomogr 9:16-18, 1985.
20. Enzmann DR, Griffin C, Rubin JB: Potential false-negative MR images of the thoracic spine in disk disease with switching of phase- and frequency-encoding gradients, Radiology 165:635-637, 1987.
21. Enzmann D, Rubin JB, Short TR: Variable flip angle, gradient echo scans of the cervical spine: comparison of 2DFT and 3DFT techniques, Neuroradiology 31:213-216, 1989.
22. Flanders AE, Schaefer DM, Doan HT et al: Acute cervical spine trauma: correlation of MR imaging findings with degree of neurologic deficit, Radiology 177:25-33, 1990.
23. Flannigan BD, Lufkin RB, McGlade C et al: MR imaging of the cervical spine: neurovascular anatomy, Am J Roentgenol 148:785-790, 1987.
24. Gelber ND, Ragland RL, Knorr JR: Gd-DTPA enhanced MRI of cervical anterior epidural venous plexus, J Comput Assist Tomogr 16:760-763, 1992.
25. Glickstein MF, Burke DL Jr, Kressel HY: Magnetic resonance demonstration of hyperintense herniated discs and extruded disc fragments, Skeletal Radiol 18:527-530, 1989.
26. Glickstein MF, Sussman SK: Time-dependent scar enhancement in magnetic resonance imaging of the postoperative lumbar spine, Skeletal Radiol 20:333-337, 1991.
27. Grenier N, Greselle J-F, Douws C et al: MR imaging of foraminal and extraforaminal lumbar disk herniations, J Comput Assist Tomogr 14:243-249, 1990.
28. Grenier N, Greselle J-F, Vital J-M et al: Normal and disrupted lumbar longitudinal ligaments: correlative MR and anatomic study, Radiology 171:197-205, 1989.
29. Grenier N, Grossman RI, Schiebler ML et al: Degenerative lumbar disk disease: pitfalls and usefulness of MR imaging in detection of vacuum phenomenon, Radiology 164:861-865, 1987.
30. Gundry CR, Heithoff KB: Epidural hematoma of the lumbar spine: 18 surgically confirmed cases, Radiology 187:427-431, 1993.

31. Hedberg MC, Drayer BP, Flom RA et al: Gradient echo (GRASS) MR imaging in cervical radiculopathy, Am J Roentgenol 150:683-689, 1988.

32. Hueftle MG, Modic MT, Ross JS et al: Lumbar spine: postoperative MR imaging with Gd-DTPA, Radiology 167:817-824, 1988.

33. Isherwood I, Prendergast DJ, Hickey DS et al: Quantitative analysis of intervertebral disc structure, Acta Radiol Suppl (Stockh) 369:492-495, 1986.

34. Jackson DE Jr, Atlas SW, Mani JR et al: Intraspinal synovial cysts: : MR imaging, Radiology 170:527-530, 1989.

35. Jinkins JR, Matthes JC, Sener RN et al: Spondylolysis, spondylolisthesis, and associated nerve root entrapment in the lumbosacral spine: MR evaluation, Am J Roentgenol 159:799-803, 1992.

36. Jinkins JR, Whittemore AR, Bradley WG: The anatomic basis of vertebrogenic pain and the autonomic syndrome associated with lumbar disk extrusion, Am J Roentgenol 152:1277-1289, 1989.

37. Jones KM, Mulkern RV, Schwartz RB et al: Fast spin-echo MR imaging of the brain and spine: current concepts, Am J Roentgenol 158:1313-1320, 1992.

38. Karnaze MG, Gado MH, Sartor KJ et al: Comparison of MR and CT myelography in imaging the cervical and thoracic spine, Am J Roentgenol 150:397-403, 1988.

39. Kato F, Mimatsu K, Kawakami N et al: Changes seen on magnetic resonance imaging in the intervertebral disc space after chemonucleolysis: a hypothesis concerning regeneration of the disc after chemonucleolysis, Neuroradiology 34:267-270, 1992.

40. Ketonen L, Totterman S, Simon JH et al: A comparison of default and reduced bandwidth MR imaging of the spine at 1.5 T, Am J Neuroradiol 11:9-15, 1990.

41. Krause D, Drape JL, Woerly B et al: Lumbar disc herniation: value of oblique magnetic resonance imaging sections, J Neuroradiol 15:305-324, 1988.

42. Larsson EM, Holtas S, Cronqvist S et al: Comparison of myelography, CT myelography and magnetic resonance imaging in cervical spondylosis and disk herniation: pre- and postoperative findings, Acta Radiol 30:233-239, 1989.

43. LeBlanc AD, Schonfeld E, Schneider VS et al: The spine: changes in T2 relaxation times from disuse, Radiology 169:105-107, 1988.

44. Liu SS, Williams KD, Drayer BP et al: Synovial cysts of the lumbosacral spine: diagnosis by MR imaging, Am J Neuroradiol 10:1239-1242, 1989.

45. Liu SS, Williams KD, Drayer BP et al: Synovial cysts of the lumbosacral spine: diagnosis by MR imaging, Am J Roentgenol 154:163-166, 1990.

46. Major NM, Helms CA, Genant HK: Calcification demonstrated as high signal intensity on T1-weighted MR images of the disks of the lumbar spine, Radiology 189:494-496, 1993.

47. Masaryk TJ, Boumphrey F, Modic MT et al: Effects of chemonucleolysis demonstrated by MR imaging, J Comput Assist Tomogr 10:917-923, 1986.

48. Masaryk TJ, Ross JS, Modic MT et al: High-resolution MR imaging of sequestered lumbar intervertebral disks, Am J Roentgenol 150:1155-1162, 1988.

49. Maupin WB, Naul LG, Kanter SL et al: Synovial cyst presenting as a neural foraminal lesion: MR and CT appearance, Am J Roentgenol 153:1231-1232, 1989.

50. Mirowitz SA, Shady KL: Gadopentetate dimeglumine-enhanced MR imaging of the postoperative lumbar spine: comparison of fat-suppressed and conventional T1-weighted images, Am J Roentgenol 159:385-389, 1992.

51. Modic MT, Herfkens RJ: Intervertebral disk: normal age-related changes in MR signal intensity, Radiology 177:332-334, 1990.

52. Modic MT, Masaryk TJ, Ross JS et al: Imaging of degenerative disk disease, Radiology 168:177-186, 1988.

53. Modic MT, Ross JS: Morphology, symptoms, and causality, Radiology 175:619-620, 1990.

54. Morano JU, Miller JD, Connors JJ: MR imaging of spinal epidural lipoma, Am J Neuroradiol 10:S102, 1989.

55. Murayama S, Numaguchi Y, Robinson AE: Degenerative lumbar spine disorders in gradient refocused echo axial magnetic resonance images, Clin Imaging 14:198-203, 1990.

56. Murayama S, Numaguchi Y, Robinson AE: The diagnosis of herniated intervertebral disks with MR imaging: a comparison of gradient-refocused-echo and spin-echo pulse sequences, Am J Neuroradiol 11:17-22, 1990.

57. Nowicki BH, Yu S, Reinartz J et al: Effect of axial loading on neural foramina and nerve roots in the lumbar spine, Radiology 176:433-437, 1990.

58. Osborn AG, Hood RS, Sherry RG et al: CT/MR spectrum of far lateral and anterior lumbosacral disk herniations, Am J Neuroradiol 9:775-778, 1988.

59. Otake S, Matsuo M, Nishizawa S et al: Ossification of the posterior longitudinal ligament: MR evaluation, Am J Neuroradiol 13:1059-1067, 1992.

60. Parizel PM, Rodesch G, Baleriaux D et al: Gd-DTPA-enhanced MR in thoracic disc herniations, Neuroradiology 31:75-79, 1989.

61. Pech P, Haughton VM: Lumbar intervertebral disk: correlative MR and anatomic study, Radiology 156:699-701, 1985.

62. Quint DJ, Boulos RS, Sanders WP et al: Epidural lipomatosis, Radiology 169:485-490, 1988.

63. Ross JS: MR imaging of the cervical spine: techniques for two- and three-dimensional imaging, Am J Roentgenol 159:779-786, 1992.

64. Ross JS, Blaser S, Masaryk TJ et al: Gd-DTPA enhancement of posterior epidural scar: an experimental model, Am J Neuroradiol 10:1083-1088, 1989.

65. Ross JS, Masaryk TJ, Modic MT: Postoperative cervical spine: MR assessment, J Comput Assist Tomogr 11:955-962, 1987.

66. Ross JS, Masaryk TJ, Modic et al: Lumbar spine: postoperative assessment with surface-coil MR imaging, Radiology 164:851-860, 1987.

67. Ross JS, Masaryk TJ, Schrader M et al: MR imaging of the postoperative lumbar spine assessment with gadopentetate dimeglumine, Am J Neuroradiol 11:711-776, 1990.

68. Ross JS, Modic MT, Masaryk TJ: Tears of the anulus fibrosus: assessment with Gd-DTPA-enhanced MR imaging, Am J Neuroradiol 10:1251-1254, 1989.

69. Ross JS, Modic MT, Masaryk TJ, et al: Assessment of extradural degenerative disease with Gd-DTPA-enhanced MR imaging: correlation with surgical and pathologic findings, Am J Neuroradiol 10:1243-1249, 1989.

70. Ross JS, Tkach J, VanDyke C et al: Clinical MR imaging of degenerative spinal disease: pulse sequences, gradient-echo techniques, and contrast agents, J Magn Reson Imaging 1:29-37, 1991.

71. Russell EJ: Cervical disk disease, Radiology 177:313-325, 1990.

72. Schellinger D, Manz HJ, Vidic B et al: Disk fragment migration, Radiology 175:831-836, 1990.

73. Schiebler ML, Grenier N, Fallon M et al: Normal and degenerated intervertebral disk: in vivo and in vitro MR imaging with histopathologic correlation, Am J Roentgenol 157:93-97, 1991.

74. Sether LA, Yu S, Haughton VM et al: Intervertebral disk: normal age-related changes in MR signal intensity, Radiology 177:385-388, 1990.

75. Silbergleit R, Gebarski SS, Brunberg JA et al: Lumbar synovial cysts: correlation of myelographic, CT, MR, and pathologic findings, Am J Neuroradiol 11:777-779, 1990.

76. Smoker WRK, Godersky JC, Knutzon RK et al: The role of MR imaging in evaluating metastatic spinal disease, Am J Roentgenol 149:1241-1248, 1987.

77. Sugimura H, Kakitsubata Y, Suzuki Y et al: MRI of ossification of ligamentum flavum, J Comput Assist Tomogr 16:73-76, 1992.

78. Sze G: Gadolinium-DTPA in spinal disease, Radiol Clin North Am 26:1009-1024, 1988.

79. Sze G, Krol G, Zimmerman RD et al: Malignant extradural spinal tumors: MR imaging with Gd-DTPA, Radiology 167:217-223, 1988.

80. Teresi LM, Lufkin RB, Reicher MA et al: Asymptomatic degenerative disk disease and spondylosis of the cervical spine: MR imaging, Radiology 164:83-88, 1987.

81. Tertti MO, Salminen JJ, Paajanen HEK et al: Low-back pain and disk degeneration in children: a case-control MR imaging study, Radiology 180:503-507, 1991.

82. Tien RD, Buxton RB, Schwaighofer BW et al: Quantitation of structural distortion of the cervical neural foramina in gradient-echo MR imaging, J Magn Reson Imaging 1:683-687, 1991.

83. Tsuruda JS, Norman D, Dillon W et al: Three-dimensional gradient-recalled MR imaging as a screening tool for the diagnosis of cervical radiculopathy, Am J Roentgenol 154:375-383, 1990.

84. Tsuruda JS, Remley K: Effects of magnetic susceptibility artifacts and motion in evaluating the cervical neural foramina on 3DFT gradient-echo MR imaging, Am J Neuroradiol 12:237-241, 1991.

85. VanDyke C, Ross JS, Tkach J et al: Gradient-echo MR imaging of the cervical spine: evaluation of extradural disease, Am J Roentgenol 153:393-398, 1989.

86. Williams MP, Cherryman GR: Thoracic disk herniation: MR imaging (letter), Radiology 167:874-875, 1988.

87. Williams MP, Cherryman GR, Husband JE: Significance of thoracic disc herniation demonstrated by MR imaging, J Comput Assist Tomogr 13:211-214, 1989.

88. Wilmink JT: Clinical relevance of cervical disk herniation diagnosed on the basis of MR imaging (letter), Am J Neuroradiol 10:1278-1279, 1989.

89. Yomashita Y, Takahashi M, Matsuno Y et al: Spinal cord compression due to ossification of ligaments: MR imaging, Radiology 175:843-848, 1990.

90. Yousem DM, Atlas SW, Goldberg HI et al: Degenerative narrowing of the cervical spine neural foramina: evaluation with high-resolution 3DFT gradient-echo MR imaging, Am J Roentgenol 156:1229-1236, 1991.

91. Yu S, Haughton VM, Ho PSP et al: Progressive and regressive changes in the nucleus pulposus. II. The adult, Radiology 169:93-97, 1988.

92. Yu S, Sether LA, Ho PSP et al: Tears of the annulus fibrosus: correlation between MR and pathologic findings in cadavers, Am J Neuroradiol 9:367-370, 1988.

18

Spinal Cord and Intradural Space

SPINAL CORD

Anatomic Variations

Thecal sac/subarachnoid space

The caudal termination of the thecal sac varies in position (Fig. 18-1). The subdural and subarachnoid spaces typically descend to the level of the second sacral vertebra, although in many individuals they terminate at lower levels.[5]

In addition, the prominence of the subarachnoid space varies among healthy individuals. Cystic dilatation of the thecal sac can be observed, particularly in the lower lumbar and sacral regions and may be associated with cystic dilatation of the sacral nerve root sheaths (i.e., Tarlov cysts) (Figs. 18-2 and 18-3). Communication of such cysts with the subarachnoid space can be verified with motion-sensitive sequences, such as steady state free precession. Signal intensity alterations indicating fluid motion within these cysts imply that they communicate with the subarachnoid space. However, similar signal changes can occasionally be caused by transmitted pulsations in noncommunicating cysts.[18] Whereas sacral meningeal cysts are common incidental findings, they may occasionally be associated with neurologic symptoms.[18] Focal prominence of the subarachnoid space occurs in some patients with spinal cord atrophy and can simulate a subarachnoid cyst.[62] The thecal sac is frequently focally dilated posteriorly in patients who have undergone previous laminectomy at the surgical site[49] (Figs. 18-4 and 18-5). Extension of the thecal sac through the laminectomy defect can result in formation of a pseudomeningocele (Fig. 18-6).[49]

Conus medullaris

The conus medullaris typically terminates at the L1 level in adults. However, the position of the conus is somewhat variable and can range from the T12 to L3 levels.[5] The conus is normally low-lying in children, and it ascends relative to the vertebral bodies during maturation.[48,78]

The precise position of the conus medullaris can be difficult to determine on sagittal T1- or T2-weighted images (Figs. 18-7 and 18-8) because the proximal cauda equina roots are often tightly clustered. Their confluent appearance can be similar to that of the conus medullaris in both diameter and signal intensity.[48,50] Close inspection of sagittal images and correlation with transaxial images usually allow the position of the conus to be determined, so that a false diagnosis of tethered cord is not made. Clumping of the cauda equina roots in patients

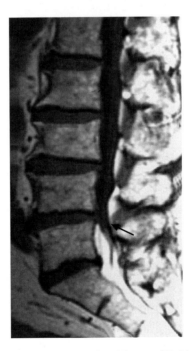

Fig. 18-1. Midsagittal T1-weighted image (TR 500, TE 12, 2 Nex) demonstrates termination of the thecal sac at the L4-5 level (*arrow*).

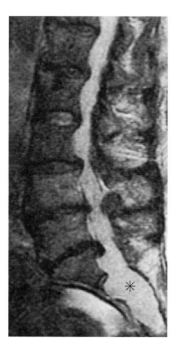

Fig. 18-2. Marked dilatation of the caudal portion of the thecal sac (*asterisk*) is demonstrated on this sagittal T2-weighted image (TR 2000, TE 74, 1 Nex). Cystic dilatation of the perineural sheaths of the sacral nerve roots was also demonstrated on additional images. Disk space narrowing and disk degeneration and herniation are noted at several lumbar levels.

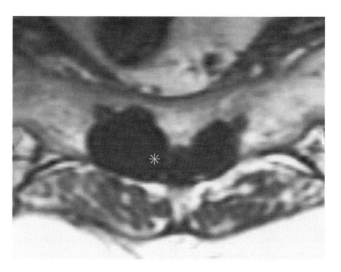

Fig. 18-3. Marked dilatation of the sacral nerve root sheaths with secondary bony remodeling (*asterisk*) is noted on this transaxial T1-weighted image (TR 400, TE 14, 4 Nex).

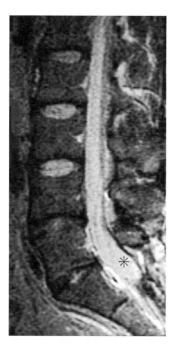

Fig. 18-4. Midsagittal T2-weighted image (TR 2000, TE 75, 1 Nex) demonstrates expansion of the posterior aspect of the thecal sac (*asterisk*) related to previous laminectomy at the L5-S1 level. Reduced signal intensity is noted at the L4-5 and L5-S1 levels because of degenerative disk disease.

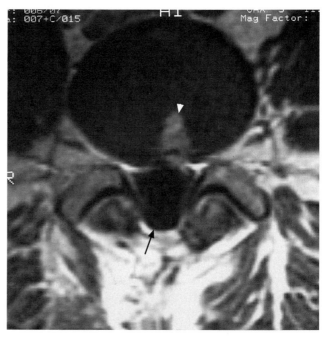

Fig. 18-5. Posterior expansion of the thecal sac (*arrow*) is noted at the level of previous laminectomy on this gadolinium chelate enhanced T1-weighted image (TR 500, TE 14, 4 Nex). Contrast material enhancement is also noted within the intervertebral disk at the site of previous curettage (*arrowhead*).

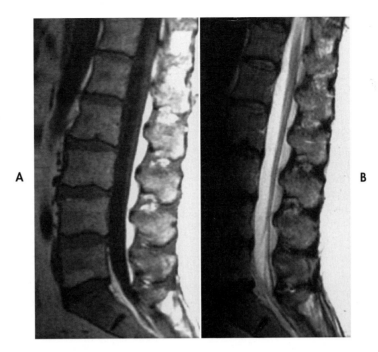

Fig. 18-6. A, Sagittal T1-weighted image (TR 500, TE 12, 2 Nex) demonstrates prominent fat within the posterior epidural space of the lumbar spine. **B,** Because of isointensity of CSF and fat, the actual dimensions of the thecal sac are difficult to determine on corresponding fast spin echo T2-weighted image (TR 4000, effective TE 102, 4 Nex, 8 echo train).

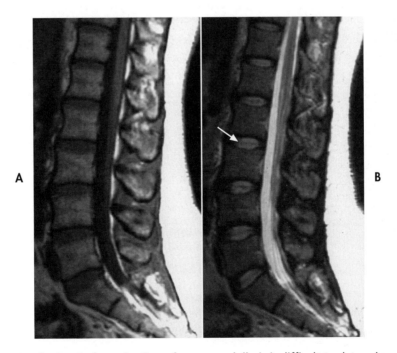

Fig. 18-7. Precise level of termination of conus medullaris is difficult to determine on **A,** sagittal T1-weighted image (TR 500, TE 12, 2 Nex) and, **B,** fast spin echo T2-weighted image (TR 4000, effective TE 102, 4 Nex, 16 echo train) because of blending of conus medullaris with proximal cauda equina nerve roots. T2-weighted image demonstrates appearance of normal intranuclear cleft of intravertebral disk (*arrow*).

Fig. 18-8. A, Midsagittal T1-weighted image (TR 500, TE 12, 2 Nex) and, **B,** T2-weighted image (TR 2000, TE 75, 1 Nex) illustrate difficulty in determining the precise level of termination of the conus medullaris because of apparent blending of this structure with the intrathecal roots of the cauda equina. Diffuse reduced signal intensity throughout all lumbar vertebral bodies on the T1-weighted image because of prominent hematopoietic bone marrow is also noted.

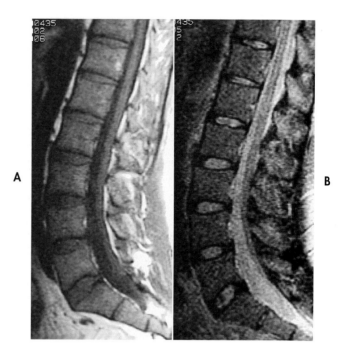

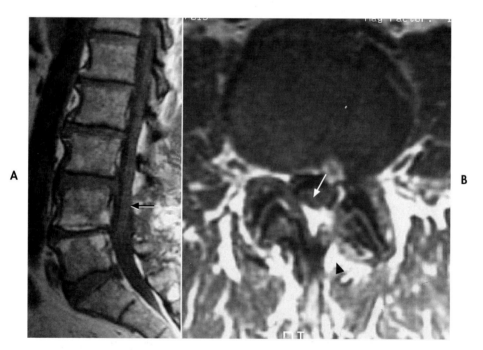

Fig. 18-9. A, The conus medullaris appears to be low-lying (*arrow*) on sagittal T1-weighted image (TR 500, TE 12, 2 Nex). This is due to clumping of cauda equina nerve roots in patient who underwent previous lumbar surgery. High signal intensity as a result of fatty marrow changes is noted within the endplates adjacent to the L4-5 interspace. **B,** The gadopentetate enhanced transaxial T1-weighted image (TR 500, TE 15, 4 Nex) demonstrates masslike clumping of the cauda equina roots (*arrow*). A left-sided laminectomy defect can be seen (*arrowhead*), with associated contrast material enhancement caused by granulation tissue. Enhancement within the intervertebral disk at the site of previous curettage is also noted, again related to granulation tissue ingrowth. Note that no abnormal contrast enhancement is associated with the inflamed cauda equina nerve roots.

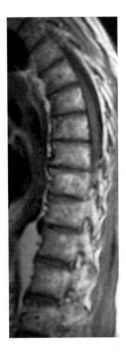

Fig. 18-10. Sagittal T1-weighted image (TR 500, TE 12, 2 Nex) provides only segmental visualization of the spinal cord because of scoliosis. Heterogeneous signal intensity throughout the marrow space of the vertebral column is also noted in this 74-year-old female.

with arachnoiditis can also contribute to difficulty in determining the location of the conus medullaris (Fig. 18-9). The clustered roots of the cauda equina along the dependent portion of the thecal sac can suggest the presence of an intradural mass lesion or hematoma on transaxial images.

Segmental visualization of the spinal cord

The spinal cord may not be visualized in continuity on sagittal images, particularly in scoliotic patients (Fig. 18-10). Rather, it is visualized segmentally on a number of images and is subject to increased partial volume effects. Reformation of sagittal images along an oblique or curved plane can allow for continuous visualization of the cord in many patients (Fig. 18-11).

Spinal nerves and ganglia

The spinal nerve roots and their associated ganglia are subject to numerous variations.[5] The dorsal nerve root is typically larger than the corresponding anterior root. Duplication of the dorsal root ganglion can be observed at the lumbar and upper sacral levels.[5] Whereas most ganglia are located within the neural foramina, the L5 through S4 ganglia are often found within the spinal canal, and some ganglia (usually sacrococcygeal) may be located within the dural sac.[5]

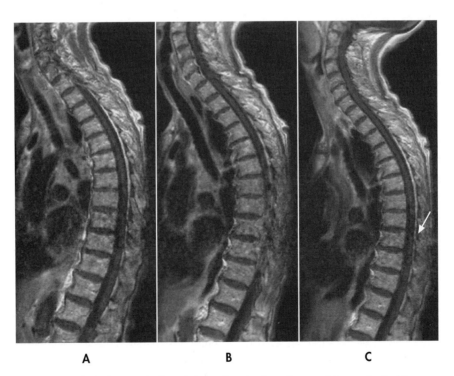

A   B   C

Fig. 18-11. A and **B,** The cervical and thoracic spinal cord cannot be evaluated in continuity on a single sagittal T1-weighted image (TR 500, TE 11, 2 Nex) because of slight scoliosis. However, retrospective reformatting of the data does allow for continuous depiction of the spinal cord and spinal column, **C.** Note that cardiac pulsation artifacts result in heterogeneous signal intensity overlying the midthoracic spinal cord (*arrow*).

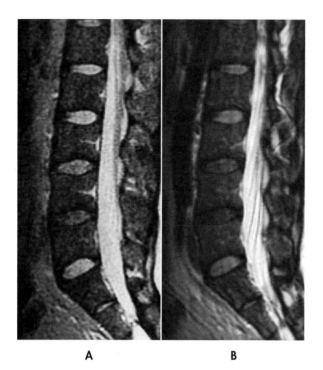

A   **B**

Fig. 18-12. A, Sagittal T2-weighted image (TR 2000, TE 75, 1 Nex) and, **B,** fast spin echo T2-weighted image (TR 4000, effective TE 102, 4 Nex, 16 echo train). The cauda equina nerve roots are depicted with improved clarity on fast spin echo image. This is attributable to improved signal-to-noise ratio (4 excitations versus 2) and increased spatial resolution (256 versus 192 phase-encoding steps). Decreased signal intensity because of degenerative disk disease is present within the L4-5 intervertebral disk and is more prominent on the fast spin echo image.

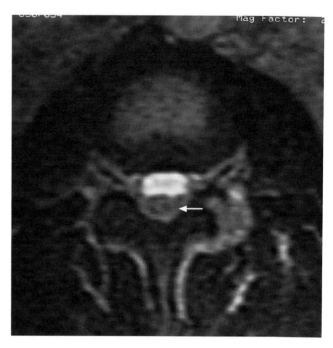

Fig. 18-13. Layering of the roots of the cauda equina within the dependent portion of the thecal sac (*arrow*) creates the appearance of an intradural low signal intensity lesion on this transaxial T2-weighted image (TR 2500, TE 75, 1 Nex).

SIMULATION OF SPINAL CORD LESIONS

- Signal alterations caused by spinal stenosis
- Partial volume averaging with cerebrospinal fluid (CSF) and fat
- Truncation artifact
- Motion artifact
- Gray matter
- Ventral median fissure
- Compact white matter pathways
- Regional variations in cord diameter

Cauda equina

The nerve roots of the cauda equina have relatively consistent patterns of branching within the dural sac, and these patterns vary according to vertebral body level.[50] Visualization of the individual roots of the cauda equina is improved when a high resolution imaging matrix is prescribed (Fig. 18-12). Clustered layering of the normal cauda equina roots within the thecal sac can simulate an intradural mass (Fig. 18-13). The cauda equina roots are normally located along the dependent aspect of the thecal sac. Although this is usually posterior, in patients who are imaged in the prone position, the roots can be observed along the anterior aspect of the sac (Fig. 18-14).

Normal patterns of cauda equina nerve root clustering must be distinguished from abnormal patterns observed in some patients with arachnoiditis.[50] In patients with arachnoiditis, the cauda equina roots can be tightly clumped into a single cluster or multiple clusters, or they may be applied along the periphery of the thecal sac[50]

(Fig. 18-9). Apparent clumping of the cauda equina roots can be observed in patients with stenosis of the central spinal canal.[50] Partial volume averaging of normal cauda equina roots with adjacent bony structures can also simulate nerve root clumping on sagittal images.

In addition to clumping, the cauda equina nerve roots can appear distorted and demonstrate abnormal contrast material enhancement in some patients with arachnoiditis.[33] There is, however, considerable variability in the enhancement pattern of inflamed nerve roots following

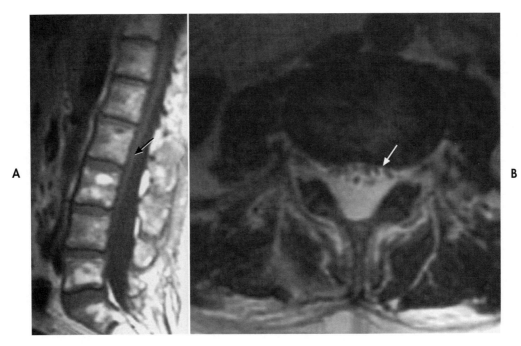

Fig. 18-14. A, Midsagittal T1-weighted image and, **B,** transaxial T2-weighted image obtained with patient in prone position. The distal spinal cord and cauda equina nerve roots (*arrows*) are displaced toward the ventral aspect of the thecal sac because of prone positioning.

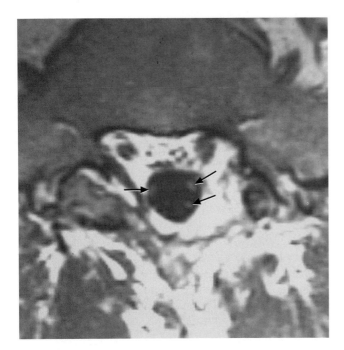

Fig. 18-15. Enhancement of the cauda equina nerve roots (*arrows*) is evident on this transaxial gadopentetate enhanced T1-weighted imaged (TR 500, TE 15, 4 Nex) in patient who underwent previous left L5-S1 laminectomy.

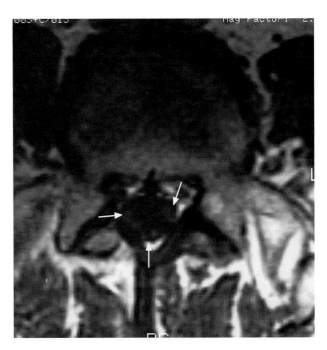

Fig. 18-16. Mild enhancement of the cauda equina nerve roots (*arrows*) is demonstrated on this gadopentetate enhanced T1-weighted transaxial image (TR 500, TE 15, 4 Nex). Absence of the right ligamentum flavum, related to previous laminectomy, is also noted.

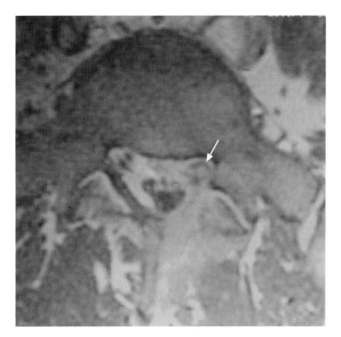

Fig. 18-17. Gadopentetate enhanced transaxial T1-weighted image (TR 500, TE 15, 4 Nex) in patient who underwent previous left L5-S1 laminectomy. The laminectomy defect is filled with enhancing soft tissue material representing granulation tissue. In addition, abnormal contrast enhancement of the ipsilateral S1 nerve root (*arrow*) as a result of postoperative inflammatory changes is noted.

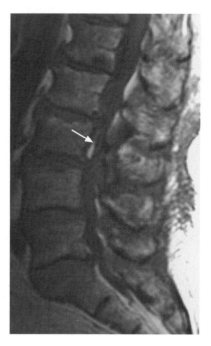

Fig. 18-18. Sagittal T1-weighted image (TR 600, TE 12, 2 Nex) performed 2 days following lumbar puncture. Linear increased signal intensity representing blood breakdown products (i.e., methemoglobin) is noted within the thecal sac at the level of the L3 vertebral body (*arrow*).

contrast material administration. In one study of 13 patients with arachnoiditis, absent, minimal, mild, and moderate enhancement of involved nerve roots was observed in nearly equal percentages of patients.[33] Thus the absence of contrast enhancement does not exclude arachnoiditis (Fig. 18-9). Abnormal contrast enhancement of nerve roots is more prominent when fat suppressed T1-weighted images are acquired.[6,73]

Mild enhancement of the intradural cauda equina roots can also be observed in some healthy individuals; this should not be interpreted as evidence of arachnoiditis.[4,33,73] More prominent nerve root enhancement can be seen in patients who have undergone previous lumbar laminectomy and diskectomy; this might represent associated inflammatory changes[6,7] (Figs. 18-15 to 18-17). Intradural nerve root enhancement can also occur following recent lumbar puncture in some patients, and hemorrhagic products are also occasionally observed within the thecal sac (Figs. 18-13 and 18-18). Contrast enhancement of thickened cauda equina roots has also been observed in patients with Guillain-Barré syndrome.[1]

Spinal cord diameter

Mild fusiform enlargement of the spinal cord at the level of the conus medullaris, as well as in the lower cervical region, can be observed in normal individuals (Figs. 18-19 and 18-20). These sites correspond to the origin of the roots of the lumbosacral and brachial plexuses, respectively, and should not be interpreted as evidence of cord swelling or infiltration. Differentiation is based on the subtle degree of cord enlargement, smooth contour, and lack of associated signal intensity alterations or abnormal contrast material enhancement.

The caliber of the spinal cord varies more subtly at different anatomic levels in normal individuals. Spinal cord area can be approximated as the product of the anteroposterior and transverse diameters of the spinal cord. Cord area measurements vary from 110 sq mm at the C2 level, to 122 sq mm at the C4 level, to 85 sq mm at the C7 level.[61] These findings emphasize the limitation of using a single value as a criterion for overall spinal cord size, since such a figure does not account for these regional variations.

The anteroposterior diameter of the spinal cord appears artifactually decreased on transaxial T2-weighted spin echo images. Truncation artifact is the major reason for such pseudoatrophy of the spinal cord, particu-

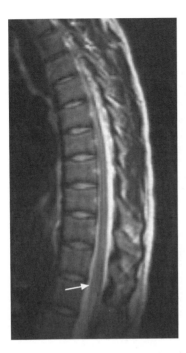

Fig. 18-19. Sagittal fast spin echo T2-weighted image (TR 4000, effective TE 96, 4 Nex, 16 echo train) demonstrates mild focal enlargement of the spinal cord in the region of the conus medullaris (*arrow*) in normal 22-year-old female.

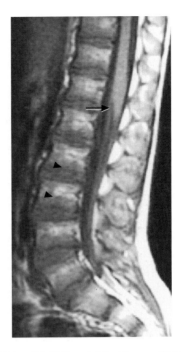

Fig. 18-20. Midsagittal T1-weighted image (TR 500, TE 12, 2 Nex) demonstrates relative enlargement of the spinal cord in the region of the conus medullaris (*arrow*) in 8-year-old female patient. High signal intensity coursing along the basivertebral veins of the vertebral bodies is also noted (*arrowheads*), representing marrow fat.

larly when images are acquired using a low resolution matrix.[17,37,57,79] Yousem et al. found that cord diameter differed by as much as 2.3 mm in patients who were imaged using 128 versus 256 phase-encoding steps.[79] Alterations in image display parameters (i.e., window width and level settings) can also influence the apparent dimension of the spinal cord on MR images. Cord diameter can vary by up to 1.5 mm when image display settings are varied.[79]

Imaging Artifacts
Congenital variations of the spinal cord

A portion of the spinal cord may be doubled or divided (diastematomyelia).[5] Duplication of the central canal of the spinal cord may also occur.[5]

Filum terminale

The filum terminale can be of variable thickness.[48] The filum terminale can also contain foci of fat as a normal variation[48] (Figs. 18-21A and B and 18-22). The presence of fat within the filum terminale or in the cord itself can simulate intradural hemorrhage or neoplasm; fat suppressed T1-weighted images will allow for distinction (Figs. 18-23A and B). Fatty filum terminale can also be associated with tethering of the spinal cord, and a

thickened fatty filum terminale can be associated with symptoms, even in patients in whom the conus medullaris is located at a normal level.[46]

Truncation artifact

Truncation artifacts are due to the inability of the Fourier transform to accurately depict high tissue contrast interfaces. This results in a series of alternating high and low signal intensity linear artifacts that are usually seen along the phase-encoding direction of the image. These artifacts are most prominent when a relatively low spatial resolution imaging matrix is used (e.g., 128 × 256) and can be made less conspicuous with use of a high spatial resolution matrix (e.g., 256 × 256) or with various filtration methods. Reorientation of the phase-encoding and frequency-encoding gradients will allow these artifacts to be redirected along a different portion of the image.

Truncation artifacts can arise at the high contrast interface between the spinal cord and adjacent CSF, particularly on sagittal T2-weighted images. These artifacts appear as longitudinally oriented linear foci of relative increased signal intensity. These findings can simulate intramedullary pathologic conditions, including syringomyelia, hydromyelia, longitudinal necrosis, or arteriove-

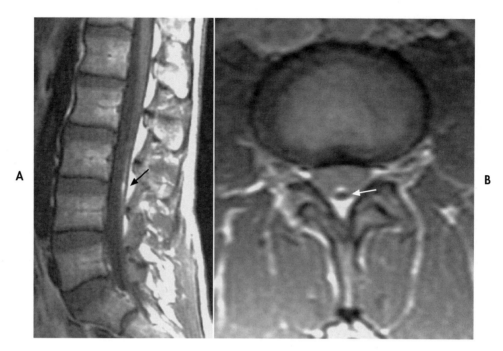

Fig. 18-21. A, Linear increased signal intensity is noted within the posterior aspect of the thecal sac (*arrow*) on sagittal T1-weighted image (TR 500, TE 12, 2 Nex), representing fat within the filum terminale. This is confirmed on **B,** transaxial proton density–weighted image (TR 500, TE 35, 2 Nex), in which chemical shift misregistration artifact (*arrow*) confirms the presence of a fat-fluid interface.

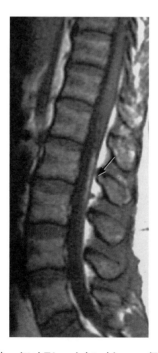

Fig. 18-22. Midsagittal T1-weighted image (TR 500, TE 12, 2 Nex) demonstrates high signal intensity caused by fat within the filum terminale (*arrow*).

nous malformation[10,37] (Figs. 18-24A and B and 18-25A and B). Because of the potential for truncation artifacts to simulate spinal cord pathologic conditions, the use of a low resolution matrix should be avoided when performing spinal MR imaging; use of an intermediate (e.g., 192 × 256) to high resolution matrix is recommended.

Simulation of syringomyelia

The ventral median fissure of the spinal cord can appear as a thin, longitudinally oriented stripe of relative decreased signal intensity on coronal T1-weighted images, simulating a syrinx[13] (Figs. 18-26A and B). Compact white matter pathways within the spinal cord can also simulate the appearance of syringomyelia.[17,64] Longitudinally oriented increased signal intensity within the spinal cord on T2-weighted images can occur in patients with poliomyelitis.[38] Hyperintensity within the ventral horns of the cord in such patients can potentially simulate syringomyelia.

Retained iophendylate (Pantopaque)

Retained iophendylate droplets may be encountered in the dural sac of patients who have had previous myelography. Because of its lipid composition, iophendylate appears as foci of relative increased signal intensity on T1-

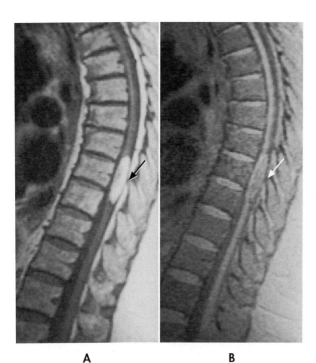

Fig. 18-23. A, Sagittal T1-weighted image (TR 500, TE 12, 2 Nex) demonstrates oval lesion measuring 5 × 3 cm centered at the T8 level (*arrow*). The lesion is of high signal intensity, indicating either blood products (i.e., hematoma) or fatty tissue. It is difficult to closely compare the signal intensity of the lesion with that of subcutaneous or posterior mediastinal fat because of varying distances from the surface coil. B, Corresponding fat suppressed image demonstrates decreased signal intensity of the lesion (*arrow*), indicating that it represents fatty tissue (lipoma or dermoid). Note incomplete suppression of subcutaneous fat because of its proximity to the surface coil.

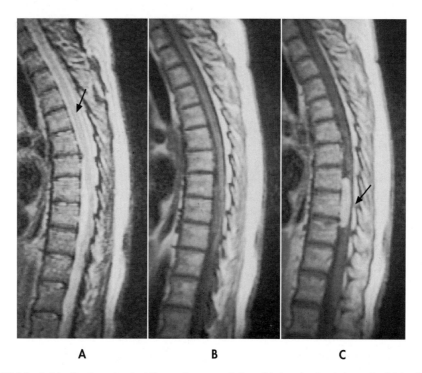

Fig. 18-24. A, Vertically oriented linear increased signal intensity is observed within the spinal cord (*arrow*) on sagittal T2-weighted image (TR 2000, TE 75, 1 Nex), representing truncation artifact. The presence of intradural extramedullary mass (presumed meningioma) is poorly depicted on unenhanced sagittal T2-weighted, **A,** and T1-weighted, **B,** (TR 500, TE 11, 2 Nex) images. However, lesion is easily visualized on T1-weighted image obtained following gadopentetate administration (*arrow*), **C.**

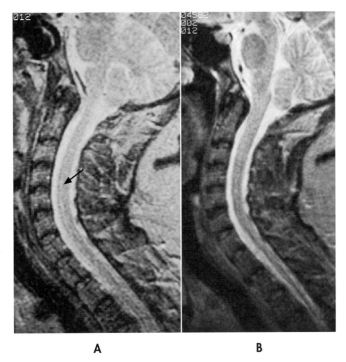

A   B

Fig. 18-25. A, Sagittal T2-weighted image (TR 2200, TE 80, 1 Nex) acquired using 192 phase-encoding steps demonstrates linear increased signal intensity (*arrow*) overlying the cervical spinal cord as a result of truncation artifact. This artifact is of reduced conspicuousness on **B,** T2-weighted image acquired using 256 phase-encoding steps (TR 2800, TE 80, 2 Nex). Also, note increased signal intensity of CSF within thecal sac as well as reduced motion artifacts on **B** because of the use of peripheral ECG gating.

weighted images. As such, it can simulate intradural lesions such as lipoma or dermoid or methemoglobin related to subacute hemorrhage.* Close inspection may indicate chemical shift misregistration surrounding the focus of increased signal intensity; this implies that fat must be present. On gradient echo images, retained iophendylate usually appears hypointense relative to CSF, and it may simulate intradural or extradural lesions, magnetic susceptibility artifact, or flow.[32]

Gray and white matter

Signal intensity variations are frequently observed within the parenchyma of the spinal cord on transaxial images in normal subjects. These signal variations can reflect differences in T1 or T2 relaxation among the gray and white matter components of the spinal cord[16,17,29] (Fig. 18-27). In the spinal cord, gray matter is located central relative to surrounding white matter, in distinction to the brain. Therefore relative increased signal in-

---

*References 3, 9, 26, 27, 32, 39, 66.

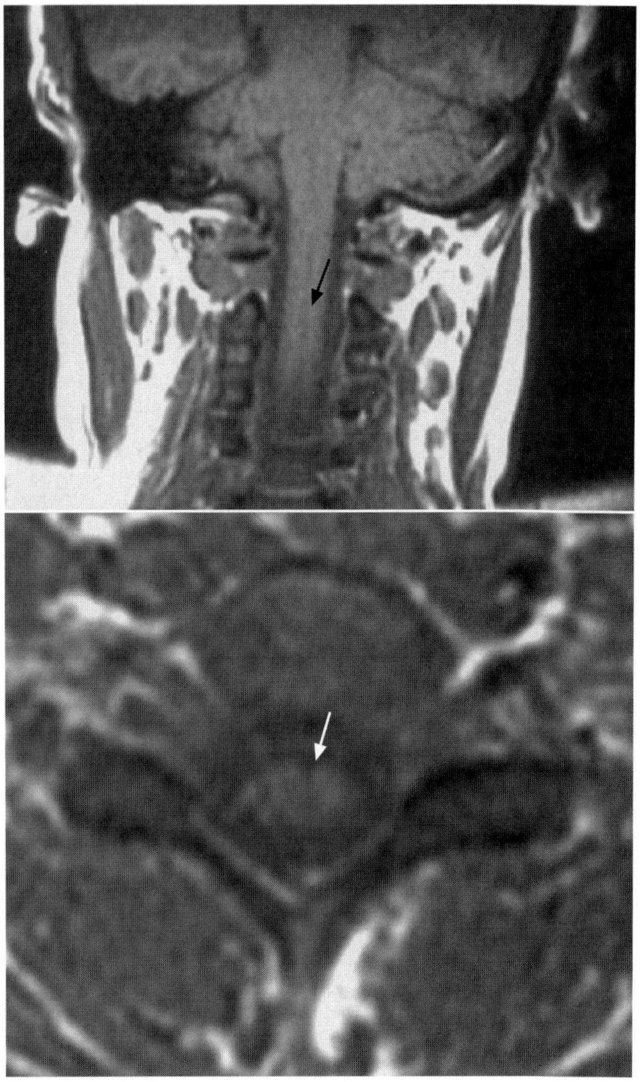

Fig. 18-26. A, Coronal T1-weighted image (TR 500, TE 11, 2 Nex) demonstrates linear decreased signal intensity (*arrow*) suggestive of syrinx involving the cervical spinal cord. However, this represents the ventral median fissure of the spinal cord, as verified on corresponding transaxial image, **B.**

tensity foci can be observed centrally within the spinal cord on T2-weighted images because of normal gray matter.[64] These signal intensity variations should be bilaterally symmetric, should have uniform moderate intensity, and may have a discernible "butterfly" configuration. Such signal intensity alterations may be apparent on transaxial gradient echo as well as spin echo images. They must be distinguished from lesions such as infarct, tumor, myelitis, and demyelination, among others. Heterotopias appear as asymmetric foci of relative increased signal intensity within the spinal cord, which are isointense with gray matter. Aberrant bundles of white matter

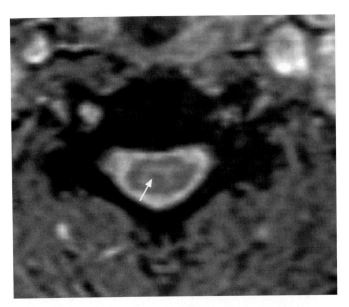

Fig. 18-27. Transaxial three-dimensional spoiled gradient echo image (TR 35, TE 15, 5-degree flip angle, 1 Nex) depicts foci of relative increased signal intensity (*arrow*) within the cervical spinal cord. These foci represent areas of gray matter and may simulate intramedullary lesions. Note the markedly reduced signal intensity of osseous structures caused by susceptibility effects resulting from variable magnetization of multiple bone components, including trabeculae, lipids, and cellular elements, on this gradient echo image.

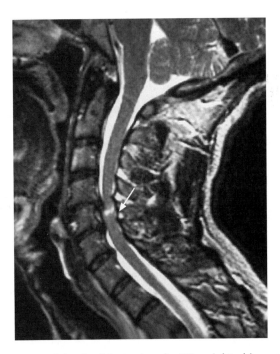

Fig. 18-28. Midsagittal fast spin echo T2-weighted image (TR 4000, effective TE 102, 4 Nex, 16 echo train) demonstrates focus of increased signal intensity within spinal cord (*arrow*), representing edema or gliosis caused by cord compression at this level.

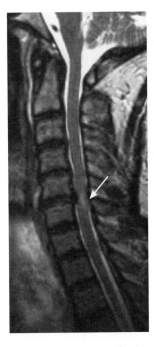

Fig. 18-29. A large disk herniation is depicted at the C5-6 level on sagittal fast spin echo T2-weighted image (TR 4000, effective TE 102, 4 Nex, 16 echo train). The disk fragment compresses the spinal cord (*arrow*) and results in increased signal intensity within the cord because of edema or gliosis.

can also occur within the spinal cord.[5] It has been observed that spinal cord white matter has a relatively decreased signal intensity as compared with its counterpart in the brain.[16]

Other entities

Foci of relative increased signal intensity on T2-weighted images within the spinal cord can be observed in patients with severe spinal stenosis[28] (Figs. 18-28 and 18-29). In one study such findings were present in more than 18% of patients with cervical spinal cord compression, and they were thought to represent myelomalacia or cord gliosis.[72] Partial volume averaging of the spinal cord with extradural fat or adjacent CSF can simulate the appearance of an intradural lesion (Fig. 18-30). Medullary lesions can also be simulated by partial volume averaging of the spinal cord with fat in the neural foramen on parasagittal images (Fig. 18-31).

Truncation artifacts arising along the spinal cord–CSF interface can lead to artifactual heterogeneous signal intensity within the spinal cord on transaxial images.[16,29,69] This entity and methods for reducing the impact of truncation artifacts have been discussed previously. Another source of artifactual signal intensity within the spinal cord is motion. This may be due to swallowing, respira-

SIMULATION OF INTRADURAL EXTRAMEDULLARY LESIONS

- Subarachnoid prominence or cysts
- Layering of cauda equina roots
- Physiologic nerve root enhancement
- Fat in filum terminale
- Retained iophendylate (Pantopaque)
- CSF pulsation artifacts
- Altered CSF flow dynamics
- Entry phenomenon
- Ferromagnetic artifact
- Postoperative alterations

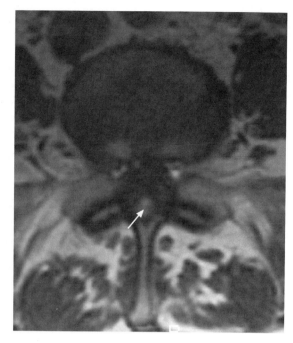

Fig. 18-30. An apparent high signal intensity intradural mass (*arrow*) is noted on transaxial T1-weighted image (TR 500, TE 15, 2 Nex). This is due to partial volume averaging of CSF with fat within the posterior epidural space, as determined by analysis of adjacent images and images acquired in additional planes.

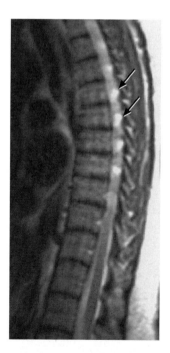

Fig. 18-31. Sagittal fast spin echo T2-weighted image of the thoracic spine (TR 4000, effective TE 96, 4 Nex, 16 echo train) demonstrates a series of high signal intensity foci (*arrows*) that appear to represent intramedullary lesions. These findings are due to partial volume averaging of the spinal cord with fat and CSF in the neural foramina, in a patient with mild scoliosis.

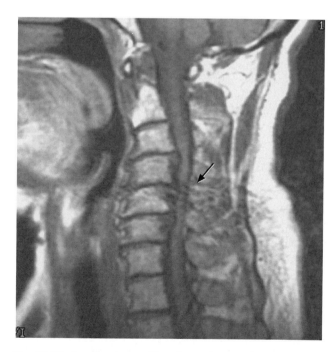

Fig. 18-32. Swallowing artifact (*arrow*) extends across the midcervical spine along the phase-encoding direction on this midsagittal T1-weighted image (TR 600, TE 19, 2 Nex). Artifact obscures detail in the region of central spinal canal stenosis.

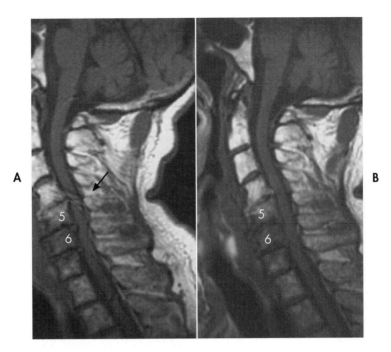

Fig. 18-33. Sagittal T1-weighted images (TR 500, TE 11, 2 Nex) of the cervical spine acquired with phase encoding along the anteroposterior, **A,** and superior-inferior, **B,** axes of the body. **A** demonstrates phase-encoding artifact (*arrow*) caused by swallowing motion projecting over the spinal cord. These artifacts are redirected with gradient reorientation. Diffuse spondylotic changes are noted, as well as marrow replacement, involving the C5 (5) and C6 (6) vertebral bodies.

tion, cardiac activity, vascular pulsation, or gross patient movement. All of these events can generate phase-encoding errors (i.e., ghosting artifacts) that will overlie the spinal cord and potentially simulate lesions (Figs. 18-32 and 18-33A and B). The available approaches for suppression of such motion artifacts are described elsewhere in this book.

Cerebrospinal fluid artifacts

CSF pulsation artifacts. Transmitted cardiac pulsations result in periodic motion of CSF within the thecal sac. This is an important cause of motion artifacts that can interfere with evaluation of the intradural space (Figs. 18-11A and B and 18-34). Pulsatile CSF motion can lead to ghosting artifacts within the dural sac, similar to those caused by other types of physiologic motion. The high signal intensity component of such artifacts can again simulate parenchymal lesions of the spinal cord.[53] More frequently, however, pulsatile CSF flow is manifested as foci of aberrant signal intensity within the intradural extramedullary space. These artifacts usually appear as foci of relative decreased signal intensity compared with surrounding high signal intensity CSF on T2-weighted spin echo or gradient echo images (Figs. 18-35 to 18-37A and B). These findings can simulate the ap-

pearance of extramedullary lesions such as neoplasm or vascular malformation.[40,42,52,53,55]

Because CSF motion is directly related to the cardiac cycle, the use of cardiac gating is often helpful in reducing such artifacts.* Adequate results can usually be achieved with use of a plethysmographic sensor on the finger, rather than the more time-consuming placement of electrocardiogram (ECG) chest leads. Cardiac gating limits the operator's choice of TR, which in turn can result in restricted tissue contrast or increased acquisition time. Gradient moment nulling is another technique that is useful for reducing CSF flow artifacts.† This involves the addition of gradient pulses, which are intended to rephase moving spins at the time of echo collection. Gradient rephasing is usually performed along the slice select and frequency encode axes, and it allows for reduction of artifacts related to motion that occurs in any direction.[20] Gradient moment nulling (also known as flow compensation) can be implemented on T2-weighted spin echo or gradient echo images and does not prolong imaging time. Optimal results can be achieved when car-

---

*References 23, 24, 52, 53, 55, 56.
†References 15, 23, 52, 53, 55, 56, 70.

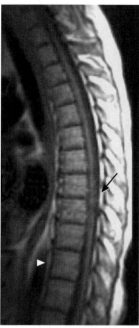

Fig. 18-34. Midsagittal T1-weighted image (TR 500, TE 10, 2 Nex) demonstrates artifactual signal intensity (*arrow*) overlying the vertebral column and spinal cord because of cardiac pulsations. Artifactual signal reduction along the lower thoracic spine (*arrowhead*) is also noted, caused by tissue extending beyond the sensitive range of the surface coil.

diac gating and gradient moment nulling are used together. Retrospective reordering of phase-encoding steps with reference to the cardiac cycle is another useful approach for decreasing CSF pulsation artifacts.[14]

CSF signal variations related to spinal stenosis. The CSF flow artifacts described above are discrete. Pulsatile CSF flow also leads to generalized mild loss of signal intensity throughout the intradural space on long TR images. This effect is not appreciable on most spinal MR examinations. However, when there is high grade stenosis of the central spinal canal, CSF distal to the stenosis often appears hyperintense as compared with CSF located proximal to the stenosis on T2-weighted images[23,52,53] (Figs. 18-38 to 18-39). This is because CSF spins distal to the stenosis are effectively shielded from the effects of pulsatile flow and therefore do not undergo related signal loss.

Other causes for aberrant CSF signal characteristics

Linear or curvilinear foci of artifactual decreased signal intensity can be observed along the surface of the spinal cord or along the course of the intradural nerve roots on T2-weighted or gradient echo images. This phenomenon is due to disruption of laminar CSF flow patterns and has been termed *boundary layer phase dispersion.*[55] Even echo rephasing is another flow phenomenon

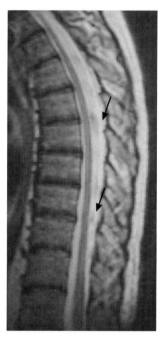

Fig. 18-35. Elongated foci of relative decreased signal intensity (*arrows*) are noted within the thecal sac on sagittal fast spin echo T2-weighted image (TR 4000, effective TE 96, 4 Nex, 16 echo train). Although these findings suggest an intradural mass or arteriovenous malformation, they are due to pulsatile flow of CSF.

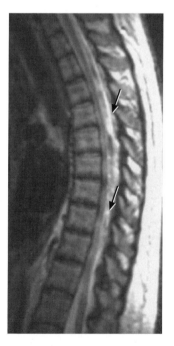

Fig. 18-36. Midsagittal fast spin echo T2-weighted image (TR 4000, effective TE 96, 4 Nex, 16 echo train) demonstrates irregular foci of relative decreased signal intensity (*arrows*) within the thecal sac caused by CSF pulsation artifacts.

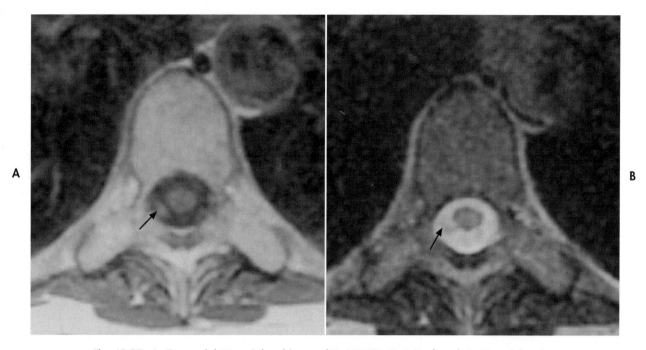

Fig. 18-37. A, Transaxial T1-weighted image (TR 467, TE 12, 2 Nex) and, **B,** T2-weighted image (TR 2250, TE 80, 1 Nex) of the thoracic spine demonstrate intradural foci of relatively increased and decreased signal intensity, respectively, (*arrows*) caused by CSF pulsation artifacts.

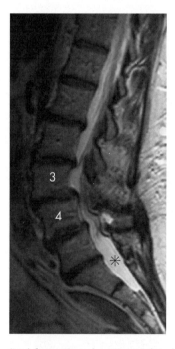

Fig. 18-38. Sagittal fast spin echo T2-weighted image (TR 4000, effective TE 102, 4 Nex, 16 echo train) of the lumbar spine in patient with severe stenosis of the spinal canal at the L3-4 level. There is relative increased signal intensity of CSF located distal to the site of stenosis (*asterisk*) as compared with CSF proximal to this level. Grade I spondylolisthesis is also noted at the L3-4 level.

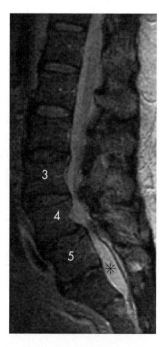

Fig. 18-39. Sagittal T2-weighted image (TR 2000, TE 75, 1 Nex) demonstrates severe stenosis of the central spinal canal at the L3-4 and L4-5 levels. CSF located distal to these levels (*asterisk*) demonstrates relative hyperintensity compared with CSF proximal to these levels.

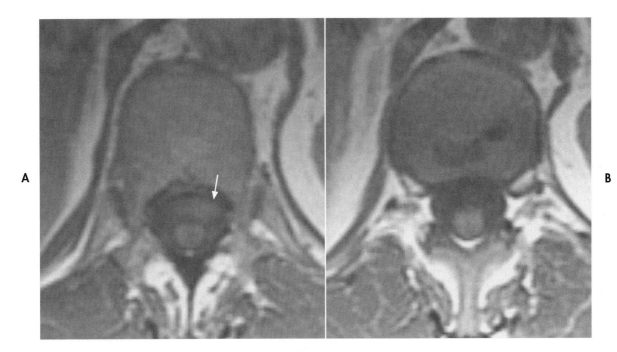

Fig. 18-40. A, Transaxial T1-weighted image (TR 550, TE 15, 4 Nex), acquired as the first section in a multisection group, depicts increased signal intensity of CSF (*arrow*) because of entry phenomenon. **B,** Image acquired from the middle of the multisection set demonstrates uniformly low signal intensity CSF.

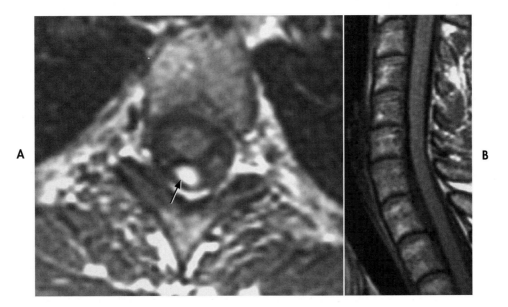

Fig. 18-41. A, Transaxial T1-weighted image (TR 600, TE 11, 4 Nex) through the upper thoracic spine demonstrates a nodular focus of increased signal intensity (*arrow*) within the posterior CSF space. This is due to entry of unsaturated CSF protons into this first image of a multisection set. This is verified by corresponding sagittal T1-weighted image, **B,** (TR 500, TE 10, 2 Nex), which demonstrates no evidence of intradural abnormality.

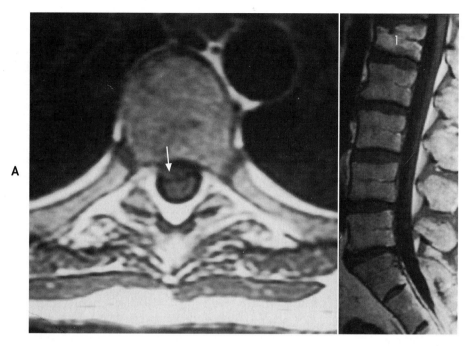

Fig. 18-42. A, Transaxial T1-weighted image (TR 400, TE 14, 4 Nex) acquired as initial section in a multisection set depicts apparent intradural mass anteriorly (*arrow*). This is due to inflow of unsaturated CSF spins, as confirmed by normal appearance of sagittal image, **B,** (TR 500, TE 12, 2 Nex). Note posttraumatic compression deformity of L1 vertebral body (1).

that can affect the CSF space.[54] This results in relative increased signal intensity of slow laminar CSF flow on even-numbered echoes of a multiecho sequence.

Artifactual increased signal intensity can be observed within the thecal sac on T1-weighted images acquired near the beginning of a multislice data set. This is due to the entry of relatively unsaturated CSF spins into the imaging section. Such spins are capable of generating increased signal intensity as compared with surrounding stationary tissues, which have encountered repeated radiofrequency pulses and have become somewhat saturated. Foci of increased signal intensity caused by this entry phenomenon can simulate intradural hemorrhage or solid lesions (Figs. 18-40A and B to 18-42A and B). In problematic cases the sequence may be repeated with the relevant section positioned near the middle rather than the periphery of the group of imaging sections. When intradural signal alterations resulting from entry phenomenon are observed on transaxial images, evaluation of corresponding sagittal images may also be useful in validating the absence of an actual pathologic condition.

High signal intensity foci within the dural sac on T1-weighted images can also arise because of slow flow or stagnation of CSF spins.[52,53] The use of radiofrequency presaturation pulses, which are prescribed above the section, will help to reduce increased CSF signal intensity caused by entry phenomenon or slow CSF flow.

Gradient echo imaging

Gradient echo imaging is often used to generate high signal intensity CSF for producing a myelographic effect. The proper combination of TR, TE, and flip angle is critical to achieving the desired uniform high signal intensity throughout the subarachnoid space. Improper choice of flip angle, in particular, can result in markedly inhomogeneous CSF signal intensity, which can simulate or obscure intradural lesions.[25]

When imaging parameters are optimized, gradient echo images can produce high quality depictions of extradural abnormalities. However, their sensitivity for depicting intramedullary lesions has been debated. In one study, gradient echo images provided equal or better depiction of intramedullary lesions than corresponding T2-weighted spin echo images in 79% of patients.[34] This was largely attributed to improved image quality, particularly regarding reduced CSF flow artifacts. However, in several other studies, gradient echo images have failed to sensitively depict intramedullary lesions.[25,29,36,75] Therefore, in patients with suspected intramedullary lesions such as neoplasms, infarcts, and demyelinating plaques, T2-weighted spin echo sequences should be performed. Intramedullary hemorrhage is one entity that is more sensitively displayed on gradient echo than spin echo images.

Susceptibility artifacts

Spin echo sequences are also preferable to gradient echo sequences in patients with metallic objects located in or near the spine,[23] because artifactual regions of signal void induced by ferromagnetic items are considerably more prominent on gradient echo images as a result of absence of a 180-degree refocusing pulse (Fig. 18-43). The region of signal void may be surrounded by peripheral hyperintensity in some cases (Figs. 18-44A and B). These susceptibility artifacts can have devastating effects on the ability to evaluate the spine. For example, in patients with metallic spinal fixation rods, the spinal cord and CSF space may be entirely obscured. When hyperintensity associated with ferromagnetic items is superimposed over the spinal cord, intramedullary lesions can also be simulated (Fig. 18-47). Ferromagnetic materials also alter local magnetic field gradients, resulting in geometric distortion of the image (Fig. 18-45). This can cause the spinal cord and thecal sac to appear to have an abnormal configuration.

Fast spin echo imaging

Fast spin echo, or RARE, sequences are used with increasing frequency for spinal MR imaging. This technique involves application of multiple 180-degree radiofrequency pulses, which are separately phase encoded, following an initial 90-degree excitation pulse. Image acquisition time is reduced proportional to the number of refocusing pulses in the echo train. The marked savings in imaging time can be used to perform sequences with longer repetition time, more excitations, and larger matrices to improve signal-to-noise ratio and spatial resolution.

Preliminary studies indicate that fast spin echo and conventional spin echo T2-weighted sequences provide similar tissue contrast for most spinal lesions. However, fast spin echo images are somewhat less sensitive in depicting signal loss because of hemorrhagic breakdown products.[44,45] Therefore intradural hematoma or tumoral hemorrhage may be more difficult to identify on fast spin echo images, and the use of supplementary gradient echo images should be considered. Fast spin echo images can also demonstrate blurring, particularly when short echo times and long echo train lengths are used.[43]

INTRADURAL SPACE LESIONS
Characterization of intradural lesions

Spinal cord cysts or cystic tumors may have signal intensity characteristics that differ from those of CSF, for reasons similar to those already described.[24] These findings can be used to help distinguish between pulsatile and nonpulsatile spinal cord cysts.[22,60] Although absence of flow-related signal loss within cystic lesions has been used to indicate their noncommunication with the CSF space, signal loss may also be observed in lesions such as arachnoid cysts on flow-sensitive sequences.[11] This is presumed to be caused by transmitted pulsations resulting in signal loss within the cyst.[18]

Isointensity of intradural cysts or cystic lesions and surrounding CSF may lead to difficulty in lesion identification, particularly when mass effect is absent.[19] Cystic and solid components of spinal cord tumors may also be difficult to distinguish using standard sequences. Heavily T2-weighted or contrast-enhanced T1-weighted images can be helpful in making this distinction. MR has been relatively insensitive for depicting extramedullary

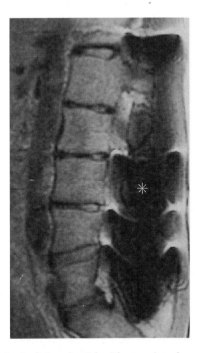

Fig. 18-43. Foci of signal void with associated areas of increased signal intensity (*asterisk*) obscure visualization of the spinal canal on sagittal proton density–weighted image (TR 2000, TE 30, 1 Nex) in patient with Harrington rods.

```
ENTITIES THAT MAY OBSCURE
INTRADURAL LESIONS
```

- Gradient echo images
- Fast spin echo images
- Susceptibility artifacts
- Isointensity with CSF or cord
- Absence of contrast material
- Inadequate spatial resolution

dermoid and epidermoid tumors[2] and has also poorly demonstrated the intraspinal component of dermal sinus tracts.[2]

Detection

Some intradural mass lesions can be difficult to visualize on the basis of altered T1 and T2 relaxation char-

acteristics.* This particularly applies to small drop metastases within the CSF space. In addition, meningiomas and neurinomas may be nearly isointense with the spinal cord parenchyma, and some cystic neurinomas can appear isointense with CSF.[64] The availability of para-

---

*References 35, 47, 65, 67, 69, 74.

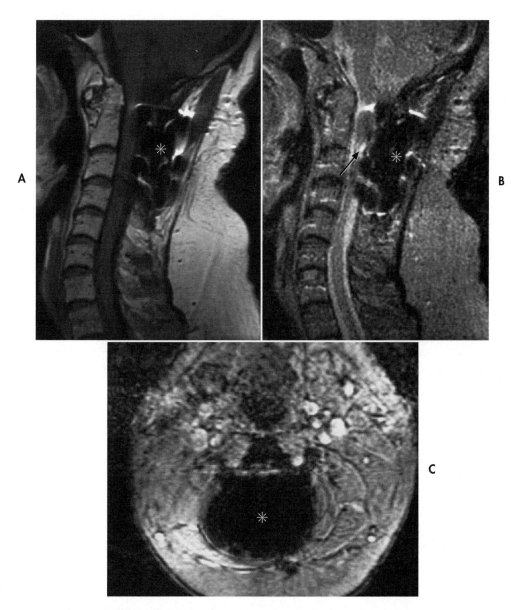

Fig. 18-44. Artifactual signal void with surrounding hyperintensity (*asterisks*) is present on **A,** T1-weighted sagittal image (TR 550, TE 19, 2 Nex) and, **B,** T2-weighted sagittal image (TR 2200, TE 80, 1 Nex) in patient who underwent previous posterior cervical fusion. The artifact is more extensive on T2-weighted than on T1-weighted images, and related hyperintensity simulates an intramedullary lesion (*arrow*) on **B.** Further accentuation of these susceptibility artifacts is noted on three-dimensional spoiled gradient echo image, **C,** (TR 35, TE 15, 5-degree flip angle, 1 Nex), (*asterisk*) where the spinal cord is completely obscured.

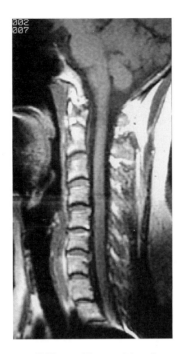

Fig. 18-45. Susceptibility artifacts arising from metallic bra snaps obscure portions of the upper thoracic spine on midsagittal T1-weighted image (TR 567, TE 19, 2 Nex). There is also associated distortion of anatomic features because of alterations in local magnetic field gradients.

magnetic contrast agents has been important in improving the conspicuousness of such lesions on MR images (Figs. 18-21A and B and 18-46A and B).

Characterization

The use of contrast material can also assist in characterizing some intradural lesions. However, contrast material enhancement is relatively nonspecific and occurs with many entities other than neoplasms.[8] Many benign spinal cord lesions that exhibit abnormal contrast enhancement can also demonstrate cord swelling and mass effect, which further simulate neoplasm. For example, spinal cord ischemia or subacute infarction can be associated with cord swelling and abnormal contrast enhancement.[21,68] Vascular congestion of the spinal cord (Foix-Alajouanine syndrome) can result in similar findings.[40,42] Abnormal contrast enhancement can be observed in patients with transverse myelitis,[46] and nodular enhancement can occur with granulomatous conditions such as tuberculosis and sarcoidosis.[68] Small foci of abnormal contrast material enhancement simulating drop metastases have been observed in children who have undergone recent surgical resection of posterior fossa tumors.[77] These findings may be due to leptomeningeal irritation caused by postoperative subarachnoid bleeding.

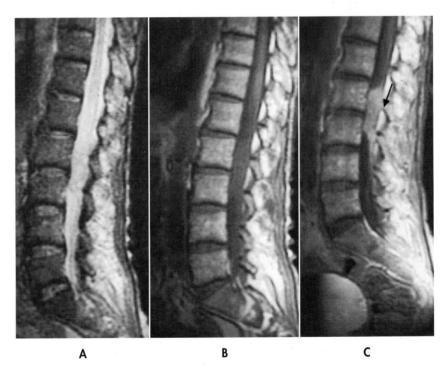

A   B   C

Fig. 18-46. A, Sagittal T2-weighted image (TR 2000, TE 75, 1 Nex) and, **B,** unenhanced sagittal T1-weighted image (TR 500, TE 12, 2 Nex) poorly depict an intradural mass lesion (*arrow*) that is clearly depicted on **C,** T1-weighted image obtained following gadopentetate administration (TR 500, TE 12, 2 Nex) in patient with lung cancer.

Patients with radiation myelopathy can present with either cord swelling or atrophy. In addition, abnormal increased signal intensity can be observed on T2-weighted images, along with focal abnormal enhancement on contrast enhanced T1-weighted images.[41,68,76,80] These findings can be observed long after therapy has been administered. Demyelinating plaques within the spinal cord, usually related to multiple sclerosis or acute disseminated encephalomyelitis, can cause considerable cord enlargement and blood-brain barrier breakdown during episodes of active demyelination.[12,68] Necrotizing myelitis is another benign entity that can simulate intramedullary neoplasm.

Distortion and clumping of intradural nerve roots caused by arachnoiditis can simulate drop metastases, particularly when associated with abnormal contrast enhancement.[50] Prominent intradural vessels related to vascular malformations can also simulate carcinomatosis.[42] Abnormal contrast enhancement can occur within the anterior horn cell regions when the spinal cord is affected by spondylotic compression.[74] Abnormal intramedullary contrast enhancement can be related to previous surgical intervention.[8] The contrast enhancement pattern of intramedullary neoplasms is highly variable and depends on lesion type and degree of cystic component.[51]

Staging

Intramedullary metastases can be associated with cord enlargement that extends far beyond the area of actual tumor involvement. In such cases, intravenous contrast material can improve delineation of the actual tumor extent.[68] Primary cord gliomas demonstrate variable enhancement; the presence of contrast enhancement cannot be relied on to delineate tumor margins.[68]

Dural arteriovenous malformations remain difficult to detect using MR imaging. These may present with focal cord enlargement and increased signal intensity on T2-weighted images as well as irregularity of the cord surface. When contrast material is given, punctate foci of contrast enhancement can be seen surrounding the cord, in addition to parenchymal cord enhancement on delayed images.[68]

Localization

It can sometimes be difficult to distinguish between extradural lesions that are closely applied to the dural sac and intradural abnormalities. Displacement of epidural fat around a lesion indicates that it is of epidural origin.[31] Lesions arising in the epidural space can secondarily enter the dural sac, creating difficulties in determining the lesion origin. For example, rare cases of herniated disk material within the dural sac have been reported.[30] Cervical schwannomas can rarely extend into the spinal cord, simulating the appearance of glioma.[71] Extradural lesions can also induce secondary alterations within the

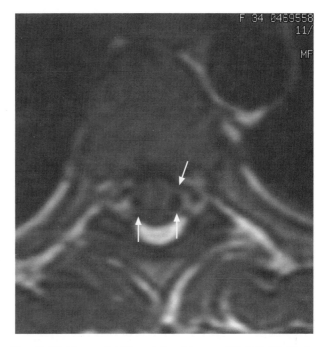

Fig. 18-47. Transaxial T1-weighted image (TR 500, TE 18, 4 Nex) of the thoracic spine demonstrates linear foci of intradural relative increased signal intensity (*arrows*), representing the dentate ligaments.

intradural space. For example, intradural morphologic and signal intensity alterations have been caused by epidural anesthesia.[63]

Normal structures located within the dural sac can simulate lesions. A midline sagittal septum can be observed within the thecal sac,[58] and the dentate ligaments can be visualized traversing the subarachnoid space (Fig. 18-47). The number of dentate ligaments varies between 18 and 22.[5]

REFERENCES

1. Baran GA, Sowell MK, Sharp GB et al: MR findings in a child with Guillain-Barré syndrome, Am J Roentgenol 161:161-163, 1993.
2. Barkovich AJ, Edwards MSB, Cogen PH: MR evaluation of spinal dermal sinus tracts in children, Am J Roentgenol 156:791-797, 1991.
3. Barsi P, Kenez J, Varallyay G et al: Unusual origin of free subarachnoid fat drops: a ruptured spinal dermoid tumour, Neuroradiology 34:343-344, 1992.
4. Beltran J, Chandnani V, McGhee RA Jr et al: Gadopentetate dimeglumine-enhanced MR imaging of the musculoskeletal system, Am J Roentgenol 156:457-466, 1991.
5. Bergman RA, Thompson SA, Afifi AK et al: Compendium of human anatomic variation: text, atlas, and world literature, Baltimore, 1988, Urban & Schwarzenberg, p 131.
6. Bobman SA, Atlas SW, Listerud J et al: Postoperative lumbar

spine: contrast-enhanced chemical shift MR imaging, Radiology 179:557-562, 1991.

7. Boden SD, Davis DO, Dina TS et al: Contrast-enhanced MR imaging performed after successful lumbar disk surgery: prospective study, Radiology 182:59-64, 1992.

8. Brant-Zawadzki M: Pitfalls of contrast-enhanced imaging in the nervous system, Magn Reson Med 22:243-248, 1991.

9. Braun IF, Malko JA, Davis PC et al: The behavior of pantopaque on MR: in vivo and in vitro analyses, Am J Neuroradiol 7:997-1001, 1986.

10. Bronskill MJ, McVeigh ER, Kucharczyk W et al: Syrinx-like artifacts on MR images of the spinal cord, Radiology 166:485-488, 1988.

11. Brooks ML, Jolesz FA, Patz S: MRI of pulsatile CSF motion within arachnoid cysts, Magn Reson Imaging 6:575-584, 1988.

12. Caldemeyer KS, Harris TM, Smith RR et al: Gadolinium enhancement in acute disseminated encephalomyelitis, J Comput Assist Tomogr 15:673-675, 1991.

13. Chen MYM, Elster AD: Simulation of syringomyelia by ventral median fissure, J Comput Assist Tomogr 14:841-842, 1990.

14. Cho MH, Kim WS, Cho ZH: CSF flow artifact reduction using cardiac cycle ordered phase-encoding method, Magn Reson Imaging 8:395-405, 1990.

15. Colletti PM, Raval JK, Benson RC et al: The motion artifact suppression technique (MAST) in magnetic resonance imaging: clinical results, Magn Reson Imaging 6:293-299, 1988.

16. Curtin AJ, Chakeres DW, Bulas R et al: MR imaging artifacts of the axial internal anatomy of the cervical spinal cord, Am J Roentgenol 152:835-842, 1989.

17. Czervionke LF, Daniels DL, Ho PSP et al: The MR appearance of gray and white matter in the cervical spinal cord, Am J Neuroradiol 9:557-562, 1988.

18. Davis SW, Levy LM, LeBihan DJ et al: Sacral meningeal cysts: evaluation with MR imaging, Radiology 187:445-448, 1993.

19. Dietemann JL, Filippi de la Palavesa MM, Kastler B et al: Thoracic intradural arachnoid cyst: possible pitfalls with myelo-CT and MR. Neuroradiology 33:90-91, 1991.

20. Duerk JL, Pattany PM: Analysis of imaging axes significance in motion artifact suppression technique (MAST): MRI of turbulent flow and motion, Magn Reson Imaging 7:251-263, 1989.

21. Dunn RS, Wiener SN: Anterior spinal artery syndrome caused by infarction of the conus medullaris (letter), Am J Roentgenol 156:1116, 1991.

22. Enzmann DR, O'Donohue J, Rubin JB et al: CSF pulsations within nonneoplastic spinal cord cysts, Am J Roentgenol 149:149-157, 1987.

23. Enzmann DR, Rubin JB: Cervical spine: MR imaging with a partial flip angle, gradient-refocused pulse sequence. I. General considerations and disk disease, Radiology 166:467-472, 1988.

24. Enzmann DR, Rubin JB, DeLaPaz R et al: Cerebrospinal fluid pulsation: benefits and pitfalls in MR imaging, Radiology 161:773-778, 1986.

25. Enzmann DR, Rubin JB, Wright A: Use of cerebrospinal fluid gating to improve T2-weighted images. I. The spinal cord, Radiology 162:763-767, 1987.

26. Gupta RK, Jena A, Kumar S: Iophendylate or spillage from epidermoid—a diagnostic dilemma on cranial MR imaging, Magn Reson Imaging 7:293-295, 1989.

27. Hackney DB, Grossman RI, Zimmerman RA et al: MR characteristics of iophendylate (Pantopaque), J Comput Assist Tomogr 10:401-403, 1986.

28. Haupts M, Haan J: Further aspects of MR-signal enhancements in stenosis of the cervical spinal canal: MRI investigations in correlation to clinical and cerebrospinal fluid (CSF) findings, Neuroradiology 30:545-546, 1988.

29. Hedberg MC, Drayer BP, Flom RA et al: Gradient echo (GRASS) MR imaging in cervical radiculopathy, Am J Roentgenol 150:683-689, 1988.

30. Holtas S, Nordstrom C-H, Larsson E-M et al: MR imaging of intradural disk herniation, J Comput Assist Tomogr 11:353-356, 1987.

31. Horner NB, Pinto RS: The fat-cap sign: an aid to MR evaluation of extradural spinal tumors, Am J Neuroradiol 10:S93, 1989.

32. Jack CR Jr, Gehring DG, Ehman RL et al: Cerebrospinal fluid-iophendylate contrast on gradient-echo MR images, Radiology 169:561-563, 1988.

33. Johnson CE, Sze G: Benign lumbar arachnoiditis: MR imaging with gadopentetate dimeglumine, Am J Neuroradiol 11:763-770, 1990.

34. Katz BH, Quencer RM, Hinks RS: Comparison of gradient-recalled-echo and T2-weighted spin-echo pulse sequences in intramedullary spinal lesions, Am J Neuroradiol 10:815-822, 1989.

35. Krol G, Sze G, Malkin M et al: MR of cranial and spinal meningeal carcinomatosis: comparison with CT and myelography, Am J Roentgenol 151:583-588, 1988.

36. Kulkarni MV, Narayana PA, McArdle CB et al: Cervical spine MR imaging using multislice gradient echo imaging: comparison with cardiac gated spin echo, Magn Reson Imaging 6:517-525, 1988.

37. Levy LM, Di Chiro G, Brooks RA et al: Spinal cord artifacts from truncation errors during MR imaging, Radiology 166:479-483, 1988.

38. Malzberg MS, Rogg JM, Tate CA et al: Poliomyelitis: hyperintensity of the anterior horn cells on MR images of the spinal cord, Am J Roentgenol 161:863-865, 1993.

39. Mamourian AC, Briggs RW: Appearance of Pantopaque on MR images, Radiology 158:457-460, 1986.

40. Masaryk TJ, Ross JS, Modic MT et al: Radiculomeningeal vascular malformations of the spine: MR imaging, Radiology 164:845-849, 1987.

41. Michikawa M, Wada Y, Sano M et al: Radiation myelopathy: significance of gadolinium-DTPA enhancement in the diagnosis, Neuroradiology 33:286-289, 1991.

42. Minami S, Sagoh T, Nishimura K et al: Spinal arteriovenous malformation: MR imaging, Radiology 169:109-115, 1988.

43. Mulkern RV, Wong ST, Winalski C et al: Contrast manipulation and artifact assessment of 2D and 3D RARE sequences, Magn Reson Imaging 8:557-566, 1990.

44. Nemoto Y, Inoue Y, Tashiro T et al: Intramedullary spinal cord tumors: significance of associated hemorrhage at MR imaging, Radiology 182:793-796, 1992.

45. Norbash AM, Glover GH, Enzmann DR: Intracerebral lesion

contrast with spin-echo and fast spin-echo pulse sequences, Radiology 185:661-665, 1992.

46. Pardatscher K, Fiore DL, Lavano A: MR imaging of transverse myelitis using Gd-DTPA, J Neuroradiol 19:63-67, 1992.

47. Parizel PM, Baleriaux D, Rodesch G et al: Gd-DTPA-enhanced MR imaging of spinal tumors, Am J Roentgenol 152:1087-1096, 1989.

48. Raghavan N, Barkovich AJ, Edwards M et al: MR imaging in the tethered spinal cord syndrome, Am J Roentgenol 152:843-852, 1989.

49. Ross JS, Masaryk TJ, Modic MT et al: Lumbar spine: postoperative assessment with surface-coil MR imaging, Radiology 164:851-860, 1987.

50. Ross JS, Masaryk TJ, Modic MT et al: MR imaging of lumbar arachnoiditis, Am J Roentgenol 149:1025-1032, 1987.

51. Rothwell CI, Jaspan T, Worthington BS et al: Gadolinium-enhanced magnetic resonance imaging of spinal tumours, Br J Radiol 62:1067-1074, 1989.

52. Rubin JB, Enzmann DR: Harmonic modulation of proton MR precessional phase by pulsatile motion: origin of spinal CSF flow phenomena, Am J Roentgenol 148:983-994, 1987.

53. Rubin JB, Enzmann DR: Imaging of spinal CSF pulsation by 2DFT MR: significance during clinical imaging, Am J Roentgenol 148:973-982, 1987.

54. Rubin JB, Enzmann DR: Optimizing conventional MR imaging of the spine, Radiology 163:777-783, 1987.

55. Rubin JB, Enzmann DR, Wright A: CSF-gated MR imaging of the spine: theory and clinical implementation, Radiology 163:784-792, 1987.

56. Rubin JB, Wright A, Enzmann DR: Lumbar spine: motion compensation for cerebrospinal fluid on MR imaging, Radiology 167:225-231, 1988.

57. Russell EJ: Cervical disk disease, Radiology 177:313-325, 1990.

58. Schellinger D, Manz HJ, Vidic B et al: Disk fragment migration, Radiology 175:831-836, 1990.

59. Schroth G, Grodd W, Guhl L et al: Magnetic resonance imaging in small lesions of the central nervous system: improvement by gadolinium-DTPA, Acta Radiol 28:667-672, 1987.

60. Sherman JL, Barkovich AJ, Citrin CM: The MR appearance of syringomyelia: new observations, Am J Roentgenol 148:381-391, 1987.

61. Sherman JL, Nassaux PY, Citrin CM: Measurements of the normal cervical spinal cord on MR imaging, Am J Neuroradiol 11:369-372, 1990.

62. Sklar E, Quencer RM, Green BA et al: Acquired spinal subarachnoid cysts: evaluation with MR, CT myelography, and intraoperative sonography, Am J Roentgenol 153:1057-1064, 1989.

63. Sklar EML, Quencer RM, Green BA et al: Complications of epidural anesthesia: MR appearance of abnormalities, Radiology 181:549-554, 1991.

64. Solsberg MD, Lemaire C, Resch L et al: High-resolution MR imaging of the cadaveric spinal cord: normal anatomy, Am J Neuroradiol 11:3-7, 1990.

65. Stimac GK, Porter BA, Olson DO et al: Gadolinium-DTPA-enhanced MR imaging of spinal neoplasms: preliminary investigation and comparison with unenhanced spin-echo and STIR sequences, Am J Neuroradiol 9:839-846, 1988.

66. Suojanen J, Wang AM, Winston KR: Pantopaque mimicking spinal lipoma: MR pitfall, J Comput Assist Tomogr 12:346-348, 1988.

67. Sze G: Gadolinium-DTPA in spinal disease, Radiol Clin North Am 26:1009-1024, 1988.

68. Sze G: MR imaging of the spinal cord: current status and future advances, Am J Roentgenol 159:149-159, 1992.

69. Sze G, Krol G, Zimmerman RD et al: Intramedullary disease of the spine: diagnosis using gadolinium-DTPA-enhanced MR imaging, Am J Roentgenol 151:1193-1204, 1988.

70. Szeverenyi NM, Kieffer SA, Cacayorin ED: Correction of CSF motion artifact on MR images of the brain and spine by pulse sequence modification clinical evaluation, Am J Neuroradiol 9:1069-1074, 1988.

71. Tabatabai A, Jungreis CA, Yonas H: Cervical schwannoma masquerading as a glioma: MR findings, J Comput Assist Tomogr 14:489-490, 1990.

72. Takahashi M, Sakamoto Y, Miyawaki M et al: Increased MR signal intensity secondary to chronic cervical cord compression, Neuroradiology 29:550-556, 1988.

73. Tien RD, Olson EM, Zee CS: Diseases of the lumbar spine: findings on fat-suppression MR imaging, Am J Roentgenol 159:95-99, 1992.

74. Valk J: Gd-DTPA in MR of spinal lesions, Am J Roentgenol 150:1163-1168, 1988.

75. VanDyke C, Ross JS, Tkach J et al: Gradient-echo MR imaging of the cervical spine: evaluation of extradural disease, Am J Roentgenol 153:393-398, 1989.

76. Wang PY, Shen WC, Jan JS: MR imaging in radiation myelopathy, Am J Neuroradiol 13:1049-1055, 1992.

77. Weiner MD, Boyko OB, Friedman HS et al: False-positive spinal MR findings for subarachnoid spread of primary CNS tumor in postoperative pediatric patients, Am J Neuroradiol 11:1100-1103, 1990.

78. Wilson DA, Prince JR: MR imaging determination of the location of the normal conus medullaris throughout childhood, Am J Neuroradiol 10:259-262, 1989.

79. Yousem DM, Janick PA, Atlas SW et al: Pseudoatrophy of the cervical portion of the spinal cord on MR images: a manifestation of the truncation artifact? Am J Neuroradiol 11:373-377, 1990.

80. Zweig G, Russell EJ: Radiation myelopathy of the cervical spinal cord: MR findings, Am J Neuroradiol 11:1188-1190, 1990.

Index